Liver Biopsy

Liver Biopsy

Edited by **Amelia Foster**

FOSTER ACADEMICS

New Jersey

Published by Foster Academics,
61 Van Reypen Street,
Jersey City, NJ 07306, USA
www.fosteracademics.com

Liver Biopsy
Edited by Amelia Foster

International Standard Book Number: 978-1-63242-256-9 (Hardback)

Printed in China.

Contents

Preface

This book presents a concise introduction to liver biopsy along with descriptive information. Liver biopsy has been a significant diagnostic procedure for the maintenance of hepatobiliary disease and the donated organ ever since it was first carried out by Paul Ehrlich in 1883. This book deals with various aspects of the biopsy procedure in detail and provides latest information on recent advances in the management of various disorders using liver biopsy. This book will provide an excellent understanding of liver biopsy to clinicians, physicians, scientists, pharmaceutics, engineers and other aspirants associated with this field.

This book has been the outcome of endless efforts put in by authors and researchers on various issues and topics within the field. The book is a comprehensive collection of significant researches that are addressed in a variety of chapters. It will surely enhance the knowledge of the field among readers across the globe.

It is indeed an immense pleasure to thank our researchers and authors for their efforts to submit their piece of writing before the deadlines. Finally in the end, I would like to thank my family and colleagues who have been a great source of inspiration and support.

Editor

Part 1

Liver Biopsy in Management of Liver Disease

1

Liver Biopsy in Transplantation: Nonalcoholic Fatty Liver Disease and the Eosinophils

Yasuhiko Sugawara, Norihiro Kokudo and Yoji Kishi
University of Tokyo,
Japan

1. Introduction

Liver biopsy is important in the perioperative management of liver transplantation with regard to the preoperative evaluation of donor liver graft, especially to rule out steatotic liver, and the postoperative diagnosis of acute cellular rejection (ACR), especially to differentiate ACR from other causes of liver dysfunction. In both situations, liver biopsy is mandatory to confirm the diagnosis.

The recent increases in metabolic syndrome and diabetes mellitus in the general population have led to an increased incidence of liver steatosis, even in donors without a history of excessive alcohol intake. Nonalcoholic fatty liver disease (NAFLD) includes a broad spectrum of liver injuries that resemble alcoholic hepatitis, ranging from simple steatosis to nonalcoholic steatohepatitis (NASH). NASH is the progressed stage of NAFLD and further progression results in fibrosis and cirrhosis, which might also be an indication for liver transplantation. ACR is one of the most serious adverse events after transplantation. It is often difficult to distinguish it from recurrent hepatitis C virus (HCV), and prompt treatment with an appropriate diagnosis is important.

In this chapter, the indications for liver biopsy and the histologic findings for the diagnosis of NAFLD and ACR are described.

2. NAFLD

The pathophysiology of NAFLD is yet to be fully elucidated, although the two-hit story proposed by James et al.[1] is widely accepted. In their hypothesis, insulin resistance is the first hit, resulting in the production and accumulation of triglycerides in the liver due to dysregulated lipogenesis and lipolysis. Further, oxidative stress and lipid peroxidation as the second hit leads to hepatic injury, inflammation, and fibrosis by multiple cytokines and adipokines. The prevalence of NAFLD is therefore associated with metabolic syndrome and will thus continue to increase in developed countries. Previous autopsy studies[2-6] in Western countries reported the incidence of NAFLD as 16% to 64% of the population. The incidence in the Asian-Pacific region is also increasing and is currently 10% to 30% [7].

Therefore, hepatectomy or transplantation for NAFLD related cirrhosis or hepatocellular carcinomas will likely increase. In addition, because NAFLD is usually asymptomatic and the diagnosis can be confirmed only by biopsy, the possibility to encounter the liver donor with NAFLD will also increase. Whether hepatic steatosis is associated with impaired liver regeneration or an increased risk of morbidity or mortality after liver surgery is controversial. Selzner and Clavien[8] showed impaired liver regeneration in steatotic livers using rat models. Similarly, impaired regeneration of steatotic liver after large hepatectomy or portal vein ligation was reported in subsequent rat model experiments.[9,10] In the clinical setting, Kooby et al.[11] evaluated the outcomes of hepatic resection in 160, 223, and 102 patients with no, mild (<30%), and marked (≥30%) steatosis, respectively, and showed that preoperative comorbidity, steatosis, blood loss, and resection of one lobe or more were independent predictors of postoperative morbidity.

Vauthey et al. [12] reported that steatohepatitis induced by irinotecan-based chemotherapy is associated with an increased risk of 90-day mortality after hepatic resection for colorectal metastases. On the other hand, Hussein et al. reported a comparable Ki-67 labeling index which is a marker of liver regeneration among three groups of patients with simple fatty liver (9 patients), NASH (13 patients), and chronic hepatitis C (25 patients), with a similar degree of inflammation. They concluded that liver regeneration in patients with NASH is not altered.[13] The number of patients included in this study was small, however, and no patients underwent hepatic resection. Further, the Ki-67 labeling index in patients with NASH was smaller than that in patients with fatty liver or HCV, although the difference was not statistically significant. Considering that NAFLD is a progressive disease ultimately resulting in liver cirrhosis, liver-related surgery must be performed with special attention to the patient's safety. Safety is the first priority in any patient, and especially in living organ donors. In general, most transplantation centers do not accept live donors with histologic liver steatosis of greater than 30%.[14,15] Actually one donor death with NASH has been reported[15]. The controversy surrounds whether all liver donor candidates should undergo liver biopsy because diagnosis of NAFLD can be made only by histopathologic examination. Body mass index (BMI) is widely regarded as a predictor of liver steatosis. Rinella et al.[16] reported that no hepatic steatosis was observed among biopsy specimens of live-liver donor candidates with a BMI of less than 25 kg/m^2, while hepatic steatosis was found in 76% of candidates with BMI greater than 28 kg/m^2. On the other hand, other studies[17,18] demonstrated that 7% to 26% of donor candidates with a BMI of less than 25 kg/m^2 had hepatic steatosis. Yamashiki et al. recently proposed the following criteria for donor biopsy: an aspartate aminotransferase/alanine aminotransferase ratio of less than 1, BMI of at least 25, and ultrasonography findings suggestive of steatosis. Based on these criteria, liver biopsy was indicated for 25% of their referred Japanese donor candidates, and hepatic steatosis of at least 10% was revealed in 12% of the donor candidates. Further, they evaluated the visceral fat area measured from a single CT slice image at the level of the umbilicus. Receiver operating characteristic curve analysis showed that a visceral fat area of at least 96 cm^2 predicted steatosis of 10% or more with a sensitivity and specificity of 78% and 87%, respectively[19].

NASH can be an indication for liver transplantation, but it also can recur or even occur de novo in the transplanted liver graft. In general, immunosuppression with corticosteroids, calcineurin inhibitors, or silorimus is associated with body weight gain, insulin resistance, and hyperlipidemia. Therefore, post-transplant patients are susceptible to developing NAFLD. Poodad et al.[20] reported de novo NAFLD that occurred within 3 months of liver transplantation in 4 of 88 patients. Later, Seo et al.[21] evaluated the incidence and predictors of de novo NAFLD among 68 recipients. De novo NAFLD was diagnosed in 12 patients (18%) based on follow-up biopsy specimens 11 to 51 months after transplantation. NASH was diagnosed in 6 patients (9%). Multivariate analyses showed that a BMI increase of more than 10% was a risk factor and the use of angiotensin-converting enzyme inhibitors was associated with reduced risk of de novo NAFLD. Although NAFLD in one of the patients in Poodad's report showed improvement following treatment with ursodeoxycholic acid (UDCA)[20], a subsequent randomized control trial[22] showed no therapeutic effect of UDCA for the treatment of NASH compared to placebo. To date, there is no established treatment to improve NASH, and prevention should be the first priority.

3. Histology

The important factor in the diagnosis of NAFLD is the differentiation of NASH from simple steatosis or steatosis with inflammation. For this purpose, several scoring systems have been proposed to date.

Histologic characteristics of NASH include (1) macrovesicularsteatosis, (2) hepatocellular ballooning and disarray, (3) intra-lobular inflammation, (4) portal tract inflammation, (5) Mallory's hyaline bodies, (6) acidophil bodies, (7) PAS-D Kupffer cells, (8) glycogenatednuclei, (9) lipogranulomas, and (10) hepatocellular iron. Brunt et al. evaluated these variables semiquantitatively and proposed three grades (mild, moderate, and severe) for necroinflammatory changes. Fibrosis was evaluated separately and scored as stage 1, zone 3 perisinusoidal/pericellular fibrosis; stage 2, zone3 perisinusoidal/pericellular fibrosis with focal or extensive periportal fibrosis; stage 3, zone 3 perisinusoidal/pericellular fibrosis and portal fibrosis with focal or extensive fibrosis; and stage 4, cirrhosis[23]. Promrat et al.[24] demonstrated the histologic improvement of NASH by pioglitazone, which is an insulin-sensitizing agent, and introduced another scoring system. In this system, six factors; steatosis, hepatocellular injury (ballooning degeneration /apoptosis/dropout cells), parenchymal inflammation, portal inflammation, fibrosis, and Mallory bodies, were evaluated and each was scored semiquantitatively from 0 to 4.

Feature	Category	Score
Steatosis grade	<5%	0
	5%-33%	1
	>33%-66%	2
	>66%	3
Lobular inflammation	No foci	0
	<2 foci	1
	2-4 foci	2
	>4 foci	3
Balooning degeneration	None	0
	Few	1
	Many	2

Table 1. Kleiner's scoring system for the diagnosis of NAFLD. The sum of the scores (ranging 0-8): 0-2, not NASH; ≧ 5, NASH

These scoring systems, however, emphasize NASH and did not encompass the entire spectrum of NAFLD. Later, the Pathology Committee of the NASH Clinical Research Network proposed a NAFLD activity scoring system that addressed the full spectrum of NAFLD and this was reported by Kleiner et al.[25] in 2005. In this study, 14 variables in 5 broad categories; steatosis, inflammation, hepatocellular injury, fibrosis, and miscellaneous features, were evaluated in 32 adult and 18 pediatric liver biopsy specimens by 9 pathologists. Based on the intra-rater and inter-rater agreement analysis and multivariate analysis for the association of the variables with a diagnosis of steatohepatitis, the NAFLD activity index was defined as the sum of the scores of three variables; steatosis, lobular inflammation, and ballooning (Table 1). Although fibrosis is considered an independent predictor, it was not included because it is less a reversible change and more a result of disease activity than a feature of injury activity.

4. Acute cellular rejection

Acute cellular rejection (ACR) is suspected when liver function tests worsen. At the University of Tokyo, liver transplant recipients undergo postoperative blood chemistry daily or every other day during hospitalization, and once every 2 weeks or once a month in the outpatient clinics. If all liver function data (aspartate aminotransferase, alanine aminotransferase, gamma-glutamyltranspeptidase, alkaline phosphatase, and total bilirubin) are elevated compared with previous levels and bile duct complications have been ruled out by ultrasound, biopsy is indicated. There are no serum markers specific for ACR and biopsy is mandatory to confirm the diagnosis. In contrast to biopsy for the donor candidates, biopsy for the diagnosis of ACR should not be delayed because ACR may result in chronic rejection, which is characterized by ductpenia or atrophy and pyknosis of the bile duct epithelium with parenchymal severe cholestasis,[26] and graft loss. Because ACR can be treated by immunosuppression, prompt and accurate diagnosis is important.

Category	Criteria	Score
Portal Inflammation	Mostly lymphocytic inflammation involving a minority of the triads.	1
	Lymphocyte infiltration to most or all of the triads.	2
	Mixed infiltration to most or all of the triads with inflammatory spillover into the periportal parenchyma.	3
Bile duct inflammation	A minority of the ducts are cuffed and infiltrated by inflammatory cells and show only mild reactive changes.	1
	Most or all of the ducts infiltrated by inflammatory cells. More than an occasional duct shows degenerative changes.	2
	As above for 2, with most or all of the ducts showing degenerative changes or focal lumenal disruption.	3
Venous endothelial inflammation	Subendothelial lymphocytic infiltration involving someportal and/or hepatic venules.	1
	Subendothelial infiltration involving most or all of the portal and/or hepatic venules.	2
	As above for 2, with moderate or severe perivenular inflammation that extends into the perivenular parenchyma and is associated with perivenular hepatocyte necrosis.	3

Table 2. Banff scheme for rejection activity index

In general, the diagnosis of ACR is confirmed and graded into four classes according to the Banff scheme[27,28] (Grade 0 [G0]: no evidence of rejection; Grade 1 [G1]: mild rejection; Grade 2 [G2]: moderate rejection; and Grade 3 [G3]: severe rejection). This grading system is based on the degree of portal infiltration of lymphocytes (P0-3), bile duct inflammation or damage (B0-3), and venous endothelial inflammation (V0-3) (Table 2).

5. Eosinophilia as an aid to diagnose ACR

To facilitate the diagnosis of ACR, the efficacy of blood and/or histologic eosinophilia has been reported in several studies[29-38] (Table 3). In these studies, sensitivity and specificity of blood eosinophilia to predict ACR before biopsy were reported to be 32% to 96% and 63% to 97%, respectively, while those of histologic eosinophilia were 54% to 92% and 65% to 98%, respectively. Further, the correlation of eosinophilia with the severity of ACR, or a decrease of blood eosinophil count in response to treatment was reported in most of these studies[39,40], although the effect of steroids alone to downregulate eosinophils cannot be ignored.

Author	Year	N (Biopsy specimens)	Blood			Histology		
			Cut off	Sensitivity/ Spefcificity	Correlation with ACR grade	Cut off	Sensitivity/ Spefcificity	Correlation with ACR grade
Foster PF	1989	283	AEC>500/mm³	96%/87%	N.A.	>7% of infiltrating cells are eosinophil	92%/98%	N.A.
Foster PF	1991	331	N.A.		N.A.	Average >2.5 cells/portal tract	82%/91%	N.A.
Ben-Ari Z	1995	92	N.A.		N.A.	N.A.		+
Manzarbeitia C	1995	43	AEC>430/mm³	35%/83%	N.A.	N.A.		N.A.
Dollinger MM	1997	55	AEC>330/mm³ on 7POD	70%/63%	N.A.	N.A.		N.A.
Hughes VF	1998	71	AEC increase >20% within 28 days prior to biopsy	81%/74%	N.A.	N.A.		N.A.
Nagral A	2001	129	AEC≧400/mm³ REC≧4%	34%/92% 43%/84%	- -	N.A. N.A.		N.A. N.A.
Barnes EJ	2003	275	AEC>400/mm³& REC>4%	32%/89%	+	N.A.		N.A.
Kishi Y	2005	314	AEC>400/mm³ REC>4%	28%/97% 33%/93%	+ N.A.	N.A. N.A.		N.A. N.A.
Kishi Y	2007	263	AEC≧82/mm³	64%/79%	N.A.	Maximal ≧2 per portal tract Proportion of portal tract with eosinophil infiltration ≧8%	54%/84% 72%/65%	+ +

Table 3. Summary of the studies evaluating blood of histologic eosinophila with the diagnosis of acute cellular rejection (ACR). AEC, absolute eosinophil count; REC, percentage of eosinophil count in the whole leukocyte count.

Notably, blood eosinophilia a few days before biopsy is associated with ACR. Although rather low sensitivity is a problem, careful monitoring of the differential leukocyte count may contribute to the early detection of ACR. On the other hand, histologic eosinophilia predicts ACR with rather high sensitivity and specificity. Gupta et al. validated the inclusion of eosinophilia in addition to portal inflammation, endothelialitis, and bile duct damage for the grading of ACR and proposed the Royal free hospital (RFH) scoring system. In this system, the highest eosinophil count in a portal tract is graded as the follows: none (score 0), 0; mild (score 1), 1-4 cells; moderate (score 2), 5-9 cells; severe (score 3), 10 or more cells.[41] Kishi et al.[38] evaluated histologic eosinophilia as the maximum eosinophil count per portal tract (Emax) and the rate of portal tracts that included at least one eosinophil (E(+) rate), and demonstrated that both were associated with ACR as well as with ACR severity. This finding was later validated in another study by Demirhan et al.[42], in which marked eosinophilia assessed as Emax and E(+) rate correlated with ACR severity and response to treatment.

6. Differentiation from HCV recurrence

Differential diagnoses of ACR include recurrent or new-onset viral hepatitis by HBV, HCV, cytomegalovirus, or Epstein-Barr virus, autoimmune hepatitis, primary biliary cirrhosis, or primary sclerosing cholangitis. Among them the differentiation from recurrent HCV is difficult especially in the early postoperative period because histologic features overlap[43], but is critical because the treatment strategy is completely opposite.

To date, several studies have evaluated the interobserver agreement for the differential diagnosis of ACR and recurrent hepatitis C. Regev et al.[43] evaluatedthe interobserver and intraobserver agreement among five experienced pathologists for the diagnosis of 102 biopsy specimens. The results indicated that both the interobserver and the intraobserver agreement were relatively low, with Kappa scores ranging from 0.20 to 0.24 for interobserver agreement and from 0.19 to 0.42 for intraobserver agreement, indicating only slight to moderate agreement[43]. Netto et al.[44] reported the results of a multiinstitutional study to evaluate the agreement on the diagnosis of 11 biopsy specimens based on the Banff schema ACR scoring system and Batts and Ludwig schema for HCV staging by 17 pathologists. The results showed a Kappa score of 0.62 to 0.76 for interobserver agreement on the diagnosis of ACR or HCV, indicating substantial or almost perfect agreement[45].

In general, pathologists tend to over diagnose ACR rather than HCV recurrence. Leung et al.[46] reported a case of histologically diagnosed ACR that improved only by interferon and ribavirin therapy, and suggested that histologic characteristics traditionally associated with ACR might represent early recurrent HCV. Barnes et al. reported that HCV-positive patients with ACR are less likely to have blood eosinophilia than HCV-negative patients with ACR. They thus proposed that the eosinophil response might be suppressed in HCV-positive patients with ACR, and that ACR might be overdiagnosed if based on histopathology in patients with normal eosinophil levels[36]. Similarly, Kishi et al.[47] reported that HCV-positive patients diagnosed with ACR had significantly higher blood eosinophil counts on the day of biopsy than HCV-positive patients without ACR. These findings indicate that measures of blood eosinophil levels might contribute to the differential diagnosis of ACR in HCV-positive recipients.

Several blood or histologic markers have been proposed to facilitate the differentiation between ACR and recurrent HCV. Unitt et al.[48] reported that minichromosome maintenance

protein-2 (Mcm-2) visualized by immunohistochemical staining in lymphocytes infiltrating into the portal tracts is more frequently expressed in ACR than in HCV recurrence. The number of Mcm-2-positive lymphocytes in the portal tract was not correlated with the ACR grade, but a cut-off of 107 positive cells per portal tract distinguished ACR from HCV with a sensitivity of 82% and a specificity of 92%. MacQuillan et al.[49] performed immunohistochemical analysis to evaluate the expression of MxA protein, which belongs to the class of guanosine triphosphatases and is a marker of activation of the type 1 interferon pathway. The findings demonstrated strong hepatocellular MxA staining in 78% of HCV recurrence and in 30% of ACR biopsy specimens.
Typical histologic features of recurrent hepatitis C include lobular disarray, Kupffer cell hypertrophy, hepatocyte apoptosis, mild sinusoidal lymphocytosis, mononuclear portal inflammation, macrovesicularsteatosis involving periportal and midzonal hepatocytes. In chronic hepatitis, lobular changes wane and portal inflammation increases. Occasionally, nodular portal-based lymphoid aggregates are formed with emerging necroinflammatory and ductular-type interface activity. Further, fibrosing cholestatic hepatitis (FCH), which is clinically featured by rapidly progressive jaundice and extremely high HCV viral loads, may occur and is fatal in most cases. The incidence of FCH among the recipients who underwent liver transplantation for HCV-related cirrhosis is reported to be 6 to 14%[50-52]. Histologically, FCH is characterized by extensive fibrosis with immature fibrous bands extending from the portal tracts to the sinusoidal spaces, prominent canalicular and hepatocellular cholestasis, ground-glass transformation, ballooning of hepatocytes with cell loss, and a mild mixed inflammatory reaction may occur[53]. A small case series[52,54,55] reported that a certain proportion of patients with FCH might respond to interferon plus ribavirin with or without conversion of tacrolimus to cyclosporine A. Increased immunosuppression as a treatment for ACR is an important cause of FCH[56].

7. References

[1] Day CP, James OF: Steatohepatitis: a tale of two "hits"? Gastroenterology 114:842-5, 1998

[2] Hilden M, Christoffersen P, Juhl E, et al: Liver histology in a 'normal' population--examinations of 503 consecutive fatal traffic casualties. Scandinavian journal of gastroenterology 12:593-7, 1977

[3] Underwood Ground KE: Prevalence of fatty liver in healthy male adults accidentally killed. Aviation, space, and environmental medicine 55:59-61, 1984

[4] Hultcrantz R, Glaumann H, Lindberg G, et al: Liver investigation in 149 asymptomatic patients with moderately elevated activities of serum aminotransferases. Scandinavian journal of gastroenterology 21:109-13, 1986

[5] Wanless IR, Lentz JS: Fatty liver hepatitis (steatohepatitis) and obesity: an autopsy study with analysis of risk factors. Hepatology 12:1106-10, 1990

[6] Daniel S, Ben-Menachem T, Vasudevan G, et al: Prospective evaluation of unexplained chronic liver transaminase abnormalities in asymptomatic and symptomatic patients. The American journal of gastroenterology 94:3010-4, 1999

[7] Chitturi S, Farrell GC, Hashimoto E, et al: Non-alcoholic fatty liver disease in the Asia-Pacific region: definitions and overview of proposed guidelines. Journal of gastroenterology and hepatology 22:778-87, 2007

[8] Selzner M, Clavien PA: Failure of regeneration of the steatotic rat liver: disruption at two different levels in the regeneration pathway. Hepatology 31:35-42, 2000

[9] Vetelainen R, van Vliet AK, van Gulik TM: Severe steatosis increases hepatocellular injury and impairs liver regeneration in a rat model of partial hepatectomy. Annals of surgery 245:44-50, 2007

[10] Hsiao IT, Lin KJ, Chang SI, et al: Impaired liver regeneration of steatotic rats after portal vein ligation: a particular emphasis on (99m)Tc-DISIDA scintigraphy and adiponectin signaling. Journal of hepatology 52:540-9, 2010

[11] 11. Kooby DA, Fong Y, Suriawinata A, et al: Impact of steatosis on perioperative outcome following hepatic resection. J Gastrointest Surg 7:1034-44, 2003

[12] Vauthey JN, Pawlik TM, Ribero D, et al: Chemotherapy regimen predicts steatohepatitis and an increase in 90-day mortality after surgery for hepatic colorectal metastases. J Clin Oncol 24:2065-72, 2006

[13] Hussein O, Szvalb S, Van den Akker-Berman LM, et al: Liver regeneration is not altered in patients with nonalcoholic steatohepatitis (NASH) when compared to chronic hepatitis C infection with similar grade of inflammation. Digestive diseases and sciences 47:1926-31, 2002

[14] Cho JY, Suh KS, Kwon CH, et al: Mild hepatic steatosis is not a major risk factor for hepatectomy and regenerative power is not impaired. Surgery 139:508-15, 2006

[15] Yamamoto K, Takada Y, Fujimoto Y, et al: Nonalcoholic steatohepatitis in donors for living donor liver transplantation. Transplantation 83:257-62, 2007

[16] Rinella ME, Alonso E, Rao S, et al: Body mass index as a predictor of hepatic steatosis in living liver donors. Liver transplantation : official publication of the American Association for the Study of Liver Diseases and the International Liver Transplantation Society 7:409-14, 2001

[17] Ryan CK, Johnson LA, Germin BI, et al: One hundred consecutive hepatic biopsies in the workup of living donors for right lobe liver transplantation. Liver transplantation : official publication of the American Association for the Study of Liver Diseases and the International Liver Transplantation Society 8:1114-22, 2002

[18] Tran TT, Changsri C, Shackleton CR, et al: Living donor liver transplantation: histological abnormalities found on liver biopsies of apparently healthy potential donors. Journal of gastroenterology and hepatology 21:381-3, 2006

[19] Yamashiki N, Sugawara Y, Tamura S, et al: Noninvasive estimation of hepatic steatosis in living liver donors: usefulness of visceral fat area measurement. Transplantation 88:575-81, 2009

[20] Poordad F, Gish R, Wakil A, et al: De novo non-alcoholic fatty liver disease following orthotopic liver transplantation. American journal of transplantation : official journal of the American Society of Transplantation and the American Society of Transplant Surgeons 3:1413-7, 2003

[21] Seo S, Maganti K, Khehra M, et al: De novo nonalcoholic fatty liver disease after liver transplantation. Liver transplantation : official publication of the American Association for the Study of Liver Diseases and the International Liver Transplantation Society 13:844-7, 2007

[22] Lindor KD, Kowdley KV, Heathcote EJ, et al: Ursodeoxycholic acid for treatment of nonalcoholic steatohepatitis: results of a randomized trial. Hepatology 39:770-8, 2004

[23] Brunt EM, Janney CG, Di Bisceglie AM, et al: Nonalcoholic steatohepatitis: a proposal for grading and staging the histological lesions. The American journal of gastroenterology 94:2467-74, 1999

[24] Promrat K, Lutchman G, Uwaifo GI, et al: A pilot study of pioglitazone treatment for nonalcoholic steatohepatitis. Hepatology 39:188-96, 2004

[25] Kleiner DE, Brunt EM, Van Natta M, et al: Design and validation of a histological scoring system for nonalcoholic fatty liver disease. Hepatology 41:1313-21, 2005
[26] Demetris AJ, Seaberg EC, Batts KP, et al: Chronic liver allograft rejection: a National Institute of Diabetes and Digestive and Kidney Diseases interinstitutional study analyzing the reliability of current criteria and proposal of an expanded definition. National Institute of Diabetes and Digestive and Kidney Diseases Liver Transplantation Database. The American journal of surgical pathology 22:28-39, 1998
[27] Banff schema for grading liver allograft rejection: an international consensus document. Hepatology 25:658-63, 1997
[28] Demetris A, Adams D, Bellamy C, et al: Update of the International Banff Schema for Liver Allograft Rejection: working recommendations for the histopathologic staging and reporting of chronic rejection. An International Panel. Hepatology 31:792-9, 2000
[29] Foster PF, Sankary HN, Hart M, et al: Blood and graft eosinophilia as predictors of rejection in human liver transplantation. Transplantation 47:72-4, 1989
[30] Foster PF, Sankary HN, Williams JW, et al: Morphometric inflammatory cell analysis of human liver allograft biopsies. Transplantation 51:873-6, 1991
[31] Ben-Ari Z, Booth JD, Gupta SD, et al: Morphometric image analysis and eosinophil counts in human liver allografts. Transpl Int 8:346-52, 1995
[32] Manzarbeitia C, Rustgi VK, Jonsson J, et al: Absolute peripheral blood eosinophilia. An early marker for rejection in clinical liver transplantation. Transplantation 59:1358-60, 1995
[33] Dollinger MM, Plevris JN, Bouchier IA, et al: Peripheral eosinophil count both before and after liver transplantation predicts acute cellular rejection. Liver Transpl Surg 3:112-7, 1997
[34] Hughes VF, Trull AK, Joshi O, et al: Monitoring eosinophil activation and liver function after liver transplantation. Transplantation 65:1334-9, 1998
[35] Nagral A, Quaglia A, Sabin CA, et al: Blood and graft eosinophils in acute cellular rejection of liver allografts. Transplant Proc 33:2588-93, 2001
[36] Barnes EJ, Abdel-Rehim MM, Goulis Y, et al: Applications and limitations of blood eosinophilia for the diagnosis of acute cellular rejection in liver transplantation. Am J Transplant 3:432-8, 2003
[37] Kishi Y, Sugawara Y, Tamura S, et al: Is blood eosinophilia an effective predictor of acute rejection in living donor liver transplantation? Transpl Int 18:1147-51, 2005
[38] Kishi Y, Sugawara Y, Tamura S, et al: Histologic eosinophilia as an aid to diagnose acute cellular rejection after living donor liver transplantation. Clinical transplantation 21:214-8, 2007
[39] Lautenschlager I, von Willebrand E, Hayry P: Blood eosinophilia, steroids, and rejection. Transplantation 40:354-7, 1985
[40] Meagher LC, Cousin JM, Seckl JR, et al: Opposing effects of glucocorticoids on the rate of apoptosis in neutrophilic and eosinophilic granulocytes. J Immunol 156:4422-8, 1996
[41] Datta Gupta S, Hudson M, Burroughs AK, et al: Grading of cellular rejection after orthotopic liver transplantation. Hepatology 21:46-57, 1995
[42] Demirhan B, Bilezikci B, Haberal AN, et al: Hepatic parenchymal changes and histologic eosinophilia as predictors of subsequent acute liver allograft rejection. Liver Transpl 14:214-9, 2008

[43] Regev A, Molina E, Moura R, et al: Reliability of histopathologic assessment for the differentiation of recurrent hepatitis C from acute rejection after liver transplantation. Liver transplantation : official publication of the American Association for the Study of Liver Diseases and the International Liver Transplantation Society 10:1233-9, 2004
[44] Batts KP, Ludwig J: Chronic hepatitis. An update on terminology and reporting. The American journal of surgical pathology 19:1409-17, 1995
[45] Netto GJ, Watkins DL, Williams JW, et al: Interobserver agreement in hepatitis C grading and staging and in the Banff grading schema for acute cellular rejection: the "hepatitis C 3" multi-institutional trial experience. Archives of pathology & laboratory medicine 130:1157-62, 2006
[46] Leung JY, Abraczinskas DR, Bhan AK, et al: Recurrent allograft HCV presenting as acute cellular rejection: successful management with interferon and ribavirin alone. Clinical transplantation 17:275-83, 2003
[47] Kishi Y, Sugawara Y, Kaneko J, et al: Blood eosinophilia after living donor liver transplantation for hepatitis C virus-related cirrhosis. Transplantation proceedings 39:1540-3, 2007
[48] Unitt E, Gelson W, Davies SE, et al: Minichromosome maintenance protein-2-positive portal tract lymphocytes distinguish acute cellular rejection from hepatitis C virus recurrence after liver transplantation. Liver Transpl 15:306-12, 2009
[49] MacQuillan GC, de Boer WB, Allan JE, et al: Hepatocellular MxA protein expression supports the differentiation of recurrent hepatitis C disease from acute cellular rejection after liver transplantation. Clinical transplantation 24:252-8, 2010
[50] Schluger LK, Sheiner PA, Thung SN, et al: Severe recurrent cholestatic hepatitis C following orthotopic liver transplantation. Hepatology 23:971-6, 1996
[51] Satapathy SK, Sclair S, Fiel MI, et al: Clinical characterization of patients developing histologically-proven fibrosing cholestatic hepatitis C post-liver transplantation. Hepatology research : the official journal of the Japan Society of Hepatology 41:328-39, 2011
[52] Cimsit B, Assis D, Caldwell C, et al: Successful treatment of fibrosing cholestatic hepatitis after liver transplantation. Transplantation proceedings 43:905-8, 2011
[53] Davies SE, Portmann BC, O'Grady JG, et al: Hepatic histological findings after transplantation for chronic hepatitis B virus infection, including a unique pattern of fibrosing cholestatic hepatitis. Hepatology 13:150-7, 1991
[54] Ong JP, Younossi ZM, Gramlich T, et al: Interferon alpha 2B and ribavirin in severe recurrent cholestatic hepatitis C. Transplantation 71:1486-7, 2001
[55] Gopal DV, Rosen HR: Duration of antiviral therapy for cholestatic HCV recurrence may need to be indefinite. Liver transplantation : official publication of the American Association for the Study of Liver Diseases and the International Liver Transplantation Society 9:348-53, 2003
[56] Testa G, Crippin JS, Netto GJ, et al: Liver transplantation for hepatitis C: recurrence and disease progression in 300 patients. Liver transplantation : official publication of the American Association for the Study of Liver Diseases and the International Liver Transplantation Society 6:553-61, 2000

2

Reversal of Liver Fibrosis: A Review

Mona H. Ismail
College of Medicine, University of Dammam, Department of Internal Medicine, Division of Gastroenterology, King Fahad Hospital of the University, Saudi Arabia

1. Introduction

Liver fibrosis is the final pathway for most chronic liver disease and is the main reason for increased mortality in affected patients. The extent of liver fibrosis displays great individual variation, even after controlling for age (at infection), gender & exogenous factors. Thus, host genetic factors are likely to play an important role in the process of liver scarring. (Weber et al., 2008). Inflammation is strongly associated with chronic liver injury, and fibrosis is part of the liver's wound-healing response. Inflammation represents the driving force for the progressive accumulation of extracellular matrix (ECM) components, eventually leading to liver cirrhosis and hepatic failure. Although even acute injury will activate mechanisms of fibrogenesis, the sustained signals of inflammation associated with chronic liver disease caused by infection, drugs, metabolic disorders, or immune attacks are required for significant fibrosis to accumulate. Cirrhosis is the result of many liver diseases and consists of fibrosis and regenerating nodules. Clinical presentations vary from asymptomatic to advanced end stage liver diseases with complications. In addition, a significant need exists for developing safe and accurate noninvasive technique for detecting progression or regression of hepatic fibrosis in patients with chronic liver disease (Fallowfield JA et al., 2006).

The past few years have seen remarkable progress in the field of liver fibrosis, including understanding the crosstalk between innate immunity and inflammatory cells & pathways regulating fibrosis regression. This article will review recent advances in this field as well as imaging and diagnostic test of liver fibrosis.

2. Advances in the mechanisms of fibrogenesis

Liver fibrogenesis is characterized by cellular activation of hepatic stellate cells (HSCs) and its mediators. HSCs have dominated studies exploring mechanisms of liver fibrosis over the last two decades. HSCs are resident vitamin A-storing cells in the perisinusoidal space of Disse between the sinusoidal endothelium and hepatocytes. Following hepatic injury, HSCs become activated into a myofibroblast-like phenotype that is contractile, proliferative and fibrogenic. Collagen and other ECM components are deposited which result in a fibrous scar eventually leading to cirrhosis and liver failure (Lee & Friedman, 2011). Liver fibrosis is a dynamic process, resulting from the equilibrium between fibrogenesis and altered matrix degradation, and may be reversible prior to the establishment of advanced architectural changes to the liver. HSC represent the final common pathway of the wound-healing response of the liver. Activation consists of two major phases, initiation (also called a 'preinflammatory stage') and perpetuation, followed by a resolution phase if the injury subsides (Friedman, 1993). Following alcohol consumption, cholestasis and iron overload, reactive oxygen species (ROS) and lipid peroxidation products are generated in large amounts leading to Kupffer cell activation. Activated Kupffer cells, infiltrating circulating monocytes, activated and aggregated platelets, and damaged hepatocytes are sources of platelet-derived growth factor (PDGF) and transforming growth factor-b1 (TGF-b1), which both trigger the initiation of intracellular signaling cascades after binding to HSC surface receptors. Activated HSC lose vitamin A droplets and increase expression of cytoskeletous proteins such as desmin and α-smooth muscle actin, which are associated with augmented contractile activity, as well as generate ECM, which includes type I and III collagen (Kawada, 2011). In addition, augmented production of the tissue inhibitor of matrix metalloproteinases (TIMP) hampers the degradation of ECM and conversely stimulates their accumulation in the inflamed liver. Activated HSC, also known as myofibroblasts (MFB), are contractile and their capacity to generate contractile force mediates the liver's injury response through modulation of sinusoidal blood flow and scar contracture.

Metalloproteinases-1 (MMP-1) is a key collagenase that metabolizes type I collagen; however, MMP activity also strictly regulates its binding partner, TIMP. Because HSC are able to generate both TIMP-1 and -2, a local balance between MMP and TIMP plays an important role in fostering the resolution of the fibrotic process (Benyon & Arthur, 2001). The liver's response to injury is an angiogenic one, with evidence of new blood vessel formation, sinusoidal remodeling, and HSC expansion (Lee et al., 2007). Neo-angiogenesis is stimulated in hepatic tissue by the progressive increase of tissue hypoxia. PDGF, vascular endothelial growth factor (VEGF), and their receptors as well as vasoactive mediators including nitric oxide and carbon monoxide are upregulated during liver fibrosis. This mechanism is strictly linked to the anatomical alterations following the establishment of periportal fibrosis with an increased contribution of the hepatic artery to the formation of sinusoidal blood. Accordingly, sinusoidal blood flow becomes increasingly arterialized with hepatocytes adjusting to an abnormally high oxygen concentration. Subsequently, the progressive capillarization of sinusoids leads to an impairment of oxygen diffusion from the sinusoids to hepatocytes with the consequent up-regulation of pro-angiogenic pathways (Pinzani et al., 2011). For example, increased VEGF concentrations may contribute to the accelerated progression of fibrosis in smokers who have hepatitis C (Dev et al., 2006).

The excess deposition of ECM proteins disrupts the normal architecture of the liver, which alters the normal function of the organ, ultimately leading to portal hypertension (PH) which is the earliest and most important consequence of cirrhosis and underlies most of the clinical complications of the disease. PH results from an increased intrahepatic resistance combined with increased portal (and hepatic arterial) blood flow.

Leptin, a key adipokine, has been implicated in fibrogenesis through a number of pathways. Leptin, a circulating adipogenic hormone, promotes stellate cell fibrogenesis and enhances TIMP-1 expression, which is associated with increased leptin signaling (Leclercq et al., 2002). Recent investigations have revealed the participation of mesenchymal cells, which originate from bone marrow, in liver fibrosis by using rodent models and damaged human livers (Forbes et al., 2004; Kisseleva et al., 2006). Similarly, fibrocytes in circulation and portal fibroblasts are acknowledged as fibrotic players (Dranoff & Wells, 2010). Furthermore, an

epithelial-mesenchymal transition (EMT) may be involved in the fibrotic process in the liver as well as in the kidney and lung (Zeisberg et al., 2007).
Perpetuation of the hepatic fibrotic process is supported by the activation of HSC and the presence of MFB, which are continuously stimulated by growth factors, cytokines and oxidative stress derived from nearby cells. Damaged hepatocytes are a source of lipid peroxides and ROS generated from hepatocytic mitochondria (Jiang et al., 2010). Macrophage chemotactic protein-1 (MCP-1) and osteopontin derived from activated Kupffer cells are involved in the infiltration of inflammatory cells into the liver (Syn et al., 2011).
Liver fibrosis is the final common pathway of the wound-healing response of the liver which can progress to liver fibrosis and eventually cirrhosis. At the cellular and molecular level, this progressive process is characterized by cellular activation of HSCs and aberrant activity of TGF-β with its downstream cellular mediators.

3. Reversibility of liver fibrosis and cirrhosis

Regression of fibrosis and cirrhosis in humans is not a novel concept. Anecdotal reports published more than forty years ago recorded an improvement in patients with cirrhosis treated for hemochromatosis and Wilson disease (Powell & Ker, 1970; Falkmer et al., 1970). Advanced fibrosis and cirrhosis has recently been described with respect to matrix turnover in trials of antiviral therapy for chronic viral hepatitis (Poynard et al., 2002). The issue of regression/reversibility of cirrhosis originates from evidence obtained in animal models upon the discontinuation of the cause of liver damage or following treatment with antifibrotic agent. In chronic liver injury, activated HSC are major source of fibrillar ECM as well as of the TIMPs which inhibit collagen degradation (Bataller & Brenner, 2005). HSC survival and apoptosis are regulated by growth factors expressed during fibrotic liver injury. Thus,HSC apoptosis plays a critical role in the recovery from biliary as well as toxic-induced liver fibrosis (Iredale et al., 1998). Moreover, the very striking improvement in the histological appearance in these reports suggests that the number of activated HSCs is reduced as well. By definition, the resolution of an injury with a return to normal histology must involve the loss or phenotypic reversal to quiescence of activated HSCs (Iredale, 2001). On the other hand, activated HSC produce the fibrolytic MMPs resulting in extracellular degradation and scar remodelling. Similarly, kuffer cells/macrophages appear instrumental in the reversal of established fibrosis when the fibrogenic stimulus is absent; while they can fuel fibrogenesis when the trigger is present (Duffield et al., 2005). Clearly, at some point (probably coinciding with the onset of the clinical symptoms of cirrhosis), fibrosis becomes irreversible. Animal models suggest that this event coincides with a significant collagen cross-linking by tissue transglutaminase, leading to the production of an insoluble matrix (Issa et al., 2004).
These observations have enhanced our understanding of the pathogenesis of liver fibrosis and defined our approach to its treatment. When hepatocyte necrosis occurs, the remaining hepatocytes undergo proliferation, leading to repair of the local environment. These processes are stimulated by growth factors derived from HSC, such as HGF, epidermal growth factor, epimorphin and pleiotrophin (Sawitza et al., 2009). It is difficult to say when cirrhosis becomes irreversible. Fibrotic deposition related to recent disease and characterized by the presence of thin reticulin fibers, often in the presence of a diffuse inflammatory infiltrate, is likely fully reversible. However, longstanding fibrosis, branded

by extensive collagen cross-linking, dense acellular/paucicellular ECM and decreased expression and/or activity of specific metalloproteinases, is likely irreversible (Issa et al., 2004; Pinzani & Rombouts, 2004). For example, cirrhosis following withdrawal of an injurious stimulus can undergo remodeling of dense micronodular cirrhosis to a more attenuated, macronodular pattern. However, some septa will persist, likely representing those laid down early in the injury, and are therefore the most "mature" (i.e., cross-linked) (Friedman, 2003).

Evidence of fibrotic regression has now been documented in chronic liver diseases, including autoimmune hepatitis, biliary obstruction, iron overload, Non-alcoholic steatohepatitis, and viral hepatitis B and C (Ismail & Pinzani, 2009). Poynard *et al., 2002* examined liver biopsy specimens taken before and after therapy from 153 patients with HCV-related cirrhosis treated with different pegylated interferon and ribavirin regimens. Using the METAVIR scoring system, they found that the extent of liver fibrosis had improved in 75 (49%) Stage-4 patients: to Stage 3 in 23 patients, to Stage 2 in 26 patients, to Stage 1 in 23 patients, and to a virtually normal histological appearance in three patients. No such improvements were recorded in the control group of patients treated with interferon monotherapy. Reversal of cirrhosis was more common among younger patients.

4. Evaluation of liver fibrosis

The accurate and early diagnosis of liver fibrosis is crucial for long-term prognosis (Castera & Pinzani, 2010). The complete evaluation of a patient with diffuse liver diseases requires clinical evaluation, laboratory tests and pathological examination. Standard liver tests (ALT, AST, Bilirubin...etc) are of limited value in assessing the degree of fibrosis. Currently, histological examination of a liver biopsy specimen is the reference standard for the diagnosis, staging, and monitoring of liver fibrosis (Bravo et al., 2001; Campbell & Reddy, 2004). Three staging systems are commonly used to classify liver fibrosis: the Knodell, METAVIR and Ishak scores (Knodell et al., 1981; Desmet et al., 1994; Anthony et al., 1978). Knodell and METAVIR score fibrosis from Stages 0 to 4, with Stage 4 as cirrhosis, whereas Ishak scores fibrosis from Stages 0 to 6, with 5 as incomplete or early cirrhosis and 6 as established cirrhosis. There are several situations in which the role of liver biopsy (LB) is being challenged. These methods are semi-quantitative which make it a poor choice when considering assessment of liver fibrosis progression or regression. Furthermore, there is the issue of sampling error, defined as variable levels of fibrosis throughout the liver, with biopsy only examining a small portion of the liver (around 1/50000th of liver mass is obtained) (Bedossa et al., 2003). In addition, histological examination is prone to intraobserver and interobserver variation, which may occur even when widely validated systems are used to assess liver damage (Regev et al., 2002). Finally, liver biopsy is an invasive procedure with associated morbidity: pain occurs in 20% of patients and major complications (such as bleeding or hemobilia) in 0.5% of patients (Huang et al., 2007; Rockey et al., 2009).

5. Noninvasive markers of fibrosis

Over the past years, several non-invasive tests have become available for clinicians to use to assess liver fibrosis and determine the best course of management for their patients, especially those with chronic hepatitis C (Afdhal, 2003; Kotlyar et al., 2008). Initial studies of noninvasive markers largely consisted of single components, but the field has evolved into combining these single components into panel markers. Several laboratory tests, scores, and indices have been proposed for noninvasive prediction of hepatic fibrosis in patients with chronic hepatitis C. Among these is the aspartate aminotransferase (AST)/alanine aminotransferase (ALT) ratio (AAR) (Saadeh et al., 2001; Giannini et al., 2003; Williams & Hoofnagle, 1988). A ratio >1 has been proposed as a test for cirrhosis. However, the test is disadvantaged by both poor sensitivity (53.2%) and a negative predictive value (80.7%). Forns fibrosis index (FFI) (Forns, 2002) was developed as a model to predict fibrosis in patients with HCV based on age, gamma glutamyl transferase (gGT), cholesterol and platelet count. The score derived from this was validated against liver histology using the METAVIR scoring system for hepatic fibrosis, and it was found to have a sensitivity of 94% & specificity of 51% for a cut-off value of >4.2 (for absence of fibrosis) and a sensitivity of 30% & specificity of 95% for a cut-off value of > 6.9 (for presence of fibrosis). Low platelet count *per se* (Ono et al., 1999) can predict advanced fibrosis. The AST-to-platelet ratio index (APRI) (Wai et al., 2003) is formulated by dividing the AST by the upper limit of normal AST divided by the platelet count and multiplied by 100. In the initial study in patients with HCV, the APRI was derived from a training set of 192 patients undergoing liver biopsy. The area under the curve (AUC) for predicting significant fibrosis (Ishak fibrosis score ≥ 3) and cirrhosis were 0.82 and 0.92, respectively, in the training set, and 0.80 and 0.89, respectively, in the validation set for 78 patients. Using optimized cut-off values, this test predicted significant fibrosis in 51% and cirrhosis in 81% of patients. Other similar scoring systems that have been applied include the cirrhosis discriminant score (Bonacini et al., 1997), age-platelet index (Poynard et al., 1997) and Pohl score (Pohl et al., 2007). These tests were compared in a study comparing AAR, CDS, AP index, Pohl score and APRI (Lackner et al., 2005). In this study of 194 patients, AUC analysis revealed similar diagnostic accuracy for CDS, AP index, APRI and platelet count for the prediction of significant fibrosis (Ishak score ≥3) (AUCs of 0.71, 0.74, 0.80 and 0.71, respectively) and cirrhosis (AUCs of 0.91, 0.91, 0.90 and 0.89, respectively). FIB-4 (Vallet-Pichard et al., 2007) is a recently described marker of fibrosis derived from a formula utilizing AST, ALT, age and platelets. In a series of 847 biopsies from HCV monoinfected patients comparing FIB-4 values to liver biopsy and FibroTest values, FIB-4 values <1.45 or >3.25 (64.6% cases) were concordant with FibroTest results in 92.1% and 76% of cases, respectively. Using the METAVIR scoring system to record fibrosis, this test had an AUC of 0.85 (95% CI 0.82–0.89) for prediction of severe fibrosis (F3–4) and 0.91 (95% CI 0.86–0.93) for prediction of cirrhosis. The FibroIndex was derived from an estimation set of 240 patients and validated in 120 subsequent patients. The test was derived from platelet count, AST and gamma globulin. Using this method, the AUC for the detection of significant fibrosis using the METAVIR histological classification of fibrosis (≥F2) was 0.83 in the estimation set and 0.82 in the validation set. Although it was calculated using best cut-offs for PPV, only 35% of patients avoided LB.

FibroTest-ActiTest (FT-AT), from BioPredictive, Paris, France, is a noninvasive blood test that combines the quantitative results of six serum biochemical markers [alfa2-macroglobulin, haptoglobin, gamma glutamyl transpeptidase, total bilirubin, apolipoprotein A1 and ALT] with patients' age and gender in a patented algorithm to generate a measure of fibrosis and necroinflammatory activity in the liver (Imbert-Bismut et al., 2001; Poynard et

Biomarker (Ref.)	Parameters	Patients	F2-3-4 (%)	AUC	Se (%)	Sp (%)	PPV/NPV (%)
Forns Fibrosis Index 2002 (Kotlyar et al., 2008)	Age, platelet count, GGTP and cholesterol.	HCV	26%	t =0.86, v =0.81	91	51	66/96
APRI Index 2003 (Giannini et al., 2003)	AST/Platelet Ratio	HCV	50	t =0.80, v =0.90	89	75	91/90
Fibrotest 2001 (Poynard et al., 1997)	α2-macroglobulin, hepatoglobulin, lipoprotein A1, bilirubin and δ-glubulin.	HCV	80	t =0.84, v =87	75	85	>90/100

Abbreviations used: GGT: g-glutamyl-transpeptidase; AST: aspartate transaminase; chronic hepatitis C: HCV; Se: sensitivity; Sp: specificity; AUC: area under the receiver operator characteristic curve; t: Training group; v: Validation group. An AUC of 1.0 is characteristic of an ideal test, where as an AUC of 0.5 or less indicates a test of no diagnostic value.

Table 1. Diagnostic performance of common non-invasive tests of liver fibrosis.

al., 2002). FT-AT provides an accurate measurement of bridging fibrosis and/or moderate necroinflammatory activity with the area under the receiver operating curve (AUROC) predictive value, between 0.70 and 0.80, when compared to liver biopsy (Sporea et al., 2008) (Table 1 summarized the diagnostic performance of noninvasive tests of liver fibrosis).

6. Limitations of serum biomarkers

One limitation of biomarkers is that none is liver-specific and they may be influenced by changes in their clearance and excretion. The inter-laboratory reproducibility of scores such as FibroTest has been shown to be satisfactory for use in clinical practice (Cales et al., 2008). Careful interpretation of each test is required e.g., when using FibroTest, the existence of haemolysis or Gilbert syndrome can lead to false-positive results (by a decrease haptoglobin or an increase in bilirubin, respectively)(Castera et al., 2011).

7. Imaging methods

Imaging techniques are an attractive way of evaluating fibrosis because they are noninvasive and have the ability to detect structural changes, which serological-based tests of fibrosis and inflammation are unable to do. Using the modalities of ultrasound, computed tomography or magnetic resonance imaging (MRI), it is possible to diagnose features of advanced chronic liver disease by recognizing surrogate markers of portal hypertension (e.g. splenomegaly, ascites..etc) with a high degree of sensitivity and specificity. However, these techniques do not reliably detect lesser degrees of fibrosis. Even diagnosis of cirrhosis is often based only on signs of advanced liver cirrhosis, e.g., signs of portal hypertension, a shrunken right liver lobe with enlargement of the caudate lobe, resulting in a high specificity but lower sensitivity of the methods (Honda et al., 1990). Ultrasound studies combining several ultrasound parameters and Doppler measurements achieved accuracies for the diagnosis of cirrhosis up to a maximum of 88% (Aubé et al., 1999). Commonly used imaging methods are discussed in the next section.

7.1 Transient elastography or fibroscan

Transient elastography (TE), or FibroScan (Echosens, Paris, France), is a novel technology for measuring liver stiffness (Ziol et al., 2005). The scan was developed on the principle that livers with increasing degrees of scarring or fibrosis have decreasing elasticity and that a shear wave propagating through stiffer material would progress faster than in a more elastic material. Thus, the stiffer the liver, the faster the sheer waves propagate. The ultrasound transducer probe is mounted on the axis of a vibrator. Pulse-echo ultrasound waves then measure the velocity of the shear wave in the liver tissue at a distance of 2.5–6.5 cm under the skin level, which corresponds to a measured distance of 4 cm in the liver tissue. TE is rapid (less than 5 minutes), highly reproducible and can easily be performed bedside or in the outpatient clinic with immediate results. Liver stiffness corresponds to the median value of ten validated measurements that range from 2.5 to 75 kPa, with normal values around 5.5 kPa (Castera et al., 2008).

TE provides clinicians with a noninvasive, accurate, and reproducible tool to estimate liver fibrosis. Numerous studies have shown that this technique is an excellent tool for the detection of advanced fibrosis or cirrhosis, but the results for the prediction of different stages of moderate fibrosis are less conclusive. Due to its noninvasive nature, simple training and ease of use, TE can be used repeatedly on patients and is optimal for large-scale studies, in which healthy patients with no indication for liver biopsy can also be included. This technique has the advantage of being safe, reproducible, and rapid. However, falsely high liver stiffness measurements might also occur during acute hepatitis, extrahepatic cholestasis, congestive heart failure, and amyloidosis (Castera et al., 2010). Failed acquisition was commonly due to obesity, particularly increased waist circumference, and limited operator experience. However, development of S and XL probes might overcome this limitation. A meta-analysis of nine studies (Talwalkar et al., 2007) showed that TE has a sensitivity of 87% (95% CI 84%-90%) and a specificity of 91% (95% CI 89%-92%) for diagnosing cirrhosis. In seven of the nine studies, Stage 2 to 4 fibrosis was diagnosed with 70% sensitivity (95% CI 67%-73%) and 84% specificity (95% CI 80%-88%). Foucher et al. reported that, in 144 chronic hepatitis C patients with fibrosis at stage 3 or 4, the cut-off values of liver stiffness measured by TE were 27.5, 49.1, 53.7 and 62.7 kPa for the appearance of esophageal varices (Stage 2/3), ascites, HCC and rupture of esophageal varices (Castéra et al., 2010).

7.2 Magnetic resonance elastography

Few studies that focus on MRI detection and quantification of liver fibrosis currently exist. More recently, a liver stiffness evaluation (LSE) by MR elastography (MRE) has been demonstrated to provide high accuracy for the noninvasive diagnosis of liver fibrosis (Talwalkar et al., 2008; Huwart et al., 2008). The technique used is similar to that used in ultrasound elastography in that it uses a vibration device to induce a shear wave in the liver. Liver elasticity is evaluated using an external probe at the back of the patient and sending low frequency vibrations (60 Hz) through the liver and measuring the MRI spin-echo sequence. With this technique, shear elasticity and viscosity maps are obtained, and a color-coded image is generated that depicts the wave velocity, and thus the stiffness, throughout the organ. A study comparing the MRE of thirty healthy volunteers and fifty patients with chronic liver disease with liver histology showed a sensitivity of 86% and a specificity of 85% for discrimination between patients with moderate and severe fibrosis (Metavir F2–F4) and those with mild fibrosis (Yin et al., 2007). However, MRE is expensive, and cost may limit its use. Thus, it may not be readily available at all hospitals.

7.3 Acoustic radiation force impulse

Acoustic radiation force impulse (ARFI) is a new technology for LSE which uses an add-on module to the standard ultrasound imaging device. It involves targeting an anatomic region for interrogation of the elastic properties with the use of a region of interest cursor while performing real-time B-mode imaging. An initial ultrasonic pulse is transmitted at diagnostic intensity levels to obtain a baseline signal for later comparison. A short-duration (approximately 0.3 s), high-intensity acoustic 'pushing pulse' is then transmitted by the same transducer and is followed by a series of diagnostic intensity pulses, which are used to track the displacement of the tissue caused by the pushing pulse (Palmeri et al., 2005). By measuring the time-to-peak displacement at each lateral location, one can reproduce the shear-wave speed of the tissue. The shear-wave propagation velocity is proportional to the square root of tissue elasticity. Results are expressed in meters per second (m/s) (range, 0.5–4.4 m/sec; ±20% accuracy over the range). In a study performed by Friedrich-Rust et al., 2009; ARFI was compared to LB and blood markers of liver fibrosis in 86 patients with chronic hepatitis (B or C). The Spearman correlation coefficients between the histological fibrosis stage and ARFI, TE, FibroTest and APRI scores indicated significant correlations: 0.71, 0.73, 0.66 and 0.45, respectively ($p<0.001$).

Newer imaging estimation of hepatic fibrosis appears promising. TE & ARFI appear to be excellent tools for early detection of cirrhosis with likely prognostic value in this setting.

8. Combination of serum markers and imaging methods

The use of sequential or combined serum tests and imaging to provide better prediction for significant fibrosis (METAVIR stages F2–F4) or cirrhosis, and thus a reduction in the need for biopsy in patients with chronic hepatitis C (CHC), is gaining support. Certainly, the stepwise concept of using a highly sensitive test to first rule out significant disease and then using a more specific test to confirm the diagnosis if the test results are positive is advantageous. One recent approach integrated a biopsy into a clinical decision algorithm by targeting patients with indeterminate or misclassified values with marker panels. The Sequential Algorithms for Fibrosis Evaluation (SAFE) biopsy study (Sebastiani et al., 2009) evaluated the APRI followed by FT-AT in 2035 CHC patients from nine clinical centers in the United States and Europe. Using this sequential approach, the number of biopsies saved at baseline was 47 and 82% with an overall accuracy of 90% for Stages F2–F4 and cirrhosis, respectively. Another study (Paggi et al., 2008) noted that the combination of APRI and a simple ultrasound assessment of the presence of liver surface nodularity could predict stages F3–F4 in 54% of CHC patients.

These techniques certainly appear to be valid approaches for reducing the need for biopsy in CHC patients. The combined use of TE and biochemical markers seems to be the most promising noninvasive techniques which can help the clinician decide whether a liver biopsy is necessary in some patients, and accordingly decide who to treat.

9. Conclusions

Our understanding of the mechanism of liver fibrosis has changed dramatically over the last decade and is no longer viewed as permanent but rather as a dynamic process. The HSC play a critical role in fibrogenesis. Reversal of fibrosis is accompanied by clearance of HSC and treatment of the primary cause of injury can allow complete resolution of fibrosis. Liver biopsy is the current reference test for the assessment of hepatic fibrosis, but because of its limitations, noninvasive markers of liver fibrosis have been developed. Although none of the currently available noninvasive marker of fibrosis are an ideal test to accurately differentiate between disease stages, the combination of serum markers, and imaging appear to have good predictive values in excluding patients with cirrhosis.

10. References

Afdhal NH (2003). Diagnosing fibrosis in hepatitis C: is the pendulum swinging from biopsy to blood tests? *Hepatology* 2003 May; 37: 972-4.

Anthony PP, Ishak KG, Nayak NC, Poulsen HE, Scheuer PJ & Sobin LH (1978). The morphology of cirrhosis. Working group sponsored by the World Health Organization. *J Clin Pathol* 1978 May; 31: 395-414.

Aubé C, Oberti F, Korali N, Namour MA, Loisel D, Tanguy JY, et al (1999). Ultrasonographic diagnosis of hepatic fibrosis or cirrhosis. *J Hepatol* 1999 Mar; 30: 472–8.

Bataller R & Brenner DA (2005). Liver fibrosis. J Clin Invest 2005 Feb; 115: 209-18.

Bedossa P, Dargere D & Paradis V (2003). Sampling variability of liver fibrosis in chronic hepatitis C. *Hepatology* 2003 Dec;38:1449-57.

Benyon RC & Arthur MJ (2001). Extracellular matrix degradation and the role of hepatic stellate cells. *Semin Liver Dis* 2001 Aug;21:373–84.

Bonacini M, Hadi G, Govindarajan S & Lindsay KL (1997). Utility of a discriminant score for diagnosing advanced fibrosis or cirrhosis in patients with chronic hepatitis C virus infection. *Am J Gastroenterol* 1997 Aug;92:1302-4.

Bravo AA, Sheth SG & Chopra S (2001). Liver biopsy. N Engl J Med 2001 Feb; 344: 495–500.

Cales P, Veillon P, Konate A, Mathieu E, Ternisien C, Chevailler A, et al (2008). Reproducibility of blood tests of liver fibrosis in clinical practice. *Clin Biochem* 2008 Jan; 41(1–2):10–8.

Campbell MS & Reddy KR (2004). Review article: the evolving role of liver biopsy. *Aliment Pharmacol Ther* 2004 Aug; 20:249-59.

Castera L, Forms X & Alberti A (2008). Non-invasive evaluation of liver fibrosis using transient elastography. *J Hepatol* 2008 May; 48: 835-47.

Castera L, Foucher J, Bernard PH, Carvalho F, Allaix D, Merrouche W, et al (2010). Pitfalls of liver stiffness measurement: a 5-year prospective study of 13,369 examinations. *Hepatology* 2010 Mar; 51:828-35.

Castera L & Pinzani M (2010). Biopsy and non-invasive methods for the diagnosis of liver fibrosis: does it take two to tango? *Gut* 2010 Jul; 59: 861-6.

Castera L (2011). Invasive and non-invasive methods for the assessment of fibrosis and disease progression in chronic liver disease. *Best Practice & Research Clinical Gastroenterology* 2011 Apr; 25(2): 291-303.

Desmet VJ, Gerber M, Hoofnagle JH, Manns M & Scheuer PJ (1994). Classification of chronic hepatitis: diagnosis, grading and staging. *Hepatology* 1994 Jun; 19: 1513–20.

Dev A, Patel K, Conrad A, Blatt LM & McHutchison JG (2006). Relationship of smoking and fibrosis in patients with chronic hepatitis C. *Clin Gastroenterol Hepatol* 2006 Jun; 4: 797–801.

Dranoff JA & Wells RG (2010). Portal fibroblasts: underappreciated mediators of biliary fibrosis. *Hepatology* 2010 Apr; 51: 1438–44.

Duffield J, Forbes S, Constandinou C, Clay S, Partolina M, Vuthoori S, et al (2005). Selective depletion of macrophages reveals distinct, opposing roles during liver injury and repair. *J Clin Invest* 2005 Jan; 115(1):56.

Falkmer S, Samuelson G & Sjolin S (1970). Penicillamine-induced normalization of clinical signs and liver morphology and histochemistry in a case of Wilson's disease. *Pediatrics* 1970 Feb; 45 :260–8.

Fallowfield JA, Kendall TJ & Iredale JP (2006). Reversal of Fibrosis: No Longer a Pipe Dream? *Clin Liver Dis* 2006 Aug; 10: 481–97.

Forbes SJ, Russo FP, Rey V, Burra P, Rugge M, Wright NA, et al (2004). A significant proportion of myofibroblasts are of bone marrow origin in human liver fibrosis. *Gastroenterology* 2004 Apr; 126: 955–63.

Forns X, Ampurdanes S, Llovet JM, Aponte J, Quinto L, Martinez- Bauer E, et al (2002). Identification of chronic hepatitis C patients without hepatic fibrosis by a simple predictive model. *Hepatology* 2002 Oct; 36: 986-92.

Friedman SL (2003). Liver fibrosis—from bench to bedside. *J Hepatol* 2003; 38: S38–53.

Friedman SL (1993). The cellular basis of hepatic fibrosis: Mechanisms and treatment strategies. *N Engl J Med* 1993 Jun; 328: 1828–35.

Friedrich-Rust M, Wunder K, Kriener S, Sotoudeh F, Richter S, Bojunga J, et al (2009). Liver Fibrosis in Viral Hepatitis: Noninvasive Assessment with Acoustic Radiation Force Impulse Imaging versus Transient Elastography. *Radiology* 2009 Aug; 252 :595-604.

Giannini E, Risso D, Botta F, Chiarbonello B, Fasoli A, Malfatti F, et al (2003). Validity and clinical utility of the aspartate aminotransferase-alanine aminotransferase ratio in assessing disease severity and prognosis in patient with hepatitis C virus-related chronic liver disease. *Arch Intern Med* 2003 Jan; 163: 218-24.

Honda H, Onitsuka H, Masuda K, Nishitani H, Nakata H & Watanabe K (1990). Chronic liver disease, value of volumetry of liver and spleen with computed tomography. *Radiat Med* 1990 Nov-Dec; 8: 222–6.

Huang JF, Hsieh MY, Dai CY, Hou NJ, Lee LP, Lin ZY, et al (2007). The incidence and risks of liver biopsy in non-cirrhotic patients: An evaluation of 3806 biopsies. *Gut* 2007 May; 56: 736-7.

Huwart L, Sempoux C, Vicaut E, Salameh N, Annet L, Danse E, et al (2008). Magnetic resonance elastography for the noninvasive staging of liver fibrosis. *Gastroenterology* 2008 Jul; 135: 32–40.

Imbert-Bismut F, Ratziu V, Pieroni L, Charlotte F, Benhamou Y, Poynard T, et al (2001). Biochemical markers of liver fibrosis in patients with hepatitis C virus infection: a prospective study. *Lancet* 2001 Apr; 357: 1069-75.

Iredale JP, Benyon RC, Pickering J, McCullen M, Northrop M, Pawley S, et al (1998). Mechanisms of spontaneous resolution of rat liver fibrosis. Hepatic stellate cell apoptosis and reduced hepatic expression of metalloproteinase inhibitors. *J Clin Invest.* Aug 1 1998 Aug;102(3):538-49.

Iredale JP (2001). Hepatic stellate cell behavior during resolution of liver injury. *Semin Liver Dis* 2001 Aug;21(3):427-36.

Ismail MH & Pinzani M (2009). Reversal of liver fibrosis. *Saudi J Gastroenterol* 2009 Jan; 15: 72-9.

Issa R, Zhou X, Constandinou CM, Fallowfield J, Millward-Sadler H, Gaca MD, et al (2004). Spontaneous recovery from micronodular cirrhosis: evidence for incomplete resolution associated with matrix cross-linking. *Gastroenterology* Jun 2004; 126(7): 1795-1808.

Jiang JX, Venugopal S, Serizawa N, Chen X, Scott F, Li Y, Adamson R, et al (2010). Reduced nicotinamide adenine dinucleotide phosphate oxidase 2 plays a key role in stellate cell activation and liver fibrogenesis in vivo. *Gastroenterology* 2010 Oct; 139: 1375–84.

Kawada N (2011). Evolution of hepatic fibrosis research. *Hepatol Res* 2011 Mar; 41: 199-208.

Kisseleva T, Uchinami H, Feirt N, Quintana-Bustamante O, Segovia JC, Schwabe RF, et al (2006). Bone marrow derived fibrocytes participate in pathogenesis of liver fibrosis. *J Hepatol* 2006 Sep; 45: 429–38.

Knodell RG, Ishak KG, Black WC, Chen TS, Craig R, Kaplowitz N, et al (1981). Formulation and application of a numerical scoring system for assessing histological activity in asymptomatic chronic active hepatitis. *Hepatology* 1981 Sep-Oct; 1: 431–5.

Kotlyar D, Blonski W & Rustgi V (2008). Noninvasive Monitoring of Hepatitis C Fibrosis Progression. *Clin Liver Dis* 2008 Aug; 12(3): 557–71.

Lackner C, Struber G, Liegl B, Leibl S, Ofner P, Bankuti C, et al (2005). Comparison and validation of simple noninvasive tests for prediction of fibrosis in chronic hepatitis C. *Hepatology* 2005 Jun; 41: 1376–82.

Leclercq IA, Farrell GC, Schriemer R & Robertson GR (2002). Leptin is essential for the hepatic fibrogenic response to chronic liver injury. *J Hepatol* 2002 Aug; 37: 206–13.

Lee JS, Semela D, Iredale J & Shah VH (2007). Sinusoidal remodeling and angiogenesis: a new function for the liver-specific pericyte? *Hepatology* 2007 Mar;45:817–25.

Lee UE & Friedman SL (2011). Mechanisms of hepatic fibrogenesis. *Best Practice & Research Clinical Gastroenterology* 2011 Apr;25(2):195-206.

Ono E, Shiratori Y, Okudaira T, Imamura M, Teratani T, Kanai F, et al (1999). Platelet count reflects stage of chronic hepatitis C. *Hepatol Res* 1999 Aug; 15: 192-200.

Paggi S, Colli A, Fraquelli M, Viganò M, Del Poggio P, Facciotto C, et al (2008). A noninvasive algorithm accurately predicts advanced fibrosis in hepatitis C: a comparison using histology with internale-external validation. *J Hepatol* 2008 Oct; 49 :564–71.

Palmeri ML, Frinkley KD, Zhai L, Gottfried M, Bentley RC, Ludwig K, et al (2005). Acoustic radiation force impulse (ARFI) imaging of the gastrointestinal tract. *Ultrason Imaging* 2005 Apr;27:75–88.

Pinzani M & Rombouts K (2004). Liver fibrosis: from the bench to clinical targets. *Dig Liver Dis* 2004 Apr; 36: 231-42.

Pinzani M, Rosselli M & Zuckermann M (2011). Liver cirrhosis. Best *Practice & Research Clinical Gastroenterology* 2011; 25(2):281-90.

Pohl A, Behling C, Oliver D, Kilani M, Monson P & Hassanein T (2001). Serum aminotransferase levels and platelet counts as predictors of degree of fibrosis in chronic hepatitis C virus infection. *Am J Gastroenterol* 2001 Nov; 96: 3142-6.

Powell LW & Ker JF (1970). Reversal of "cirrhosis" in idiopathic hemochromatosis following long-term intensive venesection therapy. *Australas Ann Med* 1970 Feb; 2: 54–7.

Poynard T, Bedossa P, METAVIR and CLINIVIR cooperative study groups (1997). Age and platelet count: a simple index for predicting the presence of histological lesions in patients with antibodies to hepatitis C virus. *J Viral Hepat* 1997 May; 4: 199-208.

Poynard T, Imbert-Bismut F, Ratziu V, Chevret S, Jardel C, Moussalli J, et al (2002). Biochemical markers of liver fibrosis in patients infected by hepatitis C virus: longitudinal validation in a randomized trial. *J Viral Hepat* 2002 Mar; 9: 128-33.

Poynard T, McHutchison J, Manns M, Trepo C, Lindsay K, Goodman Z, et al (2002). Impact of pegylated interferon alfa-2b and ribavirin on liver fibrosis in patients with chronic hepatitis C. *Gastroenterology* 2002 May; 122: 1303–13.

Regev A, Berho M, Jeffers LT, Milikowski C, Molina EG, Pyrsopoulos T, et al (2002). Sampling error and intraobserver variability in liver biopsy in patients with chronic HCV infection. *Am J Gastroenterol* 2002 Oct; 15: 945-51.

Rockey DC, Caldwell SH, Goodman ZD, Nelson RC & Smith AD (2009). American Association for the Study of Liver Diseases. Liver biopsy. *Hepatology* 2009 Mar; 49:1017–44.

Saadeh S, Cammell G, Carey WD, Younossi Z, Barnes D & Easley K (2001). The role of liver biopsy in chronic hepatitis C. *Hepatology* 2001; 33: 196-200.

Sawitza I, Kordes C, Reister S & Häussinger D (2009). The niche of stellate cells within rat liver. *Hepatology* 2009 Nov; 50: 1617–24.

Sebastiani G, Halfon P, Castera L, Pol S, Thomas DL, Mangia A, et al (2009). SAFE biopsy: a validated method for large-scale staging of liver fibrosis in chronic hepatitis C. *Hepatology* 2009 Jun; 49: 1821–7.

Sporea I, Popescu A & Sirli R (2008). Why, who and how should perform liver biopsy in chronic liver diseases. *World J Gastroenterol* 2008 Jun; 14 (21):3396-402.

Syn WK, Choi SS, Liaskou E, Karaca GF, Agboola KM, Oo YH, et al (2011). Osteopontin is induced by hedgehog pathway activation and promotes fibrosis progression in nonalcoholic steatohepatitis. *Hepatology* 2011 Jan; 53: 106–15.

Talwalkar JA, Gross JB, Venkatesh SK, Yin M, Glockner J, Takahashi N, et al (2008). Magnetic resonance elastography for the detection of moderate to severe hepatic fibrosis. *Hepatology* 2008; 48 (Suppl 1):1110A.

Talwalkar JA, Kurtz DM, Schoenleber SJ, West CP, Montori VM (2007). Ultrasound-based transient elastography for the detection of hepatic fibrosis: systematic review and meta-analysis. *Clin Gastroenterol Hepatol* 2007 Oct; 5:1214–20.

Vallet-Pichard A, Mallet V, Nalpas B, Verkarre V, Nalpas A, Dhalluin-Venier V, et al (2007). FIB-4: an inexpensive and accurate marker of fibrosis in HCV infection. comparison with liver biopsy and fibrotest. *Hepatology* 2007 Jul; 46: 32-6.

Wai CT, Greenson JK, Fontana RJ, Kalbfleisch JD, Marrero JA, Conjeevaram HS, et al (2003). A simple noninvasive index can predict both significant fibrosis and cirrhosis in patients with chronic hepatitis C. *Hepatology* 2003 Aug; 38: 518-26.

Weber S, Gressner OA, Hall R, Grünhage F & Lammert F (2008). Genetic Determinants in Hepatic Fibrosis: From Experimental Models to Fibrogenic Gene Signatures in Humans. *Clinics in liver disease* 2008 Nov; 12(4):747-57.

Williams AL & Hoofnagle JH (1988). Ratio of serum aspartate to alanine aminotransferase in chronic hepatitis. Relationship to cirrhosis. *Gastroenterology* 1988 Sep; 95 :734-9.

Yin M, Talwalkar JA, Glaser KJ, Manduca A, Grimm RC, Rossman PJ, et al (2007). Assessment of hepatic fibrosis with magnetic resonance elastography. *Clin Gastroenterol Hepatol* 2007 Oct; 5:1207–13.

Zeisberg M, Yang C, Martino M, Duncan MB, Rieder F, Tanjore H, et al (2007). Fibroblasts derive from hepatocytes in liver fibrosis via epithelial to mesenchymal transition. *J Biol Chem* 2007 Aug; 282:23337–47.

Ziol M, Handra-Luca A, Kettaneh A, Christidis C, Mal F, Kazemi F, et al (2005). Noninvasive assessment of liver fibrosis by measurement of stiffness in patients with chronic hepatitis C. *Hepatology* 2005 Jan; 41: 48-54.

3

Histopathological Diagnosis of Non-Alcoholic and Alcoholic Fatty Liver Disease

Andrea Tannapfel and Berenike Flott-Rahmel
Institute of Pathology,
Ruhr-University Bochum,
Germany

1. Introduction

Fatty liver is a common 'liver disease' often free of symptoms or complaints but might even lead to severe stages. It is characterized by lipid deposition in hepatocytes both, for alcoholic as well as and non-alcoholic fatty liver. An additional inflammatory reaction results in - alcoholic (ASH) or non-alcoholic (NASH) - steatohepatitis. Steatohepatitis is characterized by both, inflammatory infiltrates of mixed cells in the small liver lobules as well as liver cell injury in terms of ballooning. NASH resembles alcoholic liver disease, but occurs in people who consume little or no alcohol. Many people with NASH don't feel sick and are not aware of their liver problem. Nevertheless, NASH can get severe and can result in cirrhosis with permanent tissue damage.

It has long been known that the typical manifestations of alcoholic liver damage (including cirrhosis of the liver) can also be found in patients who consume no alcohol. For such persons the incorrect diagnosis of 'alcohol-related liver disease' on the basis of just histopathological findings can have grave social, legal, and insurance implications.

The term 'non-alcoholic steatohepatitis' (NASH) was established by Ludwig et al. in 1980. The terminology was later expanded (Bacon et al., 1994). Patients were described who manifested the typical histomorphological pattern of alcoholic steatohepatitis (ASH), but without or with only moderate alcohol consumption (Ludwig et al., 1997).

Diagnosis by means of biopsy is the gold standard for differentiation between reversible steatosis and progressive steatohepatitis. There are numerous publications on this topic with the aim of developing uniform standards for biopsy diagnosis or identifying reliable non-invasive or only slightly invasive alternatives to biopsy, particularly driven by the increasing prominence of alcoholic and non-alcoholic steatohepatitis.

The term non-alcoholic fatty liver (NAFL) is not restricted to adults but also used to describe the same condition in children and adolescents (Baumann, 2005). Accordingly, the term non-alcoholic steatohepatitis (NASH) is used in the paediatric age group for the more aggressive form of hepatocellular degeneration accompanied by fibrosis (Rashid & Roberts, 2000; Roberts, 2002). People at increased risk of developing a fatty liver, as well possess an increased risk of developing chemotherapy-associated steatohepatitis (CASH).

Diagnostic procedures in patients with suspected fatty liver disease should be standardized and generally accepted. The goal of this chapter is thus to delineate the current concepts of aetiology, diagnostic as well as differential diagnostic of patients with fatty liver disease

with regard to the pathohistological diagnosis and to provide expert assessment of the non-invasive alternatives.
The present book chapter is adapted from the German Leitlinie 'Histopathologische Diagnose der nichtalkoholischen und alkoholischen Fettlebererkrankung' (Tannapfel et al. 2009), under the auspieces of the 'Deutsche Gesellschaft für Pathologie', and under participation of the 'Deutsche Gesellschaft für Verdauungs- und Stoffwechselerkrankungen (DGVS) ', the 'Deutsche Diabetes Gesellschaft (DDG), the Berufsverband Deutscher Pathologen, the 'Kompetenznetz Hepatitis (HepNet) ', the 'Gesellschaft für Pädiatrische Gastroenterologie und Ernährung (GPGE) ', the 'Österreichische Gesellschaft für Pathologie (ÖGP) ', the 'Österreichische Gesellschaft für Gastroenterologie und Hepatologie (ÖGGH) ', the 'Schweizerische Gesellschaft für Pathologie (SGPath) '.

2. Definitions and diagnostic criteria

2.1 Definitions

An alcoholic (AFL) and a non-alcoholic fatty liver (NAFL) characteristically show variable amounts of lipid deposition - principally triglycerides - in hepatocytes. Involvement of more than 5% of hepatocytes is termed 'fatty degeneration'. If more than 50% of these cells are affected a 'fatty liver' is present. A subsequent inflammatory reaction with ballooning of the hepatocytes results in steatohepatitis.
NASH resembles alcoholic liver disease, but occurs in people who drink little or no alcohol. The major feature in NASH is fat in the liver, along with inflammation and damage. NASH can be severe as ASH and may lead to fibrosis or cirrhosis, in which the liver is permanently damaged.
Light-microscopically detectable deposition of lipid droplets in the cytoplasm of hepatocytes is termed steatosis. Microvesicular and macrovesicular steatosis can be distinguished; mixed forms occur (Burt et al., 1998). For the accumulation of fat in the liver four pathogenetic processes are responsible: 1. Increased uptake of free fatty acids via the portal vein (from food or body fat), 2. Increased synthesis of free fatty acids in the liver (from glucose or acetate), 3. Decreased β-oxidation of free fatty acids, 4. Decreased synthesis or secretion of very low density lipoproteins (VLDL) the pathway for elimination of lipids from the liver (Burt et al., 1998).
In the past, alcohol was usually suspected as the cause of steatosis. However, steatosis frequently can be observed in adiposity, diabetes mellitus type II and hyperlipidaemia - components of the so-called "Metabolic Syndrome". Moreover, other factors such as toxins, medications, congenital metabolic disorders (e.g. a-beta-lipoproteinaemia/hypo-betalipoproteinaemia), hormonal imbalances (as observed in polycystic ovary syndrome) or other to date unknown causes may lead to steatosis (Church et al., 2006; Dancygier, 2006; Farrell& Larter, 2006). The morphological spectrum of non-alcoholic fatty liver disease (NAFLD) stretches from simple steatosis over steatohepatitis to liver fibrosis and cirrhosis, and thus ultimately to hepatocellular carcinoma. While pure steatosis is in principle reversible, steatohepatitis represents the progressive lesion in this spectrum.
NAFLD is thought to be the most frequent liver disease in the western industrial nations and thus the commonest cause of elevated transaminases. The diagnosis of NAFLD is made on basis of clinical (exclusion of significant alcohol consumption) combined with histopathological (demonstration of steatosis or steatohepatitis) findings. Significant alcohol consumption is defined as more than 20 g alcohol per day in women and as more than 40 g/day in men (Brunt, 2001; Neuschwander-Tetri & Caldwell, 2003).

The prevalence of NAFL in the western industrial nations is assumed to be 20 - 30%, that of NASH 2 - 3% (Cortez-Pinto et al., 2006; Dancygier, 2006; Day, 2006). There is a direct relationship with body weight: In obesity (BMI >30) the prevalence of sonographically detectable steatosis is 76 - 89%, compared with 46 - 50% in alcoholics (Bellentani et al., 2004). NAFLD is increasingly being diagnosed in childhood, again predominantly in association with obesity, but occasionally with suprasellar tumours (Alfire & Treem, 2006).

The natural course of NAFLD in the individual case cannot be predicted. Only a small proportion of those affected show progression of their liver disease. The assumption is that simple steatosis will progress to NASH in around 10 - 20% of patients, and that of these, less than 5% will develop cirrhosis (Day, 2006; Kacerovsky & Roden, 2007; Mendez-Sanchez et al., 2007). Nevertheless, NAFL and NASH are currently believed to be the most important cause of so-called cryptogenic cirrhosis of the liver (Farrell& Larter, 2006; Caldwell et al., 1999).

The pathogenesis of NASH remains unclear. In the so called "two-hit" hypothesis, accumulation of free fatty acids and triglycerides in the liver (simple steatosis) represent a first hit, rendering the organ more vulnerable to a second hit that leads to steatohepatitis and ultimately, in the event of persisting or recurring damage, to fibrosis and cirrhosis (Day & James, 1998; Day, 2002).

Insulin resistance seems to play a central part (Chitturi et al., 2002). It can be observed in virtually all patients. As a consequence of elevated peripheral lipolysis and decreased glucose uptake by the musculature, uptake of free fatty acids from the bloodstream rises. This leads to an increase in hepatic triglyceride synthesis and simultaneous inhibition of triglyceride secretion in the form of VLDL as a result of decreased apoprotein synthesis. The increase in the hepatic pool of free fatty acids leads to a rise in mitochondrial and peroxisomal β-oxidation with formation of reactive oxygen species (ROS), and thus to oxidative stress and increased lipid peroxidation. Facilitated by the action of proinflammatory cytokines (via activation of NF-κB, release of TNFα), steatohepatitis develops. Via Kupffer cell activation, liver fibrosis or cirrhosis arises (Farrell & Larter, 2006; Neuschwander-Tetri & Caldwell, 2003; Cortez-Pinto et al., 2006; Kacerovsky & Roden, 2007; Mendez-Sanchez et al., 2007; Duvnjak et al., 2007; Edmison & McCullough, 2007; Medina et al., 2004). The possible direct or indirect (increased insulin resistance) role of the adipocyte hormones (leptin and adiponectin) in the pathogenesis of NASH remains largely unclear. Another factor still discussed is the influence of bacterial overgrowth in the small intestine with endogenous production of ethanol and possible direct cytokine activation (Dancygier, 2006; Edmison & McCullough, 2007; Targher et al., 2006).

2.2 Diagnostic criteria

Clinically, most patients with NAFLD exhibit no liver symptoms. The disease is often suspected merely on grounds of (mildly) raised transaminase levels and/or gamma-glutamyltranspeptidase (GGT). An ASAT/ALAT ratio of > 1 points to an alcoholic aetiology. Patients with NASH often suffer from illnesses that go hand in hand with insulin resistance. However, the presence of a metabolic syndrome does not exclude alcoholic hepatopathy (Dufour & Oneta, 2004).

In clinical practice, there is so far no means of differentiating reliably between simple steatosis and steatohepatitis solely on the basis of non-invasive (e.g. laboratory chemical) diagnostic tests (American Gastroenterological Association [AGA], 2002; Bellentani et al., 2004; Farrell & Larter, 2006). Histological demonstration of persistent liver cell damage is believed to be the best current marker for evaluation of disease progression (Gramlich et al., 2004). The question of whether transaminase levels correlate with the histological findings has still not been answered definitively (Sonsuz et al., 2000), particularly with respect to necroinflammatory activity and the degree of fibrosis. Determination of the hepatic apoptotic activity in serum (activated caspase 3, keratin 18-fragment analysis) possibly has clinical value as a non-invasive diagnostic criterion for NASH (Wieckowska et al., 2006). Furthermore, isolated reports of non-invasive scoring systems for fibrosis have been published, but their potential diagnostic and/or prognostic role in clinical practice remains unclear (Angulo et al., 2007; Farrell & Larter, 2006).

The morphological sign of non-alcoholic steatosis is a predominantly macrovesicular accumulation of lipids usually beginning at a perivenular site in the centre of a lobe. The lower limit has been set at fatty degeneration of 5% of the surface of the liver parenchyma (Kleiner et al., 2005; Neuschwander-Tetri & Caldwell, 2003). However, this does not seem to be adequately justified (Brunt & Tiniakos, 2005; Cortez-Pinto et al., 2006). Mild steatosis affects < 33% of the parenchymal surface, moderate steatosis involves 33 - 66%, and severe steatosis covers > 66% (Brunt, 2001, 2002, 2005a, 2005b; Brunt et al., 2003, 2004; Brunt & Tiniakos, 2002, 2005; Burt et al., 1998). The steatosis (of variable degree) is accompanied by usually slight mixed-cell inflammatory infiltrates (neutrophilic, granulocytic and lymphocytic cells) in the hepatic lobes. A further morphological criterion is cell ballooning, i.e. liver cell damage in the form of swelling. This can usually been seen in the vicinity of fat-laden hepatocytes and thus also typically in the centre of a lobe. Other typical, albeit not diagnostically decisive parameters are lipogranulomas and periportal glycogen containing nuclei. Mallory-Denk bodies (MDB), usually can be demonstrated in the swollen cells. The fibrosis also starts in the centre of the affected lobe, in perivenular and perisinusoidal locations. Sometimes pericellular fibrosis can be detected. As the disease progresses, portal fibrosis with formation of portoportal and portocentral bridging septa arises. No single one of these structures should be used as a so-called 'minimal criterion' without the simultaneous demonstration of ballooning (Brunt, 2001, 2002, 2005a, 2005b; Brunt et al., 2003, 2004; Brunt & Tiniakos, 2002, 2005; Burt et al., 1998 Neuschwander-Tetri & Caldwell, 2003).

The Cleveland group suggested classification of NAFLD (on prognostic grounds) into the following types:

Type 1, simple steatosis
Type 2, steatosis and inflammation
Type 3, steatosis and cell swelling (ballooning)
Type 4, steatosis, cell swelling (ballooning), and MDB or fibrosis

Progression to cirrhosis is found predominantly in types 3 and 4, both of which correspond to the typical histopathological picture of NASH (Brunt, 2001, 2002, 2005a; Brunt et al., 2003, 2004; Brunt & Tiniakos, 2002, 2005; Neuschwander-Tetri & Caldwell, 2003 Falck-Ytter et al., 2001; Matteoni et al., 1999). For morphological manifestations of paediatric NASH (see 5.3).

3. Indication for biopsy

While scientists have been searching for non invasive diagnostic procedures for confirming diagnosis and determining inflammatory activity and potential fibrosis of fatty liver disease, to date histological evaluation remains the sole method of distinguishing steatosis from advanced forms of NAFLD.

Thus, liver biopsy is the gold standard for confirmation of the diagnosis and for determination of the inflammatory activity and possible presence of fibrosis in fatty liver disease. In deciding whether biopsy is indicated, one should weigh the potential information gain and its consequences against the resources invested and the complication rate, i.e. consider the clinical context. No blanket recommendation for liver biopsy in either suspected or confirmed fatty liver disease can currently be given.

The indication for biopsy in assumed fatty liver disease depends on the clinical context. Decisive is the likelihood that the biopsy findings will have consequences for the patient's behaviour or for therapy. These possible consequences include:

Confirmation of fatty liver disease, in particular steatohepatitis, and its treatability; exclusion of steatohepatitis as cause of unexplained elevation of transaminases; exclusion or confirmation of comorbidities; ascertainment of status quo[9,35,41,44]

Deciding the appropriate treatment approach (e.g. bariatric surgery, suitability for transplantation; treatment of any comorbidity)

Motivation for behavioural modification or ascertainment of its effect (e.g. weight reduction, physical activity)

Participation in clinical studies or protocol biopsies

Special indications (e.g. assessment of explanted livers)

In this context liver biopsy must clarify the following points:

Confirmation of possible or assumed fatty liver; clarification of steatohepatitis; confirmation or exclusion of liver disease other than fatty liver disease (typing)

Extent of inflammatory activity (grading)

Degree of fibrosis and any destruction of hepatic architecture (staging)

Liver biopsy is the current "gold standard" for analysis of these issues and cannot be replaced by any non-invasive procedure (Adams & Talwalkar, 2006; Angulo & Lindor, 2002; Brunt et al., 2004; Joy et al., 2003; Neuschwander-Tetri, 2002; Wieckowska et al., 2007). It is advisable to discuss the implications of liver biopsy with the patient during the course of diagnostic clarification of possible or probable fatty liver disease. While a pronounced case of fatty liver can be diagnosed with some certainty from the findings of clinical examination and imaging procedures, particularly the extent of the fatty degeneration and the presence or absence of the many possible accompanying liver diseases cannot be determined with any certainty by non-invasive means. There are no serological tests for diagnosis or quantification of fatty degeneration of the liver parenchyma. Comparative investigations have shown that elevation of serum transaminase concentrations can point to impairment of the hepatic parenchyma, but an absence of serum transaminase elevation in fatty liver disease does not exclude inflammatory activity in liver tissue (Mofrad et al., 2003). While in principle fatty liver disease is thought to be swiftly reversible and unlikely to progress, steatohepatitis entails a significant risk of progression to severe fibrosis or cirrhosis, so that the determination of inflammatory activity has considerable prognostic relevance Matteoni et al., 1999; Teli et al., 1995; Harrison ez al., 2003; Adams & Talwalkar, 2006; Wieckowska et al., 2007).

Numerous non-invasive procedures for diagnosis of liver fibrosis have been and are being developed. Serological tests are based on algorithms, some of which are independent of fibrosis while others integrate parameters associated with hepatic fibrogenesis (Younossi et al. 2008). Currently these tests can support the diagnosis of advanced liver fibrosis, but alone, particularly in the presence of only slight to moderate changes, they can neither confirm nor exclude fibrosis with sufficient certainty; therefore, they are unsuitable for staging. Elastography is a method for determining the stiffness of the liver, which correlates with extent of fibrosis, at least during follow up. Particularly the presence or absence of severe fibrosis/cirrhosis can be assessed with high accuracy (Castera et al., 2008). The advantages of this method are its repeatability, its low inter- and intra-observer variability and its lack of side effects; its disadvantages are inadequate detection of slight and moderate fibrosis, lack of grading ability, significant interference by other liver changes (fatty degeneration, inflammatory activity, cholestasis, congestion) and by extrahepatic factors (morbid obesity, ascites) (Friedrich-Rust et al., 2008). For these reasons the diagnostic potential of elastography in fatty liver disease has been evaluated in only a few studies to date, so the method has not yet been adequately validated. In particular its role in the monitoring of the course of fatty liver disease should be further investigated. None of the tests mentioned above is suitable for assessment of destruction of hepatic architecture. Other procedures, e.g. magnetic resonance elastography for measurement of fibrosis (Bonekamp et al., 2009), are currently inadequately validated or not validated at all, and therefore cannot be recommended.

Although liver biopsy is superior to all other investigations with regard to number of relevant parameters assessed and predictive power, it cannot always be recommended as diagnostic method in possible or sufficiently confirmed fatty liver disease. Several factors affect the decision whether or not to perform biopsy:

Because biopsy is an invasive technique, the information it can be expected to yield must be balanced against the resources invested and the - albeit low - complication rate. The rate of fatal complications of liver biopsy is generally reported as 0.01%. Major intervention- or hospitalisation-related complications such as intraperitoneal haemorrhage occur in about 0.3% of cases, while more minor complications, e.g. transient pain, are observed in 20 - 30% of patients (Strassburg & Manns, 2006).

The issue of clinical consequences: The current treatment options for fatty liver disease are limited. Biopsy sampling of liver tissue for examination may be particularly useful, however, before invasive treatment measures such as bariatric surgery or liver transplantation (Tannapfel & Reinacher-Schick, 2008). In the medium term novel treatments, including medicinal approaches can be expected, entailing reassessment of the value and necessity of liver biopsy. To what extent knowledge of the findings of liver biopsy influences the patient's behaviour (weight reduction, physical activity) has to be considered on an individual basis.

Donor livers with < 30% fatty degeneration can be transplanted with no danger of primary transplant failure (Nocito et al., 2006).

4. Harvesting and processing of biopsy material / histomorphological evaluation / scoring system

The structural diagnostic criteria for NAFLD may be unevenly distributed in the liver. Thus, histological diagnosis on the basis of biopsy samples may be associated with possibly considerable sampling error (Ratziu et al., 2005). This may affect both, the diagnostic differentiation between steatosis and steatohepatitis and estimation of the extent of fibrosis (staging).

Harvesting and processing of the biopsy cylinder should observe the standard recommendations for liver biopsy. The cylinder should contain representative tissues, be about 25 mm long and or contain 15 portal fields (Rousselet et al., 2005). Fixation and

processing are routine (4% neutral buffered formalin, embedding in paraffin with the usual dehydration and preparation of routine stains such as haematoxylin and eosin, Berlin blue for demonstration of iron, PAS-diastase stain and reticulin and connective tissue staining). Sirius red staining is recommended for morphometric assessment. Immunohistological staining is not routinely required. An immunohistochemical reaction with antibodies to keratin 7 or 19 can be carried out to facilitate demonstration of gall duct lesions. Sensitive depiction of any MDB that may be present can be achieved with ubiquitin antibodies. With regard to ballooning of hepatocytes, which is included in the scoring system, demonstration of the intermediate filament cytoskeleton with antibodies against keratin 8 or 18 may be helpful, as this cytoskeletal system is reduced in cell ballooning (Lackner et al., 2008). The staging of fibrosis is shown in Table1.
The following histological criteria should be considered when interpreting and diagnosing non-alcoholic steatohepatitis: micro- or macrovesicular fatty degeneration, fibrosis, lobular inflammation - typically comprising polymorphonuclear granulocytes, lymphocytes and activated Kupffer cells - lipogranulomas, hepatocyte ballooning, acidophilic bodies, ceroid-containing macrophages and megamitochondria. Additional changes are MDB and glycogen-contaning nuclei.

Stage	Histological findings
0	No fibrosis
1a	Zone 3, perisinusoidal fibrosis, special staining (i.e. EvG) required
1b	Zone 3, perisinusoidal fibrosis, can be detected with H&E
1c	Only periportal/portal fibrosis
2	Zone 3, plus portal/periportal fibrosis
3	As above, but with bridging fibrosis
4	Cirrhosis

Table 1. Degree of fibrosis (staging)

Steatosis, inflammatory changes and hepatocytic injury can be semiquantified as a 'Brunt Score' (Brunt et al., 1999) (Table 2) or 'NAS' (NAFLD activity score; Table 3), providing the basis on which to decide whether or not steatohepatitis is present.

Activity	Steatosis	Ballooning	Inflammation
Mild: grade 1	1 - 2 (up to 66%)	Minimal	Lobular: 1 - 2 Portal: none to mild
Moderate: grade 2	2 - 3 (> 33%, occasionally > 66%)	Clear	Lobular: 2 Portal: mild to moderate
Severe: grade 3	3 (≥ 66%)	Marked	Lobular: 3 Portal: mild to moderate

Table 2. NASH activity grading. Steatosis grade 1: ≤ 33%; grade 2: > 33%, < 66%; grade 3: ≥ 66%

The NAS (NAFLD activity score) is a refinement of the Brunt score, derived by separate semiquantification of each of the three components - steatosis, hepatocyte ballooning and lobular inflammation - and addition to form a total score.

NAS	Steatosis (% fat deposition in hepatocytes)	Ballooning hepatocytes	Lobular inflammation
0	< 5% (0)	None (0)	None (0)
3	5 - 33% (1)	Few (1)	1- 2 foci per 200x field (1)
6	34 - 66% (2)	Many (2)	2 - 4 foci per 200x field (2)
8	> 66% (3)	Many (2)	> 4 foci per 200x field (3)

Table 3. NAFLD activity score (grading): The numbers in parentheses give the NAS for each histological criterion

Evaluation and semiquantitative analysis for grading (Brunt et al., 1999):

Grade of fatty degeneration:
< 5% = grade 0
5 - 33% = grade 1
34 - 66% = grade 2
More than 66% = grade 3

Grade of lobular inflammation:
Absent = grade 0
Up to 2 foci per field of view (200× magnification) = grade 1
2 to 4 foci per field of view = grade 2
More than 4 foci per field of view = grade 3
Lipogranulomas are included in the category of inflammation

Ballooning:
Absent = grade 0
Few ballooned hepatocytes = grade 1
Many ballooned hepatocytes = grade 2

This scoring system is readily reproducible and can provide the basis for deciding whether steatohepatitis should be diagnosed or not:
0 - 2 definitely no steatohepatitis
3 - 4 questionable
5 or more definite steatohepatitis

The scoring can also be applied to paediatric cases (Brunt EM, 2007; Schwimmer et al., 2005). The staging according to grade of fibrosis (Table 2b, after Kleiner et al., 2005) should also be evaluated:
Stage 1 is divided into 1a with slight central fibrosis and 1b with dense perisinusoidal fibrosis accompanied by central vein sclerosis and adjacent perisinusoidal fibrous extension. Stage 1c is used only for portal fibrosis, which may certainly occur at an early stage. Stage 2 is portal and central fibrosis. In analogy with the staging of chronic hepatitis, stage 3 is bridging fibrosis and stage 4 corresponds to cirrhosis.
The presence of MDB should also be recorded (Mendler et al., 2005).

The proposed scoring systems have not yet been generally accepted. Numerical scores alone should not replace histological diagnosis.
In Figures 1 - 4 typical images of different histopathological conditions for both, grade of steatosis and grade of fibrosis are presented.

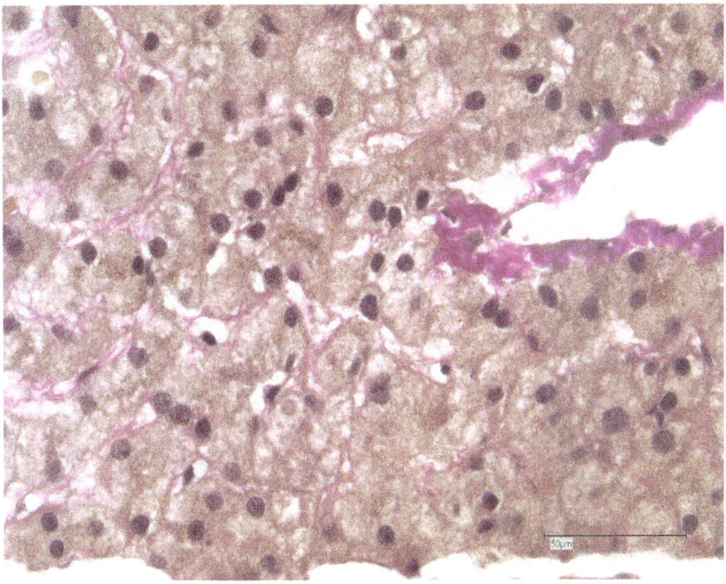

Fig. 1. Non-alcoholic steatohepatitis: fat 10 %, score: 1 plus 1 plus 1 = 3, fibrosis grade 1B

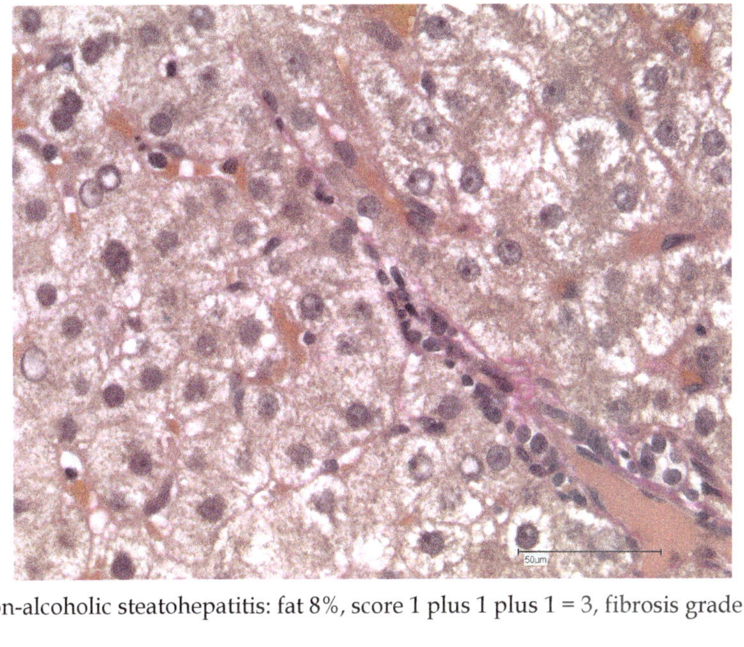

Fig. 2. Non-alcoholic steatohepatitis: fat 8%, score 1 plus 1 plus 1 = 3, fibrosis grade 1c

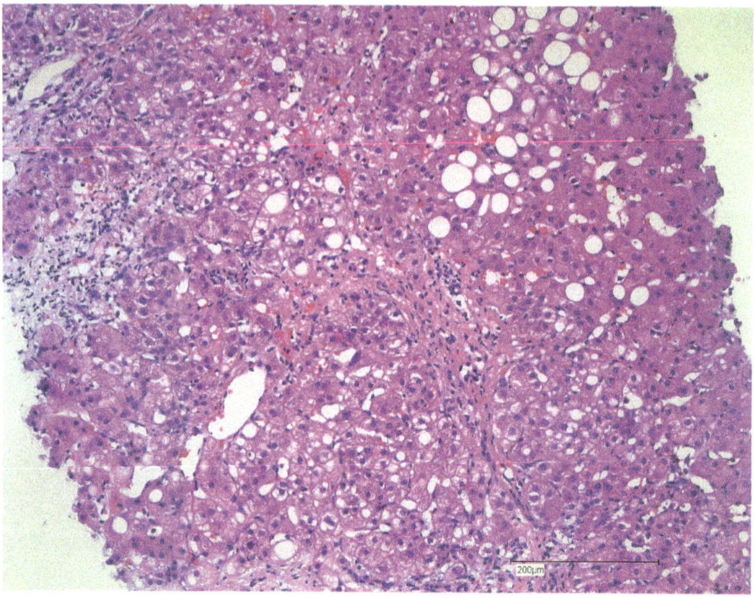

Fig. 3. Non-alcoholic steatohepatitis: fat 30%, score 1 plus 1 plus 1 = 3, fibrosis grade 3

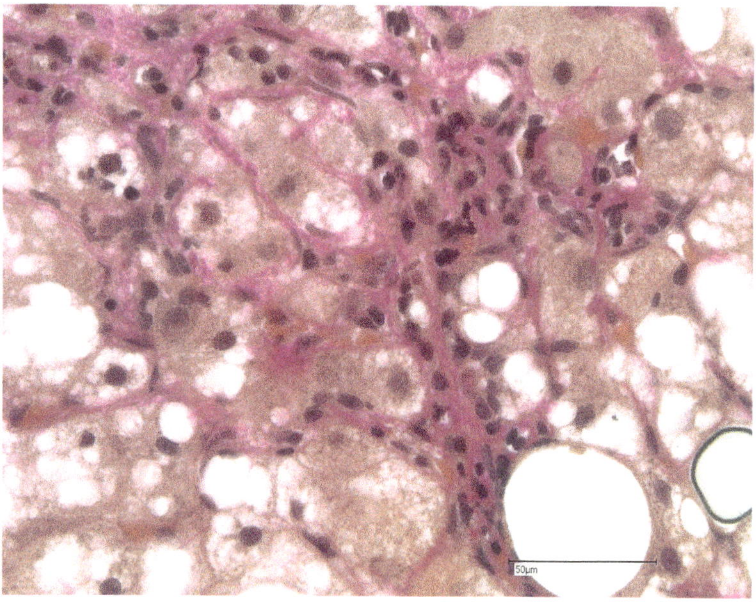

Fig. 4. Non-alcoholic steatohepatitis with cirrhosis: fat 40%, score: 2 plus 2 plus 1 = 5, fibrosis grade 4

5. Diagnosis and differential diagnosis

It is important to differentiate between ASH and NASH and also to differentiate both of them from viral hepatitides and chemotoxicity-related steatohepatitides. The histopathological peculiarities of fatty liver diseases in the paediatric age group must also be borne in mind.

The criteria used for the morphological definition of steatohepatitis are fatty degeneration of liver cells (steatosis), predominant in zone 3, lobular and/or portal field-dominant inflammatory reaction (inflammation), direct liver cell damage in the form of ballooned hepatocytes, possibly Mallory-Denk bodies (MDB), fibrosis and possibly accumulation of iron.

- Steatosis

Fatty degeneration of liver cells is documented in virtually all existing studies on ASH and NASH[4].

Macrovesicular steatosis results from the discrepancy between synthesis of lipids and their export from the hepatocytes.

Microvesicular steatosis, a possible precursor of macrovesicular steatosis, is thought to be a consequence of severe hepatocytic damage as a result of defective β-oxidation of fatty acids. The toxic effects of some medicinal drugs can also lead to microvesicular steatosis. In the course of ASH or NASH there may be complete loss of fat; thus, for example, cryptogenic cirrhosis with only slight fatty degeneration of liver cells is not infrequently ascribable to NASH (Caldwell et al., 1999; Oneta & Dufour, 2003).

- Lobular and/or portal inflammation and hepatocyte ballooning

ASH and NASH are characterised by a lobular inflammatory cell infiltrate with a variable number of leucocytes. Not infrequently the inflammatory cells are found to enclose ballooned hepatocytes. So-called lipogranulomas, i.e. inflammatory cells (including Kupffer cells and eosinophilic granulocytes) enclosing a fat-laden hepatocyte, may be seen but are not considered pathognomonic for NASH or ASH (Caldwell et al., 1999; Reid, 2001). The direct hepatocyte damage is shown by the aforementioned ballooning, which may progress to necrosis or apoptosis. Hepatocytes of zone 3 are affected most frequently (Brunt, 2005; Brunt & Tiniakos, 2005; Burt et al., 1998; Neuschwander-Tetri & Caldwell , 2003). MDB do not contribute to differentiation between ASH and NASH.

- Fibrosis

The characteristic fibrosis pattern in ASH and NASH is pericellular fibrogenesis. Collagen is found in the Disse spaces. In both ASH and NASH, zone 3 is affected first, with periportal fibrosis not infrequently observed in the liver of patients with diabetes mellitus type 1 (NASH patients). It seems that portal field fibrosis tends to predominate in ASH. Taken alone, however, this pattern of fibrosis is not a criterion for differentiation between ASH and NASH.

5.1 Differential diagnosis of alcoholic (ASH) and non-alcoholic steatohepatitis (NASH)

In general, histological criteria alone do not permit confident differentiation between ASH and NASH (Oneta & Dufour, 2003). Nevertheless, some findings may be helpful in differential diagnosis (Brunt, 2002; Brunt, 2007), although to date there is no published evidence:

- Fat

Microvesicular steatosis and "foamy" degeneration of the liver seem to indicate incipient hepatic decompensation in patients with ASH and are less common in NASH.

Patients with NASH usually exhibit more advanced fatty degeneration of liver cells than those with ASH. The affected hepatocytes, concentrated at periportal sites, more frequently display intranuclear vacuoles.

In addition to the nuclear vacuoles, patients with diabetes mellitus show fibrosis usually starting in zone 1, where MDB may also be found. Patients with NAFL who display pronounced weight increase or a jejunoileal bypass tend to exhibit portal inflammation with only slight portal fibrosis.

Only in decompensated ASH may any appreciable cholestasis occur, usually intracanalicular and sometimes with a secondary phenomenon such as pancreatitis or haemolysis as a contributory cause.

- Inflammation

As a general rule, the inflammatory infiltrate in NASH is somewhat less pronounced than in ASH. MDB are more frequent and more distinctive in ASH than they are in NASH. So-called satellitosis, granulocytic demarcation of a hepatocyte with MDB, is more frequent in ASH than in NASH.

- Fibrosis

Indicative, though not specific, for ASH are the so-called sclerosing hyaline necroses, usually in combination with obliterating vascular lesions. The latter are also considered to be responsible for the non-cirrhotic 00portal hypertension in patients with ASH. Sclerosing hyaline necroses are thought to represent a combination of liver cell necrosis and loss (predominantly in zone 3) and dense perivenular and perisinusoidal fibrosis to the point of venous obliteration (with or without MDB).

Finding	ASH	NASH
Steatosis	+	++
Ballooning	++	++
Lobular inflammation	++	+/++
Portal granulocytic inflammation	++	--/+
Mallory-Denk bodies (MDB	+++	+
Satellitosis	+++	--
Acute cholestasis	+	--
Perisinusoidal fibrosis	+	+
Sclerosing hyaline necrosis	++	--
Veno-occlusive disease (VOD)	++	--

Table 4. Criteria for differentiation of ASH and NASH

Venous or perivenular fibrosis, phlebosclerosis and (less commonly) lymphocytic phlebitis occur more frequently in ASH than in NASH. Phlebosclerosis is a frequent sign of alcohol-associated cirrhosis of the liver.

Cholestasis is found in around a third of all livers with ASH, less often in patients with NASH. Ductular proliferates are encountered more frequently in ASH than in NASH.

Criteria for differentiation of ASH and NASH see table 4.

5.2 Differential diagnosis of ASH, NASH / hepatitis / drug-induced hepatitis

The criteria for differentiation of NASH or ASH from hepatitis C virus infection are firstly the characteristic portal inflammatory infiltration pattern of HCV infection, and secondly the lack of typical hepatocyte ballooning and the intra-acinar granulocytic inflammation (Sanyal et al., 2006).

Differentiation among ASH / NASH, hepatitis C virus infection and liver damage by toxic effects of medications ('drug-induced hepatitis') is possible. In patients exhibiting signs of more than one of these diseases, discussion embracing the clinical parameters is necessary to identify the essential contributory factors.

Chronic HCV infection can also lead to macrovesicular steatosis. In particular, patients infected with HCV genotype 3 usually show more advanced fatty degeneration. However, the hepatocyte ballooning and intralobular granulocytic inflammation typical of ASH and NASH are absent.

Drug-induced hepatitis is characterised by portal and particularly intra-acinar inflammation that consists principally of neutrophilic and eosinophilic granulocytes. Cholestasis is found, and in severe cases liver cell necrosis. Steatosis does not necessarily occur in drug-induced hepatitis (exceptions include tamoxifen and amiodarone), but is often found in patients who evince certain risk factors (high BMI, diabetes mellitus). Selected drugs that may lead to steatosis are e.g Acetylsalicylic acid, Amiodarone, Didanosine (stavudine), MDMA (amphetamines).

5.3 Special form: paediatric fatty liver disease

As applies for adults both NAFLD and NASH can occur without any apparent risk factor even in children. The sole clinical manifestation is usually a persistent slight (one- to twofold) elevation in transaminases. In about 80% of the affected children and adolescents the NAFL is discovered incidentally in overweight or obese individuals. The remainder display normal weight but the majority are diabetics.

Paediatric NASH exhibits histological differences from adult NASH. The question of liver biopsy is controversial; nevertheless, there is consensus that, particularly in the event of repeated elevation of liver enzymes, chronic liver diseases such as hepatitis B and C, Wilson's disease and autoimmune hepatitides should first be ruled out. Weight reduction should be attempted. In patients who lose a moderate amount of weight over a period of six months but do not achieve normalisation of liver function, liver biopsy should be performed for definitive confirmation of the diagnosis and assessment of the prognosis. If at any time during this period evidence emerges of another disease or a competing or concurrent liver ailment (demonstration of autoantibodies, caeruloplasmin decrease), diagnosis should not be postponed until after weight reduction but ascertained immediately, with liver biopsy if necessary.

For assignment of the diagnosis of NAFLD in childhood or adolescence, fat has to make up at least 5 - 10% of the liver by weight. In analogy to the classification of fatty liver disease in adults, the steatosis is categorised as mild (less than a third of hepatocytes affected), moderate (up to two thirds of hepatocytes affected) or severe (more than two-thirds of hepatocytes affected) (Hubscher, 2004). Among adults with NAFLD, 1 - 3% go on to develop cirrhosis of the liver. If this is true for the paediatric age group, many children are at increased risk of early progressive liver fibrosis or cirrhosis.

Differences between paediatric and adult NAFLD:

To date there have been no studies on the prognosis of NAFLD. It also remains unclear what influence puberty and growth have on the time course of the disease. Adult NASH patients have a 25% risk of developing advanced liver fibrosis within 5 years and a 15% risk of cirrhosis in the same period (Neuschwander-Tetri & Caldwell, 2003). The significance of ethnicity is hotly debated. Children of Hispanic and Asiatic origin are at greater risk. In contrast to the situation in adults with non-alcoholic liver disease, males are predominantly affected in the paediatric age group (DeLeve et al., 2002; Roberts, 2007).

The first study on the histopathology of paediatric NAFLD and hepatitis found that they largely resemble the picture in adult disease, but display differing morphological aspects. With regard to inflammation and fibrosis, two subtypes can be distinguished (Schwimmer et al., 2005). In general the livers of children and adolescents with NASH reveal less lobular and more portal inflammation, and the fibrosis tends to be more portal rather than perisinusoidal (Rashid & Roberts, 2000; Roberts, 2007; Papandreou et al., 2007). This distinctive histological feature could explain the early progression of the NAFLD score in children and adolescents compared with adults. Biopsy samples exhibit more marked fatty degeneration than in adult NASH. The characteristic ballooning of hepatocytes in adults is also absent, as is the pronounced lobular inflammation with perisinusoidal fibrosis. Only in 12% of cases is paediatric NAFLD histologically comparable to the adult disease (Schwimmer et al., 2005; Schwimmer, 2007). The differential diagnoses include Wilson's disease, other disorders of hepatic metabolism (including rare diseases) and chronic inflammatory bowel diseases, which may manifest as diarrhoea with weight loss. Differentiation from hepatitis is particularly important.

5.4 Special form: chemotherapy-associated steatohepatitis (CASH)

Persons at increased risk of developing fatty liver are in greater danger of developing chemotherapy-associated steatohepatitis (CASH). Close monitoring of liver function before hepatic resection is recommended in these patients. Possible causes of elevation of liver enzymes before initiation of chemotherapy include malignant involvement of the liver and other chronic hepatic diseases as well as fatty liver disease. Liver biopsy may be necessary for differential diagnosis.

Severe liver changes have been observed following chemotherapy administered in the context of liver resection, particularly extirpation of colorectal metastases. These adverse effects of chemotherapy on the liver tissue around a tumour can lead to postoperative impairment of liver function.

The described changes resemble the histological findings after conditioning chemotherapy and subsequent allogenic stem cell transplantation in the liver. The liver damage after chemotherapy depends decisively on the degree of previous liver impairment. Neoadjuvant chemotherapy may be followed not only by sinusoidal obstruction syndrome (SOS) (DeLeve et al., 2002), but also by slight steatosis, steatohepatitis or even combined steatohepatitis and SOS (Karoui et al., 2006) . In principal, any of the cell populations in the liver can be affected by drug-induced damage. Cholangiocytes are considered to be relatively inert. Hepatocytes, followed by vascular endothelia, are the primary cell systems in which damage may also be visible on light microscopy. The changes may extend as far as fibrosis, accompanied by vascular wall damage and parenchymal bleeding.

- Fatty degeneration of liver cells

Fatty degeneration after chemotherapy with 5-fluorouracil (5-FU) is generally considered to be reversible after discontinuation of the treatment. Particularly in the case of pre-existing fatty liver, however, the rate of complications after liver resection is higher. Chemotherapy-induced fatty degeneration of liver cells can lead to functional impairment after liver resection.

- Steatohepatitis (fatty liver hepatitis)

It is known that, for example, 5-FU, taxanes or platinum-containing chemotherapeutics exert oxidative stress not only on tumour cells but also on non-neoplastic parenchymal and stromal cells (Tannapfel et al., 2001). This prompted the proposal to adopt the term "chemotherapy-associated steatohepatitis" (CASH) (Gentilucci et al., 2006; Zivkovic et al., 2007).

The metabolic pathway of some drugs is known in detail. Thus the topoisomerase-I inhibitor irinotecan (CPT11) is thought to trigger CASH even in a previously intact liver. The damage is assumed to be predominantly hepatocytic because of the glucuronidation of hepatocytes. Sublethal liver damage may be manifested by hepatocyte ballooning, microvesicular steatosis and finally inflammation with subsequent fibrosis. Like ballooning, hepatocellular cholestasis is considered to be a sign of direct cell damage. In the treatment of colorectal carcinoma irinotecan is almost always used in combination with 5-FU, so the hepatotoxic effects may be additive.

- Vascular endothelial damage

The endothelial cells can also be damaged by oxidative stress. Histologically, the vessels are occluded by connective tissue (Aloia et al., 2006; Vauthey et al., 2006; Zivkovic et al., 2007), with coexisting inflammation, fibrosis and embolic occlusion of small and larger downstream vessels. Damage of these cells in the terminal hepatic venules and sublobular veins causes on the one hand activation of the coagulation cascade (thrombosis) and on the other, hyperfibrinolysis (bleeding). These disseminated intravasal coagulations in the liver result in inflammation and subsequent fibrosis to the point of vascular occlusion. Macroscopically, the affected liver is rich in blood, spongy and livid ("blue liver"); its elasticity is diminished.

Here too the effects of various substances may be additive.

Platinum-containing chemotherapeutics (particularly oxaliplatin) also possess high hepatotoxic potential (endothelial damage, sinusoidal lesions, SOS). Resected liver tissue from patients treated with a combination of 5-FU and oxaliplatin reveal, besides sinusoidal lesions with bleeding, vascular thrombosis and vascular fibrosis, signs of CASH, with hepatocytic necrosis, fatty degeneration of liver cells and cholestasis. These changes may be visible as early as 20 days after inception of therapy.

The histological changes after administration of site-specific treatments, e.g. monoclonal antibodies against the EGF receptor or VEGF, have not yet been the subject of controlled studies.

- Classification system for staging

The precise relationship between fatty degeneration of liver cells and SOS has not yet been clearly defined. A further open question is the dose-effect relationship. Moreover, it remains unclear whether the histological changes are reversible. There seems to be no linear correlation between liver damage and elevated liver enzymes in peripheral blood. To date there is neither a clinical nor a histological classification or graduation system that would allow "staging" of the change, much less prediction of the outcome. Therefore, it can merely be recommended that liver function be closely monitored before liver resection in patients at risk of developing fatty liver (e.g. high BMI, metabolic syndrome, diabetes mellitus) (Aloia et al., 2006; Nakano et al., 2008). If the liver enzymes are elevated before initiation of chemotherapy and the cause is not tumour involvement, a full battery of laboratory tests may need to be accompanied by liver biopsy to establish the exact extent of fatty degeneration, ballooning or fibrosis. In particular, special attention should be paid to histological processing of the tissue surrounding the metastasis in specimens resected from patients who have undergone chemotherapy.

6. Genetic prevalence

At the moment, the question of genetic prevalence of NAFLD and NASH is under investigation and is obviously higher than estimated previously (Williams et al., 2011). Recently several genetic factors such as patatin-like phospholipase 3 or apolipoprotein C3 have been characterized in NAFLD (Valenti et al., 2010; Petersen et al., 2010). Even genome-wide association studies (GWASs) of liver histology in patients with non alcoholic fatty liver disease have been performed to estimate genetic susceptibility to NASH (Chalasani et al., 2010). However, these findings have to be validated.

7. Conclusion

Diagnostic procedures in patients with suspected fatty liver disease should be standardized and generally accepted. The publications on predisposition to ASH or NASH, however, cannot be uniformly interpreted because of ethnic or physiological differences among the populations analysed. It is therefore important to evaluate the situation objectively and work towards reasonable diagnostic procedures that serve the needs of these patients.

8. References

Adams, L. A. & Talwalkar, J. A. (2006). Diagnostic evaluation of nonalcoholic fatty liver disease. *J.Clin.Gastroenterol.*, Vol. 40, No. 3 Suppl 1, (March 2006), p. S34-S38, ISSN 0192-0790

AGA (2002), American Gastroenterological Association medical position statement: nonalcoholic fatty liver disease. *Gastroenterology*, Vol. 123, No. 5, (November 2002). pp. 1702-1704, ISSN 7645-6

Alfire, M. E. & Treem, W. R. (2006). Nonalcoholic fatty liver disease. *Pediatr.Ann.*, Vol. 35, No. 4, (April 2006), pp. 290-299, ISSN 0090-4481

Aloia, T., Sebagh, M., Plasse, M., Karam, V., Levi, F., Giacchetti, S., Azoulay, D., Bismuth, H., Castaing, D., & Adam, R. (2006). Liver histology and surgical outcomes after preoperative chemotherapy with fluorouracil plus oxaliplatin in colorectal cancer liver metastases. *J.Clin.Oncol.*, Vol. 24, No. 31, (1 November 2006), pp. 4983-4990, ISSN 0732-183X

Angulo, P., Hui, J. M., Marchesini, G., Bugianesi, E., George, J., Farrell, G. C., Enders, F., Saksena, S., Burt, A. D., Bida, J. P., Lindor, K., Sanderson, S. O., Lenzi, M., Adams, L. A., Kench, J., Therneau, T. M., & Day, C. P. (2007). The NAFLD fibrosis score: a noninvasive system that identifies liver fibrosis in patients with NAFLD. *Hepatology*, Vol. 45, No. 4, (April 2007), pp. 846-854, ISSN 1527-3350

Angulo, P. & Lindor, K. D. (2002) Non-alcoholic fatty liver disease. *J.Gastroenterol.Hepatol.*, Vol. 17 Suppl, (February 2002), p. S186-S190, ISSN 0815-9319

Bacon, B. R., Farahvash, M. J., Janney, C. G., & Neuschwander-Tetri, B. A. (1994) Nonalcoholic steatohepatitis: an expanded clinical entity. *Gastroenterology*, Vol. 107, No. 4, (October 1994), pp. 1103-1109, ISSN 7645-6

Baumann, U. (2005). Die kindliche Fettlebererkrankung. *Dtsch.Ärzteblatt*, Vol. 102, No. 39, p. A2634-A2639, ISSN 0012-1207

Bellentani, S., Bedogni, G., Miglioli, L., & Tiribelli, C. (2004). The epidemiology of fatty liver. *Eur.J.Gastroenterol.Hepatol.*, Vol. 16, No. 11, (November 2004), pp. 1087-1093, ISSN 0954-691X

Bonekamp, S., Kamel, I., Solga, S., & Clark, J. (2009). Can imaging modalities diagnose and stage hepatic fibrosis and cirrhosis accurately?, *J.Hepatol.*, Vol. 50, No. 1, (January 2009), pp. 17-35, ISSN 0168-8278

Brunt, E. M. (2001). Nonalcoholic steatohepatitis: definition and pathology. *Semin.Liver Dis.*, Vol. 21, No. 1, pp. 3-16, ISSN 0272-8087

Brunt, E. M. (2002). Alcoholic and nonalcoholic steatohepatitis. *Clin.Liver Dis.*, Vol. 6, No. 2, (May 2002), pp. 399-420, vii, ISSN 1089-3261

Brunt, E. M. (2005a). Nonalcoholic steatohepatitis: pathologic features and differential diagnosis. *Semin.Diagn.Pathol.*, Vol. 22, No. 4, pp. (November 2005), 330-338, ISSN 0740-2570

Brunt, E. M. (2005b). Pathology of nonalcoholic steatohepatitis. *Hepatol.Res.*, Vol. 33, No. 2, (October 2005), pp. 68-71, ISSN 1386-6346

Brunt, E. M. (2007). Pathology of fatty liver disease. *Mod.Pathol.*, Vol. 20, Suppl 1, (February 2007), p. S40-S48, ISSN 0893-3952

Brunt, E. M., Janney, C. G., Di Bisceglie, A. M., Neuschwander-Tetri, B. A., & Bacon, B. R. (1999). Nonalcoholic steatohepatitis: a proposal for grading and staging the histological lesions. *Am.J.Gastroenterol.*, Vol. 94, No. 9, (September 1999), pp. 2467-2474, ISSN 0002-9270

Brunt, E. M., Neuschwander-Tetri, B. A., Oliver, D., Wehmeier, K. R., & Bacon, B. R. (2004). Nonalcoholic steatohepatitis: histologic features and clinical correlations with 30 blinded biopsy specimens. *Hum.Pathol.*, Vol. 35, No. 9, (September 2004), pp. 1070-1082, ISSN 0046-8177

Brunt, E. M., Ramrakhiani, S., Cordes, B. G., Neuschwander-Tetri, B. A., Janney, C. G., Bacon, B. R., & Di Bisceglie, A. M. (2003). Concurrence of histologic features of steatohepatitis with other forms of chronic liver disease. *Mod.Pathol.*, Vol. 16, No. 1, (January 2003), pp. 49-56, ISSN 0893-3952

Brunt, E. M. & Tiniakos, D. G. (2002). Pathology of steatohepatitis. *Best.Pract.Res.Clin.Gastroenterol.*, Vol. 16, No. 5, (October 2002), pp. 691-707, ISSN 1521-6918

Brunt, E. M. & Tiniakos, D. G. (2005). Pathological features of NASH. *Front Biosci.*, Vol. 10, pp. 1475-1484, ISSN 1093-9946

Burt, A. D., Mutton, A., & Day, C. P. (1998). Diagnosis and interpretation of steatosis and steatohepatitis. *Semin.Diagn.Pathol.*, Vol. 15, No. 4, (November 1998), pp. 246-258, ISSN 0740-2570

Caldwell, S. H., Oelsner, D. H., Iezzoni, J. C., Hespenheide, E. E., Battle, E. H., & Driscoll, C. J. (1999). Cryptogenic cirrhosis: clinical characterization and risk factors for underlying disease. *Hepatology*, Vol. 29, No. 3, (March 1999), pp. 664-669, ISSN 1527-3350

Castera, L., Forns, X., & Alberti, A. (2008). Non-invasive evaluation of liver fibrosis using transient elastography. *J.Hepatol.*, Vol. 48, No. 5, pp. 835-847, ISSN 0168-8278

Chalasani, N., Guo, X., Loomba, R., Goodarzi, M. O., Haritunians, T., Kwon, S., Cui, J., Taylor, K. D., Wilson, L., Cummings, O. W., Chen, Y. D., & Rotter, J. I. (2010). Genome-wide association study identifies variants associated with histologic features of nonalcoholic Fatty liver disease. *Gastroenterology*, Vol. 139, No. 5, (November 2010), pp. 1567-76, 1576, ISSN 7645-6

Chitturi, S., Abeygunasekera, S., Farrell, G. C., Holmes-Walker, J., Hui, J. M., Fung, C., Karim, R., Lin, R., Samarasinghe, D., Liddle, C., Weltman, M., & George, J. (2002). NASH and insulin resistance: Insulin hypersecretion and specific association with the insulin resistance syndrome. *Hepatology*, Vol. 35, No. 2, (February 2002), pp. 373-379, ISSN 1527-3350

Church, T. S., Kuk, J. L., Ross, R., Priest, E. L., Biltoft, E., & Blair, S. N. (2006). Association of cardiorespiratory fitness, body mass index, and waist circumference to nonalcoholic fatty liver disease. *Gastroenterology*, Vol. 130, No. 7, (June 2006), pp. 2023-2030, ISSN 7645-6

Cortez-Pinto, H., de Moura, M. C., & Day, C. P. (2006). Non-alcoholic steatohepatitis: from cell biology to clinical practice. *J.Hepatol.*, Vol. 44, No. 1, (January 2006), pp. 197-208, ISSN 0168-8278

Dancygier, H. (2006). Pathogenese und Therapie der nichtalkoholischen Fettlebererkrankungen. *Dtsch.Ärzteblatt*, Vol. 103, No. 19, (12 May 2006), pp. A1301-A1307, ISSN 0012-1207

Day, C. P. (2002). Pathogenesis of steatohepatitis. *Best.Pract.Res.Clin.Gastroenterol.*, Vol. 16, No. 5, (October 2002), pp. 663-678, ISSN 1521-6918

Day, C. P. (2006). Non-alcoholic fatty liver disease: current concepts and management strategies. *Clin.Med.*, Vol. 6, No. 1, (January 2006), pp. 19-25, ISSN 1473-4893

Day, C. P. & James, O. F. (1998). Steatohepatitis: a tale of two "hits"?. *Gastroenterology*, Vol. 114, No. 4, (April 1998), pp. 842-845, ISSN 7645-6

DeLeve, L. D., Shulman, H. M., & McDonald, G. B. (2002). Toxic injury to hepatic sinusoids: sinusoidal obstruction syndrome (veno-occlusive disease). *Semin.Liver Dis.*, Vol. 22, No. 1, (February 2002), pp. 27-42, ISSN 0272-8087

Dufour, J. F. & Oneta, C. M. (2004). Alcoholic and non-alcoholic steatohepatitis. *Ther.Umsch.*, Vol. 61, No. 8, (August 2004), pp. 505-512, ISSN 0040-5930

Duvnjak, M., Lerotic, I., Barsic, N., Tomasic, V., Virovic, J. L., & Velagic, V. (2007). Pathogenesis and management issues for non-alcoholic fatty liver disease. *World J.Gastroenterol.*, Vol. 13, No. 34, (14 September 2007), pp. 4539-4550, ISSN 1007-9327

Edmison, J. & McCullough, A. J. (2007). Pathogenesis of non-alcoholic steatohepatitis: human data. *Clin.Liver Dis.*, Vol. 11, No. 1, (February 2007), pp. 75-104, ISSN 1089-3261

Falck-Ytter, Y., Younossi, Z. M., Marchesini, G., & McCullough, A. J. (2001). Clinical features and natural history of nonalcoholic steatosis syndromes. *Semin.Liver Dis.*, Vol. 21, No. 1, pp. 17-26, ISSN 0272-8087

Farrell, G. C. & Larter, C. Z. (2006). Nonalcoholic fatty liver disease: from steatosis to cirrhosis. *Hepatology*, Vol. 43, No. 2 Suppl 1, (February 2006), p. S99-S112, ISSN 1527-3350

Friedrich-Rust, M., Ong, M. F., Martens, S., Sarrazin, C., Bojunga, J., Zeuzem, S., & Herrmann, E. (2008). Performance of transient elastography for the staging of liver fibrosis: a meta-analysis. *Gastroenterology*, Vol. 134, No. 4, (April 2008), pp. 960-974, ISSN 7645-6

Gentilucci, U. V., Santini, D., Vincenzi, B., Fiori, E., Picardi, A., & Tonini, G. (2006). Chemotherapy-induced steatohepatitis in colorectal cancer patients. *J.Clin.Oncol.*, Vol. 24, No. 34, (1 December 2006), pp. 5467-5468, ISSN 0732-183X

Gramlich, T., Kleiner, D. E., McCullough, A. J., Matteoni, C. A., Boparai, N., & Younossi, Z. M. (2004). Pathologic features associated with fibrosis in nonalcoholic fatty liver disease. *Hum.Pathol.*, Vol. 35, No. 2, (February 2004), pp. 196-199, ISSN 0046-8177

Harrison, S. A., Torgerson, S., & Hayashi, P. H. (2003). The natural history of nonalcoholic fatty liver disease: a clinical histopathological study. *Am.J.Gastroenterol.*, Vol. 98, No. 9, (September 2003), pp. 2042-2047, ISSN 0002-9270

Hubscher, S. G. (2004). Role of liver biopsy in the assessment of non-alcoholic fatty liver disease. *Eur.J.Gastroenterol.Hepatol.*, Vol. 16, No. 11, (November 2004), pp. 1107-1115, ISSN 0954-691X

Joy, D., Thava, V. R., & Scott, B. B. (2003). Diagnosis of fatty liver disease: is biopsy necessary?, *Eur.J.Gastroenterol.Hepatol.*, vol. 15, no. 5, (May 2003), pp. 539-543, ISSN 0954-691X

Kacerovsky, M. & Roden, M. (2007). Nichtalkoholische Fettleber. *Diabetologe*, Vol. 3, pp. 176-183, ISSN 1860-9716

Karoui, M., Penna, C., min-Hashem, M., Mitry, E., Benoist, S., Franc, B., Rougier, P., & Nordlinger, B. (2006). Influence of preoperative chemotherapy on the risk of major hepatectomy for colorectal liver metastases. *Ann.Surg.*, Vol. 243, No. 1, (January 2006), pp. 1-7, ISSN 0003-4932

Kleiner, D. E., Brunt, E. M., Van, N. M., Behling, C., Contos, M. J., Cummings, O. W., Ferrell, L. D., Liu, Y. C., Torbenson, M. S., Unalp-Arida, A., Yeh, M., McCullough, A. J., & Sanyal, A. J. (2005). Design and validation of a histological scoring system for nonalcoholic fatty liver disease. *Hepatology*, Vol. 41, No. 6, (June 2005), pp. 1313-1321, ISSN 1527-3350

Lackner, C., Gogg-Kamerer, M., Zatloukal, K., Stumptner, C., Brunt, E. M., & Denk, H. (2008). Ballooned hepatocytes in steatohepatitis: the value of keratin immunohistochemistry for diagnosis. *J.Hepatol.*, Vol. 48, No. 5, (May 2008), pp. 821-828, ISSN 0168-8278

Ludwig, J., McGill, D. B., & Lindor, K. D. (1997). Review: nonalcoholic steatohepatitis. *J.Gastroenterol.Hepatol.*, Vol. 12, No. 5, (May 1997), pp. 398-403, ISSN 0815-9319

Ludwig, J., Viggiano, T. R., McGill, D. B., & Oh, B. J. (1980). Nonalcoholic steatohepatitis: Mayo Clinic experiences with a hitherto unnamed disease. *Mayo Clin.Proc.*, Vol. 55, No. 7, (July 1980), pp. 434-438, ISSN 0025-6196

Matteoni, C. A., Younossi, Z. M., Gramlich, T., Boparai, N., Liu, Y. C., & McCullough, A. J. (1999). Nonalcoholic fatty liver disease: a spectrum of clinical and pathological severity. *Gastroenterology*, Vol. 116, No. 6, (June 1999), pp. 1413-1419, ISSN 7645-6

Medina, J., Fernandez-Salazar, L. I., Garcia-Buey, L., & Moreno-Otero, R. (2004). Approach to the pathogenesis and treatment of nonalcoholic steatohepatitis. *Diabetes Care*, Vol. 27, No. 8, (August 2004), pp. 2057-2066, ISSN 0149-5992

Mendez-Sanchez, N., Arrese, M., Zamora-Valdes, D., & Uribe, M. (2007). Current concepts in the pathogenesis of nonalcoholic fatty liver disease. *Liver Int.*, Vol. 27, No. 4, (May 2007), pp. 423-433, ISSN 1478-3223

Mendler, M. H., Kanel, G., & Govindarajan, S. (2005). Proposal for a histological scoring and grading system for non-alcoholic fatty liver disease. *Liver Int.*, Vol. 25, No. 2, (April 2005), pp. 294-304, ISSN 1478-3223

Mofrad, P., Contos, M. J., Haque, M., Sargeant, C., Fisher, R. A., Luketic, V. A., Sterling, R. K., Shiffman, M. L., Stravitz, R. T., & Sanyal, A. J. (2003). Clinical and histologic spectrum of nonalcoholic fatty liver disease associated with normal ALT values. *Hepatology*, Vol. 37, No. 6, (June 2003), pp. 1286-1292, ISSN 1527-3350

Nakano, H., Oussoultzoglou, E., Rosso, E., Casnedi, S., Chenard-Neu, M. P., Dufour, P., Bachellier, P., & Jaeck, D. (2008). Sinusoidal injury increases morbidity after major hepatectomy in patients with colorectal liver metastases receiving preoperative chemotherapy. *Ann.Surg.*, Vol. 247, No. 1, (January 2008), pp. 118-124, ISSN 0003-4932

Neuschwander-Tetri, B. A. (2002). Evolving pathophysiologic concepts in nonalcoholic steatohepatitis. *Curr.Gastroenterol.Rep.*, vol. 4, no. 1, (February 2002), pp. 31-36, ISSN 1522-8037

Neuschwander-Tetri, B. A. & Caldwell, S. H. (2003). Nonalcoholic steatohepatitis: summary of an AASLD Single Topic Conference. *Hepatology*, Vol. 37, No. 5, (May 2003), pp. 1202-1219, ISSN 1527-3350

Nocito, A., El-Badry, A. M., & Clavien, P. A. (2006). When is steatosis too much for transplantation?, *J.Hepatol.*, vol. 45, no. 4, (October 2006), pp. 494-499, ISSN 0168-8278

Nordlinger, B., Van, C. E., Rougier, P., Kohne, C. H., Ychou, M., Sobrero, A., Adam, R., Arvidsson, D., Carrato, A., Georgoulias, V., Giuliante, F., Glimelius, B., Golling, M., Gruenberger, T., Tabernero, J., Wasan, H., & Poston, G. (2007). Does chemotherapy prior to liver resection increase the potential for cure in patients with metastatic colorectal cancer? A report from the European Colorectal Metastases Treatment Group. *Eur.J.Cancer*, Vol. 43, No. 14, (September 2007), pp. 2037-2045, ISSN 0959-8049

Oneta, C. M. & Dufour, J. F. (2003). Diagnostik, Prognose und therapeutische Möglichkeiten der nicht-alkoholischen Fettlebererkrankung. *Schweiz Med Forum*, Vol. 37, pp. 862-868, ISSN 0036-7672

Papandreou, D., Rousso, I., & Mavromichalis, I. (2007). Update on non-alcoholic fatty liver disease in children. *Clin.Nutr.*, Vol. 26, No. 4, (August 2007), pp. 409-415, ISSN 0261-5614

Petersen, K. F., Dufour, S., Hariri, A., Nelson-Williams, C., Foo, J. N., Zhang, X. M., Dziura, J., Lifton, R. P., & Shulman, G. I. (2010). Apolipoprotein C3 gene variants in nonalcoholic fatty liver disease. *N.Engl.J.Med.*, Vol. 362, No. 12, (25 March 2010), pp. 1082-1089, ISSN 0028-4793

Rashid, M. & Roberts, E. A. (2000). Nonalcoholic steatohepatitis in children. *J.Pediatr.Gastroenterol.Nutr.*, Vol. 30, No. 1, (January 2000), pp. 48-53, ISSN 0277-2116

Ratziu, V., Charlotte, F., Heurtier, A., Gombert, S., Giral, P., Bruckert, E., Grimaldi, A., Capron, F., & Poynard, T. (2005). Sampling variability of liver biopsy in nonalcoholic fatty liver disease. *Gastroenterology*, Vol. 128, No. 7, (June 2005), pp. 1898-1906, ISSN 7645-6

Reid, A. E. (2001). Nonalcoholic steatohepatitis. *Gastroenterology*, Vol. 121, No. 3, (September 2001), pp. 710-723, ISSN 7645-6

Roberts, E. A. (2002). Steatohepatitis in children. *Best.Pract.Res.Clin.Gastroenterol.*, Vol. 16, No. 5, (October 2002), pp. 749-765, ISSN 1521-6918

Roberts, E. A. (2007). Non-alcoholic steatohepatitis in children. *Clin.Liver Dis.*, Vol. 11, No. 1, (February 2007), pp. 155-72, ISSN 1089-3261

Rousselet, M. C., Michalak, S., Dupre, F., Croue, A., Bedossa, P., Saint-Andre, J. P., & Cales, P. (2005). Sources of variability in histological scoring of chronic viral hepatitis. *Hepatology*, Vol. 41, No. 2, (February 2005), pp. 257-264, ISSN 1527-3350

Sanyal, A. J., Banas, C., Sargeant, C., Luketic, V. A., Sterling, R. K., Stravitz, R. T., Shiffman, M. L., Heuman, D., Coterrell, A., Fisher, R. A., Contos, M. J., & Mills, A. S. (2006). Similarities and differences in outcomes of cirrhosis due to nonalcoholic steatohepatitis and hepatitis C. *Hepatology*, vol. 43, no. 4, (April 2006), pp. 682-689, ISSN 1527-3350

Schwimmer, J. B. (2007). Definitive diagnosis and assessment of risk for nonalcoholic fatty liver disease in children and adolescents. *Semin.Liver Dis.*, Vol. 27, No. 3, (August 2007), pp. 312-318, ISSN 0272-8087

Schwimmer, J. B., Behling, C., Newbury, R., Deutsch, R., Nievergelt, C., Schork, N. J., & Lavine, J. E. (2005). Histopathology of pediatric nonalcoholic fatty liver disease. *Hepatology*, Vol. 42, No. 3, (September 2005), pp. 641-649, ISSN 1527-3350

Sonsuz, A., Basaranoglu, M., & Ozbay, G. (2000). Relationship between aminotransferase levels and histopathological findings in patients with nonalcoholic steatohepatitis. *Am.J.Gastroenterol.*, Vol. 95, No. 5, (May 2000), pp. 1370-1371, ISSN 0002-9270

Strassburg, C. P. & Manns, M. P. (2006). Approaches to liver biopsy techniques--revisited. *Semin.Liver Dis.*, Vol. 26, No. 4, (November 2006), pp. 318-327, ISSN 0272-8087

Tannapfel, A., Geissler, F., Witzigmann, H., Hauss, J., & Wittekind, C. (2001). Analysis of liver allograft rejection related genes using cDNA-microarrays in liver allograft specimen. *Transplant.Proc.*, Vol. 33, No. 7-8, (November 2001), pp. 3283-3284, ISSN 0041-1345

Tannapfel, A. & Reinacher-Schick, A. (2008). Chemotherapy associated hepatotoxicity in the treatment of advanced colorectal cancer (CRC). *Z.Gastroenterol.*, Vol. 46, No. 5, (May 2008), pp. 435-440, ISSN 0044-2771

Tannapfel, A., Denk, H., Dienes, H.P., Langner, C., Schirmacher, P., Trauner, M., Flott-Rahmel, B. (2009). Histopathological Diagnosis of Non-alcoholic and Alcoholic Fatty Liver Disease, In: *AWMF online*, 01 November 2009, Available from: http://www.awmf.org/leitlinien/detail/ll/035-004.html

Targher, G., Bertolini, L., Rodella, S., Zoppini, G., Scala, L., Zenari, L., & Falezza, G. (2006). Associations between plasma adiponectin concentrations and liver histology in patients with nonalcoholic fatty liver disease. *Clin.Endocrinol.(Oxf)*, Vol. 64, No. 6, (June 2006), pp. 679-683, ISSN 0300-0664

Teli, M. R., James, O. F., Burt, A. D., Bennett, M. K., & Day, C. P. (1995). The natural history of nonalcoholic fatty liver: a follow-up study. *Hepatology*, Vol. 22, No. 6, (December 1995), pp. 1714-1719, ISSN 1527-3350

Valenti, L., Alisi, A., Galmozzi, E., Bartuli, A., Del Menico, B., Alterio, A., Dongiovanni, P., Fargion, S., & Nobili, V. (2010). I148M patatin-like phospholipase domain-containing 3 gene variant and severity of pediatric nonalcoholic fatty liver disease. *Hepatology*, Vol. 52, No. 4, (October 2010), pp. 1274-1280, ISSN 1527-3350

Vauthey, J. N., Pawlik, T. M., Ribero, D., Wu, T. T., Zorzi, D., Hoff, P. M., Xiong, H. Q., Eng, C., Lauwers, G. Y., Mino-Kenudson, M., Risio, M., Muratore, A., Capussotti, L., Curley, S. A., & Abdalla, E. K. (2006). Chemotherapy regimen predicts steatohepatitis and an increase in 90-day mortality after surgery for hepatic colorectal metastases. *J.Clin.Oncol.*, Vol. 24, No. 13, (1 May 2006), pp. 2065-2072, ISSN 0732-183X

Wieckowska, A., McCullough, A. J., & Feldstein, A. E. (2007). Noninvasive diagnosis and monitoring of nonalcoholic steatohepatitis: present and future. *Hepatology*, Vol. 46, No. 2, pp. 582-589, ISSN 1527-3350

Wieckowska, A., Zein, N. N., Yerian, L. M., Lopez, A. R., McCullough, A. J., & Feldstein, A. E. (2006). In vivo assessment of liver cell apoptosis as a novel biomarker of disease severity in nonalcoholic fatty liver disease. *Hepatology*, Vol. 44, No. 1, (July 2006), pp. 27-33, ISSN 1527-3350

Williams, C. D., Stengel, J., Asike, M. I., Torres, D. M., Shaw, J., Contreras, M., Landt, C. L., & Harrison, S. A. (2011). Prevalence of nonalcoholic fatty liver disease and nonalcoholic steatohepatitis among a largely middle-aged population utilizing ultrasound and liver biopsy: a prospective study. *Gastroenterology*, Vol. 140, No. 1, (January 2011), pp. 124-131, ISSN 7645-6

Younossi, Z. M., Jarrar, M., Nugent, C., Randhawa, M., Afendy, M., Stepanova, M., Rafiq, N., Goodman, Z., Chandhoke, V., & Baranova, A. (2008). A Novel Diagnostic Biomarker Panel for Obesity-related Nonalcoholic Steatohepatitis (NASH). *Obes.Surg.*, Vol 18, No. 11, (24 May 2008), pp1430-1437, ISSN 0960-8923

Zivkovic, A. M., German, J. B., & Sanyal, A. J. (2007).Comparative review of diets for the metabolic syndrome: implications for nonalcoholic fatty liver disease. *Am.J.Clin.Nutr.*, Vol. 86, No. 2, (August 2007), pp. 285-300, ISSN 0002-9165

4

Metabolic Steatosis & Fibrosis: Review of the Non-Invasive Tools for Diagnosis and Screening

Véronique Miette, Meriem Abdennour, Laurent Sandrin and Magali Sasso
Echosens,
France

1. Introduction

Hepatic steatosis affects 20% to 30% of the general adult population in affluent countries. Metabolic syndrome and its components—type 2 diabetes mellitus and central obesity—lead to the development of nonalcoholic fatty liver disease (NAFLD), in part due to insulin resistance, apoptosis and altered adipokine and cytokine pathways. Indeed, NAFLD is now considered the hepatic manifestation of metabolic syndrome. Globally, NAFLD is a common cause of chronic liver disease and, as the obesity epidemic continues, the prevalence of NAFLD is anticipated to increase. Non Alcoholic Fatty Disease (NAFLD) encompasses a histological spectrum ranging from simple steatosis to non-alcoholic steatohepatitis (NASH), the latter characterized by steatosis plus necroinflammation. NASH can have different stages of fibrosis ranging from absent (stage F0) to cirrhosis (stage F4). Currently, the technique of choice for determining hepatic fat deposition and the stage of fibrosis is liver biopsy. However, it is an invasive procedure and its use is limited. It may also be subject to sampling error. Non-invasive techniques such as ultrasound, computerized tomography (CT), magnetic resonance imaging (MRI) and proton magnetic resonance spectroscopy (1H MRS) can detect hepatic steatosis, but currently cannot distinguish between simple steatosis and steatohepatitis, or stage the degree of fibrosis accurately. Four new non-invasive methods received independent validation to assess NASH diagnosis (serologic tests) or to stage advanced fibrosis (blood tests, magnetic resonance elastography (MRE) and vibration controlled transient elastography (VCTE)).
The chapter is organized as follows: section 2 describes natural history of NAFLD and NASH. The epidemiology is detailed section 3 and the risk factors in section 4. Than the limitations of liver biopsy are explained section 5; section 6 contains a description of non invasive tools clinically used or at the contrary new development not yet clinically evaluated. Advantages and limitations of these devices are detailed. Their applications in NAFLD diseases are described. Eventually, discussion and conclusion are drawn in section 6 and section 7, respectively.

2. Natural history: NASH and NAFLD

Ludwig et al. about 30 years ago described a liver disease that resembled alcoholic hepatitis in its histopathologic features but without a history of significant alcohol consumption (Ludwig et al. 1980). Since then, literature about non-alcoholic fatty liver disease (NAFLD)

has expanded exponentially in attempts to understand its pathophysiology and treat the condition.
The term NAFLD is used to describe a condition of fat accumulation in the liver in the absence of excessive alcohol consumption and any other specific causes of hepatic steatosis (Ludwig et al. 1980; Bedogni et al. 2006). In the majority of the cases, NAFLD is of primary origin and its etiology is not yet completely understood, even if it is strictly related to the presence of insulin resistance, and thus frequently occurs as the initial part of the metabolic syndrome, and accompanies obesity, type 2 diabetes and dyslipidaemia.
NAFLD is a chronic liver condition that spans a spectrum of abnormalities ranging from simple hepatic steatosis to a predominantly lobular necroinflammation, with or without centrilobular fibrosis (termed non-alcoholic steatohepatitis or NASH), which can eventually lead to cirrhosis and its associated complications. Around 30% of NAFLD may progress to NASH (Farrell & Larter 2006). At the time of diagnosis, the presence of severe fibrosis in liver biopsies in patients with NASH has been noted in 15 to 50% of patients and 7% to 26% with cirrhosis (Angulo & Lindor 2002). Undiagnosed NASH is the most likely cause for cryptogenic cirrhosis (Bugianesi et al. 2002). Hepatocellular carcinoma is also a recognized complication of fatty liver disease and emerging evidence suggests that cardiovascular disease may also be more common.
A first phase is responsible for the accumulation of fatty acids in hepatocytes, which weakens the adaptive phase hepatocytes and makes them more susceptible to attacks. The second phase, lipid peroxidation secondary to oxidative stress, is ultimately responsible for cellular damage and the appearance of liver fibrosis.
In fact, the mechanisms and causes of the initial lesions of steatosis are less known. It is recognized that insulin resistance plays a central role in pathogenesis, occurring probably in a favorable genetic background. Adipocyte-related factors (leptin, resistin, adiponectin), particularly from the visceral fat, have been implicated in causing insulin resistance and fatty lesions. The existence of genetic factors predisposing to the development of these lesions has also been suggested (mitochondrial abnormalities, genetic polymorphism of inflammatory cytokine synthesis).

3. Epidemiology

Epidemiological studies can be separated into two categories: selected population studies and general screening population studies. The studies using highly selected populations suffer from bias but they have high specificity because histology was used to diagnose presence of NAFLD and its severity. The general population screening studies provides more representative prevalence rates but cannot identify the type of NAFLD because of the limitations of their diagnostic technique (Farrell et al. 2005).

3.1 General screening population studies

NAFLD is related to modern lifestyle and with expanded clinical importance because of the rising incidence of type 2 diabetes mellitus and obesity. In fact NAFLD affects 20-25% of the general population (Bedogni et al. 2006; Nomura et al. 1988) and 20-30% in North America and western countries (Angulo & Lindor 2002; Williams 2006), thus it is becoming one of the commonest liver disease worldwide . NAFLD continues to rise and affects about 30% of the adult population in the US now have NAFLD and 3-6 % have NASH (Torres & Harrison 2008).

In China, with the increasing pandemic of obesity, the prevalence of NAFLD has approximately doubled in the past decade. Among more affluent regions of China, the community prevalence of NAFLD is about 15% (Machann et al. 2006), the community prevalence of NAFLD in India varies from 5% to 28%, and varies from 9 to 30% in Japan (Amarapurkar et al. 2007).
The frequency of hepatic steatosis varied significantly with ethnicity (45% in Hispanics; 33% in whites; 24% in blacks), the higher prevalence of hepatic steatosis in Hispanics was due to the higher prevalence of obesity and insulin resistance in this ethnic group (Browning et al. 2004).

3.2 Selected study population

3.2.1 Obese

NAFLD occurs in the majority of subjects with severe obesity, NAFLD was present in 55-90% of severely obese patients while NASH occurred in 37% (Farrell & Larter 2006; Machado et al. 2006) and 25% has fibrosis (Gholam et al. 2007).

3.2.2 Children

NAFLD is the commonest cause of paediatric chronic liver disease in North America (Patton et al. 2010), NAFLD was observed in 10% of children in the USA (Adams) and when population of obese children are analyzed, NAFLD was found in 40% (Pacifico et al. 2010).

3.2.3 Healthy young adults

Nonalcoholic steatosis was discovered in 20% of healthy young adults who are evaluated for possible right lobe donor hepatectomy transplantation in adult-to-adult living donor transplantation (Marcos et al. 2000)

3.2.4 Patients who had random deaths

The liver of subjects died in airplane crashes or traffic accidents showed prevalence of 16% and 24% for NAFLD and 2.1% -2.4% for NASH (Hilden et al. 1977; Ground 1982).
All these are strictly selected populations, which do not reflect the true prevalence.

4. Risk factors

Nonalcoholic fatty liver disease (NAFLD) is associated with obesity and insulin resistance; it is considered the hepatic manifestation of metabolic syndrome. The metabolic syndrome is defined by the presence of 3 or more of the following criteriasummarized in Table 1: elevated waist circumference, high fasting glucose, hypertension, elevated triglycerides and decreased high density lipoprotein concentration. Features of the metabolic syndrome, Insulin resistances and systemic hypertension are independently associated with advanced forms of NAFLD. NASH is associated with obesity, diabetes mellitus and dyslipidemia.
Predictors of NASH are: a raised index of insulin resistance(odds ratio OR = 9.3, CI=3.4 -26, systemic hypertension (OR = 5.2, CI =2.0–13.5), and raised alanine aminotransferase (OR 8.6, CI = 3.1–23.5) (Dixon et al. 2001). The insulin resistance is the strongest predictor of NASH(Bugianesi et al. 2002).
Only a fraction of patient with simple steatosis will progress into the more severe NASH. This implies that other factors metabolic, environmental and genetic variables participate in the pathogenesis of the disease.

Measure	Abnormal level
Elevated waist circumference	Population- and country specific definitions
Elevated triglycerides (drug treatment for elevated triglycerides is an alternate indicator)	≥ 150 mg/dL (1.7 mmol/L)
Reduced HDL-cholesterol (drug treatment for reduced HDL-cholesterol an alternate indicator)	In Males: < 40 mg /dL (1.0 mmol/L) In Females : < 50 mg/dl (1.3 mmol/L)
Elevated blood pressure (antihypertensive drug treatment in a patient with history of hypertension in a alternate indicator)	Systolic ≥ 130 and/or diastolic ≥ 85mmHg
Elevated fasting glucose (drug treatment is alternate indicator)	≥ 100 mg/dL

Table 1. Criteria for Clinical Diagnosis of the Metabolic Syndrome from (Alberti et al. 2009).

5. Liver biopsy: a limited gold standard

In the precedent section, we saw that typical histologic features of NASH primarily include macrovesicular steatosis, a mixed lobular inflammation, and hepatocellular ballooning. Thus, for the diagnosis of NASH to be established, a liver biopsy is still required and therefore remains the gold standard. Only information from biopsy allows grading and staging of the disease.

5.1 Non-alcoholic fatty liver disease: an histological diagnosis

Non-alcoholic fatty liver disease (NAFLD) is a complex metabolic liver disease. The clinical spectrum of NAFLD ranges from benign steatosis to steatohepatitis (Farrell 2004), named NASH (non-alcoholic steatosis hepatitis). NASH defines a sub-group of NAFLD patients where steatosis coexist with liver-cell injury and inflammation (Ratziu et al. 2009). NASH is a progressive form of liver injury that may lead to liver fibrosis which can result in cirrhosis, liver failure and hepatocellular carcinoma (Farrell 2004; Ratziu et al. 2009).

The diagnosis of NAFLD is clinicopathological. NAFLD or NASH can be defined as significant steatosis or steatohepatitis not resulting from alcohol, drugs, toxins, infectious agents or other exogenous causes (Farrell 2004). NASH was first described in 1980 by Ludwig *et al.* (Ludwig et al. 1980) who described a series of patients with chronic liver disease and no history of significant alcohol intake in whom the liver histology was similar to patients with alcoholic liver disease.

The diagnosis of NAFLD is usually suspected in patients with asymptomatic and persistent elevation of aminotransferase, radiological finding of fatty liver and unexplained persistent hepatomegaly (Angulo & Lindor 2002). However the elevation of liver enzyme has a poor predictive value (Angulo & Lindor 2002; Clark et al. 2002) and no clinical or biochemical abnormality permit an accurate diagnosis of NAFLD (Angulo & Lindor 2002). Liver imaging is useful to determine the presence of fatty infiltration but cannot determine the presence and severity of liver damage (Angulo & Lindor 2002).

A liver biopsy is the gold standard to diagnose NAFLD/NASH (Nugent & Younossi 2007) and determine the stage of hepatic fibrosis (Nugent & Younossi 2007). Liver biopsy is the only way to establish definite diagnosis of NASH (Nugent & Younossi 2007) and is the only technique which can distinguish simple steatosis from steatohepatitis (Farrell 2004).

A liver biopsy can assess all liver features associated with NAFLD *e.g.* steatosis, hepatocellular injury, inflammation, fibrosis, etc. (Angulo & Lindor 2002) and can make the

distinction with chronic liver disease from other cause (Ratziu et al. 2009). Liver biopsy provides information about the stage of hepatic fibrosis which is the most crucial clinical prognostic information.
However despite all advantages of liver biopsy, its role for NAFLD patients in clinical practice remains controversial (Nugent & Younossi 2007).

5.2 When to consider a liver biopsy for NAFLD patients

A liver biopsy is essential for the diagnosis and staging of NAFLD. However given its invasiveness, its potential severe complication and the lack of treatment for NAFLD patients (Nugent & Younossi 2007), the decision for the hepatologist to refer to liver biopsy might be difficult. Furthermore, NAFLD patients are asymptomatic and are reluctant to undergo a liver biopsy (Nugent & Younossi 2007).
Decision for the hepatologist to refer to a liver biopsy is made on individual basis (Ratziu et al. 2009; Nugent & Younossi 2007). According the 2010 position statement on NAFLD/NASH of the European Association for the Study of the Liver (EASL) (Ratziu et al. 2009), a liver biopsy should be performed in patients:

- with disorders of the metabolic syndrome for whom non-invasive methods suggest advanced fibrosis or yield discordant results,
- with chronic liver disease not related to NAFLD and evidence of metabolic risk factors, insulin-resistance and steatosis at ultrasound,
- undergoing bariatric surgery and cholecystectomy.

Furthermore, in patients with disorders of the metabolic syndrome with both increased alanine transferase and steatosis at ultrasound, liver biopsy could be the first-line procedure until non-invasive methods becomes extensively and independently validated (Ratziu et al. 2009).

5.3 NAFLD liver histology

5.3.1 Histological liver lesions associated with NAFLD

The zonal location of liver lesions is an important feature for histological evaluation. Briefly, liver is histologically divided into lobules which take the shape of a hexagon (Dancygier 2010), as represented in Figure 1.

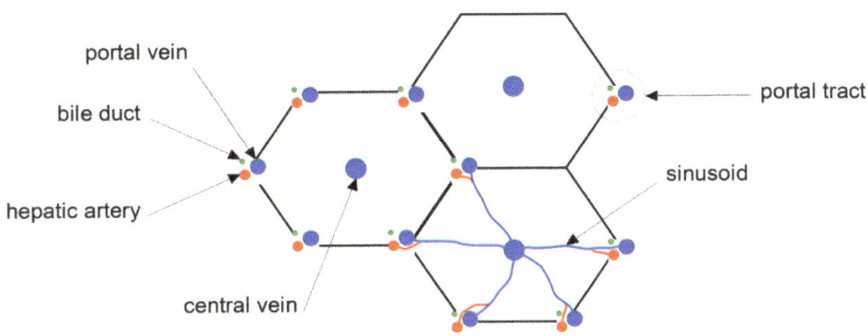

Fig. 1. Liver lobule organization.

At the centre of the lobule is the central vein. At the periphery of the lobular are portal tract. The portal tract is an island of connective tissue containing branches of the portal vein, hepatic artery and bile duct. Portal vein and hepatic artery empty into the sinusoid, from which blood flows to the central vein.

The liver lobule can be divided into three zones: the periportal zone which encircles the portal tract, the centrolobular zone which encircles the central vein and the zone in between named midlobular zone.

In NAFLD/NASH, steatosis, necroinflammation, Mallory's hyaline and fibrosis are typically concentrated in the centrolobular zone (Angulo & Lindor 2002).

5.3.1.1 Steatosis

Steatosis is characterized by the accumulation of fat droplets in the liver. Steatosis is necessary for the diagnosis of NAFLD except for patients with cirrhosis for whom steatosis can be absent. The minimal threshold to diagnose steatosis is 5% of hepatocytes containing fat droplets.

Steatosis in NAFLD patients is mainly macrovesicular (Farrell 2004) which means that fat is a single droplet that fill in the hepatocyte and displace its nucleus at the periphery of the cell. Sometimes microvesicular steatosis can also be seen but in a smaller proportion and in that case, the hepatocytes contain a large number of tinier droplets surrounding the central nucleus (Farrell 2004).

In NAFLD early or mild steatosis is seen in centrolobular zone (Farrell 2004).

Simple steatosis is a reversible condition in a matter of days to weeks (Farrell 2004).

5.3.1.2 Hepatocyte injuries

Hepatocyte injuries that frequently occur in NAFLD are: hepatocellular ballooning, liver cell death, and Mallory's hyaline (Farrell 2004).

Hepatocellular ballooning is a structural manifestation of severe cell injury (Schattner & Knobler 2008). Ballooned hepatocytes are enlarged and have a pale cytoplasm as a result of fluid retention (Farrell 2004), with a rarefaction of the cytoplasm (Schattner & Knobler 2008). Ballooning degeneration is reversible (Farrell 2004) but is likely a form of necrosis (Schattner & Knobler 2008). Hepatocellular ballooning is seen most of the time in the centri-lobular zone, mixed or adjacent to regions with steatosis (Schattner & Knobler 2008).

Liver cell death can be seen in the form of necrosis or apoptosis and is not reversible (Farrell 2004). Apoptotic hepatocytes cells are seen as shrunken cells with densely condensed nuclei (Farrell 2004). Necrotic hepatocytes are not usually prominent but mixed inflammatory infiltrate can be seen is the site where necrotic hepatocytes have disappeared (Farrell 2004).

Mallory's hyaline is seen as a ropy inclusion with the cytoplasm of hepatocytes, especially in cells showing ballooning degeneration (Farrell 2004). It develops as a result of an impaired proteosomal degradation of cytoplasmic proteins (Schattner & Knobler 2008).

Other lesions can be seen in NAFLD: glycogenated nuclei, lipogranulomas, Kupffer cells, mitochondrial abnormalities, fatty cyst, etc. (Schattner & Knobler 2008; Brunt 2005).

5.3.1.3 Inflammation

The hallmark of inflammation in NAFLD is the lobular inflammation (Schattner & Knobler 2008). Lobular inflammation is characterized by the presence of typically mild mixed inflammation, close to ballooned hepatocytes (Schattner & Knobler 2008), and includes a small number of lymphocytes, a small number of macrophages, Kupffer cells, but also a small number of polymorphonuclear leukocytes (Brunt 2005). Portal inflammation can also be seen in NAFLD (Brunt 2005).

5.3.1.4 Fibrosis

In NASH, fibrosis is first seen in the centrilobular zone (Angulo & Lindor 2002; Farrell 2004). This fibrosis is characteriscally perisinusoidal (Brunt 2005). This fibrosis can progress portal fibrosis, central-portal and portal-portal septum and eventually cirrhosis (Angulo & Lindor

2002). Around 20% of NASH patients may progress to cirrhosis (Angulo & Lindor 2002; Farrell 2004). In patients with cirrhosis, the features of steatosis and necroinflammatory activity may no longer be present (Angulo & Lindor 2002).

5.3.2 Histological description of NAFLD/NASH

There is currently no evaluation system massively admitted by experts for the evaluation of NAFLD (Angulo & Lindor 2002; Farrell 2004; Nugent & Younossi 2007; Brunt 2007). For instance, some authors (Farrell 2004; Brunt et al. 1999) but not all (Farrell 2004; Diehl 2002) consider ballooning as an absolute requisite for the diagnosis of NASH, it can be the same for other histological features such as Mallory's hyaline (Brunt 2005).

The early description of NAFLD described four subtypes: fatty liver, fatty hepatitis, fatty fibrosis and fatty cirrhosis (Adler & Schaffner 1979).

Ludwid *et al.* characterized NASH specimen by the presence of steatosis, necrosis, lobular inflammation and in most specimens Mallory's hyaline and fibrosis (Ludwig et al. 1980).

Matteoni *et al.* (Matteoni et al. 1999) proposed in 1997 the classification summarized in Table 2.

Type of NAFLD	Histological description	Prognosis
Type 1	Simple steatosis	Begnin
Type 2	Steatohepatitis : steatosis plus lobular inflammation	Probably begnin
Type 3	Steatonecrosis: steatosis and ballooning	Bad prognosis
Type 4	Steatonecrosis plus fibrosis: steatosis, lobular inflammation, ballooning, Mallory's hyaline and/or fibrosis	Bad prognosis

Table 2. Types of NAFLD according to (Matteoni et al. 1999).

Brunt *et al.* (Brunt et al. 1999) have proposed in 1999 a grading and staging system for NASH. This system includes a necroinflammatory grade and a fibrosis score. The necroinflammatory grade is a combination of features of steatosis, ballooning and inflammation since no single feature can determine activity. The three grades are summarized in Table 3.

Grade	Histological characteristics
Grade 1 - mild	Steatosis: up to 66%. Ballooning: mild, occasional Lobular inflammation: scattered and mild Portal inflammation: absent to mild
Grade 2 - moderate	Steatosis: any degree Ballooning: moderate, obvious in centrolobular zone Lobular inflammation: mild to moderate Portal Inflammation: mild to moderate
Grade 3 - severe	Steatosis: any degree Ballooning: severe, marked in centrilobular zone Lobular inflammation: severe Portal inflammation: mild to moderate

Table 3. Necroinflammatory grading system for NASH from (Brunt et al. 1999).

In addition, Brunt *et al.* (Brunt et al. 1999) proposed a staging system for fibrosis in NASH. This staging is summarized in Table 4.

Stage	Histological description
0	No fibrosis
1	Centrilobular perisinusoidal fibrosis
2	Centrilobular perisinusoidal fibrosis and portal/periportal fibrosis
3	Bridging fibrosis
4	Cirrhosis

Table 4. Staging of fibrosis for NASH, according to (Brunt et al. 1999).

Eventually, by Kleiner *et al.* from the NASH clinical research network developed (Kleiner et al. 2005) in 2005 an approach for the assessment of NAFLD. This scoring system grade three histological features: steatosis, inflammation and ballooning according to standardized histological evaluation summarized in Table 5.

Histological feature	Histological evaluation	Score
Steatosis	< 5%	0
	5-33%	1
	34-66%	2
	> 66%	3
Lobular inflammation	No foci	0
	1~2 foci per 200xfield	1
	2-4 foci per 200xfield	2
	>4 foci per 200xfield	3
Ballooning	None	0
	Few cells	1
	Many cells/prominent	2

Table 5. Scoring system for steatosis, lobular inflammation and ballooning for NAFLD (Kleiner et al. 2005).

Then, the score of each feature (steatosis, lobular inflammation and ballooning) are summed up to constitute the NAFLD activity score (NAS score) which ranges from 0-8. According to the NAS score, the diagnosis of NASH can be made or excluded as described in Table 6.

NAS score	Diagnosis
≤ 2	No NASH
3-4	Borderline
≥ 5	NASH

Table 6. Diagnosis of NASH upon the NAFLD activity score (NAS), according to (Kleiner et al. 2005).

In addition, Kleiner *et al.* (Kleiner et al. 2005) have proposed a staging system of fibrosis for NAFLD patients, which is summarized in Table 7.

Stage	Histological description
0	No fibrosis
1	Perisinusoidal or periportal fibrosis
1A	Mild centrilobular perisinusoidal fibrosis
1B	Moderate centrilobular perisinusoidal fibrosis
1C	Portal/periportal fibrosis
2	Perisinusoidal and portal/periportal fibrosis
3	Bridging fibrosis
4	Cirrhosis

Table 7. Staging of fibrosis, according to (Kleiner et al. 2005).

The Kleiner score is very fetching since it provides a standardized approach for diagnosis of NASH and this score tend to be widely used, especially for clinical studies of patients with NASH. However, despite the practical side of NAS score, it has some limitations and does not perfectly correlate with the definite diagnosis of NASH (Brunt et al. 2011).

5.4 Advantages and drawbacks of liver biopsy

5.4.1 Advantages

Despite its limitations, liver biopsy is the only method for:

- diagnosis : to distinguish simple steatosis from steatohepatitis (Farrell 2004),
- prognosis: grading and staging of NAFLD.

5.4.2 Drawbacks

Liver biopsy is invasive, often painful procedure which can result in severe complications (Grant & Neuberger 1999). Its invasiveness implies that it cannot be performed repeatedly to monitor NAFLD or NASH after intervention.

Liver biopsy can only be performed in selected patients, according to the type of liver biopsy. The mains liver biopsy procedures are summarized in the next paragraph, together with their contraindications and possible complications.

5.4.3 Type of liver biopsy: procedure, contraindication and complications

The three main types of liver biopsy are the percutaneous liver biopsy, transjugular liver biopsy and laparoscopic liver biopsy (Grant & Neuberger 1999; Bravo et al. 2001).

Laparoscopic liver biopsy is rarely used (Bravo et al. 2001) and therefore will not be described hereafter. Its complications include those of laparoscopy itself (Bravo et al. 2001).

5.4.3.1 Percutaneous liver biopsy

Percutaneous liver biopsy is the commonest liver biopsy technique.

Patients should lie in bed and are monitored for at least six hours after the biopsy (Bravo et al. 2001). Patient should be driven home from the hospital and reliable person should stay with the patient the night after the biopsy to provide care and transportation if necessary (Bravo et al. 2001). Patient should be hospitalized after liver biopsy if there is evidence of bleeding, bile leak, pneumothorax (Bravo et al. 2001).

The contraindication for a percutaneous liver biopsy include: uncooperative patients, history of unexplained bleeding, extrahepatic biliary obstruction, bacterial cholangitis, abnormal coagulation indexes, cardiac liver, ascite, blood for transfusion unavailable, suspected vascular tumor, suspected cyst in the liver (Grant & Neuberger 1999; Bravo et al. 2001).

Most of complications occur within 24 hours after the procedure (Piccinino et al. 1986) and sixty percent of complications occur within 2 hours. Commonest complications are pain and vasovagal episodes. Major complications are significant haemorrhage, haemobilia, puncture of other viscera and pneumothorax (Grant & Neuberger 1999). Mortality rate is around 0.1‰ (Bravo et al. 2001). The main cause of mortality after liver biopsy in intraperitoneal bleeding (Grant & Neuberger 1999).

5.4.3.2 Transjugular liver biopsy

Transjugular liver biopsy is recommended for most patients for whom percutaneous liver biopsy cannot be performed (Grant & Neuberger 1999) that is with cogulapathy, ascite, massive obesity, suspected vascular tumors and in patients for whom percutaneous liver biopsy failed (Bravo et al. 2001).

Procure last around on hour. A catheter is inserted in the right internal transjugular vein and guided via fluoroscopy (live X-ray) to the right hepatic vein. A needle biopsy of the liver is then performed through the catheter (Bravo et al. 2001).

Complications occurs in around 1 to 20% of patients and include: abdominal pain, neck hematoma, cardiac arrhythmias, fistula from the hepatic artery to the portal vein or biliary three and perforation of the liver capsule (Bravo et al. 2001). Mortality rate is around 0.1% to 0.5% (Bravo et al. 2001).

5.4.4 Sampling, intra/inter observer variability & effect of liver biopsy sample length

5.4.4.1 Sampling variability

A limitation of liver biopsy is its sampling variability (Ratziu et al. 2009; Qayyum et al. 2005). Sampling variability is a relevant limitation of liver biopsy due to the fact that the liver biopsy specimen represent only a very limited part of the whole liver (Bravo et al. 2001) and that histologic lesions of NAFLD/NASH are likely to have a very unevenly distribution in the liver (Brunt 2008), even at a macroscopic level.

Indeed, in Merriman *et al.* (Qayyum et al. 2005), 41 subjects underwent intraoperative liver biopsies from both right and left lobes. The κ coefficient was assessed and shown: excellent agreement for steatosis (κ = 0.88), moderate for fibrosis staging and lobular inflammation (κ = 0.53 and κ = 0.32, respectively) and slight for ballooning and portal inflammation (κ = 0.20 and κ = 0.19, respectively).

In Ratziu *et al.* (Ratziu et al. 2009), 2 samples of liver biopsy were successively collected in 51 patients. The κ reliability test was assessed and shown: substantial agreement for steatosis (κ = 0.64), moderate agreement for fibrosis staging and ballooning (κ = 0.47 and κ = 0.45, respectively), fair agreement for Mallory's hyaline (κ = 0.27) and poor agreement for lobular inflammation (κ = 0.13).

The heterogeneous distribution of histological lesions of NAFLD/NASH is particularly accentuated for lobular inflammation and ballooning that are key features in NASH diagnosis.

To avoid as much as possible potential sampling variability error, large specimen are required for reliable evaluation of NAFLD patients (Brunt 2007; Vuppalanchi et al. 2009). Usually, most of the pathologists recommend a specimen of at least 1.5 cm with at least six to eight portal tracts (Bravo et al. 2001), and preferably a specimen of at least 25 mm is preferable (Vuppalanchi et al. 2009).

5.4.4.2 Intra/inter-observer variability

Intra/inter-observer variability is an important cause of error when staging and grading liver biopsy (Ratziu et al. 2009; Marcellin et al. 2009; El-Badry et al. 2009) which can yield poor reproducibility even when performed by experts pathologists (El-Badry et al. 2009).
In the study by El-Badry *et al.* (El-Badry et al. 2009), 4 established expert pathologist from different institutions worldwide were asked to grade steatosis from 46 NAFLD patients. Concomitant computerized morphometric analysis was performed on the same slides. Poor agreement was found among pathologists for the evaluation of total steatosis: intra-class correlation agreement ICC = 0.57, macrovesicular steatosis ICC = 0.55. Failed agreement was found for the evaluation of micro-vesicular steatosis. When compared with computerized morphometic analysis, poor agreement was found for 3 pathologists (Spearman rank correlation coefficient ρ = 0.22, 0.28 and 0.38) and good agreement was found for one pathologist (ρ = 0.82). In addition, features of NASH (lobular and portal inflammation, ballooning, Mallory's hyaline) were assessed by the 4 pathologists as present or absent, as well as diagnosis of NASH, and a strong disagreement was found for all parameters including the overall diagnosis. Evaluation of NAFLD/NASH is therefore strongly observer-dependent and therefore seems weakly reproducible.
Even when performed by the same operator, variability can be important. Indeed, in Ratziu *et al.* (Ratziu et al. 2009), intra-observer variability was assessed on 50 liver biopsies and intra-observer κ reliability test yield to substantial agreement for steatosis (κ = 0.74), moderate agreement for ballooning (κ = 0.62), perisinusoidal fibrosis (κ = 0.53), fair agreement for Mallory's hyaline (κ = 0.39) and lobular inflammation (κ = 0.37). Overall staging of fibrosis was substantial (κ = 0.69) and grading of NAFLD was moderate (κ = 0.55).

5.4.4.3 Other cause of variability

Some other parameters such as tissue fixation and staining methods can also influence the evaluation and be a cause of variability in the assessment of NAFLD/NASH (DiDonato & Brasaemle 2003; Fukumoto & Fujimoto 2002).

5.4.4.4 Impact of variability

Sampling error, intra and inter-observer variability and other causes of variability may induce misdiagnosis and substantial staging inaccuracy that might have significant implication in the clinical management of NAFLD/NASH patients.

6. Non invasive tools: how to detect transition between steatosis and fibrosis?

Hepatic steatosis refers to the excessive accumulation of fat within hepatocytes. The most common form of steatosis is nonalcoholic fatty liver disease (NAFLD), which comprises a wide spectrum of liver damage, ranging from simple steatosis (`fatty liver') to nonalcoholic steatohepatitis (NASH), advanced fibrosis, and cirrhosis. Several systems of grading and staging of NAFLD have been proposed, but only a few have been validated; these typically include the degrees of steatosis, cytological ballooning, infammation, and fibrosis. To replace the biopsy, the ideal non invasive tool has to detect and quantify the same parameters than biopsy. The most important of a clinical point of view is to detect transition between simple steatosis and beginning of hepatitis. This review discusses of a part of current non invasive tools used to clinical diagnosis NAFLD and/or NASH and then these tools are compared to biopsy efficiency.

6.1 The past: non invasive tools currently used in clinical practice

6.1.1 Ultrasound

Ultrasound imaging is an established imaging modality in the diagnosis of hepatic steatosis, both clinically and in large scale studies. Several grading system have been proposed, studied, evaluated for the assessment of steatosis using ultrasound but no consensus has been achieved.

Ultrasound is the commonest technique used in clinical practice to detect fatty infiltration of the liver due to its simplicity, low cost, noninvasive nature, and widespread availability (Karcaaltincaba 2007). However, accurate quantification of steatosis is not feasible with the current technology. The basic principle underlying the sonographic detection of steatosis is that the degree of tissue brightness, the so-called echogenicity, directly depends on fat composition of the tissue (Quinn et al. 1985). Hence, a fatty liver is hyperechogenic with fine and tightly packed echoes and appears brighter on ultrasound examination (`bright liver') when compared with the echogenicity of other fat-free internal organs such as the kidneys or spleen (Joseph AE, et al.1979, Vaalls et al, 2007, ,Joy D; et al., 2003). The 'quantification' of steatosis depends on the experience of the operator: mild steatosis is characterized by 'mild' increase in liver echogenicity. Moderate steatosis can be diagnosed with increased liver echogenicity compared to the spleen for example, echogeneicity that obscures visualization of hepatic and portal vein wall. However, ultrasonographic evaluation of steatosis does not exactly match histopathologic quantification of steatosis. Furthermore, fat is less penetrable by ultrasound leading to attenuation of the signal, which causes posterior darkness (i.e., acoustic shadowing leading to hypoechogenicity in the far field) and loss of definition of the diaphragm and portal and hepatic veins, giving rise to a relatively bland and featureless appearance of the liver. It's the criteria to diagnose steatosis ≥30% (Palmentieri B. et al., 2006). Evaluation of steatosis in patients with hepatitis can be difficult due to accompanying inflammation and fibrosis. Fibrosis may also appear hyperechoic, but most of the time fibrosis and fatty infiltration co-exist in cirrhotic patients which is called fatty-fibrotic pattern (Joseph AEA, 1991). Still, despite the fact that several attempts have been made to generate scoring systems in order to provide better semi-quantitative information on the degree of steatosis (Hamaguchi M, 2007, Mehta SR 2008), ultrasonography remains largely a qualitative method for detecting NAFLD rather than a quantitative one for measuring liver fat. Several studies have examined the ability of ultrasound in recognizing fatty liver among patients suspected of having liver disease, using liver biopsy as the comparison standard, and reported sensitivity values between 60 and 94%and specificity values between 84 and 95%(Joy D. et al, 2003). the sensitivity is 55% when intrahepatic fat content is 10±20% and rises to 80% when intrahepatic fat content is greater than 30% (Ryan CK. Et al,

Hence, its ability to detect longitudinal changes is poor; it has been estimated that even a reduction of intrahepatic fat content from 40 to 20% following a successful intervention would alter the sonographic appearance of the liver by little, if any (Fishbein et al., 2005). Moreover, both the sensitivity and specificity of ultrasound decrease sharply in morbidly obese patients (Mottin CC. et al. 2004). Technical factors such as transducer frequency and instrument settings also affect the sonographic appearance of the liver, and hence the performance of ultrasound (Yeh WC et al. 2005, Garra B.S. et al.1887).

Sonography has the advantages of ease of acquisition, ability to assess the whole liver. The drawback are: subjectivity of the operator, no precise quantification, no follow-up of progression of the disease, poor agreement of intraobserver reproducibility (0.4-0.51) and interobserver (0.58) (Strauss S et al. , 2007).

We can conclude that abdominal ultrasound is a moderately specific and sensitive tool for diagnosing hepatic steatosis (> 33 %) but is not predictive for NASH.

6.1.2 Computed tomography (CT)

Noncontrast-enhanced computed tomography (CT) is widely used for the evaluation of NAFLD, by means of measuring tissue density as a function of radiographic attenuation. Tissue fat deposition results in lower attenuation (Kawata R et al., 1984), hence fatty tissues are less dense and appear darker than fat-free tissues (Piekarski J et al. 1980). Attenuation and density on CT imaging can be objectively measured on the Hounsfield scale. Fibrosis does not cause any effect on the attenuation of liver (Joy D et al. 2003). The diagnosis of fatty liver by contrast-enhanced CT imaging is more cumbersome, because contrast type and injection rate and timing of measurements can significantly influence the optimal liver-to-spleen attenuation difference for diagnosing NAFLD. Hence, unenhanced hepatic scanning remains the optimal CT technique for the detection of fatty liver (Kodama Y et al. 2007). Unenhanced CT images are used for qualitative evaluation and spleen is used as the reference organ for comparison. Spleen to liver attenuation ratio or difference between attenuation of spleen and liver can be used for the evaluation of steatosis. Studies that have evaluated CT imaging against liver biopsy have reported that the liver CT attenuation value and the ratio of liver-to-spleen CT attenuation values (Longo R et al. 1993, Oliva MR et al. 2006) correlate well with the degree of steatosis by histological analysis. Attenuation of spleen is approximately 8–10 HU less than the liver in a normal patient. Iwasaki et al. suggested cut-off value of 1.1 (spleen to liver attenuation ratio) for exclusion of moderate steatosis based on their correlative findings on 194 patients (Iwasaki M et al., 2004). The sensitivity and specificity of noncontrast-enhanced CT in the detection of moderate and severe hepatic steatosis (intrahepatic fat >30%) have been reported to range between 73% and 95%, respectively. However, at lower degrees of steatosis, the diagnostic performance of unenhanced C T for the quantitative assessment of intrahepatic fat is not clinically acceptable (Park SH et al. 2006) nor is C T able to evaluate hepatic fibrosis. In their study, liver/spleen attenuation ratio of 0.8 and difference of 9H between liver and spleen attenuation had similar sensitivity. Use of suggested criteria can be helpful in avoiding biopsy in moderately steatosic livers (Brancatelli G, 2006). In another study, Limanond et al. 2004 also concluded that unenhanced CT quantified the degree of steatosis relatively well in liver donor patients, but stated that most of the time liver biopsy is necessary to exclude fatty liver, co-existing iron deposition and parenchymal disease.

It should be noted that radiographic attenuation through the liver is non-uniform due to many factors that cannot be measured by CT, such as iron, copper, and glycogen concentrations and presence of fibrosis or oedema. For example, up to 40% of patients with NASH may have hepatic iron overload (George DK et al. 1998), which would alter hepatic CT attenuation independently of intrahepatic fat content. Recently, xenon CT, which is widely used to quantify and visualize tissue blood flow, was evaluated for its ability to assess fatty infiltration and changes in blood flow throughout the entire liver; it was found that xenon solubility was strongly and positively correlated with both grade of steatosis and each 10% range of histological fatty infiltration (r value > 0.8) and inversely associated with the liver-to-spleen CT attenuation ratio (Kobayashi M et al. 2009). Hence, xenon CT appears to provide a more objective measure of the severity of hepatic steatosis than conventional CT. However, the major limitation of CT is the exposure of patients to ionizing radiation, which makes longitudinal assessment of NAFLD impractical, especially among sensitive populations.

6.2 Magnetic resonance imaging (MRI)

Moderate-to-severe hepatic steatosis can easily be detected on T1-weighted spin-echo MRI because liver fat has very high signal intensity (Danet IM et al. 2003). This sequence can be obtained with all types of MR scanners with different Tesla power including 0.5, 1, 1.5 and 3 Tesla. In the presence of steatosis signal drop is observed on out of phase images due to phase cancellation of fat and water. However, many other factors contribute to this high signal intensity such as haemorrhage, melanin deposition, high protein content, or sinusoidal dilatation. The signal intensity is much lower for mild fatty infiltration of the liver. Therefore, in clinical practice, the most common MRI modality to evaluate NAFLD is chemical-shift imaging, which utilizes the difference in resonance frequency of water andlipidhydrogens to differentiate tissues containing only water from those containing both water and lipid (Venkataraman S et al. 2002. The spleen is generally used as the internal organ of reference for signal loss. For mild degrees of steatosis (intrahepatic fat < 15%), the signal of liver on the out-of-phase images appears nearly equal to that of spleen, although demonstrating a slightly higher signal on the in-phase images; loss of signal on out-of-phase images is progressively more prominent in moderate and severe fatty infiltration. Quantification of intrahepatic fat is made possible because of the differences in resonance frequencies between fat and water; if the out-of-phase and in-phase images are acquired by using constant calibration and other scanner settings, a quantitative fat signal fraction can be calculated from the hepatic signal intensities and this can be done pixel by pixel on the image to generate a fat signal fraction map. Many limitations of this technique (*e.g.*, time-demanding, low sensitivity, disturbed image quality due to respiratory and other bodily motions, or by magnetic field heterogeneity have been overcome by new methods, such as spoiled gradient-echo pulse sequence imaging, fast gradient echo imaging, fat-saturated fast spin-echo imaging, and fast spin-echo triple-echo Dixon imaging for example. These improved techniques have been shown to accurately quantify the hepatic fat fraction, even at low or near-normal levels. Guiu et al . 2009 recently developed a method on a breath-hold triple-echo spoiled gradient-echo sequence, which has many asserted advantages such as shorter acquisition time, measurement of fat content throughout the liver instead of in one or just a few voxels, no spatial misregistration errors, as well as easier and faster processing. Generally, the sensitivity and specificity of MRI for the detection of moderate and severe steatosis are greater than 80 and 95%, respectively; in addition, MRI has agreater than 85% sensitivity and a nearly 100% specificity for mild steatosis (intrahepatic fat 5±10%) (Mazhar et al. 2009). It was confirmed by many studies which have reported very good correlations between quantitative estimations of hepatic steatosis on MRI compared with liver biopsy (Cowin et al. 2008).

Nevertheless this technique is very expensive, not always available in hospital and does not quantify fibrosis.

6.2.1 Magnetic resonance spectroscopy (MRS)

Whereas chemical shift MRI enables the identification of steatosis within whole tissues, proton MRS facilitates the examination of the resonance frequencies of all hydrogen nuclei within a tissue region of interest (localized MRS). Although the absolute differences in resonance frequencies between protons in water and fat are quite small (3.5 ppm), they can be separated out to form a spectrum on an axis of chemical shift; spectral resolution is determined by the strength of the main magnetic field (1.5 Tesla). The intrahepatic fat values obtained by proton MRS are highly reproducible (Machann J et al., 2006) and correlate well with histological analysis of liver biopsy samples (Frimel TN et al., 2007). Moreover, the potential ability of MRS to monitor the progression of steatohepatitis by assessing saturated and unsaturated composition of fatty acyl chains in the liver has been tested in animal models, with promising results (Corbin IR, et al. 2009). MRS has been widely used in research settings for assessing the prevalence and metabolic concomitants of NAFLD among various populations including children as well as in longitudinal studies for evaluating fatty liver in response to drug treatments (Belfort R, et al. 2006) or changes in diet and physical activity.

6.3 The future: non invasive tools recently developed

6.3.1 Magnetic resonance elastography (MRE)

MR elastography (MRE) is an emerging technique for quantitatively imaging the mechanical properties of tissues. The basic approach is to generate low frequency mechanical waves (typically 20 to 200Hz) in the tissues and to use an extremely sensitive phase-contrast MR technique to quantify tissues displacements. MRE requires the addition of hardware and software to standard MR imaging system and a drumlike acoustic passive driver which is positioned against the body wall. The active driver produces acoustic vibrations which are transmitted to the passive driver, which then transmits it through the body and generate shear waves in liver. Recorded information is then processed by an inversion algorithm to generate quantitative images that depict tissues stiffness. The tissues stiffness expressed in kPa is correlated to the amount of fibrosis. Pr Ehman suggests that the increase of stiffness is a precursor of fibrosis development (Ehman et al. 2010).

A new clinical study (Talwakar et al. 2011) with 58 NAFLD patients suggests that liver stiffness evaluated with MR elastography was significantly higher in patients with NASH compared with patients with simple steatosis. Liver stiffness in patients with fibrosis (grade F>1) was significantly higher than that in patients with inflammation and no fibrosis. Liver stiffness was significantly correlated to inflammation stage and fibrosis stage. The results of this retrospective study support the hypothesis that NAFLD patients with inflammation but no fibrosis have significantly higher liver stiffness than do those with simple steatosis. Liver stiffness measured by means of MR elastography may be an accurate biomarker for detecting NASH (area under receiver operating characteristics curve, AUROC = 0.93), which suggest that MRE should be further investigated for its potential to stratify patients with NAFLD. MRE could be used to distinguish between individuals with simple steatosis and steatohepatitis.

The presence of elevated stiffness is not specific to steatohepatitis and can be generalized at all the liver disease. Moreover, this technology necessitated the use of a MR device.

6.3.2 Serologic test

The new subject of biomarkers development is to differentiate NAFLD phenotypes and to detect liver injuries (ballooning, degeneration, necrosis…) to target therapies. Several tools have been studied: biomarkers of oxidative stress, inflammation and hepatocytes apoptosis.

The most commonly used screening modality, the ALT, typically fluctuates in NAFLD and is normal in more than two-thirds of NASH patients at any given time (Wieckowska et al. 2007). For the identification of at least 5% steatosis, Poynard et al. reported that an ALT> 50 IU/L had a sensitivity and specificity of only 72% and 62% respectively (AUROC , 0.61) (Poynard et al, 2005).

Several studies explored the correlation between TBARS (thibarbituric acid-reacting substance) and steatosis (Chalasani, 2002) (Bonnefont, 2006) but there was no significant correlation. Additional studies are necessary before use in clinical context.
A new approach is the recognition of hepatocyte apoptosis. The first study correlated plasma CK-18 (cytokeratin-18) with NASH, CK-18 increased in patients with NASH compared to simple steatosis and normal biopsies (Wieckowska et al, 2006). This first study was completed recently by a cohort of 319 patients with biopsy proven NAFLD. CK-18 fragments were markedly increased in patients with NASH as compared to not NASH and borderline diagnosis (Median (Q25, Q75): 335 (196, 511), 194 (151, 270), 200 (148, 284), respectively; $P < 0.001$). On multivariable regression analysis, CK-18 fragments remained an independent predictor of NASH after adjusting for variables associated with CK-18 fragments or NASH on the univariate analysis (fibrosis, ALT, AST, age, biopsy length). AUROC curve for NASH diagnosis was estimated to be 0.83 (0.75-0.91), (Feldstein et al., 2009). The same biomarker was studied in a prospective longitudinal study with 52 patients NAFLD, with repeated biopsies at month 36. Serum cytokeratin-18 fragment level correlated well with NAS both at baseline and month 36. The change in NAS had moderate correlation with change in serum cytokeratin-18 fragment levels (r=0.51, p<0.001). Patients with increased NAS at month 36 had greater increase in serum cytokeratin-18 fragment levels (Wong et al, 2010).
Most studies would suggest that combinations of biomarkers have the highest predictive utility.

6.3.3 Composite serum markers

Several blood tests have been proposed to diagnose liver fibrosis. Some tests are simple, like the aspartate aminotransferase to platelet ratio index (APRI). Others are more complex, constructed as algorithms (regression score) like the FibroMeter (Cales et al. 2009). Most of them have been developed in chronic hepatitis C or in miscellaneous causes.

6.3.3.1 Steatosis

Bedogni *et al.* CITER developed the Fatty Liver Index (FLI) by evaluating a cohort from the Dionysos Nutrition & Liver Study. A total of 224 subjects with suspected liver disease (excluding hepatitis B and C) were selected and matched with 287 subjects without suspected liver disease. After serial analysis, four predictors (triglycerides, BMI, gamma-glutamyl transpeptidase (GGT) and waist circumference) were entered into a model to generate the FLI. The authors reported that an FLI<30 could be used to rule out and >60 to rule in hepatic steatosis. A limitation of this study is that the diagnosis of fatty liver was based on ultrasonography.
In the same way, Poynard et al. (2009) recently reported a combination of markers for steatosis referred to as the SteatoTest (BioPredictive, France) This proprietary index combines age, gender, body mass index, cholesterol, triglycerides, glucose, ALT, GGT, bilirubin, haptoglobin, alpha-2-macroglobulin, and apolipoprotein A1 in a logistic regression formula. For the prediction of steatosis ≥ 5%, the SteatoTest value had an AUROC of 0.80 in a cohort of 811 patients with NAFLD, HCV and HBV, alcoholic liver disease. Nevertheless, a substantial overlap between grades of steatosis will likely limit its widespread use; Moreover, this algorithm has yet to be externally validated. The SteatoTest (range [0-1]) was 0.14 in blood donors, 0.26 in patients without steatosis; 0.43 with [1-5%] steatosis, 0.62 with 5-33% steatosis, 0.70 with 34-66 % steatosis and 0.75 with > 66 % steatosis (Poynard et al. 2005).

6.3.3.2 NASH

Recently, Poynard and its colleaues (Poynard et al 2009)have developed a new algorithm called 'Nashtest' as a biomarker of inflammation. This proprietary tool includes the components of the SteatoTest in addition to AST, ALT, total bilirubin, height anf weight. In a study that included 257 patients with NAFLD who underwent liver biopsy, this panel was 71% sensitive and 94% specific for the diagnosis of NASH versus no NASH according to the NAFLD Activity Score. The AUROC was 0.75 (95% CI 0.67-0.82). As this index has not yet been externally validated, additional study is necessary prior its utilisation.

6.3.3.3 Fibrosis

A variety of blood tests exist to detect the NAFLD to NASH transition. For example, the NAFLD score was developed by Angulo to accurately separate patients with NAFLD with and without advanced fibrosis, rendering liver biopsy for identification of advanced fibrosis unnecessary in a substantial proportion of patients. This score was developed during a study on 733 patients (480 construction of the data basis, and 253 to validate, with NAFLD confirmed by biopsy). The NAFLD score is based on composed of routinely measured and easily available clinical and laboratory variables. The exact formula combines age, hyperglycaemia, body mass index (BMI), platelets, albumin, AST/ALT). In this study, the lower cutoff point was particularly accurate in ruling out the presence of advanced fibrosis; the NPV was 93% and 88% in the estimation and validation groups, respectively, and ranged from 87% to 98% for the prevalence of advanced fibrosis of 5% to 50%. Among these 733 patients, 439 (60%) had a negative diagnosis of advanced fibrosis, and thus a liver biopsy would have been avoided by applying the NAFLD fibrosis score; of these 439, 400 (91%) indeed had stage 0-2 fibrosis; (Angulo, 2007) However, this test was designed for severe fibrosis whereas most tests have been designed for significant fibrosis and usually for chronic hepatitis C.

Cales and its colleagues developed a regression score specifically designed to NAFLD patients called Fibrometer NAFLD (Cales et al. 2009). A study on 235 patients compared blood tests performance (NFSA (NAFLD Score of Angulo Fibrometer, Fibrometer NAFLD and APRI) and biopsy results. The score combines glucose, AST, ferritin, platelet, ALT, body weight and age. Results gave 90% negative (NPV) and positive (PPV) predictive values for significant fibrosis, when values were, respectively: FibroMeter: ≤0.611 and ≥0.715, NFSA: ≤ 0.227 and ≥0.514, APRI: ≤0.454 and ≥0.918. The ensuing proportion of patients with reliable diagnosis was: FibroMeter: 97.4%, NFSA: 86.8% ($p < 10^{-3}$ *vs* FibroMeter), APRI: 80.0% ($p < 10^{-3}$). This study thus provided an independent external validation of NFSA for significant fibrosis in a large series and for severe fibrosis. Cales and its colleagues observed a similar performance for significant fibrosis of APRI AUROC compared to the original publication in chronic viral hepatitis C. APRI AUROC was significantly inferior to that of FibroMeter and NFSA for the three diagnostic targets (except with NFSA for significant fibrosis).

All these composite serum markers are very easy to use and are able to give a first indication to the physician. But some of them are not free (Fibrometer NashTest and Steatotest for exemple) and need more external clinical validations.

6.3.4 Fibroscan® and CAP (Controlled Attenuation Parameter)

Fibroscan® (Echosens, Paris, France) is an ultrasound-based vibration-controlled transient elastography (VCTE™) device used to assess liver elasticity related to liver fibrosis (Sandrin et al. 2003). Liver stiffness is expressed in kPa. Fibroscan® shows good results for the detection of significant fibrosis and for the diagnosis of cirrhosis in hepatitis C virus (HCV) (Ziol et al. 2005), hepatitis B virus (HBV) (Marcellin et al. 2009), biliary liver disease (Corpechot et al. 2006), alcoholic liver disease (ALD) (Nahon et al. 2008) and NAFLD (Wong et al. 2010).

Fibroscan® has high degree of accuracy and reproducibility in predicting bridging fibrosis and cirrhosis in patients with viral hepatitis (Fraquelli 2007, Wong 2008). Two independent studies of 94 (Yoneda 2007) and 120 (Tamano 2007) NAFLD patients respectively concluded that VCTE™ is a non-invasive and useful method to screen possible NASH patients, who need liver biopsy, from NAFLD populations. No correlation between stiffness values and steatosis was finded. Moreover, these results are confirmed later by Wong and their colleagues (Wong, 2010) who evaluated the accuracy of VCTE™ and biochemical tests for the diagnosis of fibrosis and cirrhosis in a large cohort of 246 NAFLD patients. They wanted to determine if liver stiffness was altered by hepatic steatosis, inflammation, and obesity. The results demonstrated the usefulness of VCTE™ to quantify fibrosis: AUROC of VCTE™ for the detection of F3 fibrosis or higher and cirrhosis was 0.93 and 0.95, respectively, and was significantly higher than that of the aspartate aminotransferase-to-alanine aminotransferase ratio, aspartate aminotransferase-to-platelet ratio index, FIB-4, BARD, and NAFLD fibrosis scores (AUROC ranged from 0.62 to 0.81, $P<0.05$ for all comparisons). At a cutoff value of 7.9 kPa, the sensitivity, specificity, and positive and negative predictive values for F3 or greater disease were 91%, 75%, 52%, and 97%, respectively. Liver stiffness was not affected by hepatic steatosis, necroinflammation, or body mass index. Discordance of at least two stages between transient elastography and histology was observed in 33 (13.4%) patient but by multivariate analysis, liver biopsy length less than 20 mm and F0-2 disease were associated with this discordance. Because of high negative predictive value and modest positive predictive value, this study concluded positively for the use of VCTE™ as a screening test to exclude advanced fibrosis. In summary, Wong and colleagues have provided valuable data regarding the use of VCTE™ in patients with NAFLD. Adam *et al.* underlined that the strength of Fibroscan® appears to be for excluding advanced fibrosis and cirrhosis; however, according to Adam, there are a number of issues that need to be clarified before it is routinely used in the clinical setting: cut-off values, utility in obese and morbidly obese populations which seem to require further validation of the dedicated obese probe (called XL probe). Nevertheless de Ledinghen et al. (2010) and Rust and al. (20110) have demonstrated VCTE™ using the XL probe for obese patients can be performed with comparable diagnostic accuracy to the standard probe and enables the examination of significantly more obese patients.

So, VCTE™ based on Fibroscan® is a promising tool to quantify fibrosis but not steatosis. It's why Sasso and al. (Echosens, France) had developed a new parameter called Controlled Attenuation Parameter (CAP) based on ultrasound attenuation. This parameter can be assessed simultaneously and on the same device Fibroscan® than the liver stiffness. Knowing that fat affects ultrasound propagation, this novel attenuation parameter is based on the ultrasonic properties of the radiofrequency back-propagated signals acquired by the Fibroscan®. It is called controlled attenuation parameter (CAP) because it was devised to specifically target the liver. This control is performed by a sophisticated guidance process based on VCTE™. Therefore, CAP can be assessed by an operator who does not have any ultrasound imaging skills. Furthermore, CAP has been designed to be immediate, reproducible and operator and machine-independent. Performance of the CAP was then appraised on 115 patients, taking the histological grade of steatosis as reference. CAP was significantly correlated to steatosis (Spearman ρ=0.81, p<10^{-16}). AUROC was equal to 0.91 and 0.95 for the detection of more than 10% and 33% of steatosis, respectively. Furthermore, results show that CAP can efficiently separate several steatosis grades. These results were confirmed by a resptropsective study an 112 patients with multiple aetiologies (HBV, HCV, NAFLD/ALD) (De Ledinghen et al. 2011). These promising results suggest that CAP is a noninvasive, immediate, objective and efficient method to detect and quantify steatosis. This parameter is available on Fibroscan®, is calculated during the same acquisition than the stiffness and than gives a steatosis evaluation in the same region of interest used for the stiffness (figure 2). Future clinical evaluations on NAFLD and NASH patients will be useful to evaluate the diagnosis performance of these 2 combined non-invasive tools and the ability to detect transition between simple steatosis and steatohepatitis.

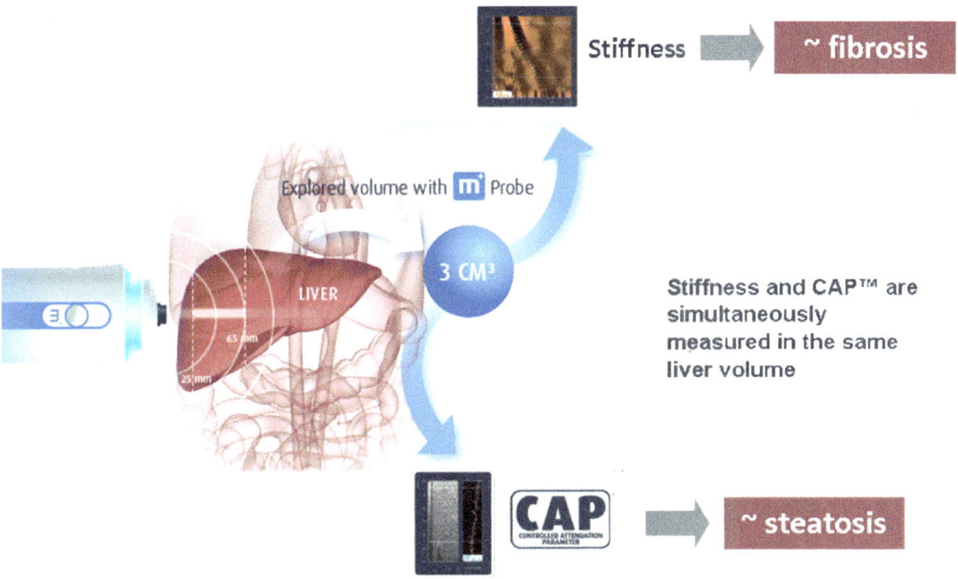

Fig. 2. Fibroscan® assess fibrosis and steatosis.

6.3.5 Discussion

According to Myers and his colleagues, the ideal non invasive tool includes 3 major goals: to diagnose NAFLD, to differentiate simple NAFLD from NASH, to determine the severity of fibrosis (Myers et al. 2009). Moreover, this ideal non invasive tool shall be:

- *Liver specific :* true for MRI, MRS, composite serum markers, serologic tests, Fibroscan® (stiffness and CAP)
- *Able to detect simple steatosis :* true for ultrasound (> 33%), CT, MRI, MRS, Fibroscan® (CAP)
- *Able to identify simple steatosis from NASH:* true for composite serum markers (shall be evaluated), Fibroscan (stiffness and CAP, shall be evaluated)
- *sensitive enough to distinguish individual stages of fibrosis:* true for serologic tests, composite serum markers, MRE, Fibroscan (stiffness)

- *easy to perform and acceptable for patients and physicians:* true for all non-invasive tools described except for CT scan cannot be repeated(ionizing)
- *Inexpensive/examination:* true for ultrasound, serologic tests, composite serum markers, Fibroscan®
- *Reproducible:* true for CT, MRI, MRS, serologic tests (shall be evaluated), composite serum markers, Fibroscan®
- *Responsive to change in disease (steatosis + fibrosis):* true for composite serum markers (shall be evaluated), Fibroscan® (stiffness and CAP, shall be evaluated)

At present only biopsy achieves most of these goals but the combination of Fibroscan® (stiffness and CAP) added with a blood marker could be a promising non invasive tool to avoid biopsy in many cases. It will be a good, simple solution, non expensive, reproducible, easy to use and very well accepted by the patients.

7. Conclusion

We have seen that NAFLD and NASH diseases are an increasing prevalence in future. The symptoms are very dangerous because of a silent, slow evolution. At present, the gold standard for the diagnosis of nonalcoholic steatohepatitis is liver biopsy; however, liver biopsy is not performed in a significant number of cases and in the absence of more-accurate imaging technologies and serum markers, the diagnosis is frequently one of exclusion. Due to the many potential errors due to sampling, inter/interobeserver variability, biopsy is the "Best" not the "Gold " standard (Bedossa & Carrat 2009) in spite of its limitations. There is also urgent need for effective and easy-to-use non-invasive methods to assess the severity of liver disease in NAFLD: while simple steatosis has a benign hepatological prognosis and may be managed with measures aiming at reducing cardio-metabolic risk, NASH may progress to end-stage liver disease and requires early hepatological referral for experimental treatment and tight follow-up. Then, the most important clinical point is to detect the transition between benign steatosis, NALD, and NASH and to be able to assess steatosis, fibrosis and inflammation. Many noninvasive tests exist to quantify either fibrosis or steatosis but few diagnose these two. Nevertheless, new technologies appear like blood markers, serologic tests, specific imaging device (MRE) or Fibroscan® device with CAP to improve the diagnosis of NAFLD and/or NASH. It is hoped that improved imaging techniques and the discovery of serum biomarkers, as well as the development of clinical algorithms, will enable a more accurate diagnosis of NASH without the need for a liver biopsy.

8. References

Adams, L. A. and A. E. Feldstein (2011). "Non-invasive diagnosis of nonalcoholic fatty liver and nonalcoholic steatohepatitis." J Dig Dis 12(1): 10-6.

Adams, L. Transient elastography in nonalcoholic fatty liver disease: making sense of echoes, Hepatology, Vol.51, No.2, (Feb), pp. 370-2

Adler, M. & Schaffner, F. (1979). Fatty liver hepatitis and cirrhosis in obese patients, Am J Med, Vol.67, No.5, (Nov), pp. 811-6

Adler, M. and Schaffner, F. (1979). Fatty liver hepatitis and cirrhosis in obese patients. *Am J Med,* Vol. 67, No. 5, pp. 811-6.

Alberti, K. G., Eckel, R. H., Grundy, S. M., Zimmet, P. Z., Cleeman, J. I., Donato, K. A., Fruchart, J. C., James, W. P., Loria, C. M. & Smith, S. C., Jr. (2009). Harmonizing the metabolic syndrome: a joint interim statement of the International Diabetes Federation Task Force on Epidemiology and Prevention; National Heart, Lung, and Blood Institute; American Heart Association; World Heart Federation; International Atherosclerosis Society; and International Association for the Study of Obesity, Circulation, Vol.120, No.16, (Oct 20), pp. 1640-5

Alberti, K. G., R. H. Eckel, et al. (2009). "Harmonizing the metabolic syndrome: a joint interim statement of the International Diabetes Federation Task Force on Epidemiology and Prevention; National Heart, Lung, and Blood Institute; American Heart Association; World Heart Federation; International Atherosclerosis Society; and International Association for the Study of Obesity." Circulation 120(16): 1640-5.

Amarapurkar, D. N., E. Hashimoto, et al. (2007). "How common is non-alcoholic fatty liver disease in the Asia-Pacific region and are there local differences?" J Gastroenterol Hepatol 22(6).

Amarapurkar, D. N., Hashimoto, E., Lesmana, L. A., Sollano, J. D., Chen, P. J. & Goh , K. L. (2007). How common is non-alcoholic fatty liver disease in the Asia-Pacific region and are there local differences?, J Gastroenterol Hepatol, Vol.22, No.6, (Jun), pp.

Angulo, P. & Lindor, K. D. (2002). Non-alcoholic fatty liver disease, J Gastroenterol Hepatol, Vol.17 Suppl, (Feb), pp. S186-90

Angulo, P. (2007). "GI epidemiology: nonalcoholic fatty liver disease." Aliment Pharmacol Ther 25(8): 883-9.

Angulo, P. and Lindor, K. D. (2002). Non-alcoholic fatty liver disease. *J Gastroenterol Hepatol,* Vol. 17 Suppl, No., pp. S186-90.

Angulo, P., J. C. Keach, et al. (1999). "Independent predictors of liver fibrosis in patients with nonalcoholic steatohepatitis." Hepatology 30(6): 1356-62.

Bedogni, G., Bellentani, S., Miglioli, L., Masutti, F., Passalacqua, M., Castiglione, A. & Tiribelli, C. (2006). The Fatty Liver Index: a simple and accurate predictor of hepatic steatosis in the general population, BMC Gastroenterol, Vol.6, pp. 33

Bedogni, G., Bellentani, S., Miglioli, L., Masutti, F., Passalacqua, M., Castiglione, A. & Tiribelli, C. (2006). The Fatty Liver Index: a simple and accurate predictor of hepatic steatosis in the general population, BMC Gastroenterol, Vol.6, pp.

Bedossa, P. and Carrat, F. (2009). Liver biopsy: the best, not the gold standard. *J Hepatol,* Vol. 50, No. 1, pp. 1-3.

Bellentani, S., G. Saccoccio, et al. (2000). "Prevalence of and risk factors for hepatic steatosis in Northern Italy." Ann Intern Med 132(2): 112-7.

Bonnefont, J., Daulhac, L., Etienne, M., Chapuy, E., Mallet, C., Ouchchane, L., Deval, C., Courade, J. P.,Ferrara, M., Eschalier, A. & Clottes, E. (2007). Acetaminophen recruits spinal p42/p44 MAPKs and GH/IGF-1 receptors to produce analgesia via the serotonergic system, Mol Pharmacol, Vol.71, No.2, (Feb), pp. 407-15

Brancatelli, G. (2006). Science to practice: Should biopsy be performed in potential liver donors when unenhanced CT shows an unacceptable degree of steatosis for transplantation?, Radiology, Vol.239, No.1, (Apr), pp. 1-2

Bravo, A. A., Sheth, S. G. & Chopra, S. (2001). Liver biopsy, N Engl J Med, Vol.344, No.7, (Feb 15), pp. 495-500

Bravo, A. A., Sheth, S. G. and Chopra, S. (2001). Liver biopsy. *N Engl J Med,* Vol. 344, No. 7, pp. 495-500.

Browning, J. D., L. S. Szczepaniak, et al. (2004). "Prevalence of hepatic steatosis in an urban population in the United States: impact of ethnicity." Hepatology 40(6): 1387-95.

Browning, J. D., Szczepaniak, L. S., Dobbins, R., Nuremberg, P., Horton, J. D., Cohen, J. C., Grundy, S. M. & Hobbs, H. H. (2004). Prevalence of hepatic steatosis in an urban population in the United States: impact of ethnicity, Hepatology, Vol.40, No.6, (Dec), pp. 1387-95

Brunt, E. M. (2005). Pathology of nonalcoholic steatohepatitis, Hepatol Res, Vol.33, No.2, (Oct), pp. 68-71

Brunt, E. M. (2005). Pathology of nonalcoholic steatohepatitis. *Hepatol Res,* Vol. 33, No. 2, pp. 68-71.

Brunt, E. M. (2007). Pathology of fatty liver disease, Mod Pathol, Vol.20 Suppl 1, (Feb), pp. S40-8

Brunt, E. M. (2007). Pathology of fatty liver disease. *Mod Pathol,* Vol. 20 Suppl 1, No., pp. S40-8.

Brunt, E. M. (2008). Do you see what I see? The role of quality histopathology in scientific study. *Hepatology,* Vol. 47, No. 3, pp. 771-4.

Brunt, E. M. (2008). Do you see what I see? The role of quality histopathology in scientific study, Hepatology, Vol.47, No.3, (Mar), pp. 771-4

Brunt, E. M., Janney, C. G., Di Bisceglie, A. M., Neuschwander-Tetri, B. A. and Bacon, B. R. (1999). Nonalcoholic steatohepatitis: a proposal for grading and staging the histological lesions. *Am J Gastroenterol,* Vol. 94, No. 9, pp. 2467-74.

Brunt, E. M., Janney, C. G., Di Bisceglie, A. M., Neuschwander-Tetri, B. A. & Bacon, B. R. (1999). Nonalcoholic steatohepatitis: a proposal for grading and staging the histological lesions, Am J Gastroenterol, Vol.94, No.9, (Sep), pp. 2467-74

Brunt, E. M., Kleiner, D. E., Wilson, L. A., Belt, P. & Neuschwander-Tetri, B. A. (2011). Nonalcoholic fatty liver disease (NAFLD) activity score and the histopathologic diagnosis in NAFLD: distinct clinicopathologic meanings, Hepatology, Vol.53, No.3, (Mar), pp. 810-820

Brunt, E. M., Kleiner, D. E., Wilson, L. A., Belt, P. and Neuschwander-Tetri, B. A. (2011). Nonalcoholic fatty liver disease (NAFLD) activity score and the histopathologic diagnosis in NAFLD: distinct clinicopathologic meanings. *Hepatology,* Vol. 53, No. 3, pp. 810-820.

Bugianesi, E., A. J. McCullough, et al. (2005). "Insulin resistance: a metabolic pathway to chronic liver disease." Hepatology 42(5): 987-1000.

Bugianesi, E., Leone, N., Vanni, E., Marchesini, G., Brunello, F., Carucci, P., Musso, A., De Paolis, P., Capussotti, L., Salizzoni, M. & Rizzetto, M. (2002). Expanding the natural history of nonalcoholic steatohepatitis: from cryptogenic cirrhosis to hepatocellular carcinoma, Gastroenterology, Vol.123, No.1, (Jul), pp. 134-40

Bugianesi, E., N. Leone, et al. (2002). "Expanding the natural history of nonalcoholic steatohepatitis: from cryptogenic cirrhosis to hepatocellular carcinoma." Gastroenterology 123(1): 134-40.

Cales, P., Boursier, J., Oberti, F., Gallois, Y., Rousselet, M. C., Moal, V., Macchi, L., Chevailler, A. & Lunel, F. (2009). [FibroMeters: a family of blood tests for liver fibrosis with high diagnostic performance and applicability in clinical practice], Pathol Biol (Paris), Vol.57, No.6, (Sep), pp. 459-62

Cales, P., Laine, F., Boursier, J., Deugnier, Y., Moal, V., Oberti, F., Hunault, G., Rousselet, M. C., Hubert, I., Laafi, J., Ducluzeaux, P. H. & Lunel, F. (2009). Comparison of blood tests for liver fibrosis specific or not to NAFLD, J Hepatol, Vol.50, No.1, (Jan), pp. 165-73

Chen, J., Talwalkar, J. A., Yin, M., Glaser, K. J., Sanderson, S. O. & Ehman, R. L. Early Detection of Nonalcoholic Steatohepatitis in Patients with Nonalcoholic Fatty Liver Disease by Using MR Elastography, Radiology, (Apr 1), pp.

Clark, J. M., Brancati, F. L. & Diehl, A. M. (2002). Nonalcoholic fatty liver disease, Gastroenterology, Vol.122, No.6, (May), pp. 1649-57

Clark, J. M., Brancati, F. L. and Diehl, A. M. (2002). Nonalcoholic fatty liver disease. *Gastroenterology*, Vol. 122, No. 6, pp. 1649-57.

Corbin, I. R., Furth, E. E., Pickup, S., Siegelman, E. S. & Delikatny, E. J. (2009). In vivo assessment of hepatic triglycerides in murine non-alcoholic fatty liver disease using magnetic resonance spectroscopy, Biochim Biophys Acta, Vol.1791, No.8, (Aug), pp. 757-63

Corpechot, C., El Naggar, A., Poujol-Robert, A., Ziol, M., Wendum, D., Chazouilleres, O., de Ledinghen, V., Dhumeaux, D., Marcellin, P., Beaugrand, M. & Poupon, R. (2006). Assessment of biliary fibrosis by transient elastography in patients with PBC and PSC, Hepatology, Vol.43, No.5, (May), pp. 1118-24

Cowin, G. J., Jonsson, J. R., Bauer, J. D., Ash, S., Ali, A., Osland, E. J., Purdie, D. M., Clouston, A. D., Powell, E. E. & Galloway, G. J. (2008). Magnetic resonance imaging and spectroscopy for monitoring liver steatosis, J Magn Reson Imaging, Vol.28, No.4, (Oct), pp. 937-45

Dancygier, H. (2010). *Clinical Hepatology: Principles and Practice of Hepatobiliary Diseases*, Springer.

Dancygier, H. (2010). Clinical Hepatology: Principles and Practice of Hepatobiliary Diseases, Springer,

Danet, I. M., Semelka, R. C. & Braga, L. (2003). MR imaging of diffuse liver disease, Radiol Clin North Am, Vol.41, No.1, (Jan), pp. 67-87

Das, K., K. Das, et al. (2010). "Nonobese population in a developing country has a high prevalence of nonalcoholic fatty liver and significant liver disease." Hepatology 51(5): 1593-602.

de Ledinghen, V.,Vergniol, J.,Foucher, J.,El-Hajbi, F.,Merrouche, W.,Rigalleau, V.,(), Feasibility of liver transient elastography with FibroScan using a new probe for obese patients, Liver Int, Vol. 30, No.7, (Aug), pp. 1043-8

DiDonato, D. & Brasaemle, D. L. (2003). Fixation methods for the study of lipid droplets by immunofluorescence microscopy, J Histochem Cytochem, Vol.51, No.6, (Jun), pp. 773-80

DiDonato, D. and Brasaemle, D. L. (2003). Fixation methods for the study of lipid droplets by immunofluorescence microscopy. *J Histochem Cytochem*, Vol. 51, No. 6, pp. 773-80.

Diehl, A. M. (2002). Liver disease in alcohol abusers: clinical perspective. *Alcohol*, Vol. 27, No. 1, pp. 7-11.

Diehl, A. M. (2002). Liver disease in alcohol abusers: clinical perspective, Alcohol, Vol.27, No.1, (May), pp. 7-11

Dixon, J. B., Bhathal, P. S. & O'Brien, P. E. (2001). Nonalcoholic fatty liver disease: predictors of nonalcoholic steatohepatitis and liver fibrosis in the severely obese, Gastroenterology, Vol.121, No.1, (Jul), pp. 91-100

Dixon, J. B., P. S. Bhathal, et al. (2001). "Nonalcoholic fatty liver disease: predictors of nonalcoholic steatohepatitis and liver fibrosis in the severely obese." Gastroenterology 121(1): 91-100.

Ehman, R. L. (2009). Science to practice: can MR elastography be used to detect early steatohepatitis in fatty liver disease?, Radiology, Vol.253, No.1, (Oct), pp. 1-3

El-Badry, A. M., Breitenstein, S., Jochum, W., Washington, K., Paradis, V., Rubbia-Brandt, L., Puhan, M. A., Slankamenac, K., Graf, R. and Clavien, P. A. (2009). Assessment of hepatic steatosis by expert pathologists: the end of a gold standard. *Ann Surg,* Vol. 250, No. 5, pp. 691-7.

El-Badry, A. M., Breitenstein, S., Jochum, W., Washington, K., Paradis, V., Rubbia-Brandt, L., Puhan, M. A., Slankamenac, K., Graf, R. & Clavien, P. A. (2009). Assessment of hepatic steatosis by expert pathologists: the end of a gold standard, Ann Surg, Vol.250, No.5, (Nov), pp. 691-7

Fabbrini, E., Conte, C. & Magkos, F. (2009). Methods for assessing intrahepatic fat content and steatosis, Curr Opin Clin Nutr Metab Care, Vol.12, No.5, (Sep), pp. 474-81

Fan, J. G. and G. C. Farrell (2009). "Epidemiology of non-alcoholic fatty liver disease in China." J Hepatol 50(1): 204-10.

Farrell, G. C. & Larter, C. Z. (2006). Nonalcoholic fatty liver disease: from steatosis to cirrhosis, Hepatology, Vol.43, No.2 Suppl 1, (Feb), pp. S99-S112

Farrell, G. C. (2004). *Fatty liver disease : NASH and related disorders* Blackwell Publishing. Malden, MA, USA.

Farrell, G. C. (2004). Fatty liver disease : NASH and related disorders Blackwell Publishing, 1405112921 (alk. paper) 1405112921 (alk. paper), Malden, MA, USA

Farrell, G. C. and C. Z. Larter (2006). "Nonalcoholic fatty liver disease: from steatosis to cirrhosis." Hepatology 43(2 Suppl 1): S99-S112.

Farrell, G. C., George, J., de la M. Hall, P. & McCullough, A. J. (2005). Fatty Liver Disease: NASH and Related Disorders,

Farrell, G. C., J. George, et al. (2005). Fatty Liver Disease: NASH and Related Disorders.

Feldstein, A. E., Wieckowska, A., Lopez, A. R., Liu, Y. C., Zein, N. N. & McCullough, A. J. (2009). Cytokeratin-18 fragment levels as noninvasive biomarkers for nonalcoholic steatohepatitis: a multicenter validation study, Hepatology, Vol.50, No.4, (Oct), pp. 1072-8

Friedrich-Rust, M., Hadji-Hosseini, H., Kriener, S., Herrmann, E., Sircar, I., Kau, A., Zeuzem, S. & Bojunga, J. Transient elastography with a new probe for obese patients for non-invasive staging of non-alcoholic steatohepatitis, Eur Radiol, Vol.20, No.10, (Oct), pp. 2390-6

Frimel, T. N., Deivanayagam, S., Bashir, A., O'Connor, R. & Klein, S. (2007). Assessment of intrahepatic triglyceride content using magnetic resonance spectroscopy, J Cardiometab Syndr, Vol.2, No.2, (Spring), pp. 136-8

Fukumoto, S. & Fujimoto, T. (2002). Deformation of lipid droplets in fixed samples, Histochem Cell Biol, Vol.118, No.5, (Nov), pp. 423-8

Fukumoto, S. and Fujimoto, T. (2002). Deformation of lipid droplets in fixed samples. *Histochem Cell Biol,* Vol. 118, No. 5, pp. 423-8.

George, D. K., Goldwurm, S., MacDonald, G. A., Cowley, L. L., Walker, N. I., Ward, P. J., Jazwinska, E. C. & Powell, L. W. (1998). Increased hepatic iron concentration in nonalcoholic steatohepatitis is associated with increased fibrosis, Gastroenterology, Vol.114, No.2, (Feb), pp. 311-8

Gholam, P. M., Flancbaum, L., Machan, J. T., Charney, D. A. & Kotler, D. P. (2007). Nonalcoholic fatty liver disease in severely obese subjects, Am J Gastroenterol, Vol.102, No.2, (Feb), pp. 399-408

Gholam, P. M., L. Flancbaum, et al. (2007). "Nonalcoholic fatty liver disease in severely obese subjects." Am J Gastroenterol 102(2): 399-408.

Grant, A. & Neuberger, J. (1999). Guidelines on the use of liver biopsy in clinical practice. British Society of Gastroenterology, Gut, Vol.45 Suppl 4, (Oct), pp. 1-11

Grant, A. and Neuberger, J. (1999). Guidelines on the use of liver biopsy in clinical practice. British Society of Gastroenterology. *Gut,* Vol. 45 Suppl 4, No., pp. 1-11.

Ground, K. E. (1982). "Liver pathology in aircrew." Aviat Space Environ Med 53(1): 14-8.

Ground, K. E. (1982). Liver pathology in aircrew, Aviat Space Environ Med, Vol.53, No.1, (Jan), pp. 14-8

Guiu, B., Petit, J. M., Loffroy, R., Ben Salem, D., Aho, S., Masson, D., Hillon, P., Krause, D. & Cercueil, J. P. (2009). Quantification of liver fat content: comparison of triple-echo chemical shift gradient-echo imaging and in vivo proton MR spectroscopy, Radiology, Vol.250, No.1, (Jan), pp. 95-102

Hilden, M., Christoffersen, P., Juhl, E. & Dalgaard, J. B. (1977). Liver histology in a 'normal' population--examinations of 503 consecutive fatal traffic casualties, Scand J Gastroenterol, Vol.12, No.5, pp. 593-7

Hilden, M., P. Christoffersen, et al. (1977). "Liver histology in a 'normal' population--examinations of 503 consecutive fatal traffic casualties." Scand J Gastroenterol 12(5): 593-7.

Iwasaki, M., Takada, Y., Hayashi, M., Minamiguchi, S., Haga, H., Maetani, Y., Fujii, K., Kiuchi, T. & Tanaka, K. (2004). Noninvasive evaluation of graft steatosis in living donor liver transplantation, Transplantation, Vol.78, No.10, (Nov 27), pp. 1501-5

Jacobs, J. E., Birnbaum, B. A., Shapiro, M. A., Langlotz, C. P., Slosman, F., Rubesin, S. E. & Horii, S. C. (1998). Diagnostic criteria for fatty infiltration of the liver on contrast-enhanced helical CT, AJR Am J Roentgenol, Vol.171, No.3, (Sep), pp. 659-64

Johnston, R. J., Stamm, E. R., Lewin, J. M., Hendrick, R. E. & Archer, P. G. (1998). Diagnosis of fatty infiltration of the liver on contrast enhanced CT: limitations of liver-minus-spleen attenuation difference measurements, Abdom Imaging, Vol.23, No.4, (Jul-Aug), pp. 409-15

Joy, D., Thava, V. R. & Scott, B. B. (2003). Diagnosis of fatty liver disease: is biopsy necessary?, Eur J Gastroenterol Hepatol, Vol.15, No.5, (May), pp. 539-43

Karcaaltincaba, M. & Akhan, O. (2007). Imaging of hepatic steatosis and fatty sparing, Eur J Radiol, Vol.61, No.1, (Jan), pp. 33-43

Kawata, R., Sakata, K., Kunieda, T., Saji, S., Doi, H. & Nozawa, Y. (1984). Quantitative evaluation of fatty liver by computed tomography in rabbits, AJR Am J Roentgenol, Vol.142, No.4, (Apr), pp. 741-6

Kleiner, D. E., Brunt, E. M., Van Natta, M., Behling, C., Contos, M. J., Cummings, O. W., Ferrell, L. D., Liu, Y. C., Torbenson, M. S., Unalp-Arida, A., Yeh, M., McCullough, A. J. and Sanyal, A. J. (2005). Design and validation of a histological scoring system for nonalcoholic fatty liver disease. *Hepatology,* Vol. 41, No. 6, pp. 1313-21.

Kleiner, D. E., Brunt, E. M., Van Natta, M., Behling, C., Contos, M. J., Cummings, O. W., Ferrell, L. D., Liu, Y. C., Torbenson, M. S., Unalp-Arida, A., Yeh, M., McCullough, A. J. & Sanyal, A. J. (2005). Design and validation of a histological scoring system for nonalcoholic fatty liver disease, Hepatology, Vol.41, No.6, (Jun), pp. 1313-21

Kobayashi, M., Suzuki, M., Ikeda, H., Takahashi, H., Matsumoto, N., Maeyama, S., Sase, S., Iino, S. & Itoh, F. (2009). Assessment of hepatic steatosis and hepatic tissue blood flow by xenon computed tomography in nonalcoholic steatohepatitis, Hepatol Res, Vol.39, No.1, (Jan), pp. 31-9

Kodama, Y., Ng, C. S., Wu, T. T., Ayers, G. D., Curley, S. A., Abdalla, E. K., Vauthey, J. N. & Charnsangavej, C. (2007). Comparison of CT methods for determining the fat content of the liver, AJR Am J Roentgenol, Vol.188, No.5, (May), pp. 1307-12

Limanond, P., Raman, S. S., Lassman, C., Sayre, J., Ghobrial, R. M., Busuttil, R. W., Saab, S. & Lu, D. S. (2004). Macrovesicular hepatic steatosis in living related liver donors: correlation between CT and histologic findings, Radiology, Vol.230, No.1, (Jan), pp. 276-80

Longo, R., Ricci, C., Masutti, F., Vidimari, R., Croce, L. S., Bercich, L., Tiribelli, C. & Dalla Palma, L. (1993). Fatty infiltration of the liver. Quantification by 1H localized magnetic resonance spectroscopy and comparison with computed tomography, Invest Radiol, Vol.28, No.4, (Apr), pp. 297-302

Ludwig, J., T. R. Viggiano, et al. (1980). "Nonalcoholic steatohepatitis: Mayo Clinic experiences with a hitherto unnamed disease." Mayo Clin Proc 55(7): 434-8.

Ludwig, J., Viggiano, T. R., McGill, D. B. & Oh, B. J. (1980). Nonalcoholic steatohepatitis: Mayo Clinic experiences with a hitherto unnamed disease, Mayo Clin Proc, Vol.55, No.7, (Jul), pp. 434-8

Ludwig, J., Viggiano, T. R., McGill, D. B. and Oh, B. J. (1980). Nonalcoholic steatohepatitis: Mayo Clinic experiences with a hitherto unnamed disease. *Mayo Clin Proc,* Vol. 55, No. 7, pp. 434-8.

Machado, M., Marques-Vidal, P. & Cortez-Pinto, H. (2006). Hepatic histology in obese patients undergoing bariatric surgery, J Hepatol, Vol.45, No.4, (Oct), pp. 600-6

Machado, M., P. Marques-Vidal, et al. (2006). "Hepatic histology in obese patients undergoing bariatric surgery." J Hepatol 45(4): 600-6.

Machann, J., Thamer, C., Schnoedt, B., Stefan, N., Haring, H. U., Claussen, C. D., Fritsche, A. & Schick, F. (2006). Hepatic lipid accumulation in healthy subjects: a comparative study using spectral fat-selective MRI and volume-localized 1H-MR spectroscopy, Magn Reson Med, Vol.55, No.4, (Apr), pp. 913-7

Marcellin, P., Ziol, M., Bedossa, P., Douvin, C., Poupon, R., de Ledinghen, V. & Beaugrand, M. (2009). Non-invasive assessment of liver fibrosis by stiffness measurement in patients with chronic hepatitis B, Liver Int, Vol.29, No.2, (Feb), pp. 242-7

Marcos, A., Fisher, R. A., Ham, J. M., Olzinski, A. T., Shiffman, M. L., Sanyal, A. J., Luketic, V. A., Sterling, R. K., Olbrisch, M. E. & Posner, M. P. (2000). Selection and outcome of living donors for adult to adult right lobe transplantation, Transplantation, Vol.69, No.11, (Jun 15), pp. 2410-5

Marcos, A., R. A. Fisher, et al. (2000). "Selection and outcome of living donors for adult to adult right lobe transplantation." Transplantation 69(11): 2410-5.

Matteoni, C. A., Younossi, Z. M., Gramlich, T., Boparai, N., Liu, Y. C. and McCullough, A. J. (1999). Nonalcoholic fatty liver disease: a spectrum of clinical and pathological severity. *Gastroenterology,* Vol. 116, No. 6, pp. 1413-9.

Matteoni, C. A., Younossi, Z. M., Gramlich, T., Boparai, N., Liu, Y. C. & McCullough, A. J. (1999). Nonalcoholic fatty liver disease: a spectrum of clinical and pathological severity, Gastroenterology, Vol.116, No.6, (Jun), pp. 1413-9

Merriman, R. B., Ferrell, L. D., Patti, M. G., Weston, S. R., Pabst, M. S., Aouizerat, B. E. and Bass, N. M. (2006). Correlation of paired liver biopsies in morbidly obese patients with suspected nonalcoholic fatty liver disease. *Hepatology,* Vol. 44, No. 4, pp. 874-80.

Nomura, H., Kashiwagi, S., Hayashi, J., Kajiyama, W., Tani, S. & Goto, M. (1988). Prevalence of fatty liver in a general population of Okinawa, Japan, Jpn J Med, Vol.27, No.2, (May), pp. 142-9

Nomura, H., S. Kashiwagi, et al. (1988). "Prevalence of fatty liver in a general population of Okinawa, Japan." Jpn J Med 27(2): 142-9.

Nugent, C. & Younossi, Z. M. (2007). Evaluation and management of obesity-related nonalcoholic fatty liver disease, Nat Clin Pract Gastroenterol Hepatol, Vol.4, No.8, (Aug), pp. 432-41

Nugent, C. and Younossi, Z. M. (2007). Evaluation and management of obesity-related nonalcoholic fatty liver disease. *Nat Clin Pract Gastroenterol Hepatol,* Vol. 4, No. 8, pp. 432-41.

Pacifico, L., Anania, C., Martino, F., Cantisani, V., Pascone, R., Marcantonio, A. & Chiesa, C. (2010). Functional and morphological vascular changes in pediatric nonalcoholic fatty liver disease, Hepatology, Vol.52, No.5, (Nov), pp. 1643-51

Pacifico, L., C. Anania, et al. (2010). "Functional and morphological vascular changes in pediatric nonalcoholic fatty liver disease." Hepatology 52(5): 1643-51.

Patton, H. M., K. Yates, et al. (2010). "Association between metabolic syndrome and liver histology among children with nonalcoholic Fatty liver disease." Am J Gastroenterol 105(9): 2093-102.

Patton, H. M., Yates, K., Unalp-Arida, A., Behling, C. A., Huang, T. T., Rosenthal, P., Sanyal, A. J., Schwimmer, J. B. & Lavine, J. E. (2010). Association between metabolic syndrome and liver histology among children with nonalcoholic Fatty liver disease, Am J Gastroenterol, Vol.105, No.9, (Sep), pp. 2093-102

Piccinino, F., Sagnelli, E., Pasquale, G. & Giusti, G. (1986). Complications following percutaneous liver biopsy. A multicentre retrospective study on 68,276 biopsies, J Hepatol, Vol.2, No.2, pp. 165-73

Piccinino, F., Sagnelli, E., Pasquale, G. and Giusti, G. (1986). Complications following percutaneous liver biopsy. A multicentre retrospective study on 68,276 biopsies. *J Hepatol,* Vol. 2, No. 2, pp. 165-73.

Qayyum, A., Goh, J. S., Kakar, S., Yeh, B. M., Merriman, R. B. & Coakley, F. V. (2005). Accuracy of liver fat quantification at MR imaging: comparison of out-of-phase gradient-echo and fat-saturated fast spin-echo techniques--initial experience, Radiology, Vol.237, No.2, (Nov), pp. 507-11

Ratziu, V., Bellentani, S., Cortez-Pinto, H., Day, C. and Marchesini, G. (2010). A position statement on NAFLD/NASH based on the EASL 2009 special conference. *J Hepatol,* Vol. 53, No. 2, pp. 372-84.

Ratziu, V., Charlotte, F., Heurtier, A., Gombert, S., Giral, P., Bruckert, E., Grimaldi, A., Capron, F. and Poynard, T. (2005). Sampling variability of liver biopsy in nonalcoholic fatty liver disease. *Gastroenterology,* Vol. 128, No. 7, pp. 1898-906.

Ratziu, V., Martin, L., Fedchuk, L. & Poynard, T. (2009). Can nonalcoholic steatohepatitis be diagnosed without liver biopsy?, Biomark Med, Vol.3, No.4, (Aug), pp. 353-61

Schattner, A. & Knobler, H. (2008). Metabolic aspects of chronic liver disease Nova Biomedical Books, New York

Schattner, A. and Knobler, H. (2008). *Metabolic aspects of chronic liver disease* Nova Biomedical Books. New York.

Torres, D. M. & Harrison, S. A. (2008). Diagnosis and therapy of nonalcoholic steatohepatitis, Gastroenterology, Vol.134, No.6, (May), pp. 1682-98

Torres, D. M. and S. A. Harrison (2008). "Diagnosis and therapy of nonalcoholic steatohepatitis." Gastroenterology 134(6): 1682-98.

Vuppalanchi, R., Unalp, A., Van Natta, M. L., Cummings, O. W., Sandrasegaran, K. E., Hameed, T., Tonascia, J. and Chalasani, N. (2009). Effects of liver biopsy sample length and number of readings on sampling variability in nonalcoholic Fatty liver disease. *Clin Gastroenterol Hepatol,* Vol. 7, No. 4, pp. 481-6.

Vuppalanchi, R., Unalp, A., Van Natta, M. L., Cummings, O. W., Sandrasegaran, K. E., Hameed, T., Tonascia, J. & Chalasani, N. (2009). Effects of liver biopsy sample length and number of readings on sampling variability in nonalcoholic Fatty liver disease, Clin Gastroenterol Hepatol, Vol.7, No.4, (Apr), pp. 481-6

Williams, R. (2006). "Global challenges in liver disease." Hepatology 44(3): 521-6.

Williams, R. (2006). Global challenges in liver disease, Hepatology, Vol.44, No.3, (Sep), pp. 521-6

5

Hepatic Oxidative Stress: Role of Liver Biopsy

Mahmoud Rushdi Abd Ellah
Department of Animal Medicine,
Faculty of Veterinary Medicine, Assiut University,
Assiut Egypt

1. Introduction

Free radicals are highly reactive substances produced continuously during metabolic processes. They participate mainly in physiological events such as the immune response, metabolism of unsaturated fatty acids, and inflammatory reaction. The balance between free radicals and antioxidants is disrupted in many diseases. This disruption may be attributed to a number of factors such as the inability of the cells to produce sufficient amounts of antioxidants, the nutritional deficiency of minerals or vitamins, and the excess production of reactive oxygen species (Abd Ellah, 2010). Free radical excess results in impairment of DNA, enzymes, and membranes and induces changes in the activity of the immune system and in the structure of basic biopolymers which, in turn, may be related to mutagenesis and aging processes (Poli, 1993).

The involvement of oxidative stress in the pathogenesis of hepatic dysfunction in human (Comporti, 1998; Poli et al.,1987; Zern et al., 1990; Poli, 1993; Tsai et al., 1993; De Maria et al., 1996; Gonzalez-Correa et al., 1997; Paradis et al., 1997; Feher et al., 1998; Wallace & Miller, 2000; Spirli et al., 2001; Alpini et al., 2002; Cesaratto et al., 2004; Jabłonowska et al., 2005) and animals (Khan et al., 1987; Mudronň et al., 1997; 1999; Spolarics, 1999; Sansinanea et al., 2000; Abd Ellah et al., 2002; 2004, 2007, 2008, 2009, 2010) has been investigated for many years.

Some of the liver diseases were associated with increase (Farinati et al., 1995; Abd Ellah et al., 2002, 2008) or decrease (Mudroň et al., 1997; Barbaro et al., 1999; Abd Ellah et al., 2004; Videla et al., 2004; Czeczot et al., 2006) antioxidants contents. Usually hepatic antioxidants increased at the beginning of hepatic disease and decreased in severe hepatic injury. The advantages of measuring hepatic oxidative status in liver biopsy are that it helps in diagnosis of hepatic dysfunction, reflects the degree of deterioration in the liver tissues, and helps to determine the severity of hepatic injury, and also, aid in recommending antioxidant's therapy in patients that had a hepatic disease with derangement in hepatic antioxidant constituents. The main purpose of the current article is to explore the value of liver biopsy as a tool for detection of hepatic oxidative stress. A focus was done on different types of free radicals, antioxidants, lipid peroxidation, and hepatic and blood oxidative status in hepatic dysfunction.

2. Free radicals

2.1 Types of free radicals

Free radicals can be defined as molecules containing a single unpaired electron in atomic or molecular orbits. These molecules have an important role in the pathogenesis of tissue damage in various disorders (Dalgic et al., 2005), such as hepatic dysfunction, mastitis, kidney damage, inflammation, immune injury and carcinogenesis (Abd Ellah, 2010). The most important free radicals include superoxide anion ($O_2^{\cdot -}$), hydroxyl radical (·OH), and hypochlorous acid (HOCL) (Stohs, 1995). HOCL is produced by the reaction of hydrogen peroxide (H_2O_2) with chloride ions and plays an important role in the leukocyte respiratory burst, which is involved in the host defense system (Lunec, 1990). Nitric oxide (NO·) acts as a free radical and as a biological mediator in biochemical reactions. Physiologically it is synthesized from L-arginine by NO synthase employing cofactor NADPH. In the host, NO· arises in some pathological situations, such as sepsis, stroke, myocardial depression, and inflammatory responses (Bredt & Snyder, 1994).

Superoxide anion induces important reducing reactions in biological materials via Fenton-like reactions, which are catalyzed by redox cycling metal ions, including iron, copper, chromium and vanadium (Stohs & Bagchi, 1995). These metal ions have the ability to accept and donate single electrons, making them important catalysts of free radical reactions, the most widely distributed and most commonly studied transition metal ions are the cations iron and copper (Stohs, 1995). Superoxide anion reduces Fe^{3+} in metalloproteins such as ferritin. The reduction of protein bound iron is an important reaction in biological material, because if there is sufficient H_2O_2 available, a reaction between the resultant Fe^{2+} and H_2O_2 occurs and gives rise to the highly reactive ·OH (Lunec, 1990). H_2O_2 traverses biological membranes and intracellularly targets phospholipids, carbohydrates, metalloproteins and DNA, and causes damage via Fenton's reaction (Samuni et al., 1981).

2.2 Sources of free radicals

Free radicals may be released in the liver as a subsequence to hepatic detoxification of drugs, chemicals and toxic materials (Feher et al., 1992; Ogino & Okada, 1995). The formation of oxygen free radicals may be physiological as in phagocytosis (superoxide and H_2O_2 are used by phagocytic cells to kill bacteria), a side effect of metabolic pathways, or may occur in pathological conditions due to toxic agents as in the case of ischemia, inflammation, disease, or due to decreased antioxidant defenses (Miller et al., 1993).

Mitochondria considered a major source for the production of $O_2^{\cdot -}$ and H_2O_2, about 2-3% of consumed oxygen is constantly converted into reactive oxygen/reactive nitrogen species (ROS/RNS) in the mitochondria, hepatocytes contain many mitochondria and therefore, generate excess ROS/RNS (Stohs, 1995).

In many liver diseases, including the wide range of neonatal hepatitis, the tissue inflammatory infiltrates are likely to be responsible for the formation of $O_2^{\cdot -}$, H_2O_2, ·OH, HOCL and the highly cytotoxic monochloramine (Southorn & Powis, 1988; McCord, 1993). In turn, the superoxide anion attracts further neutrophils to the inflammatory site by a chemotactic activity, causing an increase in tissue injury (Petrone et al., 1980). In addition, activated macrophages, Kupffer cells and vascular endothelium can generate nitric oxide, which may react with superoxide generating peroxynitrite. The latter is responsible for the inhibition of mitochondrial respiration and DNA synthesis (Moncada & Higgs, 1993).

Liver damage due to iron (hemochromatosis) and copper overload is believed, at least partially, to derive from the catalytic activity of these metals in the Fenton reaction leading to the generation of ROS and increased lipid peroxidation with consequent abnormal mitochondrial function (Bacon et al., 1993; Sokol et al., 1993; Sokol et al., 1994).

Sources of ROS in the liver are summarized in Fig. 1.

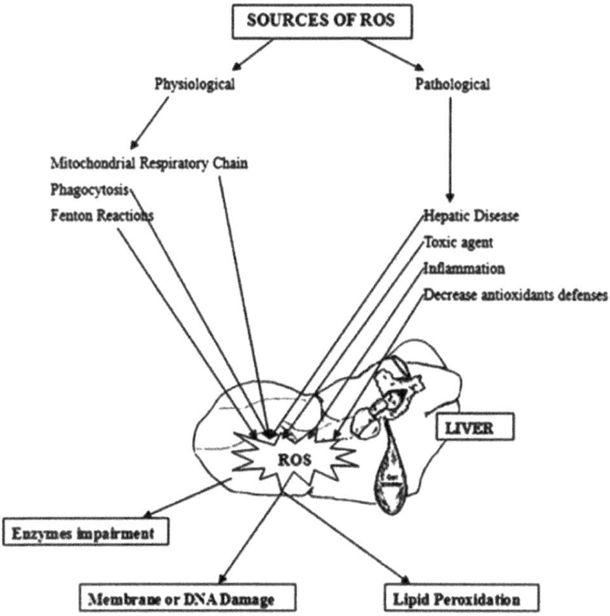

Fig. 1. Sources of reactive oxygen species (ROS) in the liver (Abd Ellah et al., 2007)

3. Antioxidants and free radicals

The cells contain a variety of antioxidant mechanisms that play a central role in the protection against reactive oxygen species (Pár & Jávor, 1984; Halliwell, 1991). The antioxidant system consists of antioxidant enzymes (superoxide dismutase (SOD), catalase (CAT) and glutathione peroxidase (GSH-Px)), glutathione, ancillary enzymes (glutathione reductase (GR), glutathione S-transferase, and glucose 6-phosphate dehydrogenase (G6PD)), metal-binding proteins (transferrin, ceruloplasmin and albumin), vitamins (α-tocopherol, ascorbate and beta-carotene), flavonoids, and urate (Halliwell, 1994).
Pathological free radical reactions do not necessarily cause cell and tissue damage, as antioxidants of cells and tissues are able to prevent free radical injury (Feher et al., 1992). On the intracellular level, ROS formation and metabolism can be summarized as shown in Fig 2.

4. Hepatic oxidative stress and lipid peroxidation

Oxidative stress results when reactive forms of oxygen are produced faster than they can be safely neutralized by antioxidant mechanisms (Sies, 1991) and/or from a decrease in antioxidant defense, which may lead to damage of biological macromolecules and disruption of normal metabolism and physiology (Trevisan et al., 2001). This condition can contribute and/or lead to the onset of health disorders (Miller et al., 1993), and play a damaging role in a number of liver disorders, for example, in anoxic and reoxygenation injury during transplantation, activated phagocytes and xanthine oxidase formed during ischemia, catalyze the formation of superoxide during reperfusion (Southorn & Powis, 1988; Nauta et al., 1990; Brass et al., 1991; Rosser & Gores, 1995).

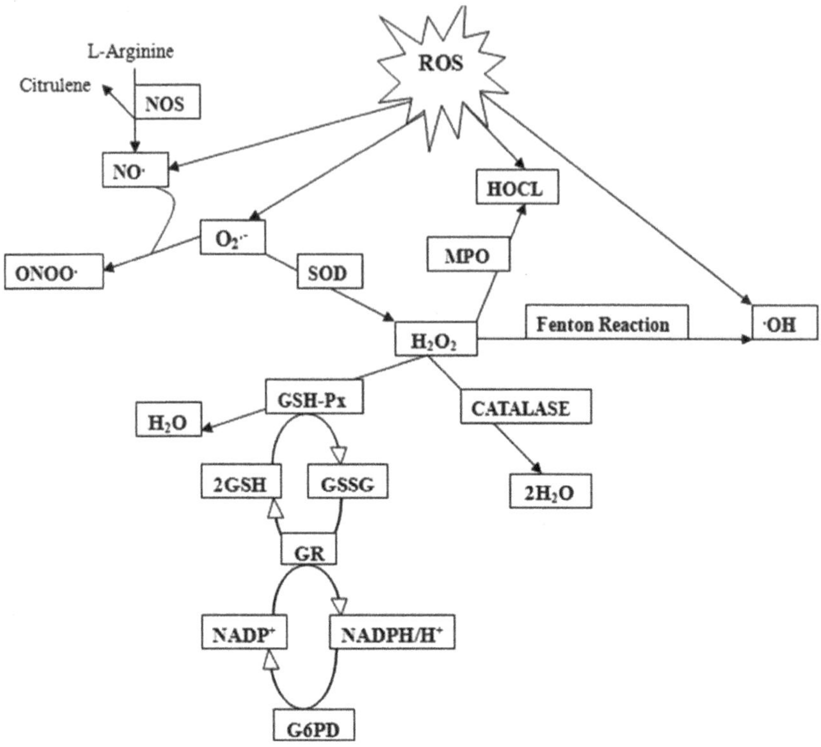

Fig. 2. Shows different types of reactive oxygen species (ROS). Abbreviations: Glutathione peroxidase (GSH-Px), Hypochlorous acid (HOCl), Hydrogen peroxide (H_2O_2), Myeloperoxidase (MPO), Nitric oxide (NO.), NO synthase (NOS), Superoxide anion (O_2·-), Hydroxyl radical (·OH), Peroxynitrite anion (ONOO·), Superoxide dismutase (SOD), Nicotinamide adenine diphosphate (NADPH), Reduced glutathione (GSH), Glutathione reductase (GR), Glucose-6-phosphate dehydrogenase (G6PD).

Lipid peroxidation is implicated in the pathogenesis of several hepatic disorders in human (Poli, 1993; Farinati et al., 1995) and animals (Mudroň et al., 1999; Abd Ellah et al., 2004). Hepatic failure in cattle was associated with decreased antioxidant mechanisms inside the cells, which led to the increase in the reactive oxygen species, especially H_2O_2. The decrease in hepatic GSH-Px activity in severe fatty degeneration, for example, results in the increase H_2O_2 (Abd Ellah et al., 2004), which can initiate free radical formation through Fenton's reaction. In addition, the decrease in hepatic vitamin E level, which is an important chain-breaking antioxidant, results in lipid peroxidation and failure to regenerate the ascorbic acid (Mudroň et al., 1997, 1999). Increased hepatic oxidative stress was also reported in cows suffering from glycogen degeneration (Abd Ellah et al., 2004), sawdust liver and liver abscesses (Spolarics, 1999; Abd Ellah et al., 2002; Sayed et al., 2003). The authors contended that the antioxidant defense was high in the case of sawdust liver, glycogen degeneration, and liver abscess, which indicated that the body can combat the increased free radical stress. Liver abscesses in fattening steers occur mainly due to intensive feeding of highly concentrated rations. Consumption of a carbohydrate-rich diet stimulates G6PD expression in endothelial and parenchymal cells (Khan et al., 1987; Spolarics, 1999). Since G6PD supports reactive oxygen metabolism, the response may represent an antioxidant pathway in the hepatic cell populations that targets sinusoid born reactive oxygen species during infections (Spolarics, 1999; Abd Ellah et al., 2002).

Underfeeding in cattle was reported to induce changes in the antioxidant systems in liver manifested by lowering hepatic G6PD and SOD activities. This result in depletion of antioxidant defense mechanisms and render the hepatocytes more susceptible to the lethal effects of endogenous or exogenous peroxides, and indicate that the generation of lipid peroxides in cattle in poor nutritional condition exceeds the antioxidant capacity of the liver cells, generating a situation of oxidative stress and peroxidation (Sansinanea et al., 2000).

The leading mechanism of free radical toxicity is the peroxidation of membrane phospholipids, which is initiated by the formation of lipid peroxide or hydroperoxides, peroxy radicals are formed in the presence of oxygen to start a chain reaction (propagation) (Arthur et al., 1985; Poli, 1993; Bianchi et al., 1997). Various pathogenic effects occur as the result of degradation of membrane lipids (Stohs, 1995). Chiefly, the hydroxyl radical and to a lesser extent the superoxide anion leads to peroxidation of membrane lipids thereby causing production of malondialdehyde (MDA) and 4-hydroxyalkenals (4HNE). These substances directly induce hepatocytes damage with generation of proinflammatory cytokines, activation of spindle cells, and fibrogenesis (Pessayre et al., 2001; Younossi et al., 2002) and may bind to various molecules, impairing their functions (Zern et al., 1990) and therefore lead to membrane damage, protein damage, enzyme dysfunction and DNA or RNA damage (Vajdovich, 2001). It is well known that persistent oxidant stress causes mutative effects on cell DNA and increases fibroblastic activity, leading to cirrhosis and carcinoma. Many studies have shown that oxidative stress takes part in the pathogenesis of cholestasis by way of cytokines (Gonzalez-Correa et al., 1997, Wallace & Miller, 2000; Spirli et al., 2001; Alpini et al., 2002) and lipid peroxidation (Tsai et al., 1993).

The role for lipid peroxidation in liver fibrosis was assessed. Lipid peroxidation products in the form of MDA adduct were detected in areas of active fibrogenesis. It has been shown that lipid peroxidation products can stimulate fibrogenesis by inducing collagen gene expression, detection and prevention of lipid peroxidation could be of major interest in preventing fibrosis and cirrhosis in this disease (Paradis et al., 1997).

Increased lipid peroxidation may be caused by inflammation related to viral infection and decreased antioxidant levels. The lipid peroxides formed may be chemotactic for the neutrophils causing increased inflammation, which further drives oxidant-mediated injury in the liver (Deutsch, 1983). Previous studies have demonstrated an increase MDA levels and decreases the antioxidant capacity in acute and chronic hepatitis (Comporti, 1985; Poli et al., 1987; Bianchi et al., 1997). Mitochondrial lipid peroxidation takes place at varying levels in liver disorders independent of etiology (Sokol et al., 1994; Mansouri et al., 1997). Increased lipid, protein, and nucleic acid peroxidation in the blood and liver biopsy specimens from patients with chronic hepatitis has been demonstrated (Farinati et al., 1995; De Maria et al., 1996; Jabłonowska et al., 2005).

5. Oxidative stress and hepatic dysfunction: Role of liver biopsy

5.1 Blood and hepatic oxidative stress

Antioxidant status of blood doesn't reflect hepatic oxidative stress only, but their levels change in a response to diseases in other organs. Studying the effect of hepatic dysfunction on blood oxidative status in cows revealed that hepatic glycogen degeneration, fatty degeneration or liver abscesses had no effect on erythrocytic oxidative status, as indicated by the insignificant changes in erythrocytes GSH-Px and G6PD activities (Abd Ellah et al., 2002, 2004). Many studies had been performed on humans to determine the effect of hepatic dysfunction on erythrocytic oxidative status, some of these studies had reported no significant changes in erythrocytes GSH-Px activity in patients suffered from liver cirrhosis and alcoholic liver disease (Johansson et al., 1986; Tanner et al., 1986; Akkus et al., 1997). Other studies had been demonstrated that a red cell GSH-Px activity significantly decreased in patients with chronic liver disease (Hadi Yasa et al., 1999; Chrobot et al., 2000; Czuczejko et al., 2003). In addition, lower activities of erythrocytes GSH-Px and SOD activities have been reported in patients with acute hepatitis B (Pak & Nikitin, 1991). The cause of such contradictory results may be related to the degree of hepatic dysfunction or the presence or absence of selenium deficiency. Significant decreases in plasma selenium level and erythrocytes GSH-Px had been reported in patients with chronic liver disease (Czuczejko et al., 2003).

Increased oxidative stress had been reported in the liver of cattle with naturally occurring fatty liver (Mudroň et al., 1999; Abd Ellah et al., 2004), with liver abscessation (Abd Ellah et al., 2002), and in animals on restricted feed intake (Sansinanea et al., 2000), without significant changes in blood oxidative status, this means that hepatic disease may present without effect on blood oxidative status, and also that detection of hepatic oxidative stress is best done through measuring oxidative stress markers in the hepatic tissues by means of liver biopsy.

5.2 Preparation of liver biopsy for antioxidants measurements

The principles for preparation of liver biopsy are: liver biopsy must be prepared directly after collection, otherwise stored at -80°C, liver biopsy must be washed twice in a cold saline or cold buffer before homogenization, blot dry and then homogenized in a cold buffer at certain pH. After centrifugation, the supernatant is harvested and used to measure hepatic antioxidant enzyme activities, which can be performed using commercial test kits (Table 1).

5.3 Liver biopsy and oxidative stress

Oxygen free radicals might play a role in the pathogenesis of tissue damage in many pathological conditions and has been implicated in a variety of liver diseases. It, therefore, may participate in the pathogenesis of toxic liver diseases and other hepatic alterations (Feher et al., 1998). Oxidative stress is a major pathogenetic event occurring in several liver disorders ranging from metabolic to proliferated ones, and is a main cause of liver damage in ischemia/ reperfusion during liver transplantation (Cesaratto et al., 2004).

The involvement of oxidative stress in the pathogenesis of liver injury has been investigated for many years (Comporti, 1985; Poli et al., 1987; Poli, 1993). Some of these studies were conducted using liver biopsy in human (Togashi et al., 1990; Ismail et al., 2010) and animals (Abd Ellah et al., 2008, 2009). But most of the studies in animals measured hepatic oxidative stress after slaughtering or euthanasia. Examples include, measuring hepatic G6PD activity in chemically induced hepatocellular carcinoma in rat liver (De Jong et al., 2001), and in liver of rat with macronodular cirrhosis induced by long-term thioacetamide administration (Sanz et al., 1997). In cattle, hepatic GSH-Px activity (Abd Ellah et al., 2004) and vitamin E (Mudroň et al., 1997, 1999) were measured in cows suffered from severe fatty degeneration. In addition, hepatic GSH-Px and G6PD activities were determined in cows suffering from glycogen degeneration (Abd Ellah et al., 2004), sawdust liver and liver abscesses (Khan et al., 1987; Spolarics, 1999; Abd Ellah et al., 2002). Furthermore, hepatic G6PD and SOD activities were measured in cows with restricted feed intake (Sansinanea et al., 2000).

Tissue preparation	Buffer used	Homogenization	Oxidative stress marker	Reference
Liver biopsy samples were washed twice in cold 0.9% salt solution	Tris–HCL (50 mM) pH 7.5	The liver biopsy was homogenized in 20 volumes of cold buffer, and then the supernatant was harvested after centrifugation at 5000 g for 30 min at 4°C.	SOD, CAT and GSH	Abd Ellah et al. (2008, 2009)
	Chilled potassium chloride (1.17%)	Liver biopsy was homogenized in chilled buffer. The homogenates were centrifuged at 800 g for 5 min at 4oC to separate the nuclear debris. The obtained supernatant was re-centrifuged at 10,500 g for 20 min at 4°C to get the post mitochondrial supernatant.	SOD, CAT and MDA	Noori et al. (2009)
	Ice-cold PBS buffer (20 mM), pH 7.3 with 10 ml of 5mM butylated hydroxyl toluene	The tissue was homogenized in 290 ml ice-cold buffer. Following this, the suspension was centrifuged and supernatant was fractioned for analysis.	LPO and AOP	Madill et al. (2009)
	Tris-HCl (50 mM), pH 7.5, 5 mM EDTA, 1 nM dithiothreitol	The tissue was homogenized in 5 ml/g cold buffer. The homogenate was centrifuged at 10,000g for 15 minutes at 4°C. The supernatant was removed for assay.	GSH-Px	Ismail et al. (2010)
	Potassium phosphate (0.05 M) and 0.1 mM EDTA, pH 7.8	The tissue was homogenized in 200µL buffer and centrifuged at 15,000g for 30 minutes at 4°C. The supernatant was used for analysis.	SOD	Ismail et al. (2010)

Table 1. Methods for preparation of liver biopsy implemented in different studies

Recently, liver biopsy was applied as a tool for detecting hepatic oxidative stress in cattle from the viewpoint of the status of hepatic antioxidant enzymes after injection of a potent hepatotoxic (DL-ethionine), data were published (Abd Ellah et al., 2008, 2009). the supernatant of liver homogenate was used to measure hepatic SOD, catalase (Abd Ellah et al., 2009), total glutathione level and glutathione reductase activity (Abd Ellah et al., 2008).
Many studies were performed to establish the importance of liver biopsy from the viewpoint of oxidative stress in a variety of liver disorders in human. Examples in human include: Oxidative stress-related parameters were investigated in liver biopsy from NAFLD patients and used to assay activities of CAT and GSH-Px (Videla et al., 2004) Oxidative stress status in children with glycogen storage disease (Ismail et al., 2009)], and with cholestatic chronic liver disease (Ismail et al., 2010) was investigated by measuring GSH-Px, SOD and CAT activities in liver biopsy samples. Activities of SOD, CAT and GSH-Px were measured in liver biopsy specimens from patients with various liver diseases, including chronic persistent hepatitis, chronic active hepatitis, non-alcoholic cirrhosis, alcoholic cirrhosis and acute hepatitis (De Jong et al., 2001).
Increased hepatic oxidative stress had also been detected in liver biopsy from patients with cirrhosis and hepatocellular carcinoma, shown by the decrease of GSH-Px activity, hepatic and blood glutathione (GSH) levels, along with an increase the oxidized glutathione/glutathione ratio in cirrhotic (Farinati et al., 1995; Barbaro et al., 1999) and liver cancer tissues (Czeczot et al., 2006), which reflects both a decrease in the synthesize capacity of liver and the antioxidant defense.
It is clear from the above review of literature that liver biopsy can be used for measuring oxidative status of the liver tissues and that significant changes were detected in different hepatic dysfunction. Antioxidant activities in liver biopsy can be used to diagnose liver disease and as a prognostic factor for the liver disease under investigation.

6. Conclusion

Most of the studies done in animals were concerned with studying the hepatic oxidative stress after slaughtering or euthanasia. Studying the hepatic oxidative status in liver biopsy are lacking in animals. In human medicine, large number of studies was implemented to achieve this goal. Hepatic disease may present without significant effect on blood oxidative status, consequently. The best way is to measure hepatic oxidants and antioxidants in liver biopsy, which reflect the actual status of the liver.

7. References

Abd Ellah, M. (2010). Involvement of free radicals in animal diseases. *Comp. Clin. Pathol.*, Vol. 19, pp. 615-619.

Abd Ellah, M., Nishimori, K., Goryo, M., Okada, K. & Yasuda, J. (2002). Glucose 6 phosphate dehydrogenase and glutathione peroxidase activities in hepatic abscesses of cattle. *Vet. Biochem.*, Vol. 39, pp. 25.

Abd Ellah, M., Nishimori, K., Goryo, M., Okada, K. & Yasuda, J. (2004). Glutathione peroxidase and glucose 6 -phosphate dehydrogenase activities in bovine blood and liver. *J. Vet. Med. Sci.*, Vol. 66, pp. 1219-1221.

Abd Ellah, M., Okada, K., Goryo, M., Kobayashi, S., Oishi, A. & Yasuda, J. (2008). Total Glutathione and Glutathione Reductase in Bovine Erythrocytes and Liver Biopsy. *J. Vet. Med. Sci.*, Vol. 70, pp. 861-864.

Abd Ellah, M., Okada, K., Goryo, M., Oishi, A. & Yasuda, J. (2009). Superoxide dismutase activity as a measure of hepatic oxidative stress in cattle following ethionine administration. *Vet. J.*, Vol. 182, pp. 336-341.

Abd Ellah, M., Yasuda, J. & Okada, K. (2007). Oxidative stress and bovine liver diseases: Role of glutathione peroxidase and glucose 6-phosphate dehydrogenase. *Jpn. J. Vet. Res.*, Vol. 54, pp. 163–173.

Akkus, I., Gultekin, F., Akoz M., Caglayan O., Bahcaci S., Gulsum C., Ay, M. & Gurel, A. (1997). Effect of moderate alcohol intake on lipid peroxidation in plasma, erythrocyte and leukocyte and on some antioxidant enzymes, *Clinical Chemistry Acta*, Vol. 266, pp. 141-147.

Alpini, G., McGill, J. & Larusso, N. (2002). The pathobiology of biliary epithelia. *Hepatology*, Vol. 35, pp, 1256-1268.

Arthur, M. J., Bentley, I. S., Tanner, A. R., Saunders, P. K., Millward-Sadler, G. H. & Wright, R. (1985). Oxygen-derived free radicals promote hepatic injury in the rat. *Gastroenterology*, Vol. 89, pp. 1114-1122.

Bacon, B., O'Neill, R. & R. Britton, (1993). Hepatic mitochondrial energy production in rats with chronic iron overload. Gastroenterology, Vol.105, pp. 1134–1140.

Barbaro, G., Di Lorenzo, G. & Ribersani, M. (1999). Serum ferritin and hepatic glutathione concentrations in chronic hepatitis C patients related to the hepatitis C virus genotype. *J. Hepatol.*, Vol. 30, pp. 774-782.

Bianchi, G., Marchesini, G., Fabbri, A., Ronchi, M., Chianese, R. & Grossi, G. (1997). Lipoperoxide plasma levels in patients with liver cirrhosis. *Hepatogastroenterology*, Vol. 44, pp. 784-788.

Brass, C., Narciso, J. & Gollan, J. (1991). Enhanced activity of the free radical producing enzyme xanthine oxidase in hypoxic rat liver. *J. Clin. Invest.*, Vol. 87, pp. 424–431.

Bredt, D. S. & Snyder, S. H. (1994). Nitric oxide, a physiological messenger molecule. *Ann. Rev. Biochem.*, Vol. 63, pp. 175-195.

Cesaratto, L., Vascotto, C., Calligaris, S. & Tell, G. (2004). The importance of redox state in liver damage. *Ann. Hepatol.*, Vol. 3, pp. 86-92.

Chrobot, A. M., Szaflarska-Szczepanik, A. & Drewa G. (2000). Antioxidant defense in children with chronic viral hepatitis B and C, *Medical Science Monitor*, Vol. 6, pp. 713-718.

Comporti, M. (1985). Lipid peroxidation and cellular damage in toxic liver injury. *Lab. Invest*, Vol. 53, pp. 599-623.

Czeczot, H., Scibior, D., Skrzycki, M. & Podsiad, M. (2006). Glutathione and GSHdependent enzymes in patients with liver cirrhosis and hepatocellular carcinoma. *Acta Biochemica Polinca*, Vol. 53, pp. 237-241.

Czuczejko, J., Zachara, B. A., Staubach-Topczewska, E., Halota, W. & Kedziora J. (2003). Selenium, glutathione and glutathione peroxidases in blood of patients with chronic liver diseases. *Acta Biochimica Polinca*, Vol. 50, pp. 1147-1154.

Dalgic, B., Nesrin, S., Gursel, B., Alev, H. & Deniz E. (2005). Evaluation of oxidant stress in Wilson's disease and non-Wilsonian chronic liver disease in childhood. *Turk. J. Gastroenterol.*, Vol. 16, pp.7-11.

De Jong, J., Frederiks, W. & Van Noorden, C. (2001). Oxygen insensitivity of the histochemical assay of glucose 6 -phosphate dehydrogenase activity for the detection of (pre) neoplasm in rat liver. *J. Histochem. Cytochem.*, Vol. 49, pp. 565-571.

De Maria, N., Colantoni, A., Fagiuoli, S., Liu, G., Rogers B., Farinati, F., Thiel, D. & Floyd, R. (1996). Association between reactive oxygen species and disease activity in chronic hepatitis C. *Free Radic. Biol. Med.*, Vol. 21, pp, 291–295.

Deutsch, J. (1983) . G 6 PD assay. In: Methods in Enzymatic Analysis. Vol. 3 , pp. 190, Bergmeyer, H. U. ed., Academic Press, New York.

Farinati, F., Cardin, R., De Maria, N., Della Libera, G., Marafin, C., Lecis, E., Burra, P., Floreania, A., Cecchetto, A. & Naccarato, R. (1995). Iron storage, lipid peroxidation and glutathione turnover in chronic anti-HCV positive hepatitis. *J. Hepatol.*, Vol. 22, pp. 449–456.

Feher, J., Lengyel, G. & Blázovics, A. (1998). Oxidative stress in the liver and biliary tract diseases. *Scand. J. Gastroenterol.*, Vol. 228, pp. 38–46.

Feher, J., Vereckei , A. & Lengyel, G.(1992). Role of free-radical reactions in liver diseases. *Acta Physiol. Hung.*, Vol. 80, pp. 351-361.

Gonzalez-Correa, J., de La Cruz, J., Martin-Aurioles, E., Lopez-Egea, M., Ortiz, P., Sanchez, de la Cuesta, F. (1997). Effects of S-adenosyl-L-methionine on hepatic and renal oxidative stress in an experimental model of acute biliary obstruction in rats. *Hepatology*, Vol. 26, pp. 121-127.

Hadi Yasa, M., Kacmaz, M., Serda Ozturk, H. & Durak, I. (1999). Antioxidant status of erythrocytes from patients with cirrhosis, *Hepatogastroenterology*, Vol. 46, pp. 2460-2463.

Halliwell, B. (1991). Reactive oxygen species in living systems: source, biochemistry and role in human disease. *Am. J. Med.*, Vol. 91, pp. 1422.

Halliwell, B. (1994). Free radicals, antioxidants, and human disease : Curiosity, cause or consequence. *Lancet*, Vol. 344, pp. 721-724.

Ismail, N., Okasha, S., Dhawan, A., Abdel Rahman A., Shaker O., Sadik N. (2009). Glutathione peroxidase, superoxide dismutase and catalase activities in hepatic tissue from children with glycogen storage disease. *Arch. Med. Sci.*, Vol. 5, pp. 86-90.

Ismail, N., Okasha, S., Dhawan, A., Abdel Rahman, A., Shaker, O. & Sadik, N. (2010). Antioxidant Enzyme Activities in Hepatic Tissue from Children with Chronic Cholestatic Liver Disease. *The Saudi Journal of Gastroenterology*, Vol. 16, pp. 90-94.

Jabłonowska, E., Tchórzewski, H., Lewkowicz, P. & Kuydowicz J. (2005). *Arch. Immunol. Ther. Exp.*, Vol. 53, pp. 529–533

Madill, J., Arendt, B., Aghdassi, E. C. Chow, M. Guindi, G. Therapondos, L. Lilly, & Allard, J. (2009). Hepatic lipid peroxidation and antioxidant micronutrients in HCV liver transplant patients with and without disease recurrence. *Transplantation Proceedings*, Vol. 41, pp. 3800.

Johansson, U., Johnsson, F., Joelsson B., Berglund, M. & Akesson, B. (1986). Selenium status in patients with liver cirrhosis and alcoholism. *Brititish Journal of Nutrition*, Vol. 55, pp. 227- 233.

Khan, A., Lovejoy, D., Sharma, A., Sharma, R., Prior, M. & Lillie, L. (1987). Effects of high dietary sulphur on enzyme activities, selenium concentrations and body weights of cattle. *Can. J. Vet. Res.*, Vol. 51, pp. 174-180.

Lunec, J. (1990). Free radicals: their involvement in disease process. *Ann. Clin. Biochem.*, Vol. 27, pp. 173-182.

Mansouri, A., Gaou, I. & Fromenty, B. (1997). Premature oxidative aging of hepatic mitochondrial DNA in Wilson's disease. *Gastroenterology*, Vol. 113, pp. 599-605.

McCord, J. (1993). Oxygen-derived free radicals. *New Horizons*, Vol. 1, pp. 70-76.

Miller, J., Brzezinska-Slebodzinska, E. & Madsen, F. (1993). Oxidative stress, antioxidants, and animal function. *J. Dairy Sci.*, Vol. 76, pp. 2812--2823.

Moncada, S & Higgs, A, (1993). The L-arginine-nitric oxide pathway. *N. Engl. J. Med.*, Vol. 329, pp. 2002–2012.

Mudroň, P., Rehage, J., Qualmann, K., Sallmann, H., Mertens., M., Scholz, H. & Kovac, G. (1997). Plasma and liver alpha tocopherol in dairy cows with left abomasal displacement and fatty liver. *Zentralblatt fur Veterinärmedizin Reihe A*, Vol. 44, pp. 91–97.

Mudroň P., Rehage, J., Qualmann, K., Sallmann, H., Scholz, H. (1999). A study of lipid peroxidation and vitamin E in dairy cows with hepatic insufficiency. *J. Vet. Med. Assoc.*, Vol. 46, pp. 219–224.

Nauta, R., Tsimoyiannis, E., Uribe, M., Walsh, D., Miller D. & Butterfield, A. (1990), Oxygen-derived free radicals in hepatic ischemia injury in the rat. *Surg. Gynecol. Obstet.*, Vol. 171, pp. 120–125.

Noori, Sh., Rehman, N., Qureshi, M. & Mahboob, T. (2009). Reduction of Carbon Tetrachloride-Induced Rat Liver Injury by Coffee and Green Tea. *Pakistan Journal of Nutrition*, Vol. 8, pp. 452-458,

Ogino T. & Okada, S. (1995). Oxidative damage of bovine serum albumin and other enzyme proteins by iron-chelate complexes. *Biochemisca et Biophysica Acta*, Vol. 1245, pp. 359-365,

Pak S. G. & Nikitin, E. V. (1991). Status of the processes of free radical oxidation and antioxidation system in patients with a severe course of hepatitis B. *Klinicheskaia Meditsina*, Vol. 69, pp. 54-57.

Pár, A. & Jávor, T. (1984). Alternatives in hepatoprotection: cytoprotection influences on mono-oxidase system--free-- radical scavengers. *Acta Physiol. Hung.*, Vol. 64, pp. 409-423.

Paradis, V., Mathurin, P., Kollinger, M., Imbert-Bismut, F., Charlotte, F., Piton, A., Opolon, P., Holstege, A., Poynard, T. & Bedossa, P. (1997). In situ detection of lipid peroxidation in chronic hepatitis C: correlation with pathological features. *J. Clin. Pathol.*, Vol. 50, pp. 401-406

Petrone, W., English, D., Wong, K. & McCord, J. (1980). Free radicals and inflammation: Superoxide-dependent activation of a neutrophil chemotactic factor in plasma. *Proc. Natl. Acad. Sci.*, Vol. 77, pp. 1159–1163.

Pessayre, D., Berson, A., Fromenty, B. & Mansouri, A. (2001). Mitochondria in steatohepatitis. *Seminars in Liver Disease*, Vol. 21, pp. 57-69.

Poli, G. (1993). Liver damage due to free radicals. *Br. Med. Bull.*, Vol. 49, pp. 604-20.

Poli, G., Albano, E. & Dianzani, M. (1987). The role of lipid peroxidation in liver damage. *Chem. Phys. Lipids*, Vol. 45, pp. 117-142.

Rosser, B. & Gores, G. (1995). Liver cell necrosis: cellular mechanisms and clinical implications. Special reports and reviews. *Gastroenterology*, Vol. 108, pp. 250–275.

Samuni, A., Chevion, M. & Czapski G. (1981). Unusual copper induced sensitization of the biological damage to superoxide radicals. *The Journal of Biological Chemistry*, Vol. 256, pp. 12632-12635.

Sansinanea, A., Cerone, S., Virkel, G., Streitenberger, S., Garcia, M. & Auza, N. (2000). Nutritional condition affects the hepatic antioxidants systems in steers. *Vet. Res. Comm.*, Vol. 24, pp. 517-525.

Sanz, N., Díez-Fernandez, C., Valverde, A. M., Lorenzo, M., Benito, M. & Cascales, M. (1997) . Malic enzyme and glucose - 6 - phosphate dehydrogenase gene expression increases in rat liver cirrhogenesis. *Br. J. Cancer*, Vol. 75, pp. 487-492.

Sayed, A. S., Abd Ellah, M. R., Ibrahim, H. A. & Yasuda, J. (2003): Hematological and Biochemical changes associating chronic localized cholangitis and sawdust liver in cattle. *Assiut Vet. Med. J.*, Vol. 49, pp. 154 -171.

Sies, H. (1991). Oxidative Stress: Oxidants and Antioxidants. Academic Press, London, San Diego.

Sokol, J., Devereaux, M., O'Brien, K., Khandwala, R. & Loehr, J. (1993). Abnormal hepatic mitochondrial respiration and cytochrome C oxidase activity in rats with long-term copper overload. *Gastroenterology*, Vol. 105, pp. 178–187.

Sokol, R., Twedt, D., McKim, J., Devereaux, M., Karrer, F. and Kam, I. (1994). Oxidant injury to hepatic mitochondria in patients with Wilson's disease and Bedlington Terriers with copper toxicosis. *Gastroenterology*, Vol. 107, pp. 1788–1798.

Southorn, P. & Powis, G. (1988). Free radicals in medicine. II. Involvement in human disease. *Mayo Clin. Proc.*, Vol. 63, pp. 390–408

Spirli, C., Nathanson, M., Fiorotto, R., Duner, E., Denson, L. & Sanz, J. (2001). Proinflammatory cytokines inhibit secretion in rat bile duct epithelium. *Gastroenterology*, Vol. 121, pp. 156-169.

Spolarics, Z. (1999). A carbohydrate-rich diet stimulates glucose- 6 -phosphate dehydrogenase expression in rat hepatic sinusoidal endothelial cells. *J. Nutr.*, Vol. 129, pp. 103-108.

Stohs, S. & Bagchi, D. (1995). Oxidative stress in the toxicity of metal ions. *Free Rad. Biol. Med.*, Vol.18, pp. 321-336.

Stohs, S. (1995). The role of free radicals in toxicity and disease. *J. Basic Clin. Physiol. Pharmacol.*, Vol. 6, pp. 205-228.

Tanner, A. R., Bantock, I., Hinks, L., Lloyd, B., Turner, N. R. & Wright, R. (1986). Depressed selenium and vitamin E levels in an alcoholic population. Possible relationship to hepatic injury through increased lipid peroxidation. *Digestive Diseases and Sciences*, Vol. 31, pp. 1307-1312.

Togashi, H., Shinzawa, H., Wakabayashi, H., Nakamura, T., Yamada, N., Takahashi, T. & Ishikawa, M. (1990). Activities of free oxygen radical scavenger enzymes in human liver. *Journal of Hepatology*, Vol. 11, pp. 200-205.

Trevisan, M., Browne, R., Ram, M., Muti, P., Freudenheim, J., Carosella, A. N. & Armstrong, D. (2001). Correlates of markers of oxidative status in the general population. *Am. J. Epidemiol.*, Vol. 154, pp. 348-356.

Tsai, L., Lee, K., Tsai, S., Lee, S. & Yu, H. (1993). Changes of lipid peroxide levels in blood and liver tissue of patients with obstructive jaundice. *Clin. Chim. Acta*, 215:41-50.

Vajdovich, P. (2001). Measurements of oxidative stress. *Vet. Clin. Pathol.*, Vol. 30, pp. 158.

Videla, L., Rodrigo, R., Orellana, M., Fernandez, V., Tapia, G., Nones, L., Varela, N., Contreras, J., Lazarte, R., Csendes, A., Rojas, J., Maluenda, F., Burdiles, P., Diaz, J., Smok, G., Thielemann, L. & Poniachik, J. (2004). Oxidative stress-related parameters in the liver of non-alcoholic fatty liver disease patients. *Clinical Science*, Vol. 106, pp. 261–268.

Wallace, J. & Miller, M. (2000). Nitric oxide in mucosal defense: A little goes a long way. *Gastroenterology*, Vol. 119, pp. 512-520.

Younossi, Z. M., Diehl, A. M. & Ong, J. P. (2002). Nonalcoholic fatty liver disease: an agenda for clinical research. *Hepatology*, Vol. 35, pp. 746-752.

Zern, M., Czaja, M. & Weiner, F. (1990). The use of molecular hybridization techniques as tools to evaluate hepatic fibrogenesis. In: Rojkind M, ed. Connective tissue in health and disease. pp. 99-122, Boca Raton: CRC Press.

6

Clinical Variants of Primary Sclerosing Cholangitis: When Does Liver Biopsy Make the Diagnosis?

Annarosa Floreani
Dept. of Surgical and Gastroenterological Sciences,
University of Padova,
Italy

1. Introduction

Primary sclerosing cholangitis (PSC) is a cholestatic disorder of unknown aetiology, characterized by inflammation and obliterative fibrosis involving the intrahepatic, extrahepatic bile ducts or both (1). It predominates among men and is frequently associated with inflammatory bowel diseases, particularly with ulcerative cholitis. Although there are animal models of PSC, pathogenesis is still poorly characterized (2). The target of the immune reaction is the medium and large bile ducts. Sensitized bile ducts are damaged by different immune cells that are activated in the gastro-intestinal tract and lymph nodes. Cholangiocytes become activated to express adhesion molecules, inflammatory and profibrogenic cytokines, together growth factors that stimulate the production of fibrous tissue.

The diagnosis of PSC is based in patients who present with an alteration of cholestatic enzymes on the basis of magnetic resonance (MRN) cholangiography or direct cholangiography (ERCP) which show the typical changes of the biliary tree with multifocal strictures and segmental dilatation (3).

PSC, however, is a heterogeneous disease characterized by at least four variants:

1. "Classical" PSC (involving the intrahepatic, extrahepatic biliary tree or both)
2. Small-duct PSC
3. PSC/autoimmune hepatitis (AIH) overlap syndrome
4. IgG4 associated cholangitis (IAC)

2. "Classical" PSC

The diagnostic approach of this variant has been changed over the last years, due to the amelioration of radiological techniques. The gold standard is the cholangiography performed with MNR or ERCP, showing the typical changes of the biliary tree (3). A recent meta-analysis including 6 manuscripts for a total 456 patients, have shown that MRN has a 86% sensitivity and 94% specificity for detecting PSC (4). The American Association for the Study of Liver Disease (AASLD) recommend against routine liver biopsy for the diagnosis of PSC in patients with typical cholangiographic findings (3). A retrospective study performed at the Mayo Clinic

in 138 patients with PSC showed that liver biopsy did not add important clinical information, with the exception of a small group of patients (1.3%) in whom liver histology was fundamental for the diagnosis of the overlap syndrome with AIH (5).
In 2002 an international group reported on the prognostic of cholangiographic abnormalities generating a scoring model based on the assumption that both intra- and extra-hepatic lesions of the biliary tree would reflect the disease severity (6). More recently, this model was validated in a large cohort of patients with PSC providing a nomogram which may be used to predict medium- and long-term prognosis in individual patients with PSC (7). Indeed, the imaging techniques have the objective to rule out secondary cholangitis and to evaluate cholangiography findings which may be associated with cholangiocarcinoma.

3. Small-duct PSC

This is a variant disease characterized by typical cholestatic and histological features of PSC but normal bile ducts on cholangiography (8). It is not clear if small-duct PSC represents an early onset of the disease or a different entity. However, studies addressing the natural history of this variant have shown a better prognosis of small-duct PSC than the large duct PSC. In particular, two multicentre studies have been published so far. The first one included 33 patients with small-duct PSC and 260 patients with large-duct PSC evaluated in Oxford and Oslo with a median follow-up of 106 vs 105 months respectively (9). More recently, another European and US study included 83 patients with small-duct PSC and 166 patients with large-duct PSC with a median follow-up of 11 years (8). Both studies report similar conclusions, showing a statistically significant better prognosis for small-duct PSC than large-duct PSC patients.
Liver biopsy is mandatory for the diagnosis of small-duct PSC in patients with a normal ERCP or MRN (3). Periductal concentric ("onion-skin") fibrosis is the classical finding of PSC, unless unspecific histological diagnosis include PSC/AIH overlap syndrome, and a number of secondary causes of sclerosing cholangitis including eosinophilic cholangitis, histiocytosis X, ischemic cholangitis, mastcell cholangiopathy, and bacterial cholangitis.

4. PSC/AIH overlap syndrome

This is a disorder mainly described in children and young adults (10-12). Its characteristics include clinical, biochemical, and histologic features typical of PSC. Gregorio et al (10) identified a 49% prevalence of PSC/AIH overlap syndrome among AIH paediatric patients, whereas in adult series it seems to be quite rare. Diagnosis of an overlap syndrome by use of the modified AIH score ranges from 1.4 to 12.5-17% (Table 1, ref. 11, 13-16). The reason of the higher rate in Italy may be explained with the inclusion in our series of a number of patients deriving from a cohort of paediatric series.
More recently, the King's group in London defines PSC with strong autoimmune features in children as autoimmune sclerosing cholangitis (ASC)(17). In contrast with the male overrepresentation in adults, over 50% of paediatric patients with ASC are girls (17). In our experience, patients with PSC/AIH overlap syndrome are significantly younger at presentation and exhibit significantly higher serum levels of transaminases and IgG than the classical PSC group (15). Association with IBD is more common in the group with "classical" PSC than PSC/AIH overlap syndrome group (46.4% vs 20%, $p<0.01$). As expected, non organ-specific autoantibodies which represent the hallmarks of autoimmunity

are positive in nearly all patients with PSC/AIH overlap syndrome. Some 50% of the patients have atypical perinuclear antineutrophil cytoplasmic antibodies (p-ANCAs). In our experience the cumulative probability of survival at 20 years was higher in PSC/AIH overlap syndrome than in the "classical" PSC (87.5% vs 73.6%) but the difference was not statistically significant (16).

Author	Country	n. of PSC patients	% with overlap
Van Buuren, 2000[13]	Netherlands	113	8%
Kaya, 2000[14]	USA	211	1.4%
Floreani, 2000[15]	Italy	41	17%
Antoniazzi, 2010[16]	Italy	79	12.6%
Al-Chalaby, 2008[11]	UK	211	6.1%

Table 1. Diagnosis of AIH/PSC overlap by use of the modified AIH score

Liver histology is mandatory for the diagnosis of PSC/AIH overlap syndrome. The main features include: piecemeal necrosis, lymphocyte rosetting, and moderate or severe periportal or periseptal inflammation (15).
The EASL guidelines recommend a medical treatment for PSC/AIH overlap syndrome with ursodeoxycholic acid and immunosuppressive therapy, but is not evidence-based due to lack of adequate studies (18).
In a retrospective study concentrating on the histological features of PSC in children, Batres et al report that 45% of 20 patients had variable degrees of interface hepatitis at diagnosis (19).

5. IgG4-associated sclerosing cholangitis

This is a distinct form of PSC recently described in the literature, of unknown aetiology and characterized by elevated serum IgG4 and infiltration of IgG4-positive plasma cells in bile ducts and liver tissue (20). Since the first observations, it became evident that IAC was highly associated to autoimmune pancreatitis (AIP) which represents a distinct form of chronic pancreatitis occasionally observed in association with Sjogren's syndrome, primary biliary cirrhosis, Crohn's disease, ulcerative cholitis or other immune-mediated disorders (21).
Kamisawa et al. reported that tissue infiltration with abundant IgG4-positive cells was a characteristic feature not only of AIP but also of other organs involved in AIP (22). The clinical profile of IAC include: 1) older age; 2) male gender (in up to 85% of cases); 3) presentation with obstructive jaundice; 4) association with AIP in more than 90% of cases; 6) abundant IgG4 infiltrate in biopsy duct specimens; 7) normalization of liver enzymes with steroids (20). A recent study found serum IgG4 in 9% in a cohort of 127 patients with PSC (23). In comparison to patients with PSC and normal levels of IgG4, the former group had significantly higher levels of alkaline phosphatise and bilirubin, in addition to higher Mayo risk prognostic score (23). Preliminary data suggest that the immunopathogenesis of IAC differs from other immune-mediated cholestatic liver disease in that T helper 2 and T regulatory cytokines were markedly overexpressed in IAC patients (24). Being apparently different from PSC and similar to AIP, sclerosing cholangitis with and without AIP shows a clinical response to steroid therapy (25). When intra-pancreatic stenosis is detected with imaging procedures, pancreatic cancer shoul be ruled out. For the diagnosis of Ig4-positive AIC a liver biopsy with IgG4 immunostaining is needed (26). If stenosis is demonstrated in the hepatic hilar region, cholangiocarcinoma should be discriminated by imaging techniques and bile duct biopsy (26).

6. Pathology findings

Liver biopsy is recommended for the diagnosis of small-duct PSC, AIH/PSC overlap syndrome and IAC. Bile duct biopsy is mandatory to rule out cholangiocarcinoma in any form of PSC. Cholangiocarcinoma should be suspected in case of dominant stenosis (common bile duct ≤1.5 mm in diameter or hepatic duct ≤1 mm)(27) or in case of "tumour" appearance in the hilar region (28).

7. Bile duct biopsy

The common characteristic in PSC is the fibro-inflammatory involvement of large ducts and the infiltration of lymphocytes in small ducts together with the "onion-like" fibrosis surrounding the small intra-hepatic ducts. The IAC type shows peculiar characteristics with dense infiltration of lymphocytes and IgG4-positive plasma cells with extensive fibrosis and obliterative phlebitis (29). In classical PSC the fibrosis is dense and older, whereas in IgG4-IAC the entire bile duct walls and periductular tissue are affected. Ghezale et al (20) reported positive and abundant IgG4 immunostaining (>10 IgG4-positive cell/HPF) of bile duct biopsy specimens of bile duct in 88% of patients. The IgG4 immunostaining needs further clarification, however; in fact, a recent study by Zhang et al (30) revealed that 23% of 98 explanted livers with PSC had periductal infiltration with abundant IgG4-positive plasma cells (>10/HPF) in the hilar area.

In the small-duct PSC large bile duct are normal and only changes in the interlobular bile ducts are seen, resulting in "normal" findings at cholangiography (31).

In the AIH/PSC overlap syndrome bile duct biopsy shows similar characteristics than "classical" PSC.

The main histopathological findings are summarized in the table 2.

	Classical PSC	Small duct PSC	AIH/PSC overlap	IgG4-ISC
LARGE BILE DUCTS	Luminal side including cholangiocytes	Normal	Similar to classical PSC	Whole bile duct walls and periductal tissue
Inflammatory Infiltrate	Mild	Absent	Mild	Abundant infiltrate of lymphocytes and IgG4-positive plasma cells
Fibrosis	Not dense	Absent	Dense	Dense
Obliterative phlebitis	-	-	-	+
SMALL BILE DUCTS				
Onion skin lesions	+	+	+	-

Table 2. Histopathologic features of bile ducts

8. Liver biopsy

Histological classification allows to score the disease in four stages (32). Stage 1 is characterized by portal oedema, mild portal inflammation, a non destructive cholangitis

with infiltration of lymphocytes in the bile duct and ductular proliferation. In stage 2 (periportal stage) the lesion extends to involve periportal fibrosis. In stage 3 (septal stage) bridging fibrous septa develop and bile ducts degenerate and disappear. Stage 4 is characterized by cirrhosis.
Liver changes, however, may be patchy and there is a sampling variability.

9. References

[1] Maggi JR, Chapman RW. An update on primary sclerosing cholangitis. Curr Opin Gastroenterol 2008; 24: 377-383.
[2] Hirschfield GM, Heathcote EJ, Gershwin EE. Pathogenesis of cholestatic liver disease and therapeutic approaches. Gastroenterology 2010; 139: 1481-1496.
[3] Chapman R, Fevery J, Kalloo A, Nagorney DM, Boberg KM, Shneider B, et al. Diagnosis and management of primary sclerosing cholangitis. Hepatology 2010; 51: 660-678.
[4] Dave M, Elmunzer BJ, Dwamena BA, Higgins PD. Primary sclerosing cholangitis: meta-analysis of diagnostic performance of MR cholangiopancreatography. Radiology 2010; 256: 387-396.
[5] Burak KW, Angulo P, Lindor KD. Is there a role for liver biopsy in primary sclerosing cholangitis? Am J Gastroenterol 2003; 98: 1155-1158.
[6] Ponsionen CY, Vrouenraets SM, Prawirodirdjo W, Rajaram R, Rauws EA, Mulder CJ, et al. Natural history of primary sclerosing cholangitis and prognostic value of cholangiography in a Dutch population. Gut 2002; 51: 562-566.
[7] Ponsionen CY. Validation Endoscopy 2010; 42: 742-747.
[8] Bjornsson E, Olsson R, Bergquist A, Lindgren S, Braden B, Chapman RW, et al. The natural history of small-duct primary sclerosing cholangitis. Gastroenterology 2008; 134: 975-980.
[9] Bjornsson E, Boberg KM, Cullen S, Fleming K, Clausen OP, Fausa O, et al. Patients with small duct primary sclerosing cholangitis have a favourable long term prognosis. Gut 2002; 51: 731-735.
[10] Gregorio GV, PortmannB, Karani J, Harrison P, Donaldson PT, Vergani D, et al. Autoimmune hepatitis/sclerosing cholangitis overlap syndrome in childhood: a 16-year prospective study. Hepatology 2001; 33: 544-553.
[11] Al-Chalabi T, Portmann BC, Bernal W, McFarlane IG, Heneghan MA. Autoimmune hepatitis overlap syndromes: an evaluation of treatment response, long-term outcome and survival. Aliment Pharmacol Ther 2008; 28: 209-220.
[12] Beuers U, Rust C. Overlap syndromes. Semin Liver Dis 2005; 25: 311-320.
[13] van Buuren HR, van Hoogstraten HJE, Terkivatan T, Schalm SW, Vleggaar FP. High prevalence of autoimmune hepatitis among patients with primary sclerosing cholangitis. J Hepatol 2000; 33: 543-548.
[14] Kaya M, Angulo P, Lindor KD. Overlap of autoimmune hepatitis and primary sclerosing cholangitis: an evaluation of a modified scoring system. J Hepatol 2000; 33: 537-542.
[15] Floreani A, Rizzotto ER, Ferrara F, Carderi I, Caroli D, Blasone L, et al. Clinical course and out come of autoimmune epatiti/primary sclerosino cholangitis overlap syndrome. Am J Gastroenterol 2005; 100: 1516-1522.

[16] Antoniazzi S, Cazzagon N, Egoue J, Lazzari R, Floreani A. The natural history of autoimmune hepatitis/primary sclerosing cholangitis (AIH/PSC) overlap syndrome. Digest Liver Dis 2010; 42, suppl.4: S312-S313 (Abstr).
[17] Mieli-Vergani G, Vergani D. Unique features of primary sclerosing cholangitis in children. Curr Opin Gastroenterol 2010; 26: 265-268.
[18] European Association for the Study of the Liver. EASL clinical practice guidelines: management of cholestatic liver diseases. J Hepatol 2009; 51: 237-267.
[19] Batres LA, Russo P, Mathews M, Piccoli DA, Chuang E, Ruchelli E. Primary sclerosing cholangitis in children: a histologic follow-up study. Pediatr Dev Pathol 2005; 8: 568-576.
[20] Ghazale A, Chari ST, Zhag L, Smyrk TC, Takahashi N, Levy MJ, et al. Immunoglobulin G4-associated cholangitis: clinical profile and response to therapy. Gastroenterology 2008; 134: 706-715.
[21] Etemad B, Whitcomb DC. Chronic pancreatitis: diagnosis, classification, and new genetic developments. Gastroenterology 2001; 120: 682-707.
[22] Kamisawa T. IgG4-positive plasma cells specifically infiltrate various organs in autoimmune pancreatitis. Pancreas 2004; 29: 167-168.
[23] Mendes FD, Jorgensen R, Keach J, Katzmann JA, Smyrk T, Donlinger J, et al. Elevated serum IgG4 concentration in patients with primary sclerosing cholangitis. Am J Gastroenterol 2006; 101: 2070-2075.
[24] Zen Y, Fujii T, Harada K, et al. Th2 and regulatory immune reactions are increased in immunoglobulin G4-related sclerosing pancreatitis and cholangitis. Hepatology 2007; 45: 1538-1546.
[25] Nishimori I, Otsuki M. Autoimmune pancreatitis and IgG4-associated sclerosing cholangitis. Best Pract Res Clin Gastroenterol 2009; 23: 11-23.
[26] Nakazawa T, Ando T, Hayashi K, Naitoh I, Ohara H, Joh T. Diagnostic procedures for IgG4-related sclerosing cholangitis. J Hepatobiliary Pancreat Sci 2010;
[27] Rudolph G, Gotthardt D, Kloeters-Plachky P, Kulaksiz H, Stiehl A. In PSC with dominant bile duct stenosis, IBD is associated with an increase in carcinomas and reduced survival. J Hepatol 2010; 53; 313-317.
[28] Kamisawa T, Takuma K, Anjiki H, Egawa N, Kurata M, Honda G, et al. Sclerosing cholangitis associated with autoimmune pancreatitis differs from primary sclerosing cholangitis. World J Gastreonterol 2009; 21: 2357-2360.
[29] Zen Y, Harada K, Sasaki M, Sato Y, Tsuneyama K, Haratake J, et al. IgG4-related sclerosing cholangitis with and without inflammatory pseudotumor, and sclerosing pancreatitis-associated sclerosing cholangitis: do they belong to a spectrum of sclerosing pancreatitis? Am J Surg Pathol 2004; 28: 1193-1203.
[30] Zhang L, Notohara K, Levy MJ, et al. IgG4-positive plasma cell infiltration in the diagnosis of autoimmune pancreatitis. Mod Pathol 2007; 20: 23-28.
[31] Karlsen TH, Schrumpf E, Boberg KM. Primary sclerosing cholangitis. Best Pract Res Clin Gastroenterol 2010; 24: 655-666.
[32] Ludwig J. Surgical pathology of the syndrome of primary sclerosing cholangitis. Am J Surg Pathol 1989; 13, suppl.1: 43-49.

7

Evaluation of Radiofrequency Ablation as a Method for Treatment of Hepatocellular Carcinoma

Heba Mohamed Abdella
Tropical Medicine, Faculty of Medicine, Ain Shams University, Cairo, Egypt

1. Introduction

Hepatocellular carcinoma is the fifth most common neoplasm in the World and the third most common cause of cancer related death (1). It accounts for 7.4% of all cancers in males and 3.2% of all cancers in females (2).

An early diagnosis of HCC is required for the institution of treatments considered to be curative. On this basis, screening of each patient with liver cirrhosis should be performed by ultrasound and by measurements of serum alphafetoprotein (AFP) at 6-months interval (3).There are different methods for active management of HCC, many factors related to the tumour itself and to the patient may make a tumour unresectable (4).

Radio frequency ablation (RFA) is the most common therapy used in patients not suitable for resection. In RFA, an electric current that is passed into the tumour tissue via an electrode tip results in heat generation and coagulative necrosis (5). The advantage of radio frequency is the small number of sessions needed to obtain tumour necrosis (6). The aim of the present study was to evaluate the radiofrequency thermal ablation as a method for treatment of hepatocellular carcinoma.

2. Patients and methods

This retrospective study was carried out at Ain-Shams University Hospital (Hepatoma unit), including patients attending the unit during the period between January 2004 to January 2006.

All patients were subjected to the following:

1. *Full history with special emphasis on* the newly developed persistent right upper abdominal pain, and unexplained hepatic decompensation
2. *Full clinical examination including:*
   A. General examination : with stress on signs of liver cell failure including jaundice, flapping tremors, plamar erythema, lower limb edema
   B. Local abdominal examination: with special stress on the presence of signs suggestive of hepatic malignancy e.g. hepatic mass and hepatic bruit.
3. *Laboratory investigations:*

Complete blood picture, liver profile, coagulation profile, hepatitis markers, serum blood glucose, and renal function tests.

Tumour markers including AFP, CA and CEA antigens for exclusion of metastasis from the GIT.

4. *Radiological evaluation:*
   a. Pelviabdominal U.S. examination;

To evaluate the number, size, and location of the hepatic focal lesions, and to exclude portal vein thrombosis, hepatic vein obstruction, porta-hepatis or coeliac lymph node enlargement, and ascites.

   b. Abdominal tri-phasic spiral C.T. scan to accurately evaluate the pattern of enhancement of the focal lesions, vascular or biliary invasion specially portal vein thombosis. The suggestive criteria for HCC were considered present when there was enhancement of the focal lesion with the I.V dye so it appeared hyperdense in the arterial phase, then it became hypodense in both portovenous and delayed phases due to the wash out of the dye from the focal lesion.

The above mentioned findings were used as a reference for evaluation of the response after ablation.

   c. Chest x-ray to exclude pulmonary metastases.

Patients were stratified according to Child-Pugh Classification (7)

Diagnosis of HCC was done based on the presence of at least 2 of 3 of the following criteria:

1. Hepatic focal lesion detected by abdominal ultrasound and has positive criteria of HCC in spiral CT scan.
2. Alphafetoprotein >200ng/ml (8).
3. Guided biopsy from the focal lesion was performed when one of the above mentioned criteria was missed.

Seventy four patients with proved hepatocellular carcinoma were selected for treatment by ultrasound-guided percutaneous radiofrequency ablation according the following inclusion criteria;

1. Patients with unresectable hepatic malignancies.
2. No evidence of extra-hepatic disease.
3. Absence of vascular or biliary invasion.
4. Presence of not more than 2 focal lesions, each is less than 5cm.
5. Child-Pugh's class A, and B.
6. Tumours in position where the electrode can be inserted and held safely.

Absolute contra-indications include:

- Sever debilitation.
- Active infection.
- Uncorrectable coagulopathy.
- Pregnancy.

After imaging study, patients were divided into 2 groups according to the number of focal lesions:

Group I: patients with single hepatic focal lesion.

Group II: patients with 2 hepatic focal lesions.

Premaneuver assessment: Patients were admitted to Tropical Medicine Department for Premaneuver assessment including cardiac and chest examination, ECG, blood pressure and blood glucose level evaluation. Ascites in ascetic patients was also controlled by diuretics and tapping if needed.

Radiofrequency ablation systems:

The two machines used in this study were:

a. The RITA model 1500RF.

b. RF 2000 system, produced by the RadioTherapeutics Corporation.

Radiofrequency ablation technique:

Patients with one focal lesion were treated in single RFA setting while patients with 2 focal lesions were treated either in single or over 2 settings separated by one week, so 80 sessions were done for 80 lesions. Percutaneous radiofrequency ablation was used to treat a total of 80 lesions which were detected by U.S and C.T in the 74 patients.

Pre-ablation assessment:

General assessment:

Medical history was revised and the laboratory test results were checked, and the ECG was interpreted with chest and cardiac examination. A peripheral I.V. line was started, and the patient was monitored for blood pressure, pulse, respiratory rate, and the peripheral oxygenation.

Ultrasound approach assessment:

Percutaneous RFA was performed with real- time US guidance by using 3.5 MHz convex probe. Pre-ablation US assessment was performed to re-evaluate the number and size of the tumours, their relationship to surrounding structures as blood vessels, bile ducts, gall bladder, diaphragm, and bowel, and to determine if a safe and adequate approach exists.

The most appropriate approach for electrode insertion was detected. For tumours located in the right lobe, an intercostal approach with the patient in the left lateral decubitus position generally was preferred. For tumours located in the left lobe, a subcostal approach was used most often. The procedure was done in the interventional radiology unit (a special sterilized unit) containing the ultrasound machine (Siemens, Toshiba), the services of general anesthesia, the radiofrequency system, and a mobile sterile table (for sterile patients and doctors' gowns, antiseptics, syringes, IV fluid, medications, and gauze). The grounding pads, representing the dispersive electrode, were placed on the patient's thighs and properly connected to the generator. The system was tested to be sure working.

Anesthesia and medications:

Local anesthesia was performed from the entry site on the skin to the liver capsule along the needle track with 10 ml of 2% xylocaine. Skin was pricked it has small sterile lancet. Most of the patients undergone RFA were treated under general intravenous anesthesia.

Needle electrode placement:

The needle electrode was introduced into the liver through the skin incision under U.S. or C.T. guidance. After verifying the positioning of the needle electrode, the multiple arrays were deployed and the needle electrode was connected to the RF generator.

Treatment strategy:

The objective in treating the tumours was to ablate the entire tumour as well as at least 1 cm-tumour- free margin of normal liver.

The deepest ablations were performed before the superficial ones to minimize the possibility of those microbubbles might obscure visualization of the deepest portions of the tumour and thus prevent completion of the ablation. The hilar portion of the tumour was ablated initially in order to destroy the inflow of blood supplying the tumour.

The needle electrode was first placed at the most posterior margin and at one side of the tumour, then to the other side. Multiple overlapping ablations were then sequentially performed progressing superficially and then laterally at 2-2.5 cm intervals within the tumour until the tumour and 1 cm-free margin had been successfully ablated.

As we start RFA session a hyper-echoic focus developed around the un-insulated portion of the electrode. This was attributed to tissue vaporization and cavitations. The area of echogenicity was round; most often progressively increased in size over the course of ablation and generally enveloped the entire tumour with variable extensions in the surrounding liver by the end of the treatment.

In some cases, the hyper-echoic focus did not develop progressively but appeared rather suddenly and was accompanied with an audible popping sound emanating from the liver.

Cool down:

When the timer runs out the generator well automatically goes into Cool Down mode for 30 seconds (5 minutes on the generator display), when the Cool Down is complete, the temperatures from all leads must be above 70°C, if not we continue ablation for another 5 minutes at target temperature, or we can rotate the device 45 degree to check temperature and continue ablation if still temp below 70°C.

Track ablation:

In most of our cases we ablate the tract before removal of the needle.

Post Ablation care:

IV antiemetic was given if needed, Strong IV analgesics were given to pain as pethidine hydrochloride 50 mg or tramadol. All patients were observed clinically for 2-3 hours in the Radiology department to detect any acute complications and to start IV fluid. Prophylactic antibiotic were started, amoxicillin-clavulanic acid (augmentin) or ceftazidine (fortum), and metronidazole (flagyl), and continued for 3 days.

Post treatment follow up

All patients underwent dynamic CT scan 1 month after completion of the therapy to detect any residual enhancing tumour tissue. If any area suspicious for viable tissue was detected, the patient was retreated by RFA of this area. Then, follow up CT was done after 3 months, then every 6 months to detect any local recurrence in the ablated tumour or de novo lesion. Alphafetoprotein level was assessed accompanying performance of CT. After 1 month if its level was still elevated, it indicated incomplete tumour ablation. Follow up after complete ablation was to detect any minor elevations which detect recurrence.

3. Results

Table 1 shows the demographic and clinical data of the studied patients.

Thirty one patients had their AFP level above the diagnostic value (200ng/ml), while the remaining 43 patients had AFP level less than 200. The (M ± SD) of serum alphafetoprotein level (AFP) was 12086 ± 7345 ng/ml and ranged between 1.8 ng/ml and 350000 ng/ml, as shown in **table 2** which illustrates also the remaining liver profile. All patients were positive for hepatitis C antibody and negative for HbsAg. HbcAb was detected in 7 patients. Abdominal ultrasound findings are shown **in table 3**. The findings of spiral CT in this study were similar to that of abdominal ultrasound as regard the number, site and diameter of the hepatic focal lesion. In this study, the spiral CT criteria suggestive for HCC were present in 63 cases (85.1%) and absent in 14 cases (14.9%) (they were proved to be HCC by biopsy.

Forty two Patients (56.8%) were within Child Pugh class A and 32 patients (43.2%) were within Child Pugh class B (patients in Child class B were with minimal and controlled ascites).

Tumour character: The seventy four patients included in the study were divided into 2 groups according to the number of focal lesions in each patient. Sixty eight patients form group I and had only one focal lesion (68 lesions) and the maximum diameter of the tumours was 3 cm or less in 42 patients and was from 3-5 cm in 26 patients. Group II formed of patients with 2 hepatic focal lesions and included 6 patients with 12 focal lesions. In group II, the maximum diameter of the tumours was 3 cm or less in 6 lesions of 6 patients and was from 3-5 cm in another 6 lesions of the same 6 patients **(Table 3).**

Age	Mean	55.5 years
	± SD	7.8 years
Gender	**No. of the patient**	%
Males	57	77%
Females	17	23%
Symptoms		
Rt. Hypochondrial pain	58	78.3%
Loss of appetite	25	33.8%
Itching	9	12.2%
Loss of weight	21	28.4%
Jaundice	23	31.1%
Ascites	11	14.9%
Fever	10	13.5%
Easy fatigability	35	47.3%
Risk factors for infection with hepatitis viruses.		
Schistosomasis & treatment with tartar emetic	40	54.1%
Blood transfusion	28	37.8%
Surgical operations	38	51.4%
Dental procedures	24	32.4%
General Examination		
Pallor	6	8.1%
Jaundice	30	40.5%
Flapping Tremors	11	14.8%
Palmar erythema	25	33.8%
Lower Limb edema	36	48.6%
Abdominal Examination		
Palpable liver	44	59.4%
Tender liver	0	0%
Ascites	10	13.5%
Splenomegaly	13	17.6

Table 1. Demographic and clinical data of the studied patients.

	Mean	**± SD**
AFP	12086	7345
ALT (IU/L)	66.8	32.5
AST (IU/L)	94.8	36.4
Albumin (gm/dL)	2.9	0.4
Bilirubin (mg/dL)	1.7	0.6

Table 2. Laboratory findings of the studied patients.

		GI (n=68), 68 lesions	GII (n=6), 12lesions
Lesion <3cm	No. of patients	42	6
	No. of lesions	42	6
Lesion 3-5cm	No. of patients	26	6
	No. of lesions	26	6

Table 3. Tumour character in the studied patients:

Results of treatment with Radiofrequency ablation:
During the first follow up done one month after ablation, 68 patients (91.9%) showed complete ablation with no evidence of residual and 6 patients (8.1 %) showed incomplete ablation [3 patients in group I and 3 patients in group II, all of them with lesion diameter 3-5cm] **(Table 4)**

	Group I (68 patients, 68 lesions)				**Group II (6 patients, 12 lesions)**			
	<3cm		3-5cm		<3cm		3-5cm	
	Number of patients	Number of lesions	Number of patients	Number of lesions	Number of patients	Number of lesions	Number of patients	Number of lesions
	42	42	26	26	6	6	6	6
Complete ablation	42 (100%)	42 (100%)	23 (88.4%)	23 (88.4%)	6 (100%)	6 (100%)	3 (50%)	3 (50%)
Partial ablation	0 (0%)	0 (0%)	3 (11.5%)	3 (11.5%)	0 (0%)	0 (0%)	3 (50%)	3 (50%)

Table 4. Results of RFA after one month

During the second follow up done after 3 months, 71 patients (95.9 %) had no evidence of local or distant recurrence. Local recurrence occurred in 3 patients in group I (4.1%).
During the third follow up done after 6 months, 70 patients (94.6%) showed no evidence of recurrence and 4 patients (5.4%) [2 patients in group I and 2 patients in group II] had a new focal lesion at distant sites of the liver.
During the fourth follow up done after 12 months, 72 patients (97.3%) showed no evidence of recurrence and 2 patients (2.7%) had a new focal lesion at other sites of the liver both were in group II **(Table 5).**

	Group I (n=68 patients)		**Group II (n=6 patients)**	
	Local recurrence	Distant recurrence	Local recurrence	Distant recurrence
3 months	3	0	0	0
6 months	0	2	0	2
12 months	0	0	0	2

Table 5. Results of 3, 6 and 12 months follow up after RFA

The residual of the tumour was managed by a second session of RFA. All local or distant recurrences were managed by a second RFA session when in suitable site except in one patients was near a biliary radicle, so managed with intralesional ethanol injection.

***Follow up of Laboratory investigation:**

As regards the liver enzymes, ALT was significantly elevated one month after RFA sessions (92.8 ± 36.4 IU/L) more than before ablation (P < 0.01), the same was noticed for AST which was also significantly higher (98 ±32.5 IU/L) (P<0.01). During the second follow up done after 3 months, ALT and AST returned to base line levels.

Three months after RFA, serum albumin was higher and ranged between 2.8-4.5 gm/dl **with (M ± SD: 0.2± 0.4gm/dl),** serum bilirubin was lower and ranged between 0.6-1.9 mg/dl with (M ± SD: 0.9±0.4gm/dL).

Before treatment with RFA serum A FP values were elevated (>200ng/mL) in 31patients (41.8%). **Table 6** shows the patients with AFP level>200 during the follow up period after ablation.

	AFP>200ng/ml	
	No. of patients	%
Before RFA	31	41.8%
One month after RFA	17	22.9%
After three months	9	12.2%
After 6 months	5	6.7%
After 12 months	3	4.1%

Table 6. Patients with AFP>200ng/ml before and after RFA.

There were no fatal complications related to RFA treatment. Nearly all the patients experienced post-ablation right hypochondrial pain that was controlled by analgesics, and nausea (70 patients, 94.5%), which was controlled by antiemetics Also, nearly all experienced post - ablation pyrexia for 1-3 days, which was controlled by antipyretics. Pneumonia occurred in only one patient (1.3%) and ascites developed in 2 patients (2.7%) . Only one patient developed pneumothorax due to ablation of Sub-diaphragmatic tumour and another 2 patients developed ascites within the first week post ablation.

At the end of this study after one year, survival analysis was evaluated. Two patients (2.7%) died as result of advanced liver disease. So, overall survival rate was 97.2% (72/74 patients). Disease free survival rate was 79.7% as thirteen patients (17.6%) survived with recurrent HCC and fifty nine patients (79.7%) were disease free over the follow up period **(Table 7).**

Survival status	**Number of patients**	%
Disease free survival patients	59	79.7%
Survived with recurrent disease	13	17.6 %
Died patients	2	2.7 %
Total number	74	100%

Table 7. Survival rates evaluation in the study

4. Discussion

Hepatocellular carcinoma (HCC) is the fifth most common neoplasm in the world and the third most common cause of cancer related death. Currently, it is the leading cause of death among cirrhotic patients (1). The studies carried out on hepatocellular carcinoma are scarce in Egypt. Nevertheless, they presumed an upward trend for HCC among chronic liver disease (CLD) patients (9).

For the last two decades several minimally invasive interventional ablative techniques aiming at providing local destruction of the tumour have been developed. Radiofrequency thermal ablation (RFA) is a more recently developed for local tissue ablation.

This retrospective study was performed on 74 patients with hepatocellular carcinoma attending Hepatoma unit of Ain Shams University during the period between January 2004 and January 2006.

In this study, it was found that the number of male patients was higher than females (57 male and 17 females) with ratio 3.4:1 and this agrees with Sherlock and Dooley 2002 who reported that in patients with HCC males exceed females in a ratio of 4-6:1(2). Also, Marrero, 2003 stated that male population both black and white is primarily affected (10).

The newly developed persistent right hypochondrial dull aching pain was the most common complaint of patients included in this study (78.3%). This is a very important finding and it meets the finding of Hillebrand and Sandowski, 2000 who found that although the percentage of patients having specific signs and symptoms differs in high-incidence and low incidence areas of HCC, the most common complaint remains abdominal pain (4). Pain is frequent but rarely severe and is felt as a non-specific, continuous dull ache in the epigastrium, right upper quadrant, or the back. Severe pain is due to perihepatitis or involvement of the diaphragm (2).

The etiology of chronic liver disease in patients of the study was hepatitis viruses' infection (HBV and/or HCV). In Egypt, HCV seroprevalence is 55% among children who had received blood transfusions and 67% among patients on renal dialysis, and is 10% among sexually transmitted disease patients (11).

In this study, 67 patients (90.5%) were positive for HCV antibody. The prevalence of HCV antibody positive patient with HCC was found to be 62% in Spain, 65% in Italy, 29% in South Africa and 29% in United States (12).

In this study all patients were negative for HBsAg but when HBcAb IgG was assessed (which indicates past infection with HBV), it was found that HBcAb IgG was positive in 7 patients (9.5%) of the study. these results agree also with El-Zayadi et al., 2001 who placed Egypt among the countries of intermediate prevalence for HBV as HBV accounts for 10-30% of CLD and HBsAg carriage was reported in 5.6% (9).

Owing to the use of ultrasound surveillance in patients with hepatic cirrhosis, HCC is diagnosed in an increasing number of patients at an early asymptomatic stage [(13)]. Patients with early stage HCC should be considered for any of the available curative treatment options including surgical resection, liver transplantation and percutaneous techniques of tumour ablation [(14)]. In the recent decade, ultrasound guided percutaneous ethanol injection (PEI), as a local therapy for hepatic tumours, has gradually been replaced by intraoperative or percutaneous RFA [(15)]. RFA was considered by many authors as superior to other existing loco regional therapies as percutaneous ethanol injection (PEI), transarterial chemoembolization (TACE) and microwave ablation [(16)].

In the present studying RFA was used to treat 80 tumours in 74 patients. The 80 tumours included 48 tumours (60%) less than 3 cm in diameter and 32 tumours (40%) 3-5cm in diameter.

Generally, a single ablation of 5cm in diameter could successfully destroy liver tumour smaller than 3cm plus the safety margin of 0.5-1cm [17]. In the present study, after one month of RFA , all the 48 tumours (100%) less than 3cm in diameter shoed complete ablation while 26/32 (81.3%) of tumours between 3-5cm showed complete ablation and 6 tumours (18.7%) showed residual viable tumour tissue (i.e. partial or incomplete ablation). In a study by Chen et al. 2005 [17], cases with tumours larger than 3.5cm in diameter accounted for 61.8% (207/335 cases) of their study population, and they got 85.9% response rate (178/207 cases), results nearly similar to the results of the present study. The whole complete response rate for all tumours was 92.5% (74/80 tumours), the 6 incompletely ablated tumours (7.5%) were larger than 3cm in diameter. These results are also near the results of Chen et al. 2005 who reported 94.8% (723/763 tumours) total ablation rate of the initial RFA. Of the 40 incompletely ablated tumours, 33 (82.5%) were larger than 3.5cm [17]. These data support the fact that the most important factor for efficacy of RFA is the size of the tumour and the RFA could successfully ablate smaller liver tumours. **Sala et al 2004** [18] supports this by the results of their study as they reported initial complete response of 96% in tumours 2cm or smaller and this figure decreased to almost 50% in multinodular or large HCC and this figure is similar to that reported by most referral groups [19].

All cohort studies assessing percutaneous ablation report the appearance of viable tumour tissue within the treated nodule or its vicinity after initial complete response [20]. This was met in our study as, three months after ablation local recurrence occurred in three patients in group I. Six months after ablation, 4 patients (2 in each group) showed distant recurrence and 2 other patients in group II showed another distant recurrence after one year. This event is heterogeneously defined (distance from the main nodule, location in the same segment) and named [21]. This is usually termed local recurrence or local tumour progression [21]. Sala et al 2004 reported local tumour progression in 76 patients in their series of 192 patients after initial complete response with a 1, 3, 5 years probability of 26%, 56%, and 74% respectively. Most were detected early in the follow up, but 34% were registered at 2 years and 13% were detected beyond 3 years [18]. Unfortunately, results of our study can not be compared with results of Sala et al 2004 as the follow up period here is only one year.

Even tumours 2cm or smaller can present with late failure and studies in resected tumours explain this: one third of tumours with 3cm or smaller present microscopic vascular invasion or satellites, which will almost likely not be affected by ablation and emerge as failure early or late during follow up [22].

At the end of the follow up period in our study (1year), the overall survival rate was 97.3% i.e. 72 patients alive and 2 patients died due to disease progression. Fifty nine patients (79.7%) represented the disease free survival while 13 patients (17.5%) lived with either local or distant recurrence.

The one year overall survival in our study was 97% which is similar to that of Shina **et al., 2005** [23] but less than **Lencioni et al., 2003**[24] which was 100%.

However our results are higher than those of **Lin et al., 2004** [25] and **Lin et al., 2005** [26] (90% , 93% respectively). At the end of the study (1 year) ,15 patients (18.9%) lived with either local recurrence or denovo lesion. **Lin et al., 2003** reported 18% local recurrence at the end of their study (2 year) while over the same period **Lncioni et al ., 2003** reported only 4% local recurrence and no report on denovo lesions.

In this series nearly all the patients experienced post-ablation minor complication as right hypochondrial pain that was controlled by analgesics and nausea, which was controlled by antiemetics Also, nearly all experienced post - ablation pyrexia for 1-3 days, which was controlled by antipyretics it agrees with **Mulier et al., 2002** [27] reported 93% of HCC patients in his study experienced post-ablation right hypochondrial pain.

Many authors have regarded low grade fever, mild right upper quadrant pain, small asymptomatic pleural effusions and transient elevation of liver functions following hepatic RFA. In reports reviewed, other minor complications included intra or peri hepatic abscess, minor hemorrhage, ascites, myoglobinuria and thrombocytopenia [28]. In the early studies of hepatic RFA, full thickness skin burns at the grounding pad sites were noted rarely and it was considered a major complication.

Another complication which deserves discussion is percutaneus ablation needle track tumour seeding but both these complications were not met in the present study.

Only one patient developed pneumothorax due to ablation of Sub-diaphragmatic tumour and another 2 patients developed ascites within the first week post ablation.

Conclusion: Radiofrequency thermal ablation is a technology that can be applied to unresectable hepatic tumours without significant morbidity when patients and treatment approach are chosen carefully.

5. References

[1] Llovet J, Fuster J and Bruix J of Barcelona Clinic Liver Cancer Group. The Barcelona Approach: Diagnosis, staging and treatment of hepatocellular carcinoma. Liver Transplantation 2004; 10:suppl.1 S115-120.

[2] Sherlock S and Dooley J. Malignant liver tumours. In Sherlock and Dooley, Diseases of the Liver and Biliary system, 11th edition, 2002; Oxford, Blackwell Scientific Publications, P. 537-561.

[3] Colombo M. Screening for cancer in viral hepatitis 2001; Clin Liver Dis; 5:109.

[4] Hillebrand D and Sandowski S. Hepatobiliary disease. In clinics in family practice 2002; Volume 2, number I.W.B Saunders Company.

[5] Rossi S, Buscarini E, Garbagnati F et al. Percutaneous treatment of small hepatic tumours by an expandable RF needle electrode. AJR Am J Roentegenol 1998; 170:1015-1022.

[6] Buscarini L, Buscarini E, Di Stasi M, et al. Percutaneous radiofrequency ablation of small hepatocellular carcinoma: long term results. Eur Radiol; 2001; 11: 914-21.

[7] Pugh R, Morray-Lyon I, Dowson J et al. Transection of the esophagus for bleeding esophageal varices. Br J Surg 1973; 60: 646-64.

[8] Igarashi H, Aoyagi Y, Suda T, et al. Studies on the correlation among the fucosylation index, concentration of alpha-fetoprotein and des-gamma-carboxy prothrombin as prognostic indicators in hepatocellular carcinoma. Hepatol Res. 2003 ; 27:280-288.

[9] El-zayadi A, Abaza H, Shawky S et al. Prevalence and epidemiological features of hepatocellular carcinoma in Egypt, a single center experience. Hepatology Research 2001; 19:170-179.

[10] Marrero J. Hepatocellular carcinoma. Curr Opin Gastroenterol 2003; 19:243-249.

[11] Yates S, Hafez M, Beld M et al. Hepatocellular carcinoma in Egyptians with and without history of hepatitis B virus infection: association with hepatitis C virus infection but not with HCV RNA level. Am J Trop Med Hyg 1999; 60:714-720.

[12] Edamoto Y, Tani M, Kurata T et al. Hepatitis C and B virus infections in hepatocellular carcinoma. Cancer 1996; 77: 1787-1791.
[13] Llovet JM, Burroughs A, Bruix J. Hepatocellular carcinoma. Lancet 2003; 362:1907-1917.
[14] Bruix J, Sherman M, Llovet JM, et al. for the EASL panel of experts on HCC. Clinical management of hepatocellular, conclusions of the Barcelona-2000 EASL conference. J Hepatol 2001; 35:421-430.
[15] Shi ML, Chun JL, Chen CL, et al. Radiofrequency ablation improves prognosis compared with ethanol injection for hepatocellular carcinoma less than 4cm. gastroenterology 2004; 127:1714-1723.
[16] Livraghi J. Radiofrequency ablation, PEIT and TACE for hepatocellular carcinoma. J Hepatobiliary Pancreat Surgery 2003; 10:67-76.
[17] Chen MH, Yang W, Yan K et al. Treatment efficacy of radiofrequency ablation of 338 patients with hepatic malignant tumours and the relevant complications. World J Gastroenterol 2005 ; 11: 6395-6401.
[18] Sala M, Llovet J, Vilana R et al. Initial response to percutaneous ablation predicts survival in patients with hepatocellular carcinoma. Hepatology 2004; 40: 1352-1360.
[19] Lencioni R, Pinto F, Armillotta N et al. Long term results of percutaneous ethanol injection therapy for hepatocellular carcinoma in cirrhosis: an European experience. Eur Radiol 1997; 7:514-519.
[20] Pompili M, Rapaccini G, Covino M et al. Prognostic factors for survival in patients with compensated cirrhosis and small hepatocellular carcinoma after percutaneous ethanol injection therapy. Cancer, 2001; 92: 126-135.
[20] Hasagawa S, Yamasaki N, Hiwaki T et al. Factors that predict intrahepatic recurrence of hepatocellular carcinoma in 81 patient initially treated by percutaneous ethanol injection. Cancer 1999; 86: 1682-1690.
[21] Goldberg S, Charboneau J, Dodd G III et al. Image guided tumours ablation proposal standardization of terms and reporting criteria. Radiology 2003; 228:335-345.
[22] Kojiro M. Focus on dysplastic nodules and early hepatocellular carcinoma: an Eastern point of view. Liver Transpl 2004; 10:S3-S8.
[23] Shiina S, Teratani T, Obi S, et al. A randomized controlled trial of radiofrequency ablation with ethanol injection for small hepatocellular carcinoma. Gastroenterology 2005; 129:122-30.
[24] Lencioni R, Allgaier H, Cioni D, et al. Small hepatocellular carcinoma in cirrhosis: randomized comparison of radiofrequency thermal ablation versus percutaneous ethanol injection. Radiology 2003; 228:235-240.
[25] Lin SM, Lin CJ, Lin CC et al. Radiofrequency ablation improves prognosis compared with ethanol injection for hepatocellular carcinoma < or =4cm. Gastroenterology 2004; 127:1714-1723.
[26] Lin SM, Lin CJ, Lin CC et al. Randomized controlled trial comparing radiofrequency thermal ablation, percutaneous ethanol injection and percutaneous acetic acid injection to treat hepatocellular carcinoma of 3cm or less. Gut 2005; 54:1151-1156.
[27] Mulier S, Mulier P, Ni Y et al. Complications of radiofrequency coagulation of liver tumours. Br J Surg 200; 89: 1206-1222.

[28] Scaife C and Curley S. Complications, local recurrence and survival rates after radiofrequency ablation for hepatic malignancies. Surg Omcol Clin N Am 2003; 12:243-255

8

Drugs and Toxins Effects on the Liver

Piero Luigi Almasio, Anna Licata and Claudia Randazzo
University of Palermo,
Italy

1. Introduction

Drug induced hepatotoxicity can be defined as a liver injury caused by drug or herbal medicines leading to liver test abnormalities or to a liver dysfunction with a reasonable exclusion of the other competing aetiologies. The liver has a central function in the metabolism of the xenobiotics, and as a result it may be susceptible to its toxic or idiosyncratic effects. While the overall incidence of drug induced liver injury (DILI) is infrequent (1 in 10.000 to 100.000 persons exposed), the impact is significant in the general population, with broad implications for patients, physicians, pharmaceutical industries and governmental regulatory agencies. DILI is the principle reason for the termination in clinical trials and the most frequent adverse event leads to drug non approvals, withdrawals or to a restriction of prescription drug use after an initial approval and post-marketing regulatory decisions. DILI has been shown to have a dose-dependent component. However, most of the cases of DILI are due to idiosyncratic reactions: over 1000 drugs and herbal products have been associated with idiosyncratic hepatotoxicity. It is difficult to establish a diagnosis of DILI. In fact, there is no single pathognomonic test to establish that a given drug in a given subject is the cause of liver injury. Furthermore, the clinical presentation of DILI may considerably vary. It can mimic other known forms of acute and chronic liver diseases and the severity may range from asymptomatic elevations of hepatic enzymes to fulminant hepatic failure. Because of these factors, a diagnosis of DILI is frequently delayed or may be entirely missed. So, the study of DILI is confounded by the heterogeneity of its clinical presentation and by the course of the injury, the delay in establishing diagnosis as it requires exclusion of other causes of liver injury, the lack of standardized criteria or specific 'gold standard' diagnostic tests and underreporting of cases of DILI or their final outcomes. The aim of this chapter is to provide a review and an update of DILI.

2. Epidemiology

Internationally, the data on the true incidence of DILI in the general population remain unknown because of the several methodological limitations of the reporting systems. Most of the epidemiological studies are retrospective and lack standardized diagnostic work-up to exclude other potential causes of the liver injury. Moreover, most studies originate from tertiary referral centres and suffer from selection bias. The underreporting of adverse drug reactions is well known and DILI is not an exception. The number of included patients in most of the clinical drug trials is less than 10.000 and hepatotoxicity has been mostly detected in the post-marketing phase. According to reporting systems, the incidence in the general population varies between 1.27 per 100.000 person a year in rural England to 2.4 in Spain and Sweden. Among medical inpatients, the incidence is 1.4 %, whereas in an outpatient setting it is 0.014 % for patient a year. In the United States (USA), approximately 2000 the cases of acute liver failure (ALF) occur annually and drugs account for over 50% of them (39% are due to acetaminophen, 13% are idiosyncratic reactions due to other medications). Drugs account for 2-5% of cases of patients hospitalized with jaundice and approximately 10% of all the cases of acute hepatitis. However, these numbers are likely underestimated. The epidemiology of DILI is influenced by geographic and cultural factors. In Western countries, the majority of cases are associated with antibiotics and psychotropic agents. In the USA, for instance, amoxicillin/clavulanate, isoniazid, nitrofurantoin and fluoroquinolones are the most frequent causes of DILI. In Asian countries, herbal and dietary supplements rather than conventional medications are often the most common causes of DILI; herbals/dietary supplements currently represent less than 10% of the cases of DILI in Western countries, although this proportion seems to increase. In the last few years, the USA Food and Drug Administration (FDA) have withdrawn two drugs from the market for causing severe liver injury: bromfenac and troglitazone. Bromfenac, a non-steroidal anti-inflammatory drug (NSAID), was introduced in 1997 as a short-term analgesic for orthopedic patients. Although approved for a dosing period of less than 10 days, patients used it for longer periods. This resulted in more than 50 cases of severe hepatic injury, and the drug had to be withdrawn in 1998. Troglitazone is a thiazolidinedione and was approved in 1997 as an antidiabetic agent. Over 3 years, more than 90 cases of hepatotoxicity were reported, which resulted in a withdrawal of this drug. Kava kava, an herb used for anxiety, was reported as being hepatotoxic and was withdrawn from the German market. The FDA has also issued a warning in this country. This demonstrates the importance of a post-marketing surveillance to identify reactions that are not reported or are underreported in drug trials. Pemoline, used for attention deficit disorder and narcolepsy is no longer available in the USA. The FDA concluded that the overall risk of liver toxicity from pemoline outweighs the benefits. Other drugs having significant use limitations because of their hepatotoxic effects are felbamate, an antiepileptic used for complex partial seizures; zileuton, indicated for asthma; tolcapone, used for Parkinson's disease; trovafloxacin, an antibiotic; benoxaprofen, a NSAID and tienilic acid, a diuretic.

3. Mechanism of hepatotoxicity

The liver is the principal organ for metabolism and elimination of many drugs. The majority of oral drugs and xenobiotics are lipophilic and water-insoluble, enabling easy absorption across cell intestinal membranes. They are rendered hydrophilic via hepatic metabolism and thus more easily excreted. Exogenous products are metabolized in the liver mainly through phase I and II reactions. The products are then excreted on either the canalicular and sinusoidal membranes (phase III reactions). During phase I metabolism, polar groups are added to lipophilic molecules by oxidation, reduction or hydrolysis to increase water-solubility. This group of reactions is catalyzed by a super family of enzymes located in the smooth endoplasmic reticulum, known as cytochrome P450 (mixed function oxidases). These membrane-bound hemoproteins carry out reactions in concert with nicotinamide adenine dinucleotid phosphate (NADPH) as a source of electrons, so they can generate toxic electrophilic chemicals and free radicals. Following phase I metabolism, most compounds are still insufficiently hydrophilic for excretion and require further processing. Phase II reactions result in the formation of readily excretable, nontoxic substances. The drug or its metabolite are conjugated in cytosol to a large water-soluble polar group, such as glutathione (GSH), glucuronic acid, sulfate, glucuronide. The enzymes responsible for this so-called phase II metabolism are glucuronosyl transferases, sulfotransferases and GSH transferases. Phase III reactions lead to the transport of drugs and metabolites out of hepatocytes. Biliary excretion is mediated by ATP-dependent transporters located in the bile canaliculi. Altered activity of these transporters can lead to hepatotoxicity. Genetic polymorphisms or environmental factors, such as concomitant drugs and alcohol, can account for differences in phase I, II and III drug metabolism among individuals and may be determinants of the susceptibility to DILI by influencing the hepatic exposure to toxic metabolites.

3.1 Mechanisms of injury

The drugs can directly have an effect on the cellular biochemistry or elicit an immune reaction. In most of the instances, the bioactivation of drug to chemically reactive metabolites or free radicals promote some chemical reactions (i.e. depletion of reduced glutathione and/or covalent bind intracellular macromolecules) leading to their changes. The reactive metabolites may induce the mitochondrial dysfunction resulting in a decrease in ATP levels; the consequential disassembly of the actin fibrils on the surface of the hepatocyte causes blebs and rupture of the membrane. Furthermore, toxic metabolites influence the transport of proteins through the canalicular membrane with the interruption of the bile flow. The stoppage of the transport pumps such as a multidrug resistance (MDR)-associated protein 3 prevents the excretion of bilirubin, causing cholestasis. Alternatively, the drugs/metabolites have the capacity to initiate immunological reactions, including both innate and adaptive immune responses. Hepatocyte stress and/or damage could result in the activation of the innate immune system. Natural killer (NK)-NKT cells in the liver modulate the innate immune response by secreting interferon (IFN)-gamma, interleukin (IL)-4, and so directly killing the cells by FasL expression. Kupffer cells, NK and NKT cells contribute to the progression of liver injury by producing pro-inflammatory mediators such as cytokines, chemokines, reactive oxygen intermediates and reactive nitrogen intermediates. These pro-inflammatory mediators can be directly cytotoxic (e.g., hydrogen peroxide, nitric oxide, peroxynitrite) and degrade the extracellular matrix (e.g., collagenase, elastase); furthermore they promote a cell adhesion and infiltration (e.g., IL-1, tumor necrosis factor-alpha, chemokines). In addition, the adaptive immune system is activated and involved in the pathogenesis of the liver injury. The reactive metabolite may covalently bind to or alter the liver proteins, such as cytochrome P450 enzymes, activating cytotoxic T cells and cytokines (immune-mediated injury). The mechanism of the immune-mediated drug reaction is not clear, but it may involve a hapten-like action. Generally, the low-molecular-weight organic chemicals are not immunogenic, but may become such when they are bound to a macromolecule, such as a protein. If a drug metabolite produced by cytochrome P450 is able to act as a hapten, it covalently binds to a liver protein, so it will perceive as foreign by the immune system, resulting in an autoimmune attack on the normal hepatocellular constituents. This hypothesis, however, does not explain many aspects of immune-mediated DILI. For instance, covalent binding (haptenation) is a regular occurrence with drugs, such as halothane, that rarely cause an immune-mediated toxicity. It is possible that a reactive metabolite also has to injure or stress the liver cells, in addition to a modification of a protein, and may cause an immune response. The outcome of the events initiated by toxic metabolites either directly affecting the cellular biochemistry or inducing immune-mediated response is the cell death. The mode of the cell death may be apoptosis or necrosis. Apoptosis involves shrinkage, organelles compaction, nuclear condensation and fragmentation of the cell into smaller bodies with the intact plasma membranes. The apoptotic cells are then rapidly removed by phagocytosis. Necrosis is characterized by a cell swelling and a membrane lysis with a release of the cytoplasmic contents. Apoptosis generally represents the activation of an enzyme-mediated autolytic cell disposal system, whereas necrosis represents a loss of osmotic regulation. Apoptosis results from the activation of a family of highly conserved proteases (caspases) through a membrane-associated death receptor. The drugs that alter the expression and function of the death receptors disrupt the mitochondrial functions and can be expected to activate apoptosis. If apoptosis occurs at a rate that exceeds the capacity of the phagocytic cells to remove the apoptotic cells, large fields of contiguous cells will swell and lyze. The selection between apoptosis versus necrosis depends on several factors, involving the ATP status. A more severe injury to mitochondria leads to a cellular energetic impaired; as a consequence the osmotic regulation is lost and the cell undergoes to swelling and lysis (necrosis), whereas a less severe injury to mitochondria without a profound ATP depletion can maintain the osmotic regulation and undergo to apoptosis. Hepatocyte death is the main event that leads to a liver injury, although the sinusoidal endothelial cells or the bile duct epithelium may also be targets.

4. Classification

DILI can be classified according to the clinical presentation and the laboratory features, the mechanism of toxicity and/or the histological findings (see section 5).

4.1 Clinical pattern

A consensus defined the liver injury as an increase of more than twice the upper limit of the normal range (ULN) in the levels of serum alanina aminotransferase (ALT) or alkaline phosphatase (Alk P) and total bilirubin, providing that one of these was more than twice the ULN. The Council for International Organizations of Medical Sciences (CIOMS) developed a series of standard designations of DILI and a classification of the injuries. According to these, the pattern distinction is based on the ratio of serum ALT results to Alk P with respect to their ULN. A ratio > 5 denotes an hepatocellular injury and a ratio < 2 denotes a cholestatic injury. Ratios between 2 and 5 are categorized as mixed. In the case in which ALT or Alk P are elevated before the medicine is started, the baseline values can be taken into account instead of the ULN.

	Type of injury		
	Hepatocellular	**Cholestatic**	**Mixed**
ALT	> twice normal	normal	> twice normal
Alk P	normal	> twice normal	> twice normal
ALT/Alk P	≥ 5	≤ 2	2 - 5
	Acetaminophen Allopurinol Amiodarone Amoxicillin-clavulanic acid Baclofen Herbals: kava kava and germander Isoniazid Ketoconazole Lisinopril Losartan Methotrexate NSAIDs Omeprazole Paroxetine Rifampin Risperidone Sertraline Statins Tetracyclines Trazodone Trovafloxacin Valproic acid	Amoxicillin-clavulanic acid Anabolic steroids Chlorpromazine Clopidogrel Oral contraceptives Erythromycins Estrogens Irbesartan Mirtazapine Phenothiazines Terbinafine Tricyclics	Amitriptyline Azathioprine Captopril Carbamazepine Clindamycin Cyproheptadine Enalapril Flutamide Nitrofurantoin Phenobarbital Phenytoin Sulfonamides Trazodone Trimethoprim-sulfamethoxazole Verapamil

Table 1. Pattern of drug-induced liver Injury

4.1.1 Hepatocellular (hepatitis) injury

The majority of drugs produce a hepatocellular pattern of injury. Most of these instances are asymptomatic and mild. When they are severe, patients on average have symptoms similar to those expected in the ones with an acute viral hepatitis. The laboratory features typically included a normal complete blood count, although a mild increase in white count may occur, and a minority of patients with immunoallergic-type reactions will show a peripheral eosinophilia. Given the fact that the underlying pathogenesis involves primarily an apoptosis and/or a necrosis of the hepatocytes, the serum aminotransferases levels are elevated. For most of the drugs producing an idiosyncratic DILI, the degree of elevation of serum aminotransferases is generally less marked than in the cases of intrinsic hepatotoxicity caused by acetaminophen, carbon tetrachloride or other halogenated hydrocarbons. The serum Alk P is generally normal or mildly elevated (less than twice the ULN). Serum total and direct bilirubin are variable. The hepatobiliary imaging shows a normal liver or a diffuse homogeneous hepatomegaly. It is very important the lack of evidence of the dilatation of the biliary tree or cholecystitis especially when patients are jaundiced. The typical findings on liver biopsy, during an acute injury, are variable and greatly dependent upon the causative drug. In most of the instances of a hepatocellular injury a rapid improvement in symptoms, signs and laboratory features can occur when the medication is discontinued.

4.1.2 Cholestatic pattern of injury

The typical manifestations of a cholestatic drug-induced hepatitis are jaundice and itching. The classic laboratory features are the elevations in serum Alk P, which is more than twice the ULN, and in the serum total and direct bilirubin. Serum aminotransferases are normal or only mildly elevated. In general, the hepatobiliary-pancreatic imaging findings show no evidence of the biliary dilatation and of the pancreatic abnormalities. The liver is usually normal or nearly normal. The typical iter of the cholestatic hepatitis is more protracted than in the hepatocellular DILI. In fact, it is not uncommon for signs and laboratory worsening to continue after the drug has been stopped, sometimes for a period of 30-60 days. There is a gradual improvement thereafter, unless the categories of the drugs are re-administered. There are rare instances in which the injury does not resolve but rather goes on to produce chronic liver diseases.

4.1.3 "Mixed" pattern of injury

The 'mixed' pattern, as the name implies, involves hepatocellular and cholestatic manifestations. The usual clinical ones are nausea, anorexia, and vomiting when severe; also jaundice and itching are present. The typical laboratory findings may include serum aminotransferase levels higher than three times the ULN and serum Alk P, total and direct bilirubin being more than twice the ULN. The biopsy features for the two types of injury are also a mixture of characteristics described above. The general course is longer than in the hepatocellular injury, but shorter than in the pure cholestatic DILI.

4.2 Mechanism of toxicity

The toxic hepatocellular injury may be classified into two groups: predictable (intrinsic) and unpredictable (idiosyncratic) reactions. The predictable drug reaction accounts for 80% of all toxicities. Intrinsic hepatotoxins cause predictably a dose-dependent hepatocellular necrosis (higher concentrations cause more liver damage) and which can be reproducible in the animal models. The latent period between the exposure and the onset of the reaction is brief (i.e. hours/days) and varies from person to person. Most cases of DILI hepatotoxicity are related to idiosyncratic reactions. The main characteristic of this type of reaction is the apparent unpredictability of the liver injury in human beings. The effects tend to be species-specific and often cannot be reproduced experimentally on the laboratory animals. There is no a constant relationship between the dose and the occurrence or severity of the drug reaction, and the latent period between the exposure to it and the sensitivity reaction is quite variable. Idiosyncrasy may be either metabolic or immunologic/allergic. In the first case, a covalent binding of drug metabolites to the cellular structures can damage the cellular functions causing the cell death. The immunologic reactions are the hypersensitivity reactions to a specific drug. The immunologic response depends upon the interaction of the drug and its metabolites with the immune system, with a resultant hepatocyte necrosis and apoptosis; this can cause the release of cytokines that can lead to the secondary cell damage or can have immune modulating effects. There is a prompt recurrence of symptoms in response to the drug re-challenge of one or two doses.

5. Histology

Specific histological patterns of liver injury caused by a drug-induced damage are discussed below.

5.1 Acute hepatocellular injury

The landmarks of an acute hepatocellular injury are the portal and the parenchyma inflammation and/or necrosis. By definition, fibrosis is absent. Regenerative features such as binucleate hepatocytes and thick cell plates are common. Prominent Kupffer cells are often present in the sinusoids. The acute hepatocellular injury can result in necrosis affecting single (spotty necrosis) or groups of hepatocytes (confluent necrosis). Hepatocellular necrosis consists of a ballooning degeneration or apoptosis associated with an infiltration of the inflammatory cells and can be zonal or nonzonal, depending upon the offending drug. Zonal necrosis is characteristic of compounds with a dose-dependent toxicity, such as carbon tetrachloride and acetaminophen (zone 3). Isolated necrosis affecting zones 1 and 2 is rare; toxins such as cocaine and ferrous sulfate or phosphorus poisoning typically affect zone 1 (periportal), while beryllium has been implicated in zone 2 necrosis. Nonzonal necrosis is more often seen with compounds that produce an idiosyncratic injury (i.e. phenytoin, methyldopa, isoniazid, and diclofenac).

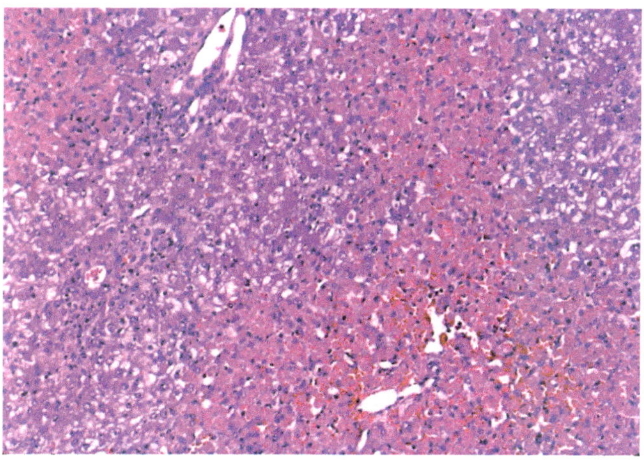

Fig. 1. Acetaminophen toxicity. Hepatocellular necrosis present in a zonal, centrilobular pattern; the inflammatory infiltration is minimal

5.1.1 Fulminant hepatitis

There are three morphological categories related to ALF. Extensive microvesicular steatosis (rare) has been observed with tetracycline and nucleoside analogues such as zidovudine. Necrosis with a marked inflammatory activity is the most common pattern seen in the idiosyncratic reactions. The confluent necrosis involves most of the liver parenchyma (massive/submassive hepatic necrosis) and the mainly implicated drugs are isoniazid, others are antimicrobial agents (sulfonamides, cotrimoxazole, ketoconazole), monoamine oxidase inhibitors and anticonvulsants (phenytoin, valproate). Necrosis with little or no inflammation is seen with acetaminophen, recreational drugs such as cocaine and 3,4-methylenedioxymethylamphetamine (MDMA; ecstasy), industrial organic compounds such as carbon tetrachloride, and some herbal preparations.

5.2 Chronic hepatocellular injury

A progression to chronicity has been reported in 5-10% of DILI and it is higher for the cholestatic/mixed injury pattern and can reveal with many forms. A chronic hepatitis with negative autoimmune markers presents histological features indistinguishable from the chronic viral hepatitis, and a progression to fibrosis can occur. Drugs associated to it include lisinopril, sulfonamide, trazodone and chemotherapeutic agents such as uracil, 5-fluorouracil pro-drug tegafur and tamoxifen. Isolated case reports implicate numerous other drugs including phenytoin and the Chinese herb Jin bu huan. Several drugs and herbs (i.e. minocycline, nitrofurantoin, diclofenac, fenofibrate, phenytoin, germander, statins, ecstasy) can cause a chronic hepatitis that is serologically and morphologically indistinguishable from de novo type I of the autoimmune hepatitis (AIH).

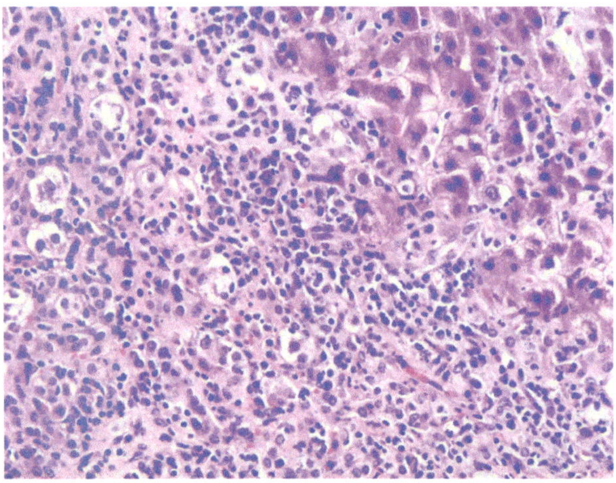

Fig. 2. Minocycline-induced autoimmune hepatitis. Necroinflammatory activity with several plasma cells

The lipofuscin pigment storage in the hepatocytes has been reported with phenothiazines, phenacetin, aminopyrine, and cascara sagrada. An hemosiderin accumulation in the liver cells may result from the excessive iron ingestion or the parenteral iron. Phospholipidosis is rare. It may develop acutely, but it is more commonly seen after a prolonged administration of the offending agent. This condition has been described in the patients taking amiodarone, amitriptyline, trimethoprim-sulfamethoxazole, chloroquine. The hepatocytes can be seen as foamy as a consequence of phospholipid accumulation in the lysosomes. These abnormal, lamellated lysosomes are visible through the electron microscopy (Figure 3).

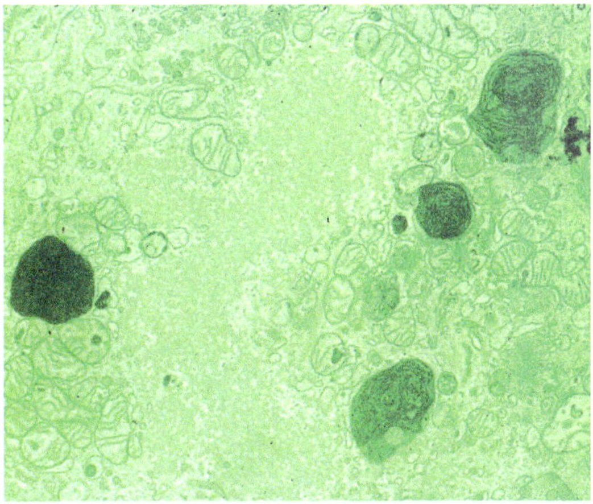

Fig. 3. Histological pattern of hepatic phospholipidosis. Presence of lysosomal inclusion bodies due to an accumulation of amiodarone

5.3 Acute cholestasis

Two forms of this histological pattern of injury can be observed. Canalicular (bland or non-inflammatory) cholestasis is characterized by bile plugs in the hepatocytes or canaliculi and it is more prominent in zone 3. Inflammation and hepatocellular injuries are not detected. Drugs causing this type of injury interfere with the hepatocyte secretion of the bile components through the bile salt excretory protein (BSEP). The degree of cholestasis is characteristic for each drug; typical examples are the anabolic steroids (Figure 4) and the oral contraceptives. Hepatocanalicular (cholangiolitic or inflammatory) cholestasis is accompanied by a portal inflammation and by only a slight hepatocytes injury, usually localized in the zones of the cholestasis. Cholestatic hepatitis is the classic pattern seen with macrolide antibiotics such as erythromycin (figure 5) and the antipsychotic agent chlorpromazine. This pattern manifests as a mixed-type injury on the liver biochemical tests.

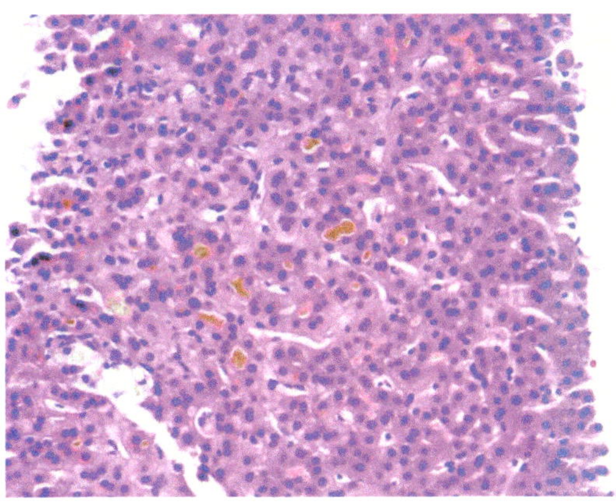

Fig. 4. Anabolic-steroid-induced cholestasis. Bile plugs present in the hepatocytes and canaliculi without inflammation or hepatocellular damage

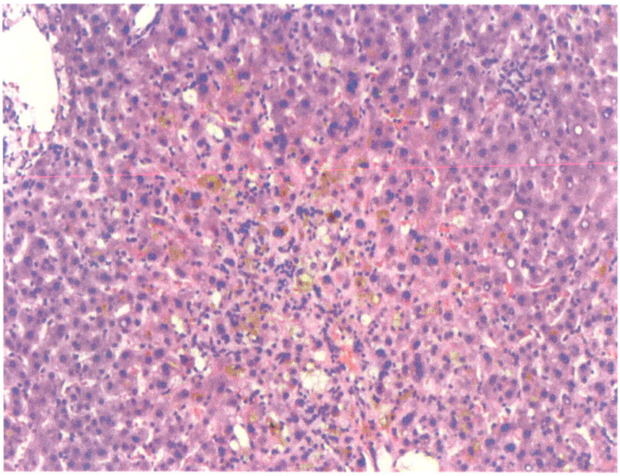

Fig. 5. Erythromycin-induced cholestatic hepatitis. Features similar to an acute hepatitis, as well as bile plugs in the hepatocytes and canaliculi

5.4 Chronic cholestasis and ductopenia

Drugs causing long-lasting cholestasis (longer than 3 months) and ductopenia include antibiotics (amoxicillin-clavulanic acid, flucloxacillin), antifungals (terbinafine), amiodarone (Figure 6). If the disease persists for a few months or further, it can occur a loss of bile ducts and an overt ductopenia termed "vanishing bile duct syndrome". A persistent inflammation and a bile ductular reaction may also be present. A vanishing bile duct syndrome can be triggered by anticonvulsants (carbamazepine, zonisamide), antipsychotics (chlorpromazine, sulpiride), NSAIDs (ibuprofen, tenoxicam) and antibiotics (amoxicillin, flucloxacillin, clindamycin, trimethoprim-sulfamethoxazole).

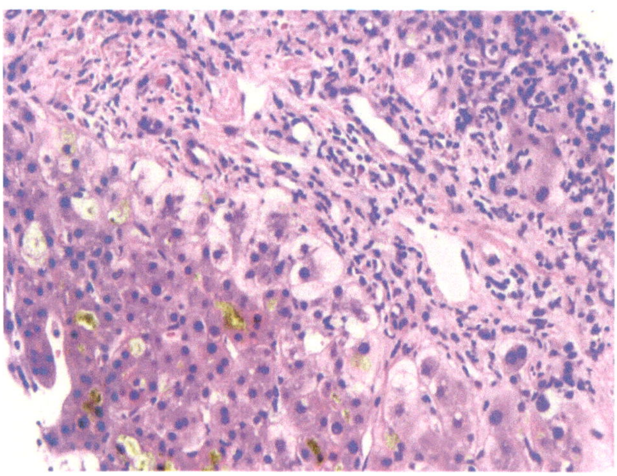

Fig. 6. Prolonged cholestasis. Persistence of canalicular bile plugs associated with a feathery degeneration of the periportal hepatocytes

5.5 Granulomatous hepatitis

At least 60 drugs have been selected to cause hepatic non-caseating granulomas, for instance allopurinol, amiodarone, diazepam, diltiazem, isoniazid, sulfonamides and sulfonylureas. Unlike in the primary biliary cirrhosis, the granulomas are habitually located in the periportal and portal tracts. They can be associated with a hepatocellular injury (granulomatous hepatitis) or cholestasis, but are more often silent and it is usually transient. The term fibrin-ring granuloma has been used for small granulomas characterized by a ring of fibrin around a central fat vacuole. Epithelioid histiocytes are present around the ring of fibrin. Fibrin-ring granulomas have been described with allopurinol, BCG vaccination and intravescical therapy for carcinoma. Gold salts may lead to the formation of lipogranulomas with black pigments.

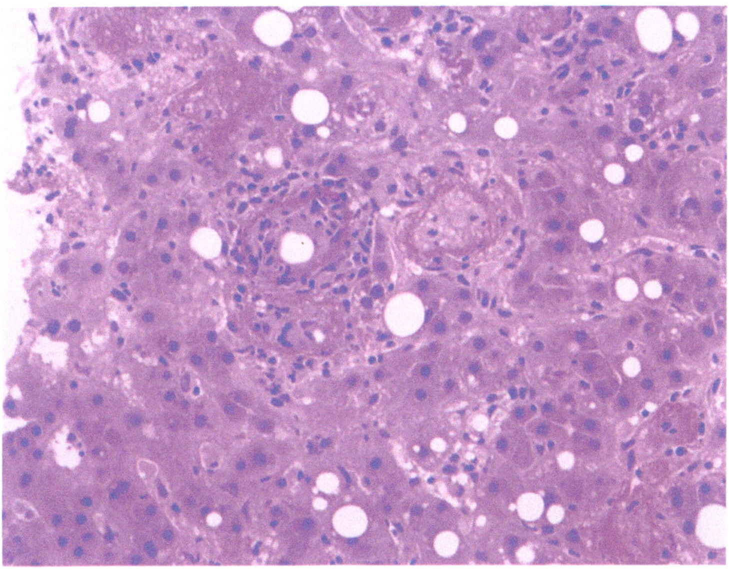

Fig. 7. Fibrin-ring granulomas. Fat vacuole surrounded by a ring of fibrin and epithelioid cells

5.6 Steatosis and steatohepatitis

Steatosis secondary to drug toxicity may be in the form of medium-sized and large droplets (macrovesicular) or small droplets (microvesicular). The term ''large droplet fat'' is used when at least half of the hepatocyte cytoplasm is full of a single lipid vacuole, while multiple lipid vacuoles are seen in the small droplet fat. Drugs that can cause macrovesicular steatosis include corticosteroids, methotrexate, nifedipine, parenteral nutrition, gold, NSAIDs (ibuprofen, indomethacin, sulindac), antihypertensives (metoprolol) and chemotherapeutic agents (5-fluorouracil, cisplatin, tamoxifen). An exclusive or predominant microvesicular steatosis is the result of mitochondrial injury and is observed with aspirin (Reye's syndrome), cocaine, high doses of tetracycline, valproic acid and zidovudine. By definition, steatohepatitis is characterized by steatosis, lobular inflammation and hepatocellular ballooning (with or without the acidophil bodies or Mallory hyaline) or pericellular fibrosis. A few drugs (particularly amiodarone and irinotecan) play a direct aetiological role in the steatohepatitis. Many other drugs exacerbate or precipitate steatohepatitis in the presence of other risk factors such as obesity and diabetes.

5.7 Vascular lesions

The drug-induced hepatic vascular disease is uncommon but can have several manifestations. Vascular lesions result from the injury of the endothelium. The hepatic sinusoidal obstruction syndrome (veno-occlusive disease) is due to the occlusion of the terminal hepatic venules and sinusoids rather than the hepatic veins and inferior vena cava that manifests histologically as an endothelial swelling and thrombosis. The resultant venous outflow obstruction leads to a sinusoidal dilatation, congestion, hepatocellular necrosis, resulting in centrilobular fibrosis. Cytotoxic/chemotherapeutic drugs (i.e. oxaliplatin) can cause injury to the sinusoidal endothelial and hepatic stellate cells. Other drugs associated with veno-occlusive diseases include pyrrolizidine alkaloids (found in herbal remedies), azathioprine, mercaptopurine, vitamin A, tetracycline.

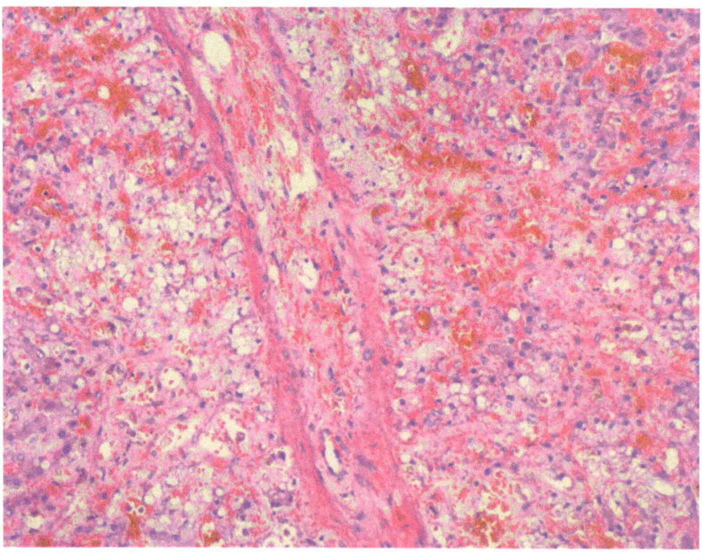

Fig. 8. Veno-occlusive disease. Endothelial injury in small hepatic venules leading to sinusoidal dilatation and congestion.

Peliosis is rare and is characterized by multiple, small, dilated blood-filled cavities without an endothelial coating in the hepatic parenchyma. It can be caused by several drugs including anabolic steroids, arsenic, azathioprine, mercaptopurine, danazol, tamoxifen, vitamin A and hydroxyurea. Lesions may resolve with a discontinuation of the offending agent. The hepatic venous outflow obstruction is a rare complication that may arise from a drug-induced thrombosis of the hepatic veins or of the inferior vena cava. The most well-known drugs associated with this syndrome are the oral contraceptives and dacarbazine. Clinically it manifests as the Budd-Chiari syndrome.

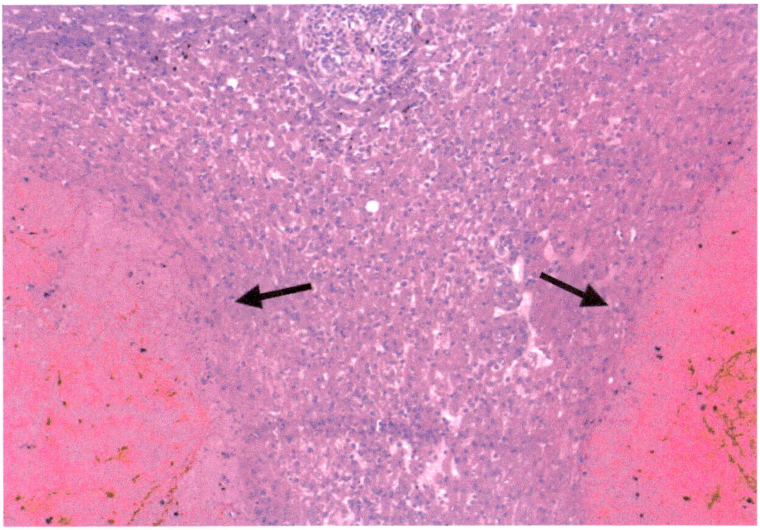

Fig. 9. Peliosis. Hepatic parenchyma containing blood-filled cavities without an endothelial lining

6. Diagnostic elements

DILI is a diagnosis of exclusion that relies on multiple elements in the medical history, presentation, laboratory results.

6.1 Time to onset

The time to onset (latency) is evaluated from the first day on which the suspected drug(s) was taken to the day on which the symptoms or the laboratory test abnormalities are manifested. A definition of the exposure to the drug and the hepatic toxicity is not always clear because the initial symptoms can be vague and are poorly remembered; the onset of the symptoms can occur days or weeks after the medication is stopped; laboratory tests are obtained at an arbitrary time. Furthermore, the drug can be stopped and started or given in several courses or in different doses and patients may take multiple medications making the identification of a single offending agent difficult.

6.2 Clinical and laboratory features

The clinical presentation varies from the asymptomatic mild liver test abnormalities to a symptomatic acute liver disease. Many drugs can induce asymptomatic high levels of the liver enzymes without producing an overt clinical disease. DILI is generally considered subclinical if the serum ALT is < 3 times the ULN; it has been described with antibiotics, antidepressants, lipid-lowering drugs, sulfonamides, salicylates, sulfonylureas and quinidine, generally in fewer than 5-10% of individuals. About 50% of patients receiving tacrine for Alzheimer's disease have shown high ALT levels. This tolerance is also observed in 25-50% of the patients taking methyldopa or phenytoin, and it is especially well described with isoniazid. When symptomatic, DILI shows a high variability and symptoms as fatigue, nausea, abdominal pain, fever, dark urine, jaundice and itching can be present. Rash, facial edema and lymphadenopathy, along with eosinophilia or atypical lymphocytosis, are important early features that, when present, point to a hypersensitivity and are typical for aromatic anticonvulsants, sulfonamides and allopurinol. Laboratory tests for patients to be made include a complete blood cell count, an hepatic and renal function, a total protein and an electrophoresis, coagulative parameters and urinalysis. Hepatitis B surface antigen, hepatitis C and hepatitis A serology should be performed to exclude an infectious aetiology. Anti nuclear antibodies (ANA) and anti smooth muscle antibodies (SMA) tests may help in the cases of a possible AIH.

6.3 De- challenge

The course of the liver injury after the ending of the suspected drug(s) is considered the de-challenge. If a medication causes DILI, its withdrawal should be followed by a clinical improvement; however, the liver injury may continue to worsen a few weeks after the causative toxic agent is stopped.

6.4 Risk factors

- Age: the adults are generally more susceptible to hepatotoxicity than children. Elderly people are at a higher risk of a hepatic injury because of the decreased clearance, the drug-to-drug interactions, the reduced hepatic blood flow, the variation of the drug binding and of the lower hepatic volume. Older age appears to be an important risk factor for the development of the hepatic injury in response to isoniazid, but younger age appears significant for the valproate-induced liver injury and for the aspirin-induced Reye's syndrome.
- Sex: the women may be more likely to develop the hepatic injury from medications, but they are also more likely to take them.
- Race: the Blacks or African American subjects appear to be more susceptible to develop anticonvulsant hypersensitivities and liver injuries, whereas Caucasian whites appear to be at an increased risk for developing a flucloxacillin-related liver injury.
- Genetic: the most important susceptibility factor for hepatotoxicity is a genetic variability. Genetic polymorphisms have a strong influence on drug metabolism, however, are largely medication-specific. For example, polymorphism of the *N*-acetyltransferase 2 (NAT-2) gene differentiates fast from slow acetylators; the latter have increased their susceptibility to isoniazid toxicity. The human leukocyte antigen (HLA)-B*5701 genotype is the major determinant of abacavir and flucloxacillin hypersensitivity reactions. Estrogen-induced cholestasis is closely linked to variants in adenosine triphosphate–binding cassette B11 (bile salt export pump), and valproate toxicity is closely linked to the variants of mitochondrial polymerase gamma (POLG1). None of these factors is, however, absolute, and hepatotoxicity can occur in patients without these specific markers.
- Alcohol: it causes depletion of glutathione (hepatoprotective) stores that make the person more susceptible to toxicity caused by drugs.
- Obesity and malnutrition: they are susceptibility factors, particularly in the case of acetaminophen, which, when used in malnourished patients, may deplete glutathione.

- Others: pregnancy, concomitantly administered medications and an history of drug reactions also increase susceptibility. Long-acting drugs may cause more injury than shorter-acting drugs. Pre-existing liver diseases and coexisting illnesses may have a greater effect on the ability of the patient to recover from the liver injury than on the likelihood that it will develop.

6.5 Exclusion of other causes of a liver injury

Most of the causality instruments for assessing DILI include results of virological, serological and radiological tests. A number of scales to codify causality of drug toxicity into objective criteria have been developed. Examples include the CIOMS Roussel-Uclaf causality assessment method (RUCAM) scale and the Maria & Victorino (M & V) clinical scale. However, they do not address all risk factors in all patients and none of these scales are used routinely in the clinical practice. A checklist of minimal required elements in the diagnosis of DILI is shown in the table 2.

Patient age (at the time of injury onset) and sex
Implicated drug, herbal or dietary supplement with generic name, dose and regimen of administration
Date on which the agent was started and stopped (or the duration of therapy)
If symptoms are present, the pattern and date of onset (or the time from the beginning of therapy), the types of symptoms
Date of the first abnormal laboratory results indicative of injury (or the time from the beginning of therapy)
Previous history or risk factors of the liver disease
Alcohol use history
Other medical conditions of importance (pertinent negatives being heart failure, shock, sepsis, and parenteral nutrition shortly before the onset of liver injury)
Other medications taken in the 2 months before the onset of the injury
Initial ALT, AST, Alk P, GGT, serum bilirubin value
Prothrombin time or INR
Eosinophils (number/mcL or %) at the onset of the injury or early in the course of the injury
Selected serial ALT (or AST) values (peak values and values demonstrating recovery)
Selected serial Alk P (or GGT) values (peak values and values demonstrating recovery)
Selected serial bilirubin values (peak values and values demonstrating recovery)
Blood test results to exclude other causes of an acute liver disease a. IgM anti-HAV (or negative anti-HAV) b. HBsAg and IgM anti-HBc (or negative anti-HBc) c. Anti-HCV and HCV RNA d. ANA and SMA (and titer if positive)
Imaging of the liver (type and results)
Abbreviations: ANA, antinuclear antibody; anti-HBc, antibody to hepatitis B core antigen; HAV, hepatitis A virus; HBsAg, hepatitis B surface antigen; IgM, immunoglobulin M; SMA, smooth muscle antibody.

Table 2. Elements necessary for reporting cases of DILI

History of previous DILI, exposure to the drug or similar agents
Results of serum ALT, Alk P and total bilirubin before the exposure to the agent or onset of DILI
Weight and height expressed as the body mass index
LDH level at the onset of the injury or early in the course of the injury
CPK level at the onset of the injury or early in the course of the injury
Serum albumin and globulin levels at the onset of the injury or early in the course of the injury
IgG level at the onset of the injury or early in the course of the injury
Anti-HEV or HEV RNA
Anti-HIV
IgM anti-CMV or CMV-DNA by PCR
Heterophil antibody or EBV-DNA by PCR
If HBsAg is present, anti-HDV and serial HBV DNA levels
Other autoantibody results such as AMA and anti-LKM
Date of resolution of the symptoms or duration of the symptoms
Liver biopsy results
Results of the re-exposure or challenge
Abbreviations: AMA, antimitochondrial antibody; CMV, cytomegalovirus; CPK, creatinine phosphokinase; EBV, Epstein-Barr virus; ERCP, endoscopic retrograde cholangiopancreatography; HBsAg, hepatitis B surface antigen; HDV, hepatitis D virus; HEV, hepatitis E virus; IgG, immunoglobulin G; IgM, immunoglobulin M; LDH, lactate dehydrogenase; LKM, liver-kidney microsomal; MRCP, magnetic resonance cholangiopancreatography; PCR, polymerase chain reaction

Table 3. Elements not always necessary but supportive of the assessment and helpful in reporting some cases of DILI

6.6 Previous reports of DILI

An important aspect in assessing DILI is whether the drug, herbal/dietary supplement have been previously reported as a causative agent of hepatotoxicity. Except for the most common medication with a characteristic pattern of injury, this information is largely unknown. A proposal was made to classify drugs with respect to their likelihood of causing a liver injury. Thus, agents were placed in five categories based on the number of published cases and case series in the literature: (A, known) > 50 cases, (B, rare) 11 to 50 cases, (C, very rare) 3 to 10 cases, (D, unproven) < 3 cases and (E, not implicated) not convincingly linked to cases of hepatotoxicity; a final category (X, insufficient information) is necessary for those agents that have not been adequately assessed (i.e. new drugs) or are too rarely used to judge their potential for hepatotoxicity.

6.7 Re-challenge

Re-challenge is defined as the intentional or inadvertent re-exposure to a drug believed to have caused either a current or a past hepatotoxicity. A positive re-challenge consists of the recurrence of the DILI, usually with a shorter latency and a greater severity. While it remains the gold standard for the diagnosis of a DILI, the re-challenge is not advised. However, a careful re-challenge might be appropriate for some cancer chemotherapeutic agents, antiretroviral or antitubercular medications.

6.8 Liver biopsy

The role of a liver biopsy in the diagnostic work-up of DILI is controversial. Although some histological features may increase the index of suspicion of DILI, there are none which can unequivocally confirm the diagnosis. If the patient demonstrates a rapid improvement in the liver tests following the ending of the drug, a routine liver biopsy is not indicated. If the patient has an underlying liver disease and /or if AIH is suspected despite negative serologies, a liver biopsy can be valuable. A liver biopsy can be helpful when the drug has not been previously implicated causing a liver injury, or when the drug reaction has a very slow regression. However, the impact of identifying some of these unusual histological patterns on management is uncertain and the indication of a liver biopsy depends on the course of the liver injury as mentioned above.

7. Grading severity in DILI

Severity in DILI can be graded as mild, moderate or severe. Most of the severity scales are based on the presence and on the number of symptoms, the height of the liver biochemistry, the presence of signs of a hepatic failure and the ultimate outcome, such as recovery, chronicity or death. In developing a prospective database of cases, Drug-Induced Liver Injury Network (DILIN) established a five-point system for grading severity.

Score	Grade	Definition
1	Mild	Elevations in serum ALT and/or Alk P levels, but the total serum bilirubin level is < 2.5 mg/dL, and INR is < 1.5
2	Moderate	Elevations in serum ALT and/or Alk P levels, and the serum bilirubin level is ≥ 2.5 mg/dL, or INR is ≥ 1.5
3	Moderate-severe	Elevations in serum ALT, Alk P, and bilirubin or INR levels, and hospitalization or ongoing hospitalization is prolonged because of a DILI episode
4	Severe	Elevations in serum ALT and/or Alk P levels, and the total serum bilirubin level is ≥ 2.5 mg/dL, and there is at least one of the following: Hepatic failure (INR ≥ 1.5, ascites, or encephalopathy) Other organ failure believed to be due to a DILI event (i.e., renal or pulmonary)
5	Fatal	Death or liver transplantation from a DILI event

Table 4. Disease severity scales used in the DILIN prospective study

8. Prognosis

The majority of the patients with a symptomatic acute DILI recover completely after the discontinuation of the drug(s). First described by Hy Zimmerman (Zimmerman, 1999), the drug-induced jaundice (total bilirubin > 2.5 mg/dL) was associated with a poor prognosis. This observation called Hy's Law is used by regulatory agencies in the evaluation of the investigational drugs showing potential hepatotoxicity during clinical trials. The outcome is obviously dependent on the severity of the liver impairment at presentation. For example, the prognosis of idiosyncratic DILI patients with ALF, coagulopathy (INR > 1.5) and encephalopathy is usually poor without a liver transplantation. Also patients with a cholestatic DILI have a significant mortality. The prognosis is also dependent on the specific compound involved. For instance, in one series, mortality ranged from 40% with a halothane-induced liver injury, whereas all patients with an erythromycin-induced liver injury survived. A longer duration of the therapy before the recognition of DILI and a continuation of the therapy despite a liver dysfunction seems to increase the risk of developing a chronic liver disease. Drugs most frequently associated with chronicity were amoxicillin/clavulanate, bentazepam and atorvastatin. Patients with a cholestatic liver injury develop more frequently a chronic liver injury. Peripheral eosinophilia has been shown to have a prognostic importance, in fact it was extremely rare in fatal DILI cases. Limited data exist on the impact of histology on the clinical outcome. Recently, in a study of patients with a disulfiram-induced liver injury, the hepatic eosinophilic infiltration is associated with a good short-term prognosis, whereas hepatocytes dropout or necrosis with a poor prognosis.

9. Treatment of DILI

Once DILI is suspected, a prompt cessation of drug(s) implicated is obviously the first step in the management. At the onset of the reaction, patients with jaundice and who also have coagulopathy and/or encephalopathy should be hospitalized. It is important to recognize the severity of the liver injury in a patient with jaundice and coagulopathy before the development of the encephalopathy. Encephalopathy is a very late sign and after its development, a rapid deterioration is often observed. Few specific therapies have been shown to be beneficial in clinical trials. Two exceptions are the use of N-acetylcysteine for acetaminophen toxicity and L-carnitine for cases of valproic acid overdose. Corticosteroids are of unproven benefit for most forms of drug hepatotoxicity, although they may have a role in the case of a hypersensitivity syndrome, in the AIH (if it is considered to be induced by drugs) and in patients with a severe or progressive liver injury, but data supporting their safety and efficacy are lacking. Patients should be followed by serial biochemical measurements.

10. Conclusion

DILI is a rare but important complication that will continue to be problematic with the new drugs coming onto the market. Recent data highlight antibiotics, central nervous system agents, herbal/dietary supplements and immunomodulatory drugs as the most common causes of DILI in the USA. The limitations of the available instruments to measure causality in DILI may be minimized by the use of expert panel opinions, while biomarkers of DILI have not been discovered yet. It is the health care system, including the physician's responsibility to monitor and report drug-induced hepatotoxicity. A systematic approach should be taken to determine the aetiology of hepatotoxicity and to remove the offending agent. New therapies for the drug-induced acute liver failure are needed.

11. References

Andrade RJ et al. (2005). Drug-induced liver injury: an analysis of 461 incidences submitted to the Spanish registry over a 10-year period. *Gastroenterology*, Vol. 129, pp. 512–521

Benichou C. (1990). Criteria of drug-induced liver disorders. Report of an international consensus meeting. J *Hepatol*, Vol. 11, pp. 272–276

Bjornsson E & Olsson R. (2005). Outcome and prognostic markers in severe drug-induced liver disease. *Hepatology*, Vol. 42, pp. 481–489

Björnsson E. (2006). Drug-induced liver injury: Hy's rule revisited. *Clin Pharmacol Ther*, Vol. 79, pp. 521

Bohan TP et al. (2001). Effect of L-carnitine treatment for valproate-induced hepatotoxicity. *Neurology*, Vol. 56, pp. 1405

Chitturi S & George J. (2002). Hepatotoxicity of commonly used drugs: nonsteroidal anti-inflammatory drugs, antihypertensives, antidiabetic agents, anticonvulsants, lipid-lowering agents, psychotropic drugs. *Semin Liver Dis*, Vol. 22, pp. 169

Dorne JL et al. (2005). Human variability in xenobiotic metabolism and pathway-related uncertainty factors for chemical risk assessment: a review. *Food Chem Toxicol*, Vol. 43, pp. 203

Farrell GC. (2002). Drugs and steatohepatitis. *Semin Liver Dis*, Vol. 22, pp. 185

Kaplowitz N. (2002). Biochemical and cellular mechanisms of toxic liver injury. *Semin Liver Dis*, Vol. 22, pp. 137

Knowles SR et al. (2000). Idiosyncratic drug reactions: the reactive metabolite syndromes. *Lancet* , Vol. 356, pp. 1587

Larrey D & Pageaux GP. (1997) Genetic predisposition to drug-induced hepatotoxicity. J *Hepatol*, Vol. 26, Suppl 2, pp. 12

Liu ZX & Kaplowitz N. (2002). Immune-mediated drug-induced liver disease. *Clin Liver Dis*, Vol. 6, pp. 755

Meier Y et al. (2005). Incidence of drug-induced liver injury in medical inpatients. *Eur J Clin Pharmacol*, Vol. 61, pp. 135

Navaro V. Hepatic adverse event nomenclature document. Available at: http://www.fda.gov/cder/livertox/presentations2005/Vic_Navaro.ppt

Park BK et al. (1995). The role of cytochrome P450 enzymes in hepatic and extrahepatic human drug toxicity. *Pharmacol Ther*, Vol. 68, pp. 385

Pauli-Magnus C & Meier, PJ. (2006). Hepatobiliary transporters and drug-induced cholestasis. *Hepatology*, Vol. 44, pp. 778

Senior R. (2007). Drug hepatotoxicity from regulatory perspective. *Clin Liver Dis*, Vol. 11, pp. 507–524

Seeff LB. (2006). Drug-induced liver injury: summary of a single topic clinical research conference. *Hepatology*, Vol. 43, pp. 618–631

Zafrani ES et al. (1983). Drug-induced vascular lesions of the liver. *Arch Intern Med*, Vol. 143, pp. 495

Zimmerman H. (1999). *Hepatotoxicity the adverse effects of drugs and other chemicals on the liver.* Lippincott, Williams & Wilkins, Philadelphia

Uetrecht J. (2009). Immune-mediated adverse drug reactions. *Chem Res Toxicol*, Vol. 22, pp. 24

USFDA Guidance for Industry. Drug-Induced Liver Injury: Premarketing Clinical Evaluation, 7507dft.htm, Available from http://www.fda.gov/cder/guidance

9

Percutaneous Liver Fiducial Implants: Techniques, Materials and Complications

David Roberge and Tatiana Cabrera
McGill University Health Centre, Canada

1. Introduction

Stereotactic body radiation therapy (SBRT) is a radiotherapy technique that utilizes precise targeting to deliver high doses of tumoricidal radiation in the course of a small number of treatment sessions. SBRT is used to treat a variety of primary and metastatic tumours of the lung, liver, pancreas, kidney, spine and prostate. These treatments are already standard for medically inoperable early lung cancer and indications are evolving for other disease sites.

In SBRT of liver lesions (Dawood *et al.*, 2009; Lo *et al.*, 2010), tumour-targeting accuracy is crucial given the radiosensitive nature of the liver, frequent proximity of the tumour to the small bowel and significant movement of the liver with breathing. Reduction of normal tissue irradiation requires the radiation to be image-guided (as opposed to relying on skin marks or body casts). This image-guidance is typically accomplished through visualization of a surrogate to the tumour. The surrogate can be the whole liver, the diaphragm or an implanted marker (Wunderink *et al.*, 2010).

Implanted markers have the advantage of being visible on planar x-ray images and fluoroscopy loops. If large enough, they can also be seen on images produced with the treatment beam. The details of the implementation of fiducial imaging vary with different radiotherapy devices but typically images of the fiducials are correlated to the position of the chest wall at different points in the breathing cycles. This gives the user knowledge of the displacement of the tumour (assumed to be at a fixed distance from the fiducials). One can then choose to turn on the beam in a specific phase of the breathing cycle or have the radiation delivery device track the movement of the tumour.

As an example, the Cyberknife system acquires up to 15 pairs of stereoscopic x-rays just before treatment. Fiducials are automatically detected by the system's image analysis software. The 3D position of the fiducials is then correlated to the position of chest wall as recorded by the movement of 3 lights on the patient's chest. The robot on which the radiation source is mounted can then use the model correlating chest wall motion and fiducial motion to mimic the movement of the tumour while the patient breathes (Figure 1). In this process, there is continuous monitoring (via cameras) of the chest wall but only intermittently imaging of the fiducials with stereoscopic x-rays. These additional x-rays are used to verify and update the correlation model.

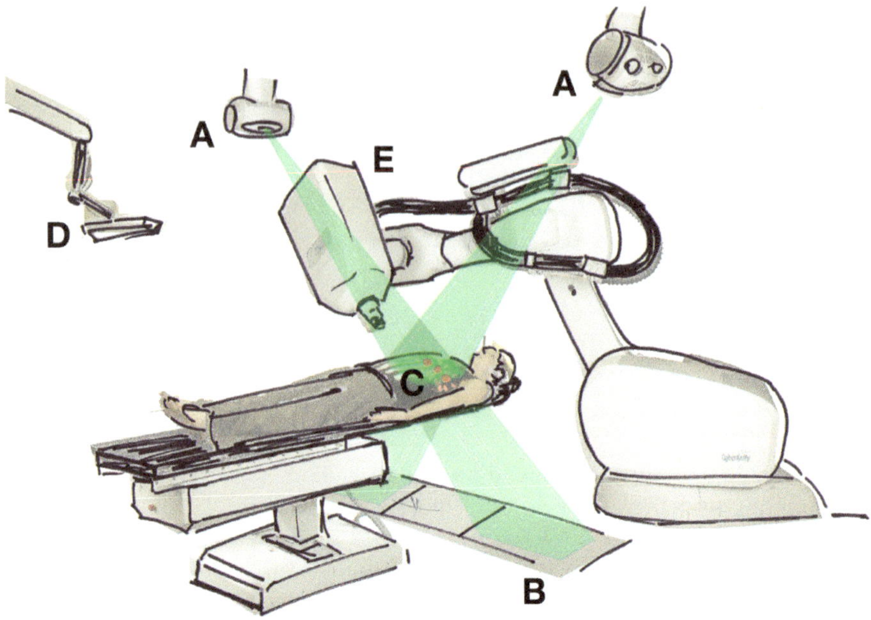

Fig. 1. Cyberknife radiosurgery device. X-ray tubes (A) are used to produce stereoscopic images recorded digitally (B) and correlated to the movement of lights on the patient's chest (C) which are monitored by two cameras (D). The model correlating the position of the chest wall to the position of the fiducials seen on the x-ray images is used to guide the miniature linear accelerator at the head of the robot (E).

2. Percutaneous fiducial implantation technique

Fiducials are inserted using image-guidance (Sotiropoulou *et al.,* 2010). Before the procedure, appropriate laboratory parameters are obtained and reviewed within an acceptable time frame, these include a complete blood count and prothrombin time with international normalized ratio. Patients with previously documented abnormalities in laboratory tests may require these to be repeated closer to the time of the procedure. Platelet transfusions are considered for platelet levels of less than 60,000/mL. Antiplatelet medications should be discontinued 7 days before the fiducial implantation; warfarin is generally discontinued 5 days before insertion, and heparin and related products discontinued 12-24 hrs prior to the procedure. Barring complications, these treatments can be restarted 24-48 hours following the procedure.

Imaging of the target lesion is reviewed with the radiation oncologist. This enables proper planning of the procedure, selection of the appropriate equipment (depending if a biopsy is required or not) and lesion(s) (it is possible that only selected lesions will be targeted for radiotherapy, and therefore for fiducial implantation).

The fiducial insertion is typically performed on an outpatient basis. The choice of imaging modality will depend on availability and operator preference. Most radiologists are comfortable with ultrasound or CT guidance. Although each modality has its advantages, certain situations may require a specific type of imaging. Typically CT is preferred for

fiducial insertion. Most patients are poor candidates for ultrasound-guided procedure because of body habitus, previous liver surgery and/or the presence of multiple lesions. CT also allows a pre-implant scan that can be acquired with contrast. This allows a better mapping of the target lesion and its neighbouring vascular structures, hopefully resulting in better fiducial placement with reduced risk of migration. This CT can also be used for treatment planning if the fiducials subsequently cause significant artefact.
Needle selection is based on the type of fiducial to be use, the number of fiducials to be placed and if a biopsy is required or not. A coaxial 19G needle is useful to perform a small-gauge core biopsy (18G), have enough tissue for histological analysis, and also allows for placement of our cylindrical gold fiducials.

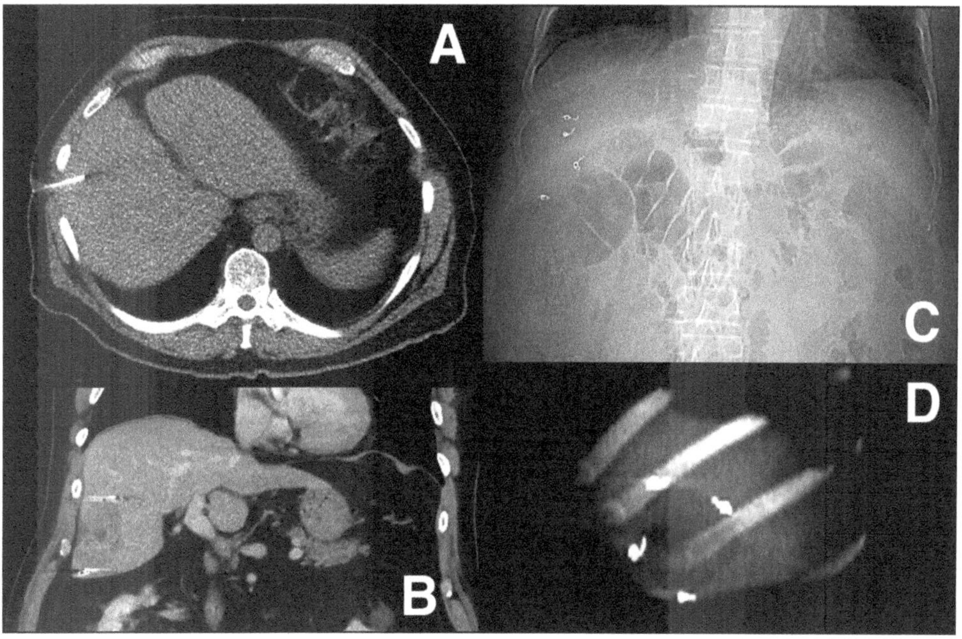

Fig. 2. A) A 22G needle is placed with a low radiation dose CT scan to place a Nester platinum coil. This case has a 6 cm lesion and 4 coils were placed at different levels (B, C, D).

With current radiotherapy systems, treatment can - if necessary - proceed with a single marker. The disadvantages of using a single marker are that movement of the marker within the liver will be difficult to detect and rotation of the target will not be reflected by the position of the marker. Geometrically, a minimum of 3 markers are required to assess rotations (as long as the fiducials are not all in a straight line). Extra markers also allow detection of migration (a constant relationship between the markers will reflect stability in their position). When there are too many markers or they are too close together (the Cyberknife system, as an example, suggests a minimum spacing of 2cm) this may lead to confusion at the time of treatment. The markers need not be within the lesion, as long as they will move in synchrony with the tumour. For example, markers can be implanted below a lesion high under the dome of the diaphragm in order to avoid the risk of pneumothorax. For small lesions, two markers placed at different sites but through the same

puncture may be sufficient; however, for bigger lesions, 3-4 markers may be preferred and the procedure may require multiple punctures.
At the end of the implant, a final scout imaging will confirm intra-hepatic fiducial placement.

2.1 Types of fiducial markers

Fiducials are typically made of a biologically inert metal with a high atomic number. These can be designed specifically for radiotherapy, repurposed devices or simple non-commercial materials. Several issues will be considered in choosing a marker. These include price, convenience, availability as well as the specific imaging system used for radiotherapy guidance.
Modern radiotherapy equipment will most often be purchased with an integrated kilovoltage imaging source dedicated to image-guidance. These systems should be able to easily resolve small gold markers with a diameter of 0.5mm (or less) but will be influenced by body habitus and overlying structures. To be visible with a megavoltage radiotherapy beam, markers will need to be thicker (this may mean 0.75-1.1mm diameter for gold) or longer (in the case of a marker which will coil up into a dense mass as it exits the needle). Images thus obtained as the treatment beam traverses the patient can be an excellent quality assurance tool.

Type of fiducial	Material	Diameter	Shape	Needle gauge	Provider
Plain / Non-commercial					
Spheres	Gold	2.0 mm	spherical	≥12 ga	varied
Cylinder / wire	Gold	varied	cylindrical	varied	varied
Repurposed					
Embolization coils	Platinum	0.889	loose coil	22 ga	Cook Medical
Commercial					
Visicoil™	Gold	0.35-1.1mm	tight linear coil	17-19 ga	Core Oncology
Best Gold Markers	Gold	0.8-1.2mm	cylindrical, available with absorbable spacer	17-18 ga	Best Medical
Cybermark™ / Align™	Gold	0.8-1.2mm	Knurled solid cylinder	17-18 ga	Civco medical solutions
Coupled™	Gold	0.8-1mm	two 3mm cylinders with absorbable spacer	17-18 ga	Civco medical solutions
FlexiMarc™	Gold	0-9-1.2mm	gold nodes along thin gold wire	17-18 ga	Civco medical solutions
FlexiCoil™	Gold	0-9-1.2mm	tight coil with solid ends	17-18 ga	Civco medical solutions
X-Mark™ / X-Mark Ultra™	Gold	0.85-1.15mm	multiple short bands along gold wire	17-18 ga	IZI Medical Products
Gold Anchor™	Gold	0.28mm	bendable notched wire	22-25 ga	Naslund Medical AB / Radiadyne
AnchorMarke®	Gold	n/a	cylinder encapsulated in bioabsorbable polymer	n/a	BrachySciences
BeamMarks®	Nickel titanium	1-1.2mm	extruded star shape	n/a	Beampoint

Table 1. Radiotherapy fiducials

The simplest markers are sterile sections of gold wire or gold spheres. Repurposed markers can include embolization coils designed for intravascular use. We have had good experience with these platinum coils as they can be placed with fine needles, are stable in the liver and are easily visualized with radiotherapy imaging. A disadvantage of these coils is that they can sometimes fail to bunch up into a tight mass – when this happens, they don't offer as precise a reference as a small solid piece of gold. Dedicated markers tend to have been designed to increase convenience and limit migration. Markers can thus be provided pre-loaded in needles or carriers. The markers can have an irregular surface or a bendable structure to "hook" into the liver. Tissue absorbable material between markers can be used to preserve marker spacing and reduce migration within the needle track. A common commercial radiotherapy fiducial (Visicoil, Core Oncology, Santa Barbara, CA) has a linear shape. As these markers can be 2-3 cm long, both ends of a single marker may be informative in resolving possible target rotation.

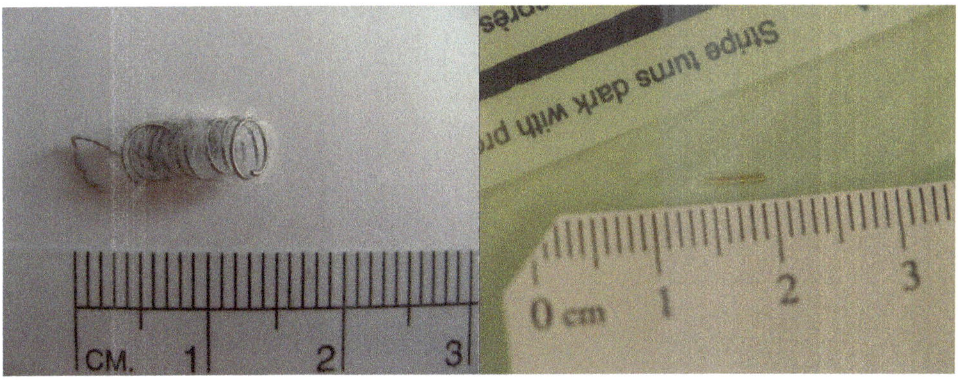

Fig. 3. Examples of a repurposed (platinum embolization coil on the left) and non-commercial (section of gold wire on the right) fiducial

3. Risks of percutaneous fiducial implantation

Fiducial placement is the source of several inconveniences. It leads to a delay in treatment – even when appointments are readily available, many clinicians will impose up to a one week delay from fiducial placement to treatment planning in order to allow the markers to "settle". The procedure is associated with additional costs and the fiducials can create significant imaging artefacts on CT. In addition, the percuteneous procedure has a variety of risks. Minor complications have been reported in 17.3% and major complications in 5% of cases (Kothary *et al.*, 2009). There are generic risks that come with introducing any needle into the liver: pain, pneumothorax, hemothorax, perforation of non target organs (the gallbladder being the most common), bile peritonitis, infection, hemobilia, neuralgia and tumour seeding. For most of these events, the biopsy literature serves as a basis of a risk estimate. Specific to fiducial placement is the risk of migration of the marker.

3.1 Pain

Pain is the most common complication on any percutaneous procedure. Up to 84% of patients will have at least mild discomfort. When present, pain can usually be managed with small amounts of narcotics (Cardella *et al.*, 2003). Is important to recognize and evaluate any moderate to severe pain, which could be related with bleeding, gallbladder or biliary puncture. When pain is severe enough to require hospitalization, radiological evaluation is warranted

3.2 Fiducial migration

Fiducial migration is a twofold problem, first because of the risk of tumour mistargeting if unrecognized migration occurs within the organ of interest, and second because of potential toxicity from the marker escaping through the hepatic veins.

3.2.1 Gross fiducial migration

Fiducials and radioactive seeds are commonly placed in the prostate. There is ample literature describing migration of these to the lung (without any serious consequence). In placing gold markers for pulmonary radiation, migration into the pleural cavity, pulmonary veins or bronchial tree will sporadically occur. For the liver, the available literature is more limited, with hepatic veins representing the potential route of fiducial migration (no cases of biliary tree migration have been reported).

In a series of 21 patients implanted with 2 mm gold spheres, one of the fiducials migrated through the inferior vena cava to a small vein at the hip where it remained lodged without apparent clinical consequence (Shirato *et al.*, 2003). In a series from Stanford University Medical Center, 33 patients underwent CT-guided placement of 0.8 mm by 5 mm hepatic fiducials. In these cases there was no gross marker migration and one patient experienced a small hemorrhagic pleural effusion (Kothary *et al.*, 2009).

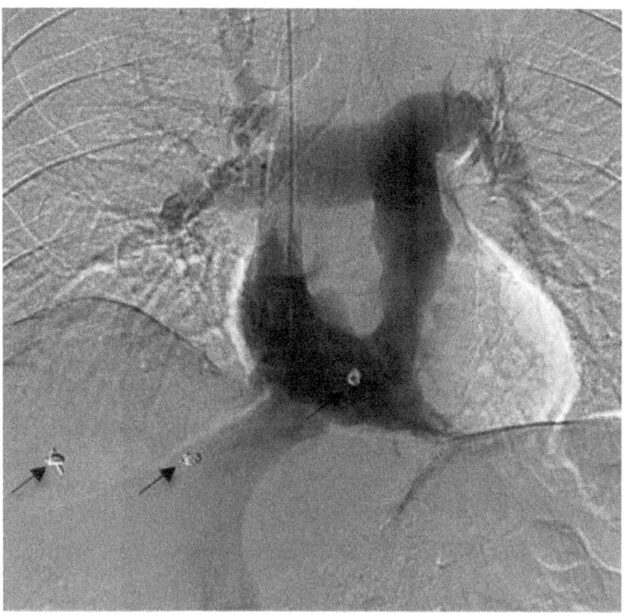

Fig. 4. Platinum coil lodged at the junction of the inferior vena cava and right atrium after migration from the liver.

In our own experience, we had a case of cardiac migration of a liver fiducial (Hennessey *et al.*, 2009). This occurred in an 81 year old patient planned for SBRT in the context of oligometastatic gastric cancer. For image-guidance, Nester embolization coils (Cook Medical Inc., Bloomington, Indiana) were planned to be implanted under CT guidance. Prior to the placement of each coil the location of the tip of the delivery needle was confirmed by CT imaging. During the procedure, the third coil unexpectedly migrated through the hepatic vein to the inferior vena cava and lodged at the vena cava/right atrial junction. The patient remained asymptomatic. He was immediately referred to angiography for extraction of the coil. Using fluoroscopic guidance, an EN Snare Retrieval System (Hatch Medical L.L.C., Snellville, GA, USA) was introduced through a jugular catheter, successfully grasped the coil and was removed. The patient was kept overnight for observation and no immediate or delayed complications were encountered due to the migration or retrieval of the coil. He subsequently went on to be treated using the remaining fiducials

3.2.2 Intra-hepatic fiducial migration

Migration of fiducials within the targeted organ has been described. Most published work concerns prostate radiotherapy with studies looking at the relative position of 3-4 prostate markers as a surrogate to migration (Sommerkamp et al., 1988). In limited experience with hepatic fiducials, intra-organ migration appears minimal – in the order of 2-3mm (Sommerkamp et al., 1988; Kitamura et al., 2002). However, quantification of movement within the liver is limited by the frequent lack of precise landmarks within this large, deformable organ. To deal with this issue, clinicians have relied on treatment margins, repeated 3D imaging and/or implantation of redundant fiducials.

3.3 Bleeding

The most important complication of liver puncture is bleeding, that can be severe when it occurs intraperitoneally. The clinical signs include changes in vital signs, imaging evidence of intraperitoneal bleeding, and subcutaneous hematoma. In this case, the patient requires hospitalization with possible transfusion, radiological intervention or surgery. Such bleeding has been estimated to occur in between 1:25,000 to 1:10,000 procedures after an intercostal percutaneous approach. Severe bleeding is evident within 2-4 hrs, but late haemorrhage can occur even up to one week after the procedure. Less severe bleeding, defined as that sufficient to cause pain or decreased blood pressure / tachycardia, but not requiring transfusion or intervention, occurs in approximately 1 in 500 procedures (Cardella *et al.*, 2003; Seeff *et al.*, 2010).

Non-symptomatic bleeding, detectable by ultrasonography may occur in 20% of patients.

3.4 Pneumothorax

Pneumothorax is critical to recognize immediately after the procedure, because it can lead to immediate catastrophic outcomes. This is the most frequent complication after lung implantation, although only 14% of these require a chest tube to resolve (Sotiropoulou *et al.*, 2010). Pneumothorax is less frequent on liver fiducal placements. An advantage of CT guidance is the easy diagnosis of pneumothorax with immediate treatment.

3.5 Tumour seeding

Although there are no reports of malignant seeding after fiducial placement, it is possible that this can occur at a similar rate than for other percutaneous diagnostic and therapeutic procedures in patients with HCC. For example, in a meta-analysis the median risk of seeding was 2.3% for the biopsy group and less than 1% for RFA with or without biopsy (Stigliano *et al.*, 2007).

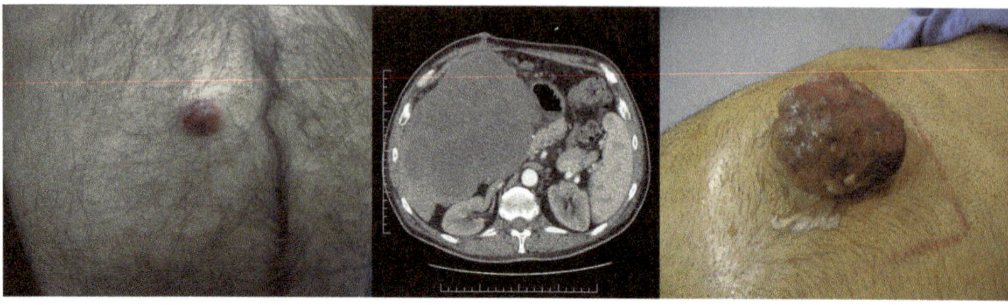

Fig. 5. Tumour seeding following percutaneous biopsy

4. Alternatives to percutaneous fiducial implantation

Fiducials are for now often a necessary evil. As radiotherapy image-guidance develops, the use of fiducials will likely decrease. This will happen faster in the lung, where the tumours can be more easily visualized on 2D and non-contrast 3D imaging. Alternatives to percutaneous fiducial placement have developed in the chest mainly in an attempt to reduce the risk of pneumothorax. In the abdomen, the need for alternatives has not been as strongly felt without common serious complications.

4.1 Endoscopic ultrasound (EUS) fiducial placement

Endoscopic ultrasound (EUS), has the advantage of proximity to structures of the mediastinum and retroperitoneum that are otherwise not easily accessible by percutaneous approaches (Varadarajulu *et al.*, 2010). Initially, the EUS technique required the use of a 19G FNA needle to deliver the fiducial, but because of the size and stiffness of the needle, the accurate placement of fiducials was compromised. The introduction of new smaller fiducial markers that can fit on a 22G needle now allows optimal placement in a variety of locations. It is minimally invasive and allows easy access to structures around the GI track. More frequently suggested for pancreatic lesions, it may also be used for retroperitoneal lymph nodes, the left adrenal gland, and the left hepatic lobe, including the caudate. The fiducials are liberated through the stomach or duodenum, commonly with prophylactic antibiotics (Ammar *et al.*, 2010; DiMaio *et al.*, 2010).

Reported success rates of EUS-guided fiducial placement are 85 to 100% with minimal complications and no migration. Failure to place a fiducial in the desired location was due to either anatomic considerations or limitations of the equipment when a 19G needle was used. The technical success using a 22G needle is reported at 97% because this type of needle does not produce the same endoscope rigidity as the 19G needle.

Despite these reports, the use of EUS for liver fiducial placement remains anecdotal and restricted to the left lobe.

4.2 Non fiducial based image-guidance

Modern radiotherapy devices often have the capability to acquire volumetric imaging at the time of treatment. These "cone-beam" CT scans typically take 30-60 seconds to acquire and thus suffer from breathing artefacts. As the technology advances, it is becoming possible to sort the images acquired during a rotation into phases of a 4D CT scan. It is also possible, in some cases, to use multiple breath holds to acquire a 3D image at a fixed point in the respiratory cycle. The volumetric image is then used to position the patient for treatment (Case *et al.*, 2009). Because the tumour will typically not be visible, the entire liver will be used as a surrogate. Although they avoid fiducial placement, these techniques have the disadvantage of not allowing monitoring of the tumour position during treatment.

4.3 Endovascular fiducial placement

In specific situations such as severe ascites, a known or suspected hemostatic defect or morbid obesity, patients can undergo intrahepatic artery coils implant. The Nester type coils (Cook, Inc; Bloomington , IN) may have a special role because its platinum structure that is radiopaque and easy to visualize during the radiotherapy. They can be liberated with a 0.035 inch catheter; microcatheters can also be used for a more selective coil placement. When possible, two or three different tumour vessels should be embolized and at the most distal position possible. The intra-arterial coil placement has the benefit of low risk of migration, and the proximity with the target lesion; it has the disadvantage of blocking an artery that could be used for further chemoembolisation.

Intravenous fiducial placement is described for lung tumour. There are no cases, to our knowledge, of this type of procedures for liver lesions, which could have a high risk of migration.

5. Conclusion

Interventional radiologist and radiation oncologist often collaborate in the implantation of radio-opaque markers for the targeting of focused radiation. Although this percutaneous fiducials placement is a useful and generally safe procedure, it carries a variety of small risks of which radiologists, radiation oncologists and patients should be aware.

6. References

Ammar, T.; Cote, G.A.; Creach, K.M.; Kohlmeier, C.; Parikh, P.J. & Azar, R.R. (2010). Fiducial placement for stereotactic radiation by using EUS: feasibility when using a marker compatible with a standard 22-gauge needle. *Gastrointest Endosc*, Vol. 71, No. 3, (Mar 2010), pp. 630-633, 1097-6779

Cardella, J.F.; Bakal, C.W.; Bertino, R.E.; Burke, D.R.; Drooz, A.; Haskal, Z., et al. (2003). Quality improvement guidelines for image-guided percutaneous biopsy in adults. J *Vasc Interv Radiol*, Vol. 14, No. 9 Pt 2, (Sep 2003), pp. S227-230, 1051-0443

Case, R.B.; Sonke, J.J.; Moseley, D.J.; Kim, J.; Brock, K.K. & Dawson, L.A. (2009). Inter- and intrafraction variability in liver position in non-breath-hold stereotactic body radiotherapy. *Int J Radiat Oncol Biol Phys*, Vol. 75, No. 1, (Sep 1 2009), pp. 302-308, 1879-355X

Dawood, O.; Mahadevan, A. & Goodman, K.A. (2009). Stereotactic body radiation therapy for liver metastases. *Eur J Cancer*, Vol. 45, No. 17, (Nov 2009), pp. 2947-2959, 1879-0852

DiMaio, C.J.; Nagula, S.; Goodman, K.A.; Ho, A.Y.; Markowitz, A.J.; Schattner, M.A. & Gerdes, H. (2010). EUS-guided fiducial placement for image-guided radiation therapy in GI malignancies by using a 22-gauge needle (with videos). *Gastrointest Endosc*, Vol. 71, No. 7, (Jun 2010), pp. 1204-1210, 1097-6779

Hennessey, H.; Valenti, D.; Cabrera, T.; Panet-Raymond, V. & Roberge, D. (2009). Cardiac embolization of an implanted fiducial marker for hepatic stereotactic body radiotherapy: a case report. *J Med Case Reports*, Vol. 3, No. 2009), pp. 140, 1752-1947

Kitamura, K.; Shirato, H.; Shimizu, S.; Shinohara, N.; Harabayashi, T.; Shimizu, T., et al. (2002). Registration accuracy and possible migration of internal fiducial gold marker implanted in prostate and liver treated with real-time tumor-tracking radiation therapy (RTRT). *Radiother Oncol*, Vol. 62, No. 3, (Mar 2002), pp. 275-281, 0167-8140

Kothary, N.; Heit, J.J.; Louie, J.D.; Kuo, W.T.; Loo, B.W., Jr.; Koong, A., et al. (2009). Safety and efficacy of percutaneous fiducial marker implantation for image-guided radiation therapy. *J Vasc Interv Radiol*, Vol. 20, No. 2, (Feb 2009), pp. 235-239, 1535-7732

Lo, S.S.; Dawson, L.A.; Kim, E.Y.; Mayr, N.A.; Wang, J.Z.; Huang, Z. & Cardenes, H.R. (2010). Stereotactic body radiation therapy for hepatocellular carcinoma. *Discov Med*, Vol. 9, No. 48, (May 2010), pp. 404-410, 1944-7930

Seeff, L.B.; Everson, G.T.; Morgan, T.R.; Curto, T.M.; Lee, W.M.; Ghany, M.G., et al. (2010). Complication rate of percutaneous liver biopsies among persons with advanced chronic liver disease in the HALT-C trial. *Clin Gastroenterol Hepatol*, Vol. 8, No. 10, (Oct 2010), pp. 877-883, 1542-7714

Shirato, H.; Harada, T.; Harabayashi, T.; Hida, K.; Endo, H.; Kitamura, K., et al. (2003). Feasibility of insertion/implantation of 2.0-mm-diameter gold internal fiducial markers for precise setup and real-time tumor tracking in radiotherapy. *Int J Radiat Oncol Biol Phys*, Vol. 56, No. 1, (May 1 2003), pp. 240-247, 0360-3016

Sotiropoulou, E.; Stathochristopoulou, I.; Stathopoulos, K.; Verigos, K.; Salvaras, N. & Thanos, L. (2010). CT-guided fiducial placement for cyberknife stereotactic radiosurgery: an initial experience. *Cardiovasc Intervent Radiol*, Vol. 33, No. 3, (Jun 2010), pp. 586-589, 1432-086X

Stigliano, R.; Marelli, L.; Yu, D.; Davies, N.; Patch, D. & Burroughs, A.K. (2007). Seeding following percutaneous diagnostic and therapeutic approaches for hepatocellular carcinoma. What is the risk and the outcome? Seeding risk for percutaneous approach of HCC. *Cancer Treat Rev*, Vol. 33, No. 5, (Aug 2007), pp. 437-447, 0305-7372

Sommerkamp, H.; Rupprecht, M. & Wannenmacher, M. (1988). Seed loss in interstitial radiotherapy of prostatic carcinoma with I-125. *Int J Radiat Oncol Biol Phys*, Vol. 14, No. 2, (Feb 1988), pp. 389-392, 0360-3016

Varadarajulu, S.; Trevino, J.M.; Shen, S. & Jacob, R. (2010). The use of endoscopic ultrasound-guided gold markers in image-guided radiation therapy of pancreatic cancers: a case series. *Endoscopy*, Vol. 42, No. 5, (May 2010), pp. 423-425, 1438-8812

Wunderink, W.; Mendez Romero, A.; Seppenwoolde, Y.; de Boer, H.; Levendag, P. & Heijmen, B. (2010). Potentials and limitations of guiding liver stereotactic body radiation therapy set-up on liver-implanted fiducial markers. *Int J Radiat Oncol Biol Phys*, Vol. 77, No. 5, (Aug 1 2010), pp. 1573-1583, 1879-355X

10

Adverse Effects of Drugs and Toxins on the Liver

Jan Schjøtt
Regional Drug Information Centre (RELIS Vest), Haukeland University Hospital, Norway

1. Introduction

More than 1000 drugs and toxins are suspected to induce liver damage, but only for a few are causality proven. Preclinical studies of drugs cannot predict hepatotoxicity due to the low incidence of such events, and postmarketing data are difficult to interpret. This is due to the fact that the clinical presentation of drug-induced liver injury is highly variable from asymptomatic, reversible elevation of liver enzymes to a fulminated hepatic failure. Furthermore, in most cases the clinical, biochemical and pathological pictures are indistinguishable from that seen with other causes of liver disease. Thus, suspected drug-induced hepatic injury is often a diagnosis made by exclusion of other causes. These include among others infectious, inflammatory and neoplastic diseases in the liver as well as complications in the organ due to systemic diseases. A common diagnostic challenge is a situation where patients who develop acute liver disease use several drugs, together with alcohol, recreational and illegal compounds. Moreover, even excipients present in drug formulations cannot always be ruled out as causative agents. Furthermore, due to the increasing popularity of complementary and alternative medicine, several new substances have been suspected of liver injury. These toxins are associated with ingredients of herbal medicine and nutritional-based therapies. The common belief that these substances and therapies are only beneficial to humans is challenged by an increasing number of reports of adverse effects including hepatic injury. As a general rule, drug- and toxin-induced liver injury is usually benign with full recovery after withdrawal of the offending agent. However, this implies that a drug or a toxin must be recognized as a possible causative agent. Furthermore, drug- and toxin-induced liver injury is a frequent cause of liver failure, and represents a health problem in our society. The present chapter summarizes the main principles of adverse effects of drugs and toxins on the liver, in particular examples of adverse effects of herbal medicine and nutritional-based therapies in the literature as well as cases submitted to drug information centres and pharmacovigilance units in Norway.

1.1 Epidemiology and demographics of drug-induced liver injury

The risk of serious liver damage is small compared to the number of patients who use drugs, but drug-induced hepatic injury is currently one of the most important reasons for

exclusion of drugs for further clinical development, and withdrawal of drugs from the market (Bakke et al., 1995). Furthermore, prescribed drugs have been shown to account for about 30-50% of cases of acute liver failure with risk of death or liver transplantation (Ostapowicz et al., 2002; Larrey & Pageaux 2005). The true incidence of drug-induced liver injury is not known because most of the data comes from retrospective studies. An important exception is single prospective study of the incidence of drug-induced adverse effects in the liver for a general population, performed over 3 years in France (Sgro et al., 2002). It was found to be 14/100 000 persons, and this incidence is 16 times higher than that collected by pharmacovigilance centres. Thus, spontaneously reported cases analysed in a retrospective fashion are not useful to predict or compare hepatotoxic potential of various drugs. A retrospective study from the UK showed that among 800 jaundiced patients referred to a single centre, 3.5% had drug-induced liver injury. The annual incidence rate of drug-induced liver injury in this study was estimated to 1.27 per 100 000 inhabitants per annum (Hussaini et al., 2007). A Swiss study found that approximately 1 in 100 patients developed drug-induced liver injury during hospitalisation in a department of medicine. Incidences were highest for antineoplastic agents and tuberculostatics (Meier et al., 2005).
Demographic data have suggested several risk or host factors for drug-induced liver injury. Typical examples are female sex, old age, use of alcohol, genetic factors, comorbidities, large body mass index, and several others. However, susceptibility of an individual varies with the drug in question, and drug properties (chemical structure) represent a separate risk factor (Lucena et al., 2008). Although drug-induced liver injury is in general rare in children, salicylates and valproic acid are associated with hepatic damage in this population. Chronic liver disease is thought to be of minor importance as a risk factor, but liver injury to isoniazid is seen in patients with viral hepatitis or Human Immunodeficiency Virus (HIV). Furthemore, chronic alcohol ingestion, fasting and malnutrition can increase the risk of serious paracetamol (acetaminophen) toxicity (Metha et al., 2010). Data on the risk of liver injury for specific drugs is not known. Although asymptomatic rises in liver enzymes are common for several drugs, the more clinically relevant forms of liver damage are thought to occur with a frequency between 1 in 1000 and 1 in 10,000. Liver injury associated with overdose is frequently due to ingestion of paracetamol. Non-steroidal anti-inflammatory drugs (NSAIDs), along with antimicrobial agents and antiepiletics, are the most frequent causes of liver injury with conventional doses (Andrade et al., 2005; Andrade et al., 2007; Lucena et al. 2008). These drugs are consumed massively worldwide, and for NSAIDs a estimated incidence of 0,3-9/100 000 have been suggested (Bessone, 2010). Amoxicillin-clavulanate was the single agent responsible for the highest number of incidences in a report from a Spanish registry (Andrade et al., 2005).

1.2 Main types of drug-induced liver injury

Drugs can cause liver injury in several ways, but three main types are usually referred: dose-dependent (or intrinsic) toxicity, dose-independent (or idiosyncratic metabolic) toxicity and drug allergy (or idiosyncratic immunological). Overdose of most drugs can represent a threat to the liver, and psychotropic drugs are often involved. Increased use of antiepileptics, like lamotrigine, against depressive periods in bipolar disorder, are reflected by an increasing number of reports of deliberate overdose. Intrinsic toxicity is predictable and often caused by high concentrations of parent drug and/or a metabolite when the liver`s defence systems against toxic damage are overwhelmed. Most people ingesting large amounts of a drug are affected, and liver injury is apparent within a few days. Injury is usually reversible within days to weeks if liver failure does not develop. A randomized, placebo-controlled trial where transaminases were monitored in healthy adults receiving therapeutic doses (4 g daily) of paracetamol, showed that more than 50% of the subjects who received drug showed an increase of alanine aminotransferase (ALT) more than 5 times baseline. Furthermore, this was in particular associated with subjects with Latin American background who showed two-fold increased risk of increase of ALT more than 3 times that of upper limit of the normal range (ULN) (Watkins et al., 2006). Thus, overdose is not always necessary to induce liver injury when using drugs with intrinsic toxicity in susceptible subjects.

With chronic high dose of a drug with intrinsic toxicity, like methotrexate, liver injury can manifest itself first after months or years. In the case of idiosyncratic metabolic toxicity, host factors that may enhance susceptibility to drugs, are of particular importance. Inherited defects in drug metabolism can give abnormal reactions to drugs, but liver injury can take weeks to years to develop. After drug withdrawal, reversibility is gradual over weeks and new injury develops slowly with rechallenge. It has been questioned if these reactions are dose-independent after all. A study showed that when drugs that caused idiosyncratic hepatotoxicity were given at a daily dose of 100 mg or higher, they were more likely to induce liver injury than when administered at a dose below 10 mg per day (Walgren et al., 2005). Therefore, the difference between intrinsic and idiosyncratic toxicity are not sharp, and liver injury in an individual depends on a complex relationship between susceptibility and drug factors. Besides dose-dependent and idiosyncratic toxicity, drug allergy may also cause liver disease, though it is supposed to be more uncommon. In these cases the liver is injured by inflammation caused by the immune system, and extrahepatic signs of hypersensitivity reactions like fever, rash and periphere eosinophilia can be present. Clinical characteristics like a relatively short period of therapy (1-4 weeks) before onset, rapid onset on rechallenge, and risk of cross-reactions to related drugs are associated with this type. After drug withdrawal, the injury is reversible within weeks. Thus, time-course of onset and reversibility of idiosyncratic immunological or metabolic liver injury is closely associated with adaptive reactions in the immune system and accumulation/elimination of toxic metabolites, respectively. However, the difference between these two types of idiosyncratic injury is not distinct. There are cases of idiosyncratic immunological reactions without fever, rash and eosinophilia, and there is growing evidence that immune cells or immune mechanisms are more important for both predictive and idiosyncratic liver injury than previously thought (Adams et al., 2010).

1.3 Main mechanisms of drug-induced liver injury

The liver has a central role as a detoxifying organ towards xenobiotics and chemicals. However, biotransformation to less toxic substances can actually involve production of molecules that can induce liver injury through various pathways. Important mechanisms involved in non-allergic drug-induced hepatic injury can be divided into (Han et al, 2010): (1) drug metabolism and reactive metabolite formation, (2) covalent binding, (3) reactive oxygen species generation, (4) activation of signal transduction pathways that modulate cell death or survival and (5) mitochondrial damage. Furthermore, immunological mechanisms can be triggered by these reactions. Most of the current knowledge of mechanisms for drug-induced liver injury is associated with basic studies, and the clinical relevance of the present models of damage needs to be defined. In the following, only the main principles of injury are summarized. Because of the liver's capacity to regenerate, full recovery is possible even if drug-induced liver injury has caused extensive hepatocyte death.

1.3.1 Drug metabolism and reactive metabolite formation

Biotransformation of lipophilic xenobiotics to more hydrophilic substances before excretion in urine or bile is an important function in the liver. Phase I enzyme reactions involve among other cytochrom-P450 (CYP-450) reactions which converts xenobiotics to reactive metabolites. The metabolites can via Phase II enzymes be conjugated to hydrophilic molecules (glucuronide conjugation-most important reaction among several) before excretion. The reactive metabolite N-acetyl-p-benzo-quinone imine (NAPQI) is produced via CYP1A2 and CYP2E1 (CYP-450) enzymes. However, the majority of paracetamol is metabolized by glucuronidation (Phase II reaction), and the small amount (approximately 10% of a paracetamol dose) of NAPQI that is produced is immediately inactivated by conjugation with glutathione (GSH). With an overdose of paracetamol, glucuronidation is saturated and detoxifying pathways described above are overwhelmed. The reason why reactive metabolites can induce damage through idiosyncratic liver injury is based on a complex interplay between several factors. Age, sex, liver function and disease, environmental (enzyme induction and inhibition) and genetic (polymorphism) can influence the level or function of CYP-450, and thereby production of reactive metabolites. Inherent toxicity of these, their distribution and accumulation within the organ, cells and subcellular organelles together with the status of defence systems are likely to be of additional importance (Grattagliano et al., 2009).

1.3.2 Covalent binding

Bioactivation of drugs through Phase I reactions can produce electrophilic metabolites with intrinsic chemical reactivity toward several cellular macromolecules. Covalent binding of short-lived reactive metabolites to cellular components includes proteins, peptides, lipids and nuclear acids, and this modification is thought of as essential in hepatotoxicity of drugs (Kemper, 2008). An important pathway for bioactivation of many acidic NSAIDs involves formation of reactive acylglucuronides (Bailey & Dickinson, 2003). Thus, Phase II reactions of bioactivation, usually thought of as a detoxifying process, can also produce reactive metabolites associated with hepatotoxicity. Furthermore, covalent modification of cellular components can initiate both toxic and/or immunological mechanisms of liver injury (Bailey & Dickinson, 2003).

1.3.3 Reactive oxygen species generation

Metabolic activation of drugs can involve production of reactive oxygen species. Through chemical modification of cellular macromolecules they can induce hepatocellular injury. Reactive oxygen species can initiate protein and lipid peroxidation, and deplete antioxidant defences like reduced glutathione (GSH), and modify sulphydryl (SH) groups on cellular components. These non-covalent reactions represent additional toxic mechanisms to covalent reactions. Depletion of GSH, and oxidation of SH groups on Ca^{2+}-ATPases are related to damage induced by NAPQI in the case of paracetamol overdose.

The subsequent increased cellular stress and uncontrolled increase in cytosolic Ca^{2+} concentration stimulate Ca^{2+}-activated degradative enzymes with further cellular injury. Disruption of membranes of cells, subcellular organelles including mitochondria, can affect energy production and further disrupt ionic homeostasis, and initiate cell death pathways.

1.3.4 Activation of signal transduction pathways

The stress in hepatocytes induced by reactive metabolites, including reactive oxygen species, can activate several signal transduction pathways. Several endogenous signal substances modify signal transduction including various cytokines. The pathways activate prodeath or survival proteins that determines the fate of the cell. Even in necrotic liver injury, associated with paracetamol, such pathways could be of relevance (Han et al., 2010). Important for liver injury is c-Jun N-terminal protein kinases (JNK). JNK can be activated with many stresses including reactive oxygen species, and represents a common mechanism of cellular injury associated with several diseases (Han et al., 2010).

1.3.5 Mitochondrial damage

Mitochondria have a central role in liver injury. Cytotoxic drugs and/or metabolites can attack the organelle directly or through pathways described above. Important pathological mechanisms are mitochondrial permeability transition (MTP) through opening of MPT pore in the membranes of the organelle, and activation of signals, death receptors and proapototic pathways. As a result acute necrosis, apoptosis and autophagic cell death can occur (Kass, 2006). Mitochondrial dysfunction is involved in most forms of drug-induced liver injury, and through dysfunction of the organelle more subacute or chronic injury can develop. Valproic acid can inhibit mitochondrial fatty oxidation, uncouple mitochondrial respiration and induce MTP (Pessayre et al., 2010).

1.3.6 Immunological mechanisms

Various types of immune cells, including lymphocytes, reside in the liver, and other leukocytes are distributed to this organ during inflammation (Adams et al., 2010). Furthermore, antidrug antibodies and autoantibodies can be detected during liver injury (Liu & Kaplowitz, 2002). A drug-modified protein formed due to reactions described previously (reactive metabolite formation and covalent binding) can initiate either classic immune responses against the drug or an autoimmune response against a modified protein. The classic immune response is characterized with short time period to onset of symptoms and a memory component, while the autoimmune response develops after a long time period with no memory. The different courses are based on interaction with different T helper cells, but involvement of B cells and other immune cells could be of importance (Adams et al., 2010). Drug-induced allergic hepatitis are usually thought of as mediated by type IV immunological reactions, and eosinophilia, atypical lymphocytosis and liver infiltrate are frequently observed together with the presence of sensitized T lymphocytes. Type II hypersensitivity reactions with circulating specific antibodies occur, but to a lesser extent. Halothane is associated with antibodies directed against CYP2E1 (Andrade et al., 2007). Due to a complex interplay with drug factors and individual susceptibility, an immunological reaction or tolerance to the drug can develop. Typical examples of drugs that can cause allergic hepatitis are sulphonamides.

1.3.7 Cell death, cell involvement and other targets of injury

In most cases, hepatocyte injury and death is the critical step leading to the clinical manifestations of drug-induced liver injury. However, in certain circumstances, cholangiocytes or endothelial cells may be the principle target cell (e.g., ductopenic cholestasis and sinusoidal obstruction syndrome) (Han et al., 2010). Non-parenchymal hepatic tissue like Kupffer and endothelial cells are also involved in causing injury, and can be activated by chemotactic factors. In immunological reactions different leukocytes are involved as mentioned earlier. Furthermore, besides mitochondria, microsomes and nuclear components can be targets for injury. Modification of cellular function by down- or up-regulation of genes can also mediate drug-induced hepatic damage. The modifying role of several cytokines and other signal substances in pathways of necrosis, apoptosis or survival are emerging, as is the relevance of various risk factors for the clinical course of the injury (acute liver failure, full recovery or development of chronic disease) (Russmann et al., 2009).

Figure 1 summarizes adverse effects of drugs and toxins on the liver.

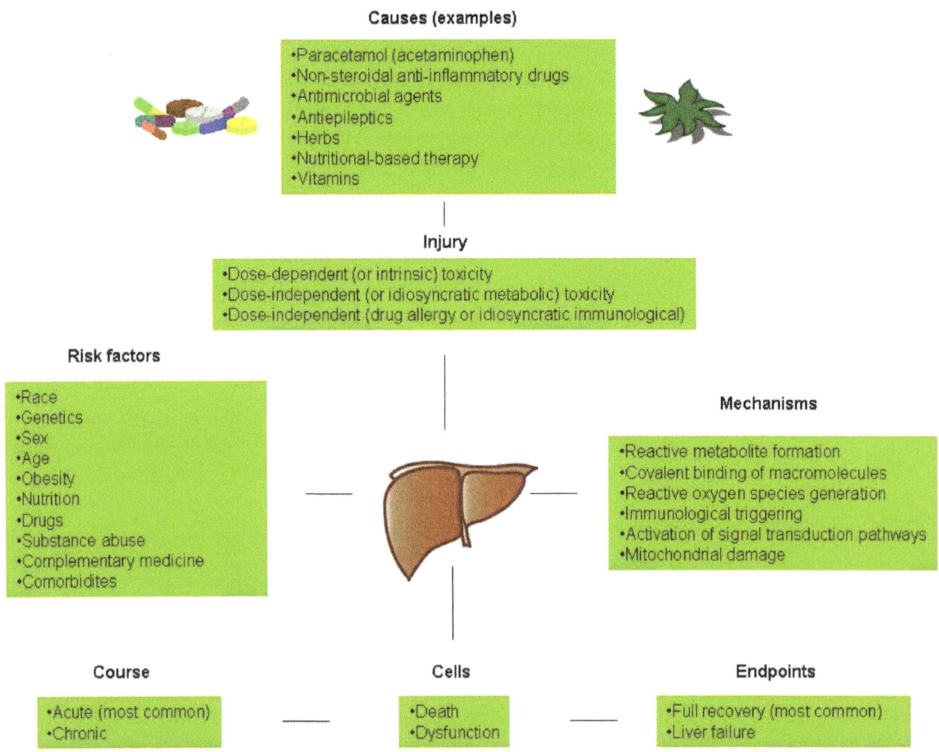

Fig. 1. Adverse effects of drugs and toxins on the liver. Notice that idiosyncratic forms of liver injury are associated with a complex interplay between individual risk factors (inborn, physiologic or environmental) and mechanisms of injury. In an individual this interplay determines if a threshold for disease is reached. Increased dose of the offending agent increases the likelihood of disease in most individuals in the case of drugs with intrinsic toxicity.

1.4 Diagnosis and clinical presentation of drug-induced liver injury

Suspected drug-induced hepatic injury is often based on an exclusion of alternative diagnosis. These include among others infectious, inflammatory and neoplastic diseases in the liver as well as complications in the organ due to systemic diseases, either aquired or inherited. Several diagnostic tools are available, but it is difficult to prove causality related to a specific drug. Notice, that as a general rule, drug-induced liver injury is usually benign with full recovery after withdrawal of the offending agent. However, in some cases acute liver failure due to massive necrosis or end-stage disease with cirrhosis due to chronic injury can be the result.

1.4.1 Liver enzymes, other laboratory data and imaging techniques

Measurement of liver enzymes remains the most practical tool to diagnose liver damage, and includes mainly alanine aminotransferase (ALT), an enzyme present in hepatocytes, and alkaline phosphatase (ALP), an enzyme in the cells lining the biliary ducts of the liver. Based on elevation of, and ratio between elevation of, these enzymes, hepatocellular, cholestatic or mixed liver injury is diagnosed (Benichou, 1990; Danan, 1993). Acute hepatocellular liver injury is defined by ALT > 2 ULN or an ALT/ALP ratio ≥ 5. Acute cholestatic injury is defined as an increase in serum ALP > 2 ULN or by an ALT/ALP ratio ≤ 2. Mixed hepatic injury features an intermediate between hepatocellular and cholestatic patterns, and features of either type may predominate. By definition, the ALT/ALP ratio is between 2 and 5, while ALT > 2 ULN and ALP increased. With already elevated ALT or ALP, increase from baseline rather than ULN is often used. Liver enzymes like aspartate aminotransferase (AST), lactate dehydrogenase (LDH), gamma glutamyl transpeptidase (GGT) and bilirubin are of less importance, but can give additional information about the type and extent of liver damage.

The most frequent type of drug-induced liver injury is acute hepatocellular. To exclude alternative causes, viral and bacterial serology and screening for autoimmune hepatitis are often performed. The lymphocyte transformation test, which measures the proliferation of T cells of a suspected sensitized patient when exposed to the causative drug in vitro, could be a consistent test for identifying a drug suspected of causing allergic hepatitis, but it is not fully reliable and associated with methodological problems (Andrade et al., 2007). Furthermore, in more specific cases complications in the liver due to systemic diseases, either inborn or acquired, could involve additional laboratory and other examinations. Abdominal ultrasound, computer tomography and other imaging techniques cannot discriminate drug-or toxin-induced hepatic injury from other causes. However, they can exclude benign or malign mechanical obstruction in the case of cholestatic or mixed hepatic injury, and visualize biliary tracts and main blood vessels (Andrade et al., 2007).

1.4.2 Liver biopsy and histological findings in drug-induced liver injury

There are no histological findings specific for drug-induced liver injury. Some drugs usually cause one clinical or pathological (signature) injury like estrogens with cholestasis, but other drugs can cause a variety of pictures. An illustrating example is a recent published case series of suspected liver injury to duloxetine where several patterns of hepatic injury occurred, including hepatocellular and cholestatic features with highly variable liver histology (Vuppalanchi et al., 2010). Liver biopsy is seldom performed do to these arguments, and is not regarded as essential in all cases of suspected drug-induced liver injury. There is also risk of error in sampling of tissue, or time of sampling due to different courses of clinical disease. However, in spite of low specificity of liver biopsy it represents the most important tool for defining the pattern of hepatotoxicity. Furthermore, liver biopsy could be of prognostic value in the case of chronic liver disease, when progression is poorly reflected by other laboratory and clinical assessments (Andrade et al., 2007). Moreover, a biopsy can also be used to stage the severity of hepatotoxicity if a patient is dependent on a drug that may have to be continued (Kleiner, 2009).

Hepatitis, with or without cholestasis, is the most common histological pattern of drug-induced liver injury. The most serious is acute liver failure which shows necrosis with or without signs of inflammation, or microvascular steatosis with little or no inflammation. Chronic hepatitis can show signs of autoimmunity or not. Cholestasis, granulomatous hepatitis and different patterns of steatosis are other examples together with vascular abnormalities (Ramachandran et al., 2009). There are three types drug-induced acute cholestatic drug injury. Bland cholestasis is the result of abnormal biliary secretion without significant hepatocellular damage. In cholestatic hepatitis (mixed type) there is parenchymal damage; and the third form of acute cholestasis is defined by the presence of bile duct injury or cholangiolitis. Drugs may cause chronic cholestasis through two additional mechanisms: through the obliteration of bile ducts, also known as the vanishing bile duct syndrome, or by extrahepatic biliary obstruction, known as secondary sclerosing cholangitis (David & Hamilton, 2010). Cirrhosis, as a sign of advanced scarring of the liver, is a late finding. Importantly, a mixed liver injury is far more characteristic of drug-induced hepatotoxicity than of viral hepatitis. Almost all drugs that produce cholestatic injury are also capable of inducing a mixed pattern. Although drug-induced cholestatic and mixed lesions progress to acute liver failure less frequently than hepatocellular types, their resolution is generally slower. For example, a long-term follow-up of a large cohort in a registry demonstrated a significantly higher trend towards becoming chronic in cholestatic/mixed cases compared to hepatocelullar-type disease (Andrade et al., 2006).

1.4.3 Clinical suspicion and drug history

Onset and course of the reaction, response to drug withdrawal or reintroduction are examples of clinical factors to assess causality of drug-induced liver injury. Furthermore, the level of documentation for the type, frequency and other characteristics of liver injury associated with the suspected drug are important. The temporal profile between drug and reaction is crucial to establish the diagnosis of drug-induced liver injury, as the onset of liver disease follows drug ingestion (Lucena et al. 2008). However, the manifestation of liver toxicity may occur weeks or months after drug ingestion and even after the drug has been stopped. A toxic metabolite with a much longer half-life than the parent compound could accumulate during a treatment period, and liver injury could be unmasked some time after drug withdrawal. Notice that enzyme elevations can persist for months after the drug has been discontinued. In some instances, measurement of serum levels of the drug or its metabolite can be helpful; an example is diagnosis and treatment of toxicity due to paracetamol. Since the list of drugs capable of causing liver injury is long, a systematic literature search for each drug that the patient has been taking is necessary. Keeping in mind that patients frequently use several prescription drugs, over the counter drugs, and herbal and nutritional products means that finding the offending agent can be a difficult task. The case for drug-induced liver injury is strengthened if the reported pattern of injury in the literature is similar to the observed clinical and histological picture (Lucena et al. 2008). Rechallenge with the drug can help to establish a drug etiology, but it is often not done due to the inherent risk involved (Fontana et al., 2010). Since diverse histological patterns of drug-induced liver injury can mimic virtually any primary liver disease, appropriate imaging and laboratory tests are necessary to exclude other etiologies before the diagnosis of drug-induced liver injury can be accepted. Figure 2 summarizes diagnosis of drug- and toxin-induced liver injury.

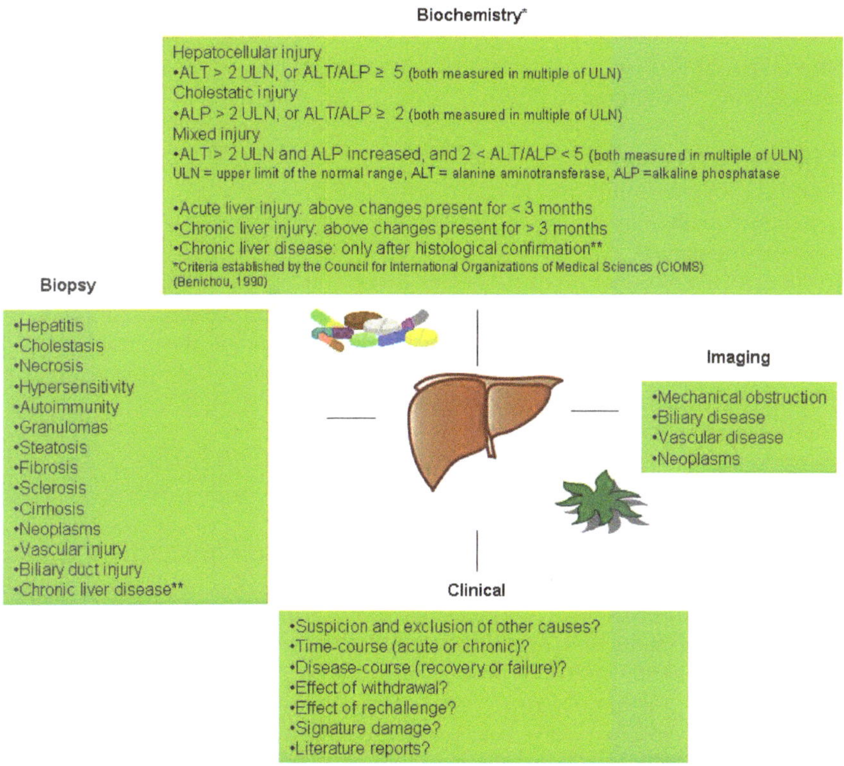

Fig. 2. Diagnosis of drug- and toxin-induced liver injury. Notice that due to the highly variable clinical presentation of this form of liver injury, that can be indistinguishable from other causes, causality is often based on circumstantial evidence.

1.4.4 Algorithms or scales, and clinical networks

More objective, systematic approaches with criteria for having an adverse effect (all types) or a more specific adverse effect (drug-induced liver injury) have been proposed. Three examples of these algorithms or scales are the Council for International Organizations of Medical Sciences (CIOMS) (Benichou, 1990; Danan, 1993), the Clinical Diagnostic Scale (CDS) or the Maria and Victorino (M&V) scale (Maria & Victorino, 1997) and the Digestive Disease Week-Japan (DDW-J) scale (Takikawa et al., 2003). The main principle of these scales is an evaluation of several criteria (numerical weighted), sum of scores or decision trees to assess the probability that a liver disease is drug-induced. All of them use several diagnostic factors mentioned earlier in this chapter. A major problem is validation of the scales when there is no accepted gold standard, and lower reliability when the number of experts who evaluate the same cases increases (García-Cortés et al., 2011). Furthermore, sensitivity to various individual risk, drug and diagnostic factors can be limited when applying such categorical scales. To increase our knowledge of drug-induced liver injury in a more homogenous and standardized fashion, collaborating clinical networks in Europe (Andrade et al., 2005; Andrade et al., 2006) and the United States (Hoofnagle, 2004) have been established. The purpose of these networks is to study prospectively new cases to improve our understanding of etiology, pathogenesis and risk of drug-induced liver injury (Fontana et al., 2009). A promising task is development of more drug-specific assessment tools for causality (Fontana et al., 2010).

1.5 Liver disease and drugs

As a general rule liver injury has to be extensive before metabolism of drugs are reduced. Thus, patients with existing liver disease without cirrhosis often can use drugs in conventional therapeutic doses. However, there is no specific test to predict liver function with respect to the elimination of particular drugs. Liver function tests are often used to evaluate liver capacity with relevance to hepatic clearance of drugs. The level of albumin, and coagulation factors, through measurement of international normalized ratios (INR), are of importance for both pharmacokinetics (protein binding, metabolism and distribution), but also pharmacodynamics (increased risk of bleeding with anticoagulants). Furthermore, advanced liver disease can change both pharmacokinetics and -dynamics in the organ as well as systemic. Development of renal failure and hepatic encephalopathy in advanced liver disease are two examples. Increased volume of distribution of water-soluble drugs in ascites can require increased loading dose, while shunting of drugs due to cirrhosis can reduce presystemic elimination (first-pass effect) with high bioavailability as a result. Crucial to understanding of the pharmacokinetics of a drug is that the unbound fraction is available for either distribution or clearance, and this fraction is at the same time responsible for the pharmacodynamic effect. Liver disease can be associated with reduced protein binding and reduced metabolism, and an increased unbound fraction of a drug can be associated with toxic effects. With advanced liver disease, and extrahepatic effects as mentioned above, the net result can be difficult to predict (Verbeeck, 2005). Furthermore, drug concentration levels usually reflect the sum of bound and unbound drug, but not the ratio. Thus, dosing and monitoring of drugs in advanced liver disease must include these implications. Acute liver injury preferently gives parenchymal damage, but with little change in metabolic capacity similar to autoimmune hepatitis. Chronic liver diseases are associated risk of reduction in drug-metabolizing activities. However, it affects the two main phases of biotransformation differently. Phase II reactions is often considered to be affected to a lesser extent than Phase I, but can also be substantially impaired in patients with advanced cirrhosis. Some drug monographs give advice on dosage of drugs in liver disease in relation to the semi-quantitative Child-Pugh score (Verbeeck, 2005). The score employs five clinical measures of liver disease, and is frequently used to assess the severity of liver function impairment. However, it represents only a rough guidance for dosage adjustment because data on how the liver metabolizes individual drugs is missing.

1.6 Withdrawal of drug and treatment of drug-induced liver injury

Drug-induced liver injury can range from asymptomatic and reversible elevations of liver enzymes to a fulminant hepatic failure. Between these two manifestations, the clinician is faced with the question of withdrawal of a drug or continuation of therapy. A liver injury can develop into liver failure if the offending drug is not withdrawn despite symptoms and signs of hepatic disease. Risk factors like old age, preexisting cirrhosis, fasting, malnutrition, chronic alcohol abuse, may all increase the risk of liver injury, as the dose of a drug in case of dose-dependent toxicity. However, elevation of liver enzymes does not always predict the risk for acute liver failure of drugs (Larrey & Pageaux, 2005, Lewis, 2006), and this raises the controversial question of which drugs where regular monitoring of liver enzymes are of clinical value. The approval authorities are motivated by risk reduction, and the drug industry adds to this the economy of keeping drugs on the market while the clinician wants to reduce irrelevant alerts in practice. An illustrating example of the challenge this represent for physicians is the commonly prescribed statins, where mild elevation of liver enzymes is thought of as a pharmacodynamic effect of altered lipid homeostasis, and not a toxic damage of the drug (Onusko, 2008, Bader, 2010).

Elevations of ALP > 2-3 or ALT > 3-5 ULN is suggested as a general thumb rule for evaluation of drug withdrawal, while long-time (months) elevation of liver enzymes irrespective of magnitude, can be a warning sign with therapy of drugs like valproic acid, methyldopa and methotrexate. However, for several drugs initial elevation of liver enzymes does not progress despite continuing the drug and the elevation can return to baseline. This phenomenon (often called tolerance in this context) is seen in up to 50% of patients taking tacrine, and is thought of as an adaptive process in the liver perhaps due to upgrading of protective pathways (Lewis, 2006). The choice of continued therapy despite significant elevation of liver enzymes is of course modified by how important the drug is for treatment of the patient. However, ALT > 8 ULN requires immediate drug withdrawal (Tajiri et al., 2008). Notice that withdrawal of the suspected drug is the most important therapeutic action in drug-induced liver injury, and there are currently no specific antidotes with the exception of N-acetylcysteine used to replenish GSH in paracetamol intoxication (David & Hamilton, 2010). Due to the fact that depletion of GSH could be associated with hepatotoxic effect of several other drugs than paracetamol, new animal and clinical studies emerge that describe treatment of drug-induced liver injury with this antidote (Baniasadi et al., 2010; Said & El-Agamy, 2010). Furthermore, modifying important signal pathways for liver injury could represent a therapeutic option in the future. Today, treatment of most cases of drug-induced liver injury is mainly symptomatic.

1.7 Further studies and prevention

Every aspect of drug-induced liver injury discussed so far is currently a subject of intense research. Both epidemiological studies and establishment of cooperative networks could give us valuable information and new understanding about relevant drugs, risk factors and diagnostic measures. To reveal the basic mechanisms of liver damage, further studies in genomics, proteomics, biochemistry and histopathology are essential. They can hopefully refine our current classification and reveal new predictive biomarkers to detect liver pathology or host factors associated with risk. Identifying genetic factors is difficult due to the low incidence of drug-induced liver injury, and the current thought that genetic associations with liver injury are generally drug specific (Daly, 2010). A recently identified association between drug-induced liver injury due to flucloxacillin and the HLA-B*5701 allele, is the strongest reported association between any gene and drug-induced liver injury, with an observed odds ratio for disease development of approximately 80 (Daly et al., 2009; Daly, 2010). HLA genotype can also be associated with the type of liver injury. An illustrating example is the finding that particular types of liver injury (cholestatic/mixed liver injury) might be linked at least in part to an inherited HLA genotype (Andrade et al., 2004). The HLA class molecules are associated with immunological processes, and a relevant question discussed earlier in this chapter concerns the current classification in idiosyncratic toxic or immunological types of injury. The hapten hypothesis (Castella et al., 2006) postulates that drugs, or reactive moieties derived from the drugs (toxic compunds), can react with cell proteins forming covalent drug-protein adducts (immunological triggering), and as mentioned earlier there is growing evidence that immune cells or immune mechanism are more important for both predictive and idiosyncratic liver injury than previously thought (Adams et al., 2010).

Pharmaceutical companies have traditionally used cell lines or subcellular fractions (microsomes) for in vitro safety (toxicology) studies, but recent evidence suggest that co-cultures of primary hepatocytes and Kuppfer cells are a useful supplement (Sahi et al., 2010). Hepatocytes in culture retain hepatic key functions compared to cell lines, and represent a more relevant model to study metabolism, transport and toxicity for extrapolation to humans. Thus, initial studies in cultures can then be supplemented with subsequent studies in cell lines to evaluate particular toxic mechanisms (Gómez-Lechón et al., 2010). Pharmaceutical companies in collaboration with medical agencies in Europe and USA are eager to find what combination of "omics" technologies that best can predict hepatotoxity. Both of concern for preclinical drug development, but also by the fact that non-clinical data at the time of marketing of some drugs indicated potential risk of liver injury (Hughes, 2008). However, as will be discussed later, assessment of retrospective data from clinical reports can still be of value to formulate useful hypotheses of causative mechanisms, and risk factors of relevance, to be tested in basic studies.

2. Toxins from herbal medicine and nutritional-based therapies

Due to the increasing popularity of complementary and alternative medicine, several new substances have been suspected to induce liver injury. These include among others ingredients from herbal products, vitamins and minerals. Consumption of these forms of complementary medicine is not unusual. A study from the UK showed that 44% of patients on warfarin, a drug with a low therapeutic index and highly sensitive to interactions, used nutritional-based therapy on a weekly basis or more often (Leung et al., 2009). Furthermore, more than 90% of the patients did not discuss use of complementary medicine with their physician (Nutescu et al., 2006). The common belief that these substances and therapies are only beneficial to humans is challenged by an increasing number of reports of adverse effects including hepatic injury. Currently the mechanisms behind these effects are poorly described, but there is no reason to believe that they are different from the principles of drug-induced liver injury described above. Thus, toxins from these products represent xenobiotics that the liver is exposed to, and potentially damaged by, in much the same way as conventional drugs. However, problems with formulations, standardization, epidemiology and current research on the products makes causality of liver injury even more complicated in comparison to that of conventional drugs.

2.1 Problems with formulation and standardization of complementary products

Most herbal medicines are classified as dietary supplements, and together with nutritional-based therapies they are not subjected to the safety, quality assessment and standardization which we associate with conventional drugs supplied by the pharmaceutical industry (Stickel et al., 2005). Herbal medicines often contain several active ingredients, and composition of the product (quantity and purity) is often poorly described. Furthermore, the quality and strength of the individual ingredients depends on climate, growth, collection, preparation and extraction of plant material. Thus, geographical location, part of the season for which the material is collected, and routines for extraction and processing can show considerable variation for different products with the same ingredients (Chang et al., 2006). Moreover, this variation indicates that batch to batch or lot differences of the same product can be expected (Gurley et al., 2000). A serious safety problem is the fact some medicines contain synthetic drugs not declared by the package, or that the content does not reflect label claims. Examples of such adulteration are stimulating substances like caffeine and ephedrine, but also steroids have been found in complementary products after patients developed signs of Cushings syndrome (Byard, 2010). Importantly, the product or ingredients could be contaminated by lead, other toxic metals, pollutants, pesticides, bacterias and mold (Stickel et al, 2005; Byard, 2010). The product could also contain allergens that can mediate hypersensitivity reactions in susceptible persons. Similar to the case with conventional drugs where excipients cannot be ruled out as causative agents, solvents like ethanol and acetone could contribute to damaging effects. Some of these solvents were not present in traditional preparations of the plants. Thus, essential when using complementary medicine is that the product contains a clear definition of ingredients with extensive description of the production process together with statements of potential adverse effects and interactions. However, the complicated terminology of complementary medicine with use of several synonyms and botanic names confuse both health care professionals and patients.

2.2 Problems with epidemiology of liver injury of complementary products

Complementary products lack the rigorous process of toxicology and safety assessment we associate with clinical testing of conventional drugs. Thus, preclinical data on potential for liver injury is not available in most cases (De Smet, 2002). Furthermore, the products usually contain a mixture of several ingredients, and to determine the safety of each would be a rigorous task. There are examples of clinical trials to study the effects of herbal medicines, but most of our knowledge of adverse effects comes from case reports and reviews (Smith & Dillon, 2009). Keeping in mind that use of complementary medicine often remain unknown to clinicians, the suspicion of ingredients in these medicines as causative agents for liver injury can be ignored. Thus, the true incidence of adverse effects due complementary products is not known (Smith & Dillon, 2009; Shaw, 2010). The available epidemiologic data of adverse reports is also influenced by the fact that selected populations with risk factors that increase the potential for liver injury are in particular exposed. Complementary products are proposed as effective against aging, obesity, liver disease, hypersensitivity, and psychiatric diseases as examples. Patients with such diseases already use several conventional drugs with their own risk of liver injury, and interactions with complementary medicine could be the final trigger to elicit acute hepatic damage. The retrospective and partial nature of our knowledge makes detection of liver injury from complementary medicine even more challenging than for conventional drugs. Medical agencies and poison units in several countries as well as the serious part of the industry are well aware of this problem, and initiatives like establishment of databases and public information against under-reporting are emerging, besides strategies for licensing of herbal medicine (Stickel et al., 2005).

2.3 Examples of toxins

To mention all the examples of toxins from complementary medicine suspected of causing liver injury is beyond the purpose of this chapter. However, a few examples will illustrate how difficult it is to establish a causative relationship, in particular which ingredient in a product that actually represent the offending toxin. Furthermore, the problem with extrapolation from basic studies in cells and animals to the clinical situation is described.. Lack of relevant dose-effect or -toxicity data from preclinical assessment faces the basic scientist with the question if clinically relevant quantities are used in the model, while the clinical scientist wonders if the clinical situation of liver injury is due to a therapeutic dose or an overdose. There is often abundant data of in vitro cytotoxicity of substances, yet evidence is lacking of in vivo hepatotoxicity in animal models under conditions similar to human use. Finally, the quality of the individual test substance in such studies should ideally be identical to compare studies, but this is not always the case. The following examples are chosen based on herbs and toxins known to induce liver injury in the last two decades, and where studies have emerged that suggest the plausible mechanisms involved.

2.3.1 Kava

Kava (kava kava, awa, or kew), derived from the plant Piper methysticum, has been used in the South Pacific as a ceremonial aqueous beverage since ancient times. Kava has been marketed as an anxiolytic and mood enhancer (Singh & Singh, 2002). Products containing derivates from the plant has been implicated in a number of human liver failure cases, which led to its ban in Germany, France, Switzerland, Australia, and Canada (Lim et al., 2007). This was a surprise due to the long history of safe use of the Kava beverage as a part of the culture in the South Pacific. The principle pharmacological activities of Kava are due to kavalactones, where kavain is the most important. Kavalactones can form electrophilic, quinone metabolites, potentially leading to GSH depletion and oxidative stress (Zhou et al., 2010). Furthermore, kavalactones inhibit CYP-450 enzymes in vitro (Mathews et al., 2002). Studies in isolated rat livers suggest that kavain (a major kavalactone) is associated with ultrastructural damage (Fu et al., 2008). However, these in vitro and ex vivo data were not supported by the in vivo observation that rats fed with aqueous kava root extracts containing as much as 500 mg kavalactones/kg body weight for 4 wk exhibited no noticeable toxicity (Singh & Devkota, 2003). Recently it was reported that a piperidine alkaloid, pipermethystine (PM), induces apoptosis in human hepatoma HepG2 cells (Nerurkar et al., 2004), but fails to induce hepatic toxicity in vivo (Lim et al., 2007). Furthermore, pipermethystine is not present in significant quantities in roots and rhizomes from the plant used in herbal medicines (Zhou et al., 2010). A new report suggest that the principle damaging substituent is flavokawain B, a lipohophilic chalcone (Zhou et al. 2010). The authors suggest that flavokawain B can through induction of oxidative stress and depletion of GSH modulate signalling pathways including JNK to induce cellular apoptosis. However, a critical review summarizing the current evidence for the possible offending agents in Kava, dismiss kavalactones, pipermethystine, and flavokawain B as a cause of liver injury. The authors instead suspect contamination of products by aflatoxins or other mould hepatotoxins (Teschke et al., 2011).

2.3.2 Chaparral

Chaparral (Larrea tridentate) is a desert shrub traditionally used by Native Americans for treatment of aging and obesity. The herbal preparation was used for its antioxidant properties (Gordon et al., 1995). A study of 18 reports of illnesses associated with the ingestion of chaparral, found evidence of hepatotoxicity in 13 cases. Clinical presentation, characterized as jaundice with a marked increase in serum liver enzymes, occurred 3 to 52 weeks after the ingestion of chaparral, and it resolved 1 to 17 weeks after most individuals stopped their intake of the product. The predominant pattern of liver injury was characterized as toxic- or drug-induced cholestatic hepatitis; in 4 individuals, there was progression to cirrhosis; and in 2 individuals, there was acute fulminant liver failure that required liver transplants (Sheikh et al., 1997). The mechanism of chaparral toxicity involves its active ingredient, nordihydroguaiaretic acid (NDGA). NDGA is described as an antioxidant which several proposed toxic effects including inhibition of lipo- and cyclooxygenase, reduction of cellular ATP, increase in intracellular Ca^{2+} and inhibition of CYP-450 (Arteaga et al., 2005; Stickel et al., 2005).

2.3.3 Ma Huang

A common herbal ingredient in weight loss products is Ma Huang (Ephedra sinica). Ma Huang contains ephedrine alkaloids, although not so potent CNS stimulant as the pharmaceutical ephedrine. Ephedrine is structurally related to amphetamine. In traditional Chinese medicine, this is seen as useful herb for treating asthma, cough and wheezing. However, content of ephedrine alkaloids is supposed to induce liver injury in susceptible persons. A retrospective study reviewed the records of 12 patients, who had hepatotoxicity thought to be related to the ingestion of herbal weight loss compounds from various ingredients, including Ma Huang (Neff et al., 2004). A problem with Ma Huang was suspicion of misuse, and the substance was banned by the Food and Drug Administration (FDA) in 2004 (Shaw, 2010). Several adverse reaction reports included serious psychiatric effects combined with a history of substance abuse (Maglione et al., 2005). A problem with products with ephedrine alkaloids is development of tolerance with risk of increasing doses. Although obese patients used Ma Huang, ephedrine alkaloids were also popular among young healthy people due to proposed effects like appetite suppression, increased sport performance and energy. Given the fact that Ma Huang is often mixed with other ingredients (potentially hepatoxic) in products, increased dose could represent additional risk of liver injury.

2.3.4 Particular liver toxins and mechanisms

The three examples described above illustrate several aspects of complementary products and liver injury. The difficult extrapolation from toxicity observed in vitro to animal studies when the products and ingredients in question lack standardization. Furthermore, the intriguing problem of how to explain idiosyncratic, rare, reports of toxicity with traditional products used apparently safe for hundred of years. Moreover, ingredients that are similar to substances of misuse add a risk of dose-dependent toxicity of such products. Notably, individual herbal liver toxins with some documentation are the unsaturated pyrrolizidine alkaloids. They occur in several plants, including Senecio and Symphytum species, and chronic use results in a very specific liver injury, veno-occlusive disease, with occlusion of the central and sublobular hepatic veins which can progress to cirrhosis (Shaw, 2010). Pyrrolizidine alkaloids are absorbed in the intestine and transported to the liver where they are metabolized to pyrroles. Pyrroles are very reactive chemically and cross link with double stranded DNA. They bind both proteins and nucleic acids within hepatocytes, but also damage sinusoidal endothelial cells by depletion of GSH and increased oxidative stress (Chen & Huo, 2010). Toxins from the herb Germander (Teuchrium chamaedrys) are an example of liver damage caused by the formation of reactive compounds by metabolism (Shaw, 2010). Reactive metabolites are generated by metabolism of its constituent neoclerodane diterpenoids. Neoclerodane diterpenoids is metabolised by CYP3A4, and electrophilic metabolites are believed to deplete GSH and damage cells through reduced defence system. However, depletion of cellular SH groups, binding to cytoskeleton of hepatocytes with altered cell membranes, and apoptosis are part of hepatoxic damage as studied in rat hepatocytes (Chitturi & Farrell, 2008). Interestingly, immune-mediated pathways in initiating liver injury were also associated with ingestion of Germander. When rechallenged with the herb, a rapid rise of serum transaminases was observed in some of the patients. Furthermore, autoantibodies (antinuclear, smooth muscle and antimitochondrial) were present in sera from patients who drank germander teas (Polymeros et al., 2002). In particular, a specific autoantibody (antimicrosomal epoxide hydrolase) was identified from sera of long-term drinkers of germander tea (De Berardinis et al., 2000). The target for this autoantibody is an epoxide hydrolase on the hepatocyte surface. These examples demonstrates the use of clinical experience (veno-occlusive disease, effect of rechallenge) to generate, examine and test mechanistic hypotheses in basic studies.

2.3.5 Vitamins

Daily use of vitamins and dietary supplements is common. In 2007, vitamin C, vitamin E, and multivitamins were among the five best-selling supplements, and most people consider vitamins and supplements safe (Rosenbloom, 2010). However, liver injury related to excessive doses of vitamins has been described for decades. The clinical picture of liver injury ranges from mild elevations of serum liver enzymes to cirrhosis. In the case of vitamin A, toxicity does not usually occur with standard doses below 50 000 international units (IU) per day as contained in common multivitamin preparations, but individual tolerability may vary (Stickel et al., 2011). Comorbidity, liver disease and chronic alcohol consumption can be associated liver injury with doses as low as 20 000 IU/day. A study in cultured HepG2 cells and freshly isolated rat hepatocytes, polar retinol metabolites caused marked cytotoxicity in a concentration- and time-dependent manner in both cell types with injury mainly caused by apoptosis (Dan et al., 2005). Alcohol-induced CYP2E1 is supposed to transform retinoids into highly reactive and toxic polar metabolites, and points to caution with supplements of vitamin A combined with chronic ingestion of ethanol. The above example is just one of several ingredients in nutritional-based therapies that can cause liver injury, and often use of excessive doses of the products can be the reason. However, the interaction with alcohol is of particular relevance due to the high prevalence of ethanol ingestion in the public. Nutritional-based therapies advertised against a multitude of diseases on the Internet are often a mixture of vitamins, proteins, herbs, salts and other ingredients. However, their composition can be far from the evidenced based nutritional therapies in hospitals, and they are in principle associated with all the problems mentioned earlier (aldulteration, contamination, etc). Based on the experience that fasting and malnutrition can increase the risk of serious paracetamol toxicity, there is a risk of liver injury due to irrational use of such supplements rather than the accepted diet in a community.

2.4 Further studies and use of retrospective data

The previous sections have clearly demonstrated that toxins from herbal medicine and nutritional-based therapies potentially can damage the liver in much the same way as conventional drugs. However, due to the aforementioned problem with formulation, standardization and epidemiology in complementary medicine, this type of liver injury is even more challenging to sort out than that of conventional drugs. Preventive measures in the form of information to health care professionals and the public about risk, regulative measures by medicinal agencies, and involvement by the industry itself are of paramount importance. Secondly, retrospective data from human cases should ideally include a thorough description of the product, chemical analysis of the quality and amount of the ingredients, history of the clinical course (effect of rechallenge? particular risk factors?), histopathological samples (signature injury?) from liver biopsy with other laboratory and clinical information. To test different hypotheses of basic mechanisms, a standard test substance should be formulated and then subsequently tested in established in vitro, ex vivo, and animal models. To effectively share knowledge between research groups this requires cooperation between the scientific communities in collaborating clinical networks as described previously for drug-induced liver injury (Andrade et al., 2005; Andrade et al., 2006; Hoofnagle, 2004).

Collection of tissue specimen during liver injury should not be discarded as a valuable biobank and ideas for subsequent studies of mechanisms and causality. A clinical pharmacologist would like to have relevant drug concentrations of suspected drug or toxins with metabolites if analytical assays were available. This would provide information on compliance (is the drug or toxin actually present in the blood?), and furthermore on exposure (is the substance found in a high concentration-higher than expected)? Although methodologically difficult, comparison of such data with drug or toxin concentrations in the offending organ would be an ideal tool to study tissue accumulation of substance. This could give clues to inherited (genetically defect cell transporters?) or environmental (other drug or toxin block a cell transporter?) risk factors of relevance. Liver biopsy during drug- and toxin-induced liver injury is of course not commonly used for this purpose. However, development of liquid chromatography-mass spectrometric (LC-MS/MS) assays for tissue specimens of tacrolimus from liver biopsy have been shown to be better correlated to histopathologic rejection scores than conventional immunoassays of ordinary blood concentrations (Capron et al., 2007). With further development of highly sensitive LC-MS/MS assays, specific determination of substances with metabolites can hopefully be useful in the context of drug- and toxin-induced liver injury. Development of imaging techniques (like nuclear magnetic resonance, NMR) and contrast agents for non invasive evaluation of substances and/or injury in the organ represent additional tools. Based on the experience that current methods for early detection and prediction of drug-induced liver injury in patients are not optimal, applications of analytical technologies such as NMR and LC-MS/MS to profile individual metabolite formation in biofluids (plasma and urine) after conventional dosing are suggested (O'Connell & Watkins, 2010). The hope is that alterations in the profiles of endogenous metabolites ("the metabolome") may precede development of clinically overt drug-induced liver injury.

3. Case reports and drug information centres

Drug information centres (DICs) have been established in Europe and other parts of the world in order to give health professionals, i.e. physicians, dentists, nurses, midwives and pharmacists, non-commercial information about drug treatment, drug problems and pharmaceuticals (Hedegaard & Damkier, 2009; Schjøtt et al. 2002). The RELIS network is today made up by the four regional drug information centres (DICs) in Norway. The centres are organised in close collaboration with the departments of clinical pharmacology at four university hospitals. Pharmacists and clinical pharmacologists answer problem-oriented drug-related queries from health care professionals. The queries are published along with the answers and reference sources in a web-based, full-text query-answer database (the RELIS database), which is accessed through the RELIS homepage. Question-answer pairs are indexed, and can be retrieved form the database through a search function. Furthermore, each RELIS function as a regional pharmacovilance unit processing spontaneous adverse drug reaction reports in cooperation with the Norwegian Medical Agency. Reports are retrievable from the Norwegian Adverse Drug Reaction database, and relevant information about drug and toxin associated liver injury are published on the RELIS homepage, in newsletters to physicians and in national and international journals. Of importance is the close collaboration between RELIS and clinical pharmacologists. Thus, analytical pharmacological competence and skills in laboratory diagnostics are supplemented with knowledge of practical pharmacokinetic tools in the diagnosis of adverse effects. As a problem-oriented DIC, RELIS believe that presentation of clinically relevant examples instead of more general warnings and alerts are a useful medium to inform health care professionals about risk of drug- and toxin-induced liver injury. In the last section of this chapter, we present two illustrating examples of information about such liver injury from RELIS.

3.1 Green tea and the quality of a case report

In 2009, RELIS published as an adverse drug reaction report about Lotus-f3 (Bergman & Schjøtt, 2009). Lotus-f3 contains an extract of green tea, which has been associated with hepatotoxicity. The presentation of the case followed the guidelines for submitting adverse event reports for publication (Kelly et al., 2007). The guidelines were developed because deficiencies in vital information in published cases can often limit the value of such reports by failing to provide enough details for either (i) a differential diagnosis or provisional assessment of cause-effect association, or (ii) a reasonable pharmacological or biological explanation. Importantly, the authors (Kelly et al., 2007) claim that properly described, a published report of one or more adverse events can provide a useful signal of possible risks associated with the use of a drug or medical product which might warrant further exploration. Through communication with the reporting physician and the local hospital, RELIS was able to obtain relevant clinical information including successful withdrawal of

Lotus-f3, liver biopsy, laboratory data and subsequent successful rechallenge with a concomitant drug. Importantly, RELIS had previously received several questions concerning the possible association between natural products and hepatitis or jaundice since 1995. Moreover, in five of these questions, the suspected natural products contained green tea, among other constituents. Thus, availability of relevant documentation based on previous suspicion was retrievable from the RELIS database which was valuable during the processing of this case description.

3.2 Fortodol and fatal addulteration

Fortodol was marketed in Norway as nutritional-based product, containing curcumin from Turmeric (Curcuma longa) as the active ingredient. Curcumin is proposed as an analgetic and anti-inflammatory agent. From 2007, RELIS received several queries and adverse reaction reports associated with Fortodol. In several of these, increase in liver enzymes and suspicion of liver injury was related to ingestion of the product. Five cases of liver failure, including three women (47-65 year) and two men (67-69 year), where reported. The case of the oldest man was fatal and this prompted RELIS in 2009 to retrieve capsules of the product from the relatives of the diseased. The capsules were subsequently analysed, and contained a mean of 42 mg of nimesulid per capsule. Nimesulid is a NSAID, not registrated or marketed as a legal drug in Norway. The drug has been withdrawn from the market of several European countries due to suspicion of liver injury. The European Medical Agency (EMEA) recommends that nimesulid should be used for up to 15 days at a daily maximum dose of 100 mg x 2. Fortodol was sold in packages containing 100 capsules, with recommended daily dose of 1-2 as needed. RELIS together with the Norwegian Medical Agency warned health care professionals and the public through interviews and articles in the media. The Norwegian Food Safety Authority subsequently contacted the importer of the product, and Fortodol was withdrawn from the market. In Sweden, four cases of serious liver injury was known with one fatal (Kechagias et al., 2010). The Swedish Medical Agency analysed Fortodol, and found nimesulid in two out of nine packages. This example demonstrates consequences of adulteration and the important role of DICs in the process of detection of and information about a health problem.

4. Conclusion

The present chapter summarizes damaging effects of drugs and toxins on the liver, in particular adverse effects of herbal medicine and nutritional-based therapies. It has been emphazised that toxins from complementary medicine can damage the liver in much the same way as conventional drugs. Liver injury due to drugs or toxins represents a diagnostic challenge for the clinician and a complex research issue for the scientist. Both pre-marketing and post-marketing data associated with a drug are of importance to describe potential for liver injury and risk factors of relevance. The search for relevant predictors of liver injury during pre-clinical and clinical phases of drug testing (chemical properties that increase the potential for drug-induced liver injury?) as well as risk factors (inherited, environmental or acquired characteristics that increase the likelihood of clinical liver disease?) in individuals prescribed legal drugs continues. Future studies are associated with "omics" technologies (genomics, proteomics, metabolomics) and "the metabolome" (variation in the profiles of endogenous metabolites) to describe new predictive biomarkers. However, cooperation in clinical networks represents a significant contribution to our understanding of etiology, pathogenesis and risk of drug-induced liver injury. Furthermore their aim at developing more drug-specific assessment tools for evaluation of causality is promising. In the case of toxin-induced liver injury, preventive measures in the form of information to health care professionals and the public about risk, regulative measures by medicinal agencies, and involvement by the industry itself are of importance. Due to the idiosyncratic nature of drug-or toxin-induced liver injury, case reports provided by DICs represent a source of signal generation of risk and formulation of hypotheses of relevance to explain clinical events.

5. References

Adams, D.H.; Ju, C.; Ramaiah, S.K.; Uetrecht, J. & Jaeschke, H. (2010). Mechanisms of immune-mediated liver injury. *Toxicological Sciences*, Vol.115, No.2, (June 2010), pp. 307-321, ISSN 1096-6080

Andrade, R.J.; Lucena, M.I.; Alonso, A.; García-Cortes, M.; García-Ruiz, E.; Benitez, R.; Fernández, M.C.; Pelaez, G.; Romero, M.; Corpas, R.; Durán, J.A.; Jiménez, M.; Rodrigo, L.; Nogueras, F.; Martín-Vivaldi, R.; Navarro, J.M.; Salmerón, J.; de la Cuesta, F.S. & Hidalgo, R. (2004). HLA class II genotype influences the type of liver injury in drug-induced idiosyncratic liver disease. *Hepatology*, Vol.39, No.6, (June 2004), pp. 1603–1612, ISSN 0270-9139

Andrade, R.J.; Lucena, M.I.; Fernández, M.C.; Pelaez, G.; Pachkoria, K.; García-Ruiz, E.; García-Muñoz, B.; González-Grande, R.; Pizarro, A.; Durán, J.A.; Jiménez, M.; Rodrigo, L.; Romero-Gomez, M.; Navarro, J.M.; Planas, R.; Costa, J.; Borras, A.; Soler, A.; Salmerón, J. & Martin-Vivaldi, R; Spanish Group for the Study of Drug-Induced Liver Disease. (2005). Drug-induced liver injury: an analysis of 461 incidences submitted to the Spanish registry over a 10-year period. *Gastroenterology*, Vol.129, No.2 (August 2005), pp. 512–521, ISSN 0016-5085

Andrade, R.J.; Lucena, M.I.; Kaplowitz, N.; García-Muņoz, B.; Borraz, Y.; Pachkoria, K.; García-Cortés, M.; Fernández, M.C.; Pelaez, G.; Rodrigo, L.; Durán, J.A.; Costa, J.; Planas, R.; Barriocanal, A.; Guarner, C.; Romero-Gomez, M.; Muņoz-Yagüe, T.; Salmerón, J. & Hidalgo, R. (2006). Outcome of acute idiosyncratic drug-induced liver injury: long-term follow-up in a hepatotoxicity registry. *Hepatology*, Vol. 44, No.6, (December 2006), pp.1581-1588, ISSN 0270-9139

Andrade, R.J.; Robles, M.; Fernández-Castañer, A.; López-Ortega, S.; López-Vega, M.C. & Lucena, M.I. (2007). Assessment of drug-induced hepatotoxicity in clinical practice: a challenge for gastroenterologists. *World J Gastroenterol*, Vol.13, No.3, (January 2007), pp. 329-340, ISSN 1007-9327

Arteaga, S.; Andrade-Cetto, A. & Cárdenas, R. (2005). Larrea tridentata (Creosote bush), an abundant plant of Mexican and US-American deserts and its metabolite nordihydroguaiaretic acid. *J Ethnopharmacol*, Vol.98, No.3, (April 2005), pp. 231–239, ISSN 0378-8741

Bader, T. (2010). Liver tests are irrelevant when prescribing statins. *Lancet*, Vol.376, No. 9756, (December 2010), pp. 1882-1883, ISSN 0140-6736

Bailey, M.J. & Dickinson, R.G. (2003). Acyl glucuronide reactivity in perspective: biological consequences. *Chemico-Biological Interactions*, Vol.145, No.2, (May 2003), pp. 117-137, ISSN 0009-2797

Bakke, O.M.; Manocchia, M.; de Abajo, F.; Kaitin, K.I. & Lasagna, L. (1995). Drug safety discontinuations in the United Kingdom, the United States, and Spain from 1974 through 1993: a regulatory perspective. *Clinical Pharmacology & Therapeutics*, Vol.58, No.1, (July 1995), pp. 108-117, ISSN 0009-9236

Baniasadi, S.; Eftekhari, P.; Tabarsi, P.; Fahimi, F.; Raoufy, M.R.; Masjedi, M.R. & Velayati, A.A. (2010). Protective effect of N-acetylcysteine on antituberculosis drug-induced hepatotoxicity. *Eur J Gastroenterol Hepatol*, Vol. 22, No. 10, (October 2010), pp. 1235-1238, ISSN 0954-691X

Benichou, C. (1990). Criteria of drug-induced liver disorders. Report of an international consensus meeting. *J Hepatol*, Vol.11, No.2, (September 1990), pp. 272-276, ISSN 0168-8278

Bergman, J. & Schjøtt, J. (2009). Hepatitis caused by Lotus-f3? *Basic Clin Pharmacol Toxicol*, Vol.104, No.5, (May 2009), pp. 414-416, ISSN 1742-7835

Bessone, F. (2010). Non-steroidal anti-inflammatory drugs: what is the actual risk of liver damage? *World J Gastroenterol*, Vol.16, No.45, (December 2010), pp. 5651-5661, ISSN 1007-9327

Byard, R.W. (2010). A review of the potential forensic significance of traditional herbal medicines. *J Forensic Sci*, Vol. 55, No. 1, (January 2010), pp. 89-92, ISSN 0022-1198

Capron, A.; Lerut, J.; Verbaandert, C.; Mathys, J.; Ciccarelli, O.; Vanbinst, R.; Roggen, F.; De Reyck, C.; Lemaire, J. & Wallemacq, P.E. (2007). Validation of a liquid chromatography-mass spectrometric assay for tacrolimus in liver biopsies after hepatic transplantation: correlation with histopathologic staging of rejection. *Ther Drug Monit*, Vol.29, No.3, (June 2007), pp. 340-348, ISSN 0163-4356

Castell, J.V. & Castell, M. (2006). Allergic hepatitis induced by drugs. *Curr Opin Allergy Clin Immunol*, Vol.6, No.4, (August 2006), pp. 258–265, ISSN 1528-4050

Chang, W.T.; Thissen, U.; Ehlert, K.A.; Koek, M.M.; Renger, H.; Jellema, R.H.; Hankemeier, T.; van der Greef, J. & Wang, M. (2006). Effects of growth conditions and processing on Rehmannia glutinosa using fingerprint strategy. *Planta Med*, Vol.72, No.5, (April 2006), pp. 458-467, ISSN 0032-0943

Chen, Z. & Huo, J.R. (2010). Hepatic veno-occlusive disease associated with toxicity of pyrrolizidine alkaloids in herbal preparations. *Neth J Med*, Vol.68, No.6, (June 2010), pp. 252-260, ISSN 0300-2977

Chitturi, S. & Farrell, G.C. (2008). Hepatotoxic slimming aids and other herbal hepatotoxins. *J Gastroenterol Hepatol*, Vol.23, No.3, (March 2008), pp. 366-373, ISSN 0815-9319

Daly, A.K.; Donaldson, P.T.; Bhatnagar, P.; Shen, Y.; Pe'er, I.; Floratos, A.; Daly, M.J.; Goldstein, D.B.; John, S.; Nelson, M.R.; Graham, J.; Park, B.K.; Dillon, J.F.; Bernal, W.; Cordell, H.J.; Pirmohamed, M.; Aithal, G.P. & Day, C.P.; DILIGEN Study; International SAE Consortium. (2009). HLA-B*5701 genotype is a major determinant of drug-induced liver injury due to flucloxacillin. *Nat Genet*, Vol.41, No.7, (July 2009), pp. 816-819, ISSN 1061-4036

Daly, A.K. (2010). Drug-induced liver injury: past, present and future. *Pharmacogenomics*, Vol.11, No.5 (May 2010), pp. 607-611, ISSN 1462-2416

Dan, Z.; Popov, Y.; Patsenker, E.; Preimel, D.; Liu, C.; Wang, X.D.; Seitz, H.K.; Schuppan, D. & Stickel, F. (2005). Hepatotoxicity of alcohol-related polar retinoid metabolites involves apoptosis via loss of mitochondrial membrane potential. *FASEB J*, Vol.19, No.7, (May 2005), pp. 845–847, ISSN 0892-6638

Danan, G. & Benichou, C. (1993). Causality assessment of adverse reactions to drugs-I. A novel method based on the conclusions of international consensus meetings: application to drug-induced liver injuries. *J Clin Epidemiol,* Vol.46, No.11, (November 1993), pp. 1323-1330, ISSN 0895-4356

David, S. & Hamilton, P.J. (2010). Drug-induced liver injury. *US Gastroenterology and Hepatology Review,* Vol.6, No.8, (December 2010), pp. 73–80, ISSN 1758-3934

De Berardinis, V. ; Moulis, C. ; Maurice, M. ; Beaune, P. ; Pessayre, D. ; Pompon, D. & Loeper, J. (2000). Human microsomal epoxide hydrolase is the target of germander-induced autoantibodies on the surface of human hepatocytes. *Mol Pharmacol,* Vol.58, No.3 (September 2000), pp. 542-551, ISSN 0026-895X

De Smet, P.A. (2002). Herbal remedies. *N Engl J Med,* Vol.347, No.25, (December 2002), pp. 2046-2056, ISSN 0028-4793

Fontana, R.J.; Watkins, P.B.; Bonkovsky, H.L.; Chalasani, N.; Davern, T.; Serrano, J. & Rochon, J.; DILIN Study Group. (2009). Drug-Induced Liver Injury Network (DILIN) prospective study: rationale, design and conduct. *Drug Safety,* Vol.32, No.1, (January 2009), pp. 55-68, ISSN 0114-5916

Fontana, R.J.; Seeff, L.B.; Andrade, R.J.; Björnsson, E.; Day, C.P.; Serrano, J. & Hoofnagle, J.H. (2010). Standardization of nomenclature and causality assessment in drug-induced liver injury: summary of a clinical research workshop. *Hepatology,* Vol.52, No.2, (August 2010), pp. 730-742, ISSN 0270-9139

Fu, S.; Korkmaz, E.; Braet, F.; Ngo, Q. & Ramzan, I. (2008). Influence of kavain on hepatic ultrastructure. *World J Gastroenterol,* Vol.14, No.4, (January 2008), pp. 541-546, ISSN 1007-9327

García-Cortés, M.; Stephens, C.; Lucena, M.I.; Fernández-Castañer, A. & Andrade, R.J. (2011). Causality assessment methods in drug induced liver injury: strengths and weaknesses. *Journal of Hepatology,* (February 2011), Epub ahead of print, ISSN 0168-8278

Gómez-Lechón, M.J.; Castell, J.V. & Donato, M.T. (2010). The Use of Hepatocytes to Investigate Drug Toxicity. In: *Hepatocytes: Methods and Protocols. Methods Molecular Biology,* P. Maurel, (Ed.), 389-415, Humana Press, ISBN 9781607616870, New York, USA

Gordon, D.W.; Rosenthal, G.; Hart, J.; Sirota, R. & Baker, A.L. (1995). Chaparral ingestion. The broadening spectrum of liver injury caused by herbal medications. *JAMA,* Vol. 273, No.6, (February 1995), pp. 489-490, ISSN 00987484

Grattagliano, I.; Bonfrate, L.; Diogo, C.V.; Wang, H.H.; Wang, D.Q. & Portincasa, P. (2009). Biochemical mechanisms in drug-induced liver injury: certanties and doubts. *World J Gastroenterol,* Vol.15, No.39, (October 2009), pp. 4865-4876, ISSN 1007-9327

Gurley, B.J.; Gardner, S.F. & Hubbard, M.A. (2000). Content versus label claims in ephedra-containing dietary supplements. *Am J Health Syst Pharm,* Vol.57, No. 10, (May 2000), pp. 963-969, ISSN 1079-2082

Han, D.; Shinohara, M.; Ybanez, M.D.; Saberi, B. & Kaplowitz, N. (2010). Signal Transduction Pathways Involved in Drug-Induced Liver Injury, In: *Adverse Drug Reactions. Handbook of Experimental Pharmacology,* J. Uetrecht, (Ed.), 267-310, Springer, ISBN 978-3-642-00662-3, Heidelberg, Germany.

Hedegaard, U. & Damkier, P. (2009). Problem-oriented drug information: physicians' expectations and impact on clinical practice. *Eur J Clin Pharmacol*, Vol.65, No.5, (May 2009), pp. 515–522, ISSN 0031-6970

Hoofnagle, J.H. (2004). Drug-induced liver injury network (DILIN). *Hepatology*, Vol.40, No.4, (October 2004), pp. 773-773, ISSN 0270-9139

Hughes, B. (2008). Industry concern over EU hepatotoxicity guidance. *Nature Reviews Drug Discovery*, Vol.7, No.9, (September 2008), pp. 719-719, ISSN 1474-1776

Hussaini, S.H.; O'Brien, C.S.; Despott, E.J. & Dalton, H.R. (2007). Antibiotic therapy: a major cause of drug-induced jaundice in southwest England. *Eur J Gastroenterol Hepatol*, Vol.19, No.1, (January 2007), pp. 15–20, ISSN 0954-691X

Kass, G.E.N. (2006). Mitochondrial involvement in drug-induced hepatic injury. *Chemico-Biological Interactions*, Vol.163, No.1-2, (October 2006), pp. 145-159, ISSN 0009- 2797

Kechagias, S.; Hägg, S. & Lotfi K. (2010). Drug-induced liver injury from the dietary supplement Fortodol. A manipulated preparation delayed the diagnosis (Article in Swedish). Lakartidningen, Vol.107, No.4, (Jan –Feb 2010), pp. 186-188, ISSN 0023-7205

Kelly, W.N.; Arellano, F.M.; Barnes, J.; Bergman, U.; Edwards, R.I.; Fernandez, A.M.; Freedman, S.B.; Goldsmith, D.I.; Huang, K.A.; Jones, J.K.; McLeay, R.; Moore, N.; Stather, R.H.; Trenque, T.; Troutman, W.G.; van Puijenbroek, E.; Williams, F. & Wise, R.P.; International Society for Pharmacoepidemiology; International Society of Pharmacovigilance. (2007). Guidelines for submitting adverse event reports for publication. *Drug Saf*, Vol.30, No.5, (May 2007), pp. 367-373, ISSN 0114-5916

Kemper, R.A. & Lai, G. (2008). Hepatic Bioactivation and Drug-Induced Liver Injury. In: *Advances in Bioactivation Research*, A.A. Elfarra (Ed.), 291-323, Springer, ISBN 978-0-387-77299-8, New York, USA.

Kleiner, D.E. (2009). The pathology of drug-induced liver injury. *Semin Liver Dis*, Vol. 29, No.4, (November 2009), pp. 364-372, ISSN 0272-8087

Larrey, D. & Pageaux, G.P. (2005). Drug-induced acute liver failure. *Eur J Gastroenterol Hepatol*, Vol.17, No.2, (February 2005), pp. 141–143, ISSN 0954-691X

Leung, V.W.; Shalansky, S.J.; Lo, M.K. & Jadusingh, E.A. (2009). Prevalence of use and the risk of adverse effects associated with complementary and alternative medicine in a cohort of patients receiving warfarin. *Ann Pharmacother*, Vol.43, No.5, (May 2009), pp. 875–881, ISSN 1060-0280

Lewis, J.H. (2006). 'Hy's Law,' the 'Rezulin Rule,' and other predictors of severe drug-induced hepatotoxicity: putting risk-benefit into perspective. *Pharmacoepidemiology and Drug Safety*, Vol.15, No.4, (April 2006) pp. 221–229, ISSN 1053-8569

Lim, S.T.S.; Dragull, K.; Tang, C.S.; Bittenbender, H.C.; Efird, J.T. & Nerurkar, P.V. (2007). Effects of Kava alkaloid, pipermethystine, and kavalactones on oxidative stress and cytochrome P450 in F-344 Rats. *Toxicological Sciences*, Vol.97, No.1, (May 2007), pp. 214–221, ISSN 1096-6080

Liu, Z.X. & Kaplowitz, N. (2002). Immune-mediated drug-induced liver disease. *Clin Liver Dis*, Vol.6, No.3, (August 2002), pp. 755-774, ISSN 1089-3261

Lucena, M.I.; García-Cortés, M.; Cueto, R.; Lopez-Duran, J.L. & Andrade, R.J. (2008). Assessment of drug-induced liver injury in clinical practice. *Fundamental & Clinical Pharmacology*, Vol.22, No.2, (April 2008), pp. 141-158, ISSN 07673981

Maglione, M.; Miotto, K.; Iguchi, M.; Jungvig, L.; Morton, S.C. & Shekelle, P.G. (2005). Psychiatric effects of ephedra use: an analysis of Food and Drug Administration reports of adverse events. *Am J Psychiatr*, Vol.162, No.1, (January 2005), pp. 189-191, ISSN 0002-953X

Maria, V.A. & Victorino, R.M. (1997). Development and validation of a clinical scale for the diagnosis of drug-induced hepatitis. *Hepatology*, Vol.26, No.3, (September 1997), pp. 664-669, ISSN 0270-9139

Mathews, J. M.; Etheridge, A. S. & Black, S. R. (2002). Inhibition of human cytochrome P450 activities by kava extract and kavalactones. *Drug Metab Dispos*, Vol.30, No.11, (November 2002), pp. 1153–1157, ISSN 0090-9556

Meier, Y.; Cavallaro, M.; Roos, M.; Pauli-Magnus, C.; Folkers, G.; Meier, P.J. & Fattinger, K. (2005). Incidence of drug-induced liver injury in medical inpatients. *Eur J Clin Pharmacol*, Vol.61, No.2, (April 2005), pp. 135-143, ISSN 0031-6970

Metha, N.; Ozick, L. & Gbadehan, E. (April 2010). Drug-induced hepatotoxicity. In: *Emedicine.medscape.com*, (March 2011). Available from: http://emedicine.medscape.com

Neff, G.W.; Reddy, K.R.; Durazo, F.A.; Meyer, D.; Marrero, R. & Kaplowitz, N. (2004). Severe hepatotoxicity associated with the use of weight loss diet supplements containing ma huang or usnic acid. *J Hepatol*, Vol. 41, No.6, (December 2004), pp. 1062–1064, ISSN 0168-8278

Nerurkar, P. V.; Dragull, K. & Tang, C. S. (2004). In vitro toxicity of kava alkaloid, pipermethystine, in HepG2 cells compared to kavalactones. *Toxicol Sci*,Vol.79, No.1, (May 2004), pp. 106–111, ISSN 1096-6080

Nutescu, E.A.; Shapiro, N.L.; Ibrahim, S. & West, P. (2006). Warfarin and its interactions with foods, herbs and other dietary supplements. *Expert Opin Drug Saf*, Vol.5, No.3, (May 2006), pp. 433–451, ISSN 1474-0338

O'Connell, T.M. & Watkins, P.B. (2010). The application of metabonomics to predict drug-induced liver injury. *Clin Pharmacol Ther*, Vol.88, No. 3, (September 2010), pp. 394-399, ISSN 0009-9236

Onusko, E. (2008). Statins and elevated liver tests: whats´s the fuss? *J Fam Pract*, Vol.57, No.7, (July 2008), pp. 449-452, ISSN 0094-3509

Ostapowicz, G.; Fontana, R.J.; Schiødt, F.V.; Larson, A.; Davern, T.J.; Han, S.H.; McCashland, T.M.; Shakil, A.O.; Hay, J.E.; Hynan, L.; Crippin, J.S.; Blei, A.T.; Samuel, G.; Reisch, J. & Lee, W.M.; Acute Liver Failure Study Group. (2002). Results of a prospective study of acute liver failure at 17 tertiary care centers in the United States. *Ann Intern Med*, Vol.137, No.12, (December 2002), pp. 947-954, ISSN 0003-4819

Pessayre, D.; Mansouri, A.; Berson, A. & Fromenty, B. (2010). Mitochondrial Involvement in Drug-Induced Liver Injury. In: *Adverse Drug Reactions. Handbook of Experimental Pharmacology*, J. Uetrecht, (Ed.), 311-365, Springer, ISBN 978-3-642-00662-3, Heidelberg, Germany.

Polymeros, D.; Kamberoglou, D. & Tzias, V. (2002). Acute cholestatic hepatitis caused by Teucrium polium (golden germander) with transient appearance of antimitochondrial antibody. *J Clin Gastroenterol*, Vol.34, No.1, (January 2002), pp. 100–101, ISSN 0192-0790

Ramachandran, R. & Kakar, S. (2009). Histological patterns in drug-induced liver disease. *J Clin Pathol*, Vol.62, No.6, (June 2009), pp. 481–492, ISSN 0021-9746

Rosenbloom, M. (February 2011). Vitamin Toxicity. In: *Emedicine.medscape.com*, (March 2011), Available from: http://emedicine.medscape.com

Russmann, S.; Kullak-Ublick, G.A. & Grattagliano, I. (2009). Current concepts of mechanisms in drug-induced hepatotoxicity. *Curr Med Chem*, Vol.16, No.23 (August 2009), pp. 3041-3053, ISSN 0929-8673

Sahi, J.; Grepper, S. & Smith, C. (2010). Hepatocytes as a tool in drug metabolism, transport and safety evaluations in drug discovery. *Curr Drug Discov Technol*, Vol.7, No.3, (September 2010), pp. 188-98, ISSN 1570-1638

Said, S.A. & El-Agamy, D.S. (2010). Prevention of sodium valproate-induced hepatotoxicity by curcumin, rosiglitazone and N-acetylcysteine in rats. *Arzneimittelforschung*, Vol.60, No.11, (November 2010), pp. 647-653, ISSN 0004-4172

Schjøtt, J.; Pomp, E. & Gedde-Dahl, A. (2002). Quality and impact of problem-oriented drug information: a method to change clinical practice among physicians? *Eur J Clin Pharmacol*, Vol.57, No.12, (February 2002), pp. 897–902, ISSN 0031-6970

Shaw, D. (2010). Toxicological risks of Chinese herbs. *Planta Med*, Vol.76, No.17, (December 2010), pp. 2012–2018, ISSN 0032-0943

Sheikh, N.M.; Philen, R.M. & Love, L.A. (1997). Chaparral-associated hepatotoxicity. *Arch Intern Med*, Vol.157, No.8, (April 1997), pp. 913-919, ISSN 0003-9926

Singh, Y. N. & Singh, N. N. (2002). Therapeutic potential of kava in the treatment of anxiety disorders. *CNS Drugs*, Vol.16, No.11, (June 2002), pp. 731–743, ISSN 1172-7047

Singh, Y. N. & Devkota, A. K. (2003). Aqueous kava extracts do not affect liver function tests in rats. *Planta Med*, Vol.69, No.6, (June 2003), pp. 496–499, ISSN 0032-0943

Sgro, C.; Clinard, F.; Ouazir, K.; Chanay, H.; Allard, C.; Guilleminet, C.; Lenoir, C.; Lemoine, A. & Hillon, P. (2002). Incidence of drug-induced hepatic injuries. A French population-based study. *Hepatology*, Vol.36, No.2, (August 2002), pp. 451–455, ISSN 0270-9139

Smith, A. & Dillon, J. (September 2009). Acute liver injury associated with the use of herbal preparations containing glucosamine: three case studies. In: *BMJ Case Reports*, (March 2011), ISSN 1757-790X, Available from: http://casereports.bmj.com

Stickel, F.; Patsenker, E. & Schuppan, D. (2005). Herbal hepatotoxicty. *Journal of Hepatology*, Vol.43, No.5, (November 2005), pp. 901–910, ISSN 0168-8278

Stickel, F.; Kessebohm, K.; Weimann, R. & Seitz, H. K. (2011). Review of liver injury associated with dietary supplements. *Liver International*, (January 2011), Ahead of print, ISSN1478-3223

Tajiri, K. & Shimizu, Y. (2008). Practical guidelines for diagnosis and early management of drug-induced liver injury. *World JGastroenterol*, Vol.14, No.44, (November 2008), pp. 6774–6785, ISSN 1007-9327

Takikawa, H.; Takamori, Y.; Kumagi, T.; Onji, M.; Watanabe, M.; Shibuya, A.; Hisamochi, A.; Kumashiro, R.; Ito, T.; Mitsumoto, Y.; Nakamura, A. & Sakaguchi, T. (2003). Assessment of 287 Japanese cases of drug induced liver injury by the diagnostic scale of the International Consensus Meeting. *Hepatol Res*, Vol.27, No.3, (November 2003), pp. 192-195, ISSN 1386-6346

Teschke, R.; Qiu, S.X. & Lebot, V. Herbal hepatotoxicity by kava: update on pipermethystine, flavokavain B, and mould hepatotoxins as primarily assumed culprits. *Dig Liv Dis*, (March 2011), Epub ahead of print, ISSN 1590-8658

Verbeeck, R.K. (2008). Pharmacokinetics and dosage adjustment in patients with hepatic dysfunction. *Eur J Clin Pharmacol*, Vol.64, No.12, (September 2008), pp.1147–1161, ISSN 0031-6970

Vuppalanchi, R.; Hayashi, P.H.; Chalasani, N.; Fontana, R.J.; Bonkovsky, H.; Saxena, R.; Kleiner, D. & Hoofnagle, J.H; Drug-Induced Liver Injury Network (DILIN). (2010). Duloxetine hepatotoxicity: a case-series from the drug-induced liver injury network. *Aliment Pharmacol Ther*, Vol.32, No.9, (November 2010), pp. 1174–1183, ISSN 0269-2813

Walgren, J.L.; Mitchell, M.D. & Thompson, D.C. (2005). Role of metabolism in drug-induced idiosyncratic hepatotoxicity. *Crit Rev Toxicol*, Vol.35, No.4, (April-May 2005), pp. 325-361, ISSN 1040-8444

Watkins, P.B.; Kaplowitz, N.; Slattery, J.T.; Colonese, C.R.; Colucci, S.V.; Stewart, P.W. & Harris, S.C. (2006). Aminotransferase elevations in healthy adults receiving 4 grams of acetaminophen daily: a randomized controlled trial. *JAMA*, Vol.296, No.1, (July 2006), pp. 87-93, ISSN 1590-8658

Zhou, P.; Gross, S.; Liu, J.H.; Yu, B.Y.; Feng, L.L.; Nolta, J.; Sharma, V.; Piwnica-Worms, D. & Qiu, S.X. (2010). Flavokawain B, the hepatotoxic constituent from kava root, induces GSH-sensitive oxidative stress through modulation of IKK/NF-kappaB and MAPK signaling pathways. *FASEB J*, Vol.24, No.12, (December 2010), pp. 4722-4732, ISSN 0892-6638

Part 2

Liver Biopsy in Transplantation

11

The Liver Biopsy During Organ Procurement

Johannes W. Rey[1] and Jochen W.U. Fries[2]
[1]*University Hospital of Mainz, Department of Internal Medicine I,*
[2]*University Hospital of Cologne, Institute of Pathology,*
Germany

1. Introduction

Hepatic steatosis is a commonly noticed and most prevalent condition among donated liver grafts. The pressing demand for organs and increased patient death rates while awaiting organ transplantation has led to the use of cadaveric livers with hepatic steatosis for transplantation. Recent data reported the use of steatotic liver grafts in 71% of cases (Noujaim et al., 2009). Moreover, to meet the organ shortage, the criteria for donation have been broadened to include donors with advanced age, hepatitis B and C viruses, neoplasms, and benign underlying diseases (Fondevila et al., 2009). The use of expanded-criteria donors (ECDs) and the donor risk index (DRI) are strategies that have been proposed to increase the donor pool (Feng et al., 2006). The Donor Risk Index (DRI) lists seven donor characteristics, together with cold ischemia time and location of the donor as risk factors for graft failure. DRI >1.7 is reported to be associated with shorter survival after liver transplantation (Palmiero et al., 2010). It is hypothesized that donor hepatic steatosis is an additional independent risk factor (Spitzer et al., 2010). It remains unclear which value micro and/or macrovesicular steatosis have for the short and long term results after liver transplantation. Therefore, different papers report a safe use of grafts with a severe microvesicular steatosis (Fishbein et al., 1997; McCormack et al., 2007). However, steatosis is one of the most important factors affecting liver allograft function. Steatosis is common in several situations, including: obesity, diabetes, and alcohol abuse (Durand et al., 2008). Organ donation predictive factors for recipient survival were: age, viral status, and degree of liver steatosis. Liver transplantation for alcoholic liver disease showed the highest complication rate. Chronic liver rejection occurred more frequently in the AIH transplanted group. The most useful predictive factors for 1-year survival were urea/creatinine and liver function tests. (Patkowski et al., 2009). In addition, transplantation of a liver with >25% steatosis was a risk factor for the development of a biliary complication (Baccarani et al., 2009). Nevertheless, macrovesicular steatosis is known as a risk factor for early graft dysfunction and graft failure. Most transplantation centres consider 60% the value limit for transplantability, while others have adopted 30% as a cut-off limit (D'Alessandro et al., 2010).

Organ donor shortage continues to pose a significant problem. To ensure fair and transparent allocation of too few post-mortem grafts, the model of end-stage liver disease (MELD)-based allocation was implemented in the Eurotransplant area in December 2006. This has decreased the waiting list mortality rate from 20 to 10 %, but at the same time has reduced post OLT survival (1-year survival from almost 90% to below 80%), which is largely due to patients with a labMELD score >30. Following MELD introduction, the regular allocation threshold increased from a matchMELD of initially 25 to a current value of 34. At the same time, the quality of donor organs has seen a continuous deterioration over the last 10 - 15 years, e.g., 63% of organs have a donor risk index of > 1.5 (Schlitt et al., 2011). Among the several reasons that might play an important contributing role are the pressing organ demand and the increasing percentage of elderly donors with co-morbidities, such as steatosis hepatis, combined with a high MELD-Score of the recipient at the point of transplantation. MELD >30 currently represents a major risk factor for outcome after liver transplantation. However, risk factors differ in individual patient subgroups (Weismuller et al., 2011). There has been data supporting the use of ECD organs in good-risk recipients. These include grafts from donors that are 60 years old, with prolonged hypotension, or with mild to moderate macrovescicular steatosis (Amin et al., 2004). The frozen-section histological evaluation of biopsies from cadaveric liver donors is an accurate, time-effective, and predictive method for the assessment of graft suitability. Nevertheless, it is discussed controversially if frozen-section histological evaluation of biopsies is a safe and efficient method in detection of macro- and microvesicular steatosis. Therefore, it is reported that validated pretransplant frozen-section analysis is a reliable technique when the maximum value for organ transplantation was 60% steatosis. Thus, the usefulness of another technique to support a more precise steatosis evaluation is recommended (D'Alessandro et al., 2010).

2. Brain death, permission and intensive care treatment

When brain death is determined according to actual guidelines, donors are selected for potential organ donation after permission is given. The diagnosis of brain death requires the absence of brain-stem reflexes and respiratory drive in a normothermic, non-drugged, comatose patient with a known irreversible brain lesion and no contributing metabolic derangements. Permission for organ donation has to be given considering the current transplantation law in the procurement country. While the donor liver is allocated further intensive care treatment is still necessary. Hepatic function is impaired after brain death. There is depletion of hepatic glycogen and a reduction in hepatic sinusoidal perfusion that occurs because of leukocyte activation and accumulation in the microcirculation (Smith, 2004). It is unclear if the application of cortisone reduces the leukocyte activation in the liver tissue. Maintenance of cardiovascular, pulmonary and endocrinological stability is important for successful organ transplantation. The goals in managing the hemodynamic status of the donor are: to achieve normovolemia, maintain blood pressure, and optimize cardiac output, so as to achieve gradients of perfusion pressure and blood flow that promote organ function with the use of the least amount of vasoactive-drug support. Diabetes insipidus results from the absence of vasopressin after the destruction of the posterior pituitary gland. It contributes to hyperosmolarity, hemodynamic instability, and electrolyte abnormalities (e.g. hypernatremia) as a consequence of an excessive loss of free water. These effects should be prevented, because hypernatremia leads to osmotic gradients at the liver cell with consecutive cell swelling in the recipient after liver transplantation. However, recent data suggests that transplant measures of early liver function and risk of failure, up to 1-year post-transplant, do not differ significantly based on peak or terminal donor serum sodium levels. These results indicate that donor serum sodium level likely has little clinical impact on post-transplant liver function. (Dictus et al., 2009; Kutsogiannis et al., 2006; Mangus et al., 2010; Shah, 2008; Wood et al., 2004).

3. Surgical procurement

The surgical technic of organ procurement has been reported earlier by Rosenthal et al. in 1983. The following chapter briefly resumes the major important aspects. The necessary technical details, depending especially on the combination of organs to be removed, are: wide exposure, dissection of each organ to be removed up to disconnection from the circulation while the heart is still beating, placement of cannulas for in-situ cold perfusion, orderly removal of the organs with cold perfusion protection of the organs to be removed last. In instances of liver and kidney procurement only, a midline sternal splitting incision is not routinely used, but can provide immediate access to the heart if there is any instability and can help to remove the liver more gently. After wide abdominal exposure, liver mobilization is carried out first, since this is the most meticulous dissection and attention to hemostasis is strict. Careful inspection of the arterial anatomy is done first; any anomalous arteries must be preserved. A branch to the left lobe is sometimes seen arising from the left gastric artery and can be seen in the superior portion of the gastrohepatic ligament. A branch to the right lobe arises from the superior mesenteric artery. This artery has occasionally been the entire arterial supply to the liver. The hepatic artery is dissected from the aorta. The common bile duct is exposed at its entrance to the pancreas and transected. The portal vein is dissected after transection of the pancreas to facilitate exposure. The inferior mesenteric and coronary veins are ligated; the splenic and superior mesenteric veins are mobilized. The junction of the inferior caval vein and right heart is identified, to provide maximal length of upper cuff of the vena cava. The liver is essentially ready for removal at this point. Cannulas are then placed for in-situ perfusion and crushed ice is immediately applied for cooling the external abdomen. First, cannulas are placed in the vena cava and aorta at their respective bifurcations and the vessels divided distally. Heparin 300 units/Kg is given to prevent clotting (Rosenthal et al., 1983). Today, liver procurement is mostly performed by local surgeons experienced in at least ten organ donations as required. Liver preservation is realised using Histidine-Tryptophan-Ketoglutarate solution (Custodiol®) or University of Wisconsin solution (Viaspan®) as preservative.

4. Surgical evaluation

A successful evaluation of a liver graft for transplantation is based on several essential criteria: donor medical history, laboratory data on liver function, virological analysis, sonography, as well as intraoperative liver exploration particular for colour and palpation. Identifying marginal from good donor livers is one of the most difficult surgical tasks. Thus, surgical experience and evaluation criteria have increased importance in liver transplantation. Visual inspection and palpation are the most commonly used methods for surgeons to establish liver quality. The positive predictive value of a surgical appraisal of liver steatosis has been reported to be 71% for severe; 46% for moderate; and 17% for mild steatosis (Adam et al., 1991). When donor surgeons suspect steatosis by inspection of a liver graft, a frozen section is only performed in 38% to 47% of cases (Nocito et al., 2006). However, for a successful evaluation and consequent transplantation, reliable and objective means are needed to assess the liver before transplantation. Histopathological examination should provide a helpful decision for the transplant surgeon whether or not the organ is suitable for transplantation. Therefore, in all cases of organ procurement a wedge biopsy of 1-cm side length should be performed in two liver segments, one for each liver lobe (i.e., segments 3 and 6 or 7) (Frankel et al., 2002; Rey et al., 2009).

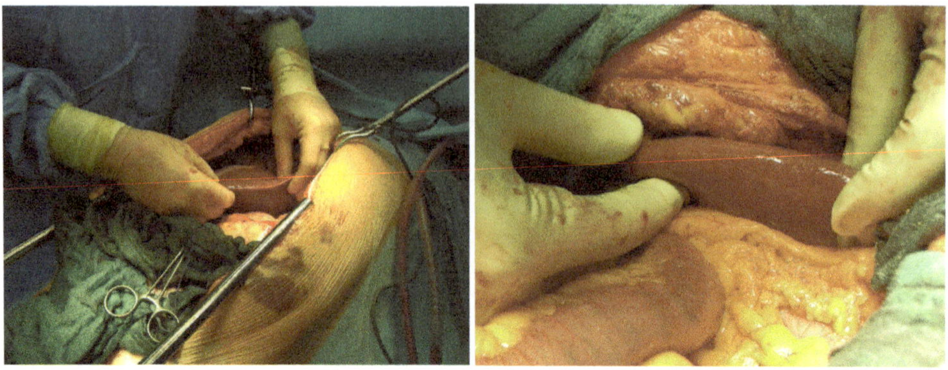

Fig. 1. The surgical evaluation of organ donor livers before preservation in situ.

To evaluate liver quality is one of the most difficult surgical challenges during organ procurement. Therefore visual inspection and palpation are the most commonly used methods in situ before liver preservation. At this time liver biopsy is mostly required.

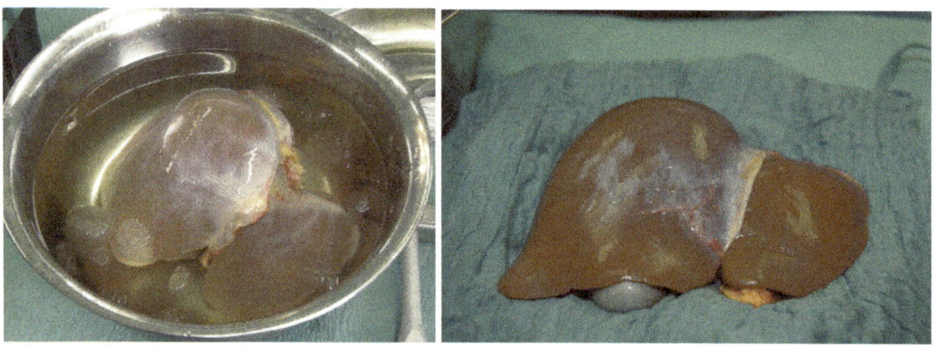

Fig. 2. After liver preservation and procurement surgical evaluation of graft quality will be repeated.

After liver procurement the graft´s quality will be evaluated again by the donor surgeon. Surgical and anatomical characteristics are documented and communicated to the transplant coordinator and transplant surgeon. So far the liver biopsy results should be available. Finally, the graft is packaged into three bags of aseptic fluid.

5. Frozen section

Frozen section examination is useful in excluding donor organs which may become dysfunctional after transplantation. It has been shown that primary non-function has significantly decreased using frozen section examination (Markin et al., 1993).

If a frozen section is required, the procedure consists of the following principal steps: the surgeon should take a wedge biopsy of 1-cm side length. The wedge will be split lengthwise; one half is snap frozen in liquid nitrogen from which 3 - 4-µm-thick sections are cut, briefly fixed in 4% buffered formalin (pH 7.4), rinsed, and counterstained with H&E. After dehydration in rising concentrations of alcohol, the section is coverslipped and analyzed by routine light microscopy.

In order to obtain a frozen section of high enough quality, a number of important aspects have to be considered in frozen section technique of liver tissue, being outlined in the following passage, even though we assume that any pathologist will be familiar with the principle of frozen section cutting. Once the wedge is split longitudinally, the obtained section should be placed with its cauterized side down, flatly upon the frozen section chuck. When placing the sectioned tissue, this thickness should guarantee cauterization artifacts extending to the freshly cut surface. This is increasingly important, if the actual tissue area is small, being crucial in wedges with less than 0.5cm wedge length. Irrespective of the actual wedge length, the area of the section should not extend beyond 1.0 cm^2. If the wedge is bigger, splitting it into two should be considered and each piece analyzed by frozen section separately to obtain a picture of the entire area. A biopsy is considered to be sufficiently large, if it contains at least 10 cross sections of portal tracts. The number of portal tracts has to be documented to ensure a sufficient quality control. In addition, at least 4 sections of 3 - 5 µm each should be cut and stained with H&E, to be able to analyze tissue alterations on several sections in sequence and in order to evaluate their importance. This will help to properly identify artifacts due to the procedure itself, such as uneven cuts, folds, shattering or rips of the section.

The problems of inadequate equilibration to the correct temperature are several fold (Fig. 3). The temperature of the equipment, i.e. the knife, the chuck, and the cutting table itself as well as that of the frozen tissue should be at least -20^{0}C and kept constant. This means equilibration time for the frozen tissue and the newly introduced section blade. Ideally, the "optimal" temperature is reached, when the cut section flows over the knife in a smooth uniform sheet with minimal curling. This, however, may mean taking the time to make adjustments to the cryostat temperature, which is time well spent to optimize the outcome, considering the consequences of rejection due to bad sectioning technique. A block that is too cold will quickly curl in an unmanageable way or shatter, creating a Venetian blind-like artefact. The tissue can be condensed if it is too cold, and it will even be tougher to cut, resulting in thick and thin sections. In contrast, if the block is too warm it results in a crumpled section. Thus, when placing the section itself, a layer of freezing compound with a flat surface has to be provided on the pre-cooled, and well cleaned chuck first, on which the freshly cut section is placed and completely covered by freezing compound medium. To obtain optimal freezing results, either a pre-cooled (at -20 ^{0}C) metal block is placed on top of the section or a freezing spray can be used. The former is helpful when larger tissue sections need to be frozen, the latter is best when the tissue section is small. Care has to be taken to avoid compression. Larger sections will not be satisfactorily frozen by spray, which may lead to uneven freezing with subsequent shattering of the section taken. In addition, using a spray leads to creation of an aerosol, which can be detrimental when the fumes are inhaled (i.e. cardiac arrythmia etc). To prevent inhalation, the lid of the cryostat compartment should be closed transiently to let the fumes settle.

Cutting into the frozen tissue block is best done when the block is placed in such a way that the knife starts cutting at one of the corners of the wedge, since the liver capsule is normally harder than the parenchyma, leading to the compression of the softer hepatic tissue, shattering or ripping of the section, if the capsule is transected longitudinally first. In addition, the frozen tissue should be well cut into with several sections before using any for analysis, in order to avoid freezing artefacts and guarantee that the entire area is well exposed and sectioned.

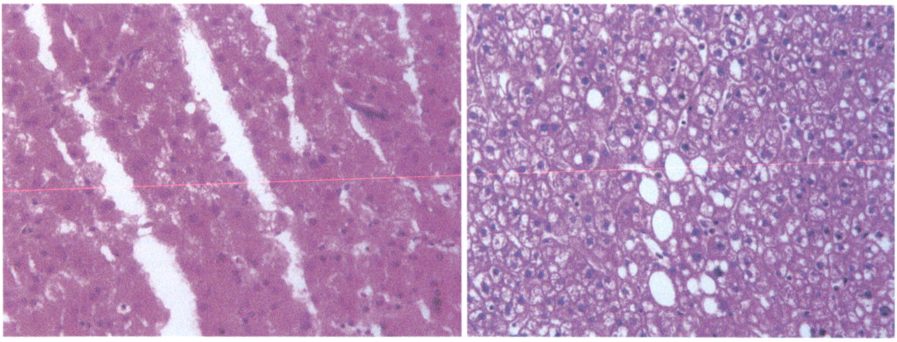

Fig. 3. Problems in cutting frozen section. Venetian blind - like artefacts (left), and sub-optimally preserved liver parenchyma (right) do not allow proper evaluation, particularly microvesicular steatosis

Besides technical problems, cutting a frozen liver section may cause unexpected trouble based on primary parenchymal alterations, such as increased hepatocellular fat deposition. In this case, lower cryostat temperatures of -25 ^{0}C can be helpful, provided there is time for equilibrating the equipment, the knife and the tissue to this temperature first, which may take about 20-30 minutes depending on the size of the frozen tissue specimen. This delay in processing being worthwhile on one hand, may be problematic on the other, when the allotted time for pathologic evaluation is short due to logistical problems of time consuming transport for the frozen section material or the delivery of the liver specimen.

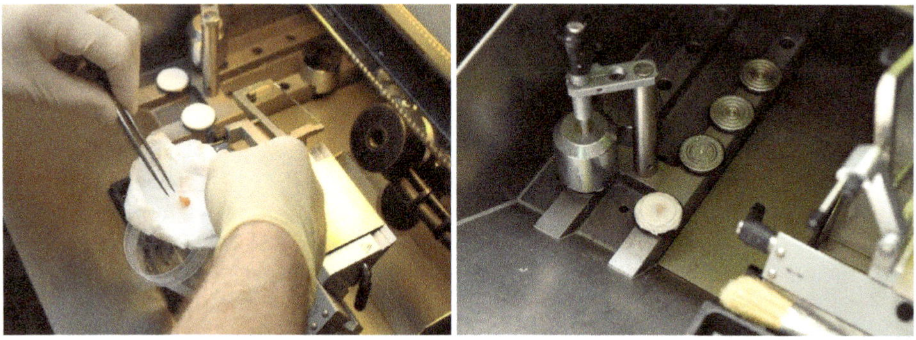

Fig. 4. A wedge biopsy of 1-cm side length. The wedge will be split lengthwise; one half was snap frozen in liquid nitrogen.

For subsequent analysis of the frozen tissue, it is post-fixed in 4% buffered formalin and paraffin embedded. For that purpose, the frozen tissue should be taken out of the cryostat and allow to thaw just enough to be taken safely from the chuck. The majority of the compound medium starting to thaw should be removed and the tissue placed immediately into formalin. The remaining rest of the compound medium does not effect the subsequent fixation procedure. The procedure of subsequent analysis is equal to that of the rest of the wedge, namely being immediately fixed and paraffinized. It is prudent to wait with the fixation of the rest of the wedge tissue, in case a second frozen section is needed, which should not be a problem, if the wedge is of sufficient size. Meanwhile, the wedge tissue should be kept on ice.

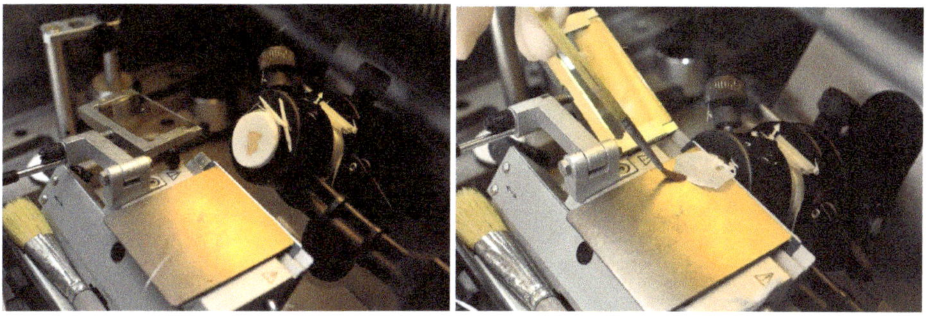

Fig. 5. Several 3-4 µm thick sections are cut after the tissue block is well cut in to expose flatly its entire surface.

The most frequently encountered problem is the evaluation of hepatocellular, microvesicular steatosis (Fig. 6). If the tissue is not well preserved or suboptimally frozen, the subsequent frozen section may prove uncuttable at the thickness of 3 µm, which would allow optimal identification but instead has to be cut thicker. This setting will prevent meaningful analysis of the percentage of microvesicular steatosis. In contrast, macrovesicular steatosis is less influenced by section thickness, unless it exceeds 5 µm, but the accuracy of prediction will be lower, posing a possible problem in cases where the extend of steatosis reaches a critical level, potentially even leading to the rejection of the transplant in question. Staining methods for fat accumulation are available for frozen section as well as for paraffinized material. However, in a paraffin section, good (and thin) section quality is sufficient in our opinion to reliably recognize the degree of steatosis, while there is the danger that usually buffered, 4% formalin fixation and subsequent paraffin embedding will dissolve many fat droplets, particularly if they are of the microvesicular kind so that the fat stain will not show the true amount of deposition. The problem in frozen section lies again in the section's thickness: while thicker sections give better staining results, they do not allow good identification of the degree of microvesicular fat deposition, while macrovesicular fat deposition does not require a fat stain. In addition, the staining solution should be used within a week after preparation, which means that frequently the solution will have to be freshly made.

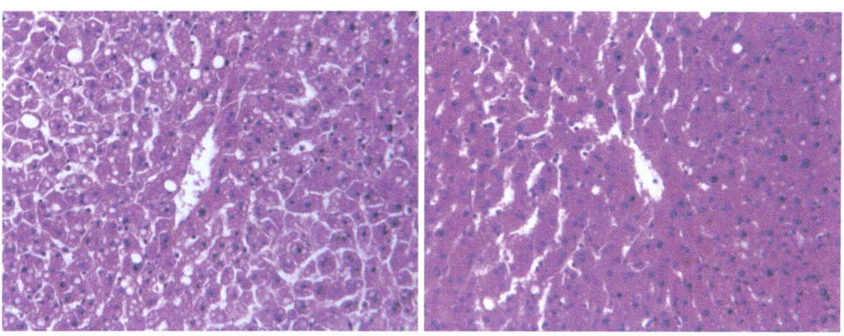

Fig. 6. Microvesicular steatosis: 3 µm thick sections on the left allow optimal evaluation, while the 5µm thick section on the right will lead to under estimation of steatosis. 250X; HE Stain

The other main finding in frozen section liver biopsies concerns the evaluation of parenchymal fibrosis. Here, an increased section thickness will lead to over estimation of the degree if fibrosis as well as potential misjudgement of the width of the liver sinus versus the hepatic trabeculae. While the sinuses will appear small, the trabeculae seem broader than is actually the case. This deception may be important to keep in mind, when the question of liver congestion with potential hemosiderin deposition arises.

In case focal, nodular lesions are encountered on an otherwise normal appearing liver, a frozen section is mandatory, if the organ is principally regarded as transplantable by the surgeon. Here, it is helpful when the entire lesion is excised such that the surrounding normal liver tissue is part of the excision, in order to be able to evaluate the edge of the lesional process (infiltrative or smooth). However, this resection is not sufficient for the histopathological evaluation: besides the excisional biopsy, the regularly taken biopsies from segment 3 and 6 or 7 should be also be performed, because they enable the pathologist to analyse the quality of the liver and its alterations independently from the lesion.

6. Histopathological evaluation during organ procurement

Standards for histopathological evaluation of liver biopsies are still lacking. We recommend, based on our experience that frozen section should be taken within a side length of 1 cm minimum and not only from the liver surface. The pathologist needs sufficient clinical and surgical data for diagnosis. The frozen section should be evaluated when material is post-fixed by a second pathologist for quality standard reasons. These results must be communicated to the transplantation center immediately. The pathologic evaluation, however, should not only include histopathologic findings, but also be extended to other primarily macroscopic findings such as: arteriosclerotic damage to the vessels, subcapsular cysts, and tumors, as well as bile duct abnormalities, since those findings may prevent transplantability despite a well preserved liver parenchyma.

One of the most frequently encountered problems is the size of the wedge itself. Occasionally, not a wedge but a crescent-like slice of hepatic tissue parallel to the surface is taken, and is almost always the only tissue for frozen section and only from the left liver lobe. This procedure is inadequate in several ways: (i) the amount of hepatic tissue is too small; (ii) there are clearly less than 10 portal tracts in this small excision; (iii) the closeness to the capsule may incorrectly suggest a fibrotic process, leading to rejection of the organ; (iv) a biopsy of only one (mostly left) liver lobe is insufficient; it cannot be assumed that the unbiopsied (mostly right) lobe is of equal quality or shows the same pathologic process. By analysing explanted but not-transplanted livers over the past 5 years, we encountered the practice of taking a crescent-like slice in several cases. In almost all cases, the evaluation resulted in rejection of the transplant organ, which after a complete work-up with histologic evaluation of all liver segments, could not be supported from the pathological analysis. The risk of prolonged bleeding with additional measures from the surgeon has been cited as a reason for taking a cresent-like slice in individual cases. While any procedure complicating the evaluation of the transplant should be principally avoided, this reasoning appears unacceptable since there should be sufficient time for arrest of bleeding while the frozen section is performed.

As far as differences between the liver lobes are concerned, we have learned from our study of explanted livers that in all but one case (out of 50) the degree of fibrosis or steatosis did not significantly vary among the different liver segments or the liver lobes (Rey et al., 2009). However, our single case with focal biliary cirrhosis in the right, but nor the left liver lobe, (Fig. 7) supports the concept of taking a wedge biopsy from both liver lobes.

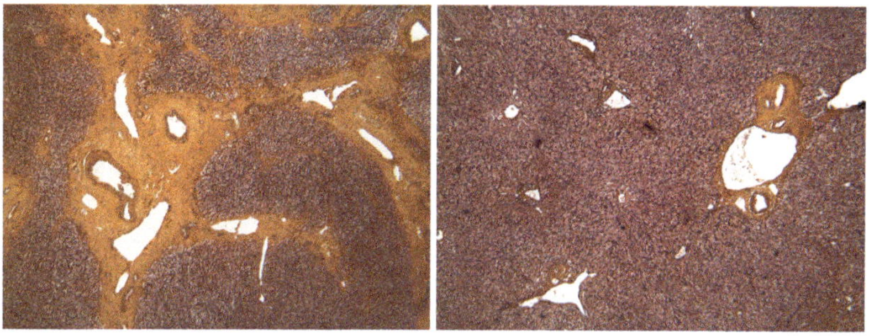

Fig. 7. Differences between liver lobes: Originating from the same liver, the left picture shows the parenchyma of the right lobe with bridging fibrosis and widened bile ducts due to focal bile duct obliteration, while the right picture shows a section from the left lobe with well preserved parenchyma. The liver was rejected from the surgeon with the argument that since the right lobe representing two thirds of the liver was "cirrhosed", (with no additional frozen section done), the "remaining" unchanged left lobe was not sufficient to transplant the organ. 40x; Gomori stain.

Similarly, a focal fat accumulation in alcoholic livers may be taken for an increased steatosis not present in the remaining liver. This opinion is in contrast to current literature which has demonstrated that a single liver biopsy adequately represents the histologic characteristics of the liver (Lo et al., 2008). It has been reported that left and right lobe biopsies obtained during diagnostic laparoscopy have a highly significant histologic correlation for necrosis, steatosis, inflammation, and fibrosis (Picciotto et al., 1983). Nevertheless, the overall importance for adequate histopathological characteristic of the liver parenchyma during organ procurement requires a wedge biopsy with at least 10 portal tractions, and not a superficial biopsy from the liver surface.

As we reported earlier, the colour of the liver surface is insufficient as major criteria in making the decision of transplantation or rejection. The quality of perfusion, the light quality of the operating room, the surgeons experience as well as different degrees of steatosis may greatly diminish the reliability of these criteria. Thus, if the quality of the organ appears doubtful, a frozen section is mandatory.

When a liver is biopsied in order to evaluate it's transplantability, several crucial questions have to be answered by the evaluating pathologist. The most important question is whether the tissue has a lesion or not. The answer depends largely on the quality of the tissue and particularly on the quality of the frozen section, as previously outlined. While highly abnormal lesions, such as a diffuse macrovesicular fat deposition or complete liver cirrhosis, pose hardly any problem even if the frozen section is suboptimal. In contrast, the so called marginal organ lesions, such as mild fibrosis or microvesicular fat deposition, will be under diagnosed (because the bad quality of the section does not allow identification of these changes) and regarded as transplantable without restriction. This could pose a problem in posttransplant management. On the other hand, changes that are over diagnosed lead to a premature rejection.

Once the pathologist decides that there is a lesion, the question arises whether this lesion is focal or diffuse. Diffuse processes are expected to appear in all liver segments alike, as we could appreciate from our study from explanted, but not allocated livers, in which all segments were investigated histologically. The nature of these processes, such as: alcoholic damage, hepatitis B, or C, cannot be evaluated with certainty by frozen section.

Most important is the evaluation of focal lesions. As table 1 lists, there are several with different pathophysiology to be considered. The information from the primary evaluating surgeon is of great importance. It should state whether there is indeed a single focal lesion, its location (subcapsular; right versus left liver lobe), its macroscopic appearance (colour, size, tissue density), and most importantly, whether the excised tissue encompasses the entire lesion or only a part.

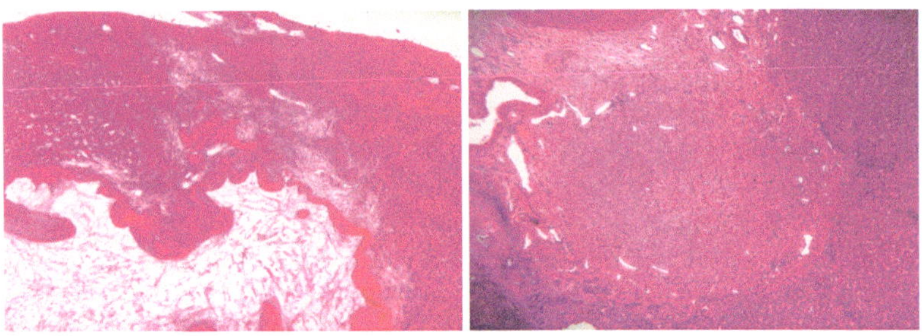

Fig. 8. Focal lesions: on the left, a thick walled cyst, differentially a simple cyst as well as an echinococcal cyst may be considered. On the right, a typical sclerosed lesion with a potentially difficult differential between a (rare) sclerosed malignant process or - as revealed itself on consecutive sections - a (frequently encountered) sclerosed hemagioma. 40x; H&E stain.

In the following section, the main focal lesions which may be encountered in a frozen section are briefly listed and their relevance outlined. At first, the pathologist must differentiate between malignant and benign focal lesions. Among the malignant lesions, the most important ones are *metastatic foci*, which may originate from a large variety of different sources, among them the gastrointestinal, the urogenital, and the respiratory tract. In women, breast and ovary have to be considered. However, in the biopsy these differentials cannot be made. Currently, such livers are regarded as non transplantable, but in the future with the tendency of increasing organ demands, the question to transplant a liver with a metastatic or malignant lesion may be reconsidered depending on the lesion and the clinical evaluation. The other differential of a focal malignant lesion arising in an otherwise normal liver is a *hepatocellular carcinoma (HCC)*. Albeit rare, the identification of such a lesion in a frozen section may be challenging or even impossible, if no normal liver tissue is included for comparison. While the typically thickened plates (being often more than 4 cells wide) are easily identified, the nuclear changes (increased size and nucleoli) can be hard to discern due to artificial swelling of the frozen tissue. Here, the transition from the tumour to the normal surrounding liver as well as plentiful mitoses is helpful. Rare tumour entities encountered are sarcomas, such as: *angiosarcoma, leiomyosarcoma, fibrosarcoma, rhabdomyosarcoma, as well as malignant fibrous histiocytoma.*

Simple cysts vs. Echinococcal cyst Congenital cystic disease Cystic mesenchymal hamartoma Hemangioma (capillary vs cavernous) Hemangioendothelioma Biliary hamartoma Lymphangiomatosis Angiomyolipoma Focal fatty change Heterotopia	prolonged ischemia (cold/warm) Focal nodular hyperplasia Liver Cell Adenoma Nodular, regenerative Hyperplasia Peliosis hepatis Biliary adenoma HCC in normal liver Sarcomas

Table 1. Focal lesions in the liver as important differential diagnosis in frozen section

Benign focal lesions are numerous, but differ in the frequency that they are encountered. Among the most frequent are benign, simple cysts, hemangiomas and biliary hamartomas. All lesions can be found in subcapsular localization. *Non-paracytic cysts* are typically filled with a clear liquid, having an almost transparent wall and often a flat, sometimes a cuboidal or columnar epithelial lining. They are composed of mature connective tissue and are occasionally calcified. Macroscopically, they can be viewed as problematic when they are bled in. Differentially, an *echinococcal cyst* should be considered, although remnants of scolices may be undetectable. *Congenital autosomal dominant or recessive cystic disease* can be found in some cases; here the identification of renal and pancreatic cysts is important. Depending on the degree of cyst formation, even those organs may be considered transplantable (Rey et al., 2009). In children, a *cystic mesenchymal hamartoma of childhood* should be considered, whenever a pediatric liver transplant is in question. This occurs typically in the right liver lobe at the age of 16 months to 5 years. These hamartomas are mainly composed of connective tissue with small foci of remnants of liver cells, duct cells, even portal tissue.

Among angiomatous lesions, the *capillary and the cavernous hemagioma* are the most frequently accounted subcapsular lesions. Here, a predilection of the right liver lobe, and the female gender is found for the cavernous subtype. Histologically, the typical appearance is multiple, dilated blood-filled spaces lined with mature flat epithelium, separated by fibrous tissue. Problems arise from the tendency of these lesions to undergo regression and fibrosis, which may make it difficult to differentiate them from potential malignant lesions.

Hemangioendotheliomas can be found as focal lesions in childhood as well as in adult livers, although multiple foci throughout the liver may be encountered in childhood. Their histologic appearance is characterized by vascular spaces variable size, lined by immature plump endothelial cells.

Regarding the number of cases, the most difficult decisions to be made are those in which a sclerosing hemangioma has to be differentiated from hemangioendothelioma or bile duct adenocarcinoma. While the evidence of erythrocytes is helpful, all lesions are prone to bleeding and the evaluation of nuclear and cytoplasmic atypia can be severely hampered by the sub-optimal quality of a frozen section. Here, a series of sections should be taken. However, in the few cases encountered with some uncertainty left inspite of a frozen section, the liver was rejected as transplant organ. Subsequent analysis of these livers revealed that the lesion was a sclerosing hemangioma.

Biliary hamartomas, also called cholangiohamartoma or von Meyenburg complexes, are congenital lesions of a disturbed restructuring of the ductal plate (Chung, 1970). They represent cystic spaces lined by bile duct epithelium and fibrotic obliteration of intrahepatic bile ducts (Woolf&Vierling, 1993). Depending on the localisation and prevalence of cystic ectasia and fibrotic obliteration, several disease entities can be differentiated ranging from the congenital hepatic fibrosis to the Caroli syndrome (Caroli, 1968). The lesions can be found as single or multiple subcapsular foci sharply demarcated and firm, being of grey-white colour and wedge-shaped; their size ranging from 0.5 to 1.0 cm. Cellular atypias are missing. Occasionally, small microhamartomas have to be differentiated from fibrotic portal tracts. However, the presence or absence of portal veins and arteries should enable the correct diagnosis.

Rarely, a *lymphangiomatosis* is found (Van Steenbergen et al., 1985). This solitary lesion is normally located intrahepatically and thus will normally not present itself to the evaluating surgeon. It has to be differentiated from a cavernous hemangioma since it can contain blood, besides cell debris and protein-rich fluid. If it is encountered, a systemic form (present in different organs) has to be recognized versus a sporadic, exclusively hepatic form.

Another benign but tumour-appearing lesion is a *nodule with focal fat accumulation* typically observed in livers from patients with high alcohol consumption (Brawer et al., 1980). This lesion can also be rarely found after tetracycline intake (Peters et al., 1967). Histologically, intrahepatic fat deposition and regional necrotic hepatocytes with inflammatory demarcation is seen.

An *angiomyolipoma* is yet another, mostly unexpected solitary finding, consisting of vessels, smooth muscle and fat tissue as well as medullary marrow. Normally of small size, it may be enlarged up to 20cm (Nonomura et al., 1994).

Ischemic transplant damage or damage to suboptimal organ perfusion, hypotonia and shock of the donor should be considered, if liver cell necrosis, hepatic fat deposition and cholestasis are observed. Prolonged cold ischemia will damage the sinusoidal cells; prolonged warm ischemia the hepatocytes (Schon et al., 1998).

Two other lesions can be challenging in frozen sections: *focal nodular hyperplasie (FNH)* versus adenoma (table 2). In ¾ of all cases, FNH represents an unexpected finding (Goodman, 1987) in women between the age of 20 and 50 years. Typically it is a solitary lesion (80%) and less frequently a multiple lesion (10% two foci, 10% >2 foci) predominantly in the right liver lobe. Star-like fibrotic strands have given the lesion the misnomer "focal cirrhosis". Thus, only a biopsy will be able to differentiate between this and genuine fibrotic/cirrhotic lesions. The picture is characterized by fibrovascular and ductular areas radiating from the septa, accompanied by an expanding periphery of normal-appearing hepatocytes . While cells may appear polymorph, no dysplasia is seen. Glycogen and fat deposition is present. Intracanalicular bile cylinders can be found as well as bile duct proliferation. In contrast, a *liver cell adenoma* is a lesion almost exclusively found in women in their 3rd to 4th decade. Partially surrounded by a pseudo-capsule made from compacted liver cells, it consists exclusively of hepatocytes 2-3 layers wide lined with regular sinusoids, but without any portal tracts or bile ducts. If focal areas of immature connective tissue are found, a mesenchymal hamartoma should be considered instead.

Nodular regenerative hyerplasia or nodular transformation are small nodules, up to 0.6cm, which represent parenchymal regeneration present in non-cirrhotic livers versus multiacinar nodules without (type 1) or with (type 2) epithelial dysplasia mostly occurring in cirrhotic livers (Nakanuma, 1990).

	Focal Nodular Hyperplasia (FNH)	Liver Cell Adenoma
Location	right liver lobe, subcapsular; ev. multiple	subcapsular; solitary 80%
Central scar	present	absent
Fibrous septae	frequent	rare
Bile ducts and portal tracts	present	absent
Parenchymal lesion	nodular	homogenous
Hemorrhage and necrosis	rare	frequent
Cholestasis	mild	enhanced
Capsule	absent	Partial to ample encapsulation
Vascularity	Vessel with broadened walls	Thin walled vessels (sinusoids)

Table 2. Relevant findings for frozen section evaluation between FNH and liver cell adenoma

A *biliary adenoma* is a small, firm, white appearing nodule of less than 1 cm in diameter consisting of proliferating bile duct epithelium in subcapsular location. Focal inflammatory obliteration of a bile duct by may even lead to a cirrhotic alteration of an entire liver subsegment, which being located under the capsule, can be taken as a pars pro toto change of the entire liver. In our particular case, this resulted in rejection by the surgeon, again without further liver biopsy of other segments, which would have revealed the focality of the process.

Peliosis hepatis, often a 0.3 to 3.0 cm large lesion represents blood-filled, cystically dilated sinusoids without cellular lining (Zak, 1950). They are randomly distributed throughout the liver. Thus, the decision to transplant will largely depend on their size and number as well as their potential negative effect on liver function, particularly since etiologically different infectious diseases have to be considered (Bartonella Henselae, tuberculosis, HIV, S. aureus). Two subtypes are important (Yanoff&Rawson, 1964): the parenchymatous subtype is associated with hemorrhagic necroses, while the phlebic subtype is characterized by dilated sinusoids. However, peliosis has to be differentiated from other lesions such as biliary hamartomas, liver cysts and most frequently from all lesions resulting from acute congestion due to acute right heart insufficiency. Here, the lesion's pericental accentuation, and the lack of cystic structures are important in the diagnosis.

Heterotopias in the liver are rarely encountered, such as ectopic pancreatic tissue within heterotopic duct cysts (Schaefer et al., 1989).

Again, in most cases, a frozen section of the lesion after total excision will bring a satisfactory answer. However, livers were rejected on the ground of such a lesion described by the transplant surgeon, which were not biopsied as part of the decision process, although the subsequent histological evaluation of this liver (analyzing all 8 segments, and the vessels/bile ducts of the hilar region histopathologically) clearly indicated that this had been a benign process, which should not have led to transplant rejection. There may have been other reasons unknown to us leading to the rejection of the liver. Considering the organ shortage and cost and effect of a frozen section, potentially supporting a decision of rejection, we would advise to perform a frozen section of such lesions in most cases, even if it would be only for providing an irrevocable proof of non-transplantability to the relatives of the decreased. Any rejection has to be seen as disregarding the last wish of the deceased or the relatives, which in our opinion should be well justified. Furthermore, for future efforts to improve the transplantation rate it seems prudent that the transfer of information potentially leading to a decision of rejection are becoming more transparent and accessible in an epidemiologic databank for future analysis.

Once the histopathological evaluation is performed, the result should be documented on the appropriate transplant form, including the number of frozen sections taken, the quality of the tissue and whether it is sufficient for analysis, the actual histologic evaluation separately for each frozen section/each segment, and the final assessment, whether or not the liver is good/acceptable/poor as transplant organ from a histopathological perspective. This last addendum is important in cases in which the evaluation between transplant surgeon and pathologist differs to the point that the organ is rejected. Pathological evaluations may result in transplantable appearing organs; however, several other reasons may prevent the surgeon from following this advice. Among them are problems with the donor organ concerning the reconstruction of the hilar vessels (anomalies) and the bile ducts (major bile duct too small, anomalies) as well as problems concerning the transplant acceptor. Thus, in the databank regarding the evaluation sheet from a rejected organ, the reasons and the person responsible for the rejection should be clearly stated.

7. Histopathological evaluation after organ procurement

Once the histologic evaluation of the frozen section is concluded, the remaining tissue is postfixed overnight as is the remaining part of the wedge biopsy in buffered, 4% formalin, pH 7.4. The pH of the formalin used should be pre-monitored: commercially available formalin solution may differ in its pH from highly acidic to basic values, all of which being sold as "buffered". The day after paraffin embedding, 3 to 4-µm-thick sections should be cut and routinely stained. A typical standard series of stains (besides H&E) should include: a Gomori's stain (as fibrotic marker), a PAS stain (for best histologic resolution of hepatocytes and sinuses) , and an iron stain such as Berlin blue (for iron deposition). An elastic van Gieson stain may be added, however, it does not provide any advantage; in contrast, it proves less sensitive in detecting fibrosis. If microvesicular staetosis is a major feature - at least if it was one major reason for rejection – a Sudan stain for fat should be included in the list.

One should carefully select the tissue sections to be stained. It seems unnecessary to stain every single one with all stains to be considered. Instead, a representative postfixed section from the primarily frozen tissue as well as one of the primarily formalin-fixed tissue should be selected for this purpose. The remaining tissue (mostly rest tissue from the wedge) should be evaluated primarily by H&E. If there is any question, one still has the opportunity to analyse these tissue portions by additional stains as well.

A discrepancy between the frozen sections analysis and the histopathologic analysis after organ procurement should be reported immediately to the transplant centre. In our experience, this is a very rare occasion: in revaluating the biopsy sites of previous frozen section excisions, we found only one out of 50 biopsies, whose basic diagnosis and evaluation mismatched distinctly. In this case, however, the diagnosis of a major degree of steatosis was made on biopsy, which could neither be found by re-evaluating the former (single!) biopsy site in the third liver segment nor by analysing all other segments of the rejected liver. Unfortunately, the biopsy could not be retrieved to be re-analysed as well, which should be the recommendation in such cases so as to learn more about the reason.

Another aspect of evaluation is the analysis of hepatocellular iron deposition. By frozen section and without further stains, the differential of hemosiderin (containing iron), and hematoidin (containing no iron) is impossible. Therefore, we recommend a Berliner blue reaction, which will provide a blue precipitate in cases of hemosiderin, but not with hematoidin deposition.

8. Conclusion

Continuously collecting clinical, surgical, and histopathologic data in a central registry of all transplanted livers may provide valuable information as to whether the evaluation at time of transplantation was correct. If a posttransplant biopsy is taken after liver transplantation, the results of its histopathologic evaluation should likewise be collected in the same registry. This measure will improve our knowledge of the importance of morphological alterations and their significance at the time of transplantation. If the liver is rejected as transplant organ, these pieces of information may provide the basis for consoling relatives of the deceased about the reasons for not transplanting the organ and thus acting against his or her last will.
Furthermore, routine control biopsies, in intervals such as 12 months, three years and beyond, may provide valuable information whether or not organs regarded as marginally suitable due to histologic alterations, especially microvesicular versus macrovesicular fat accumulation, are able to recover. In case of death of the transplant recipient, liver evaluation by biopsy or autopsy should become a routine investigation in order to retrospectively control the transplant decision.

9. Addendum

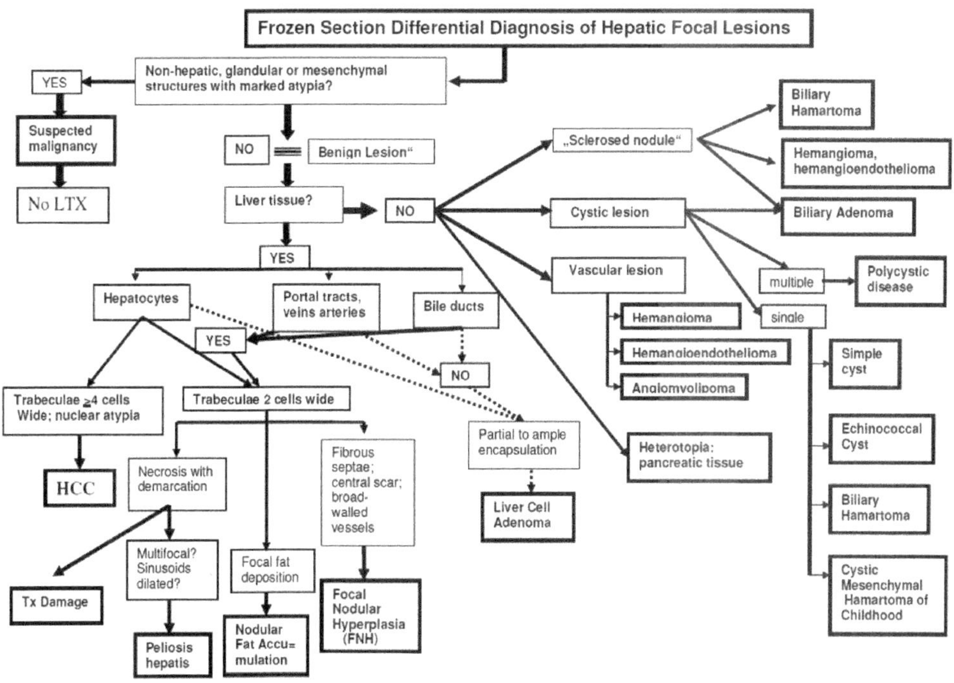

Fig. 9. Flow sheet: "Frozen Section Differential Diagnosis of Hepatic Focal Lesions"

10. References

Adam, R., Reynes, M., Johann, M., Morino, M., Astarcioglu, I., Kafetzis, I., Castaing, D. & Bismuth, H. (1991). *The outcome of steatotic grafts in liver transplantation*, Transplant Proc, Vol. 23, No. 1 Pt 2, (Feb 1991), pp. 1538-40

Amin, M. G., Wolf, M. P., TenBrook, J. A., Jr., Freeman, R. B., Jr., Cheng, S. J., Pratt, D. S. & Wong, J. B. (2004). *Expanded criteria donor grafts for deceased donor liver transplantation under the MELD system: a decision analysis*, Liver Transpl, Vol. 10, No. 12, (Dec 2004), pp. 1468-75

Baccarani, U., Adani, G. L., Isola, M., Avellini, C., Lorenzin, D., Rossetto, A., Curro, G., Comuzzi, C., Toniutto, P., Soldano, F., Bresadola, V., Risaliti, A. & Bresadola, F. (2009). *Steatosis of the graft is a risk factor for posttransplantation biliary complications*, Transplant Proc, Vol. 41, No. 4, (May 2009), pp. 1313-5

Brawer, M. K., Austin, G. E. & Lewin, K. J. (1980). *Focal fatty change of the liver, a hitherto poorly recognized entity*, Gastroenterology, Vol. 78, No. 2, (Feb 1980), pp. 247-52

Caroli, J. (1968). *Diseases of intrahepatic bile ducts*, Isr J Med Sci, Vol. 4, No. 1, (Jan-Feb 1968), pp. 21-35

Chung, E. B. (1970). *Multiple bile-duct hamartomas*, Cancer, Vol. 26, No. 2, (Aug 1970), pp. 287-96

D'Alessandro, E., Calabrese, F., Gringeri, E. & Valente, M. (2010). *Frozen-section diagnosis in donor livers: error rate estimation of steatosis degree*, Transplant Proc, Vol. 42, No. 6, (Jul-Aug 2010), pp. 2226-8

Dictus, C., Vienenkoetter, B., Esmaeilzadeh, M., Unterberg, A. & Ahmadi, R. (2009). *Critical care management of potential organ donors: our current standard*, Clin Transplant, Vol. 23 Suppl 21, No. (Dec 2009), pp. 2-9

Durand, F., Renz, J. F., Alkofer, B., Burra, P., Clavien, P. A., Porte, R. J., Freeman, R. B. & Belghiti, J. (2008). *Report of the Paris consensus meeting on expanded criteria donors in liver transplantation*, Liver Transpl, Vol. 14, No. 12, (Dec 2008), pp. 1694-707

Feng, S., Goodrich, N. P., Bragg-Gresham, J. L., Dykstra, D. M., Punch, J. D., DebRoy, M. A., Greenstein, S. M. & Merion, R. M. (2006). *Characteristics associated with liver graft failure: the concept of a donor risk index*, Am J Transplant, Vol. 6, No. 4, (Apr 2006), pp. 783-90

Fishbein, T. M., Fiel, M. I., Emre, S., Cubukcu, O., Guy, S. R., Schwartz, M. E., Miller, C. M. & Sheiner, P. A. (1997). *Use of livers with microvesicular fat safely expands the donor pool*, Transplantation, Vol. 64, No. 2, (Jul 27 1997), pp. 248-51

Fondevila, C., Jimenez-Galanes, S. & Garcia-Valdecasas, J. C. (2009). *[How can the number of liver transplantations be increased?]*, Gastroenterol Hepatol, Vol. 32, No. 7, (Aug-Sep 2009), pp. 519-30

Frankel, W. L., Tranovich, J. G., Salter, L., Bumgardner, G. & Baker, P. (2002). *The optimal number of donor biopsy sites to evaluate liver histology for transplantation*, Liver Transpl, Vol. 8, No. 11, (Nov 2002), pp. 1044-50

Kutsogiannis, D. J., Pagliarello, G., Doig, C., Ross, H. & Shemie, S. D. (2006). *Medical management to optimize donor organ potential: review of the literature*, Can J Anaesth, Vol. 53, No. 8, (Aug 2006), pp. 820-30

Lo, I. J., Lefkowitch, J. H., Feirt, N., Alkofer, B., Kin, C., Samstein, B., Guarrera, J. V. & Renz, J. F. (2008). *Utility of liver allograft biopsy obtained at procurement*, Liver Transpl, Vol. 14, No. 5, (May 2008), pp. 639-46

Mangus, R. S., Fridell, J. A., Vianna, R. M., Milgrom, M. L., Chestovich, P., Vandenboom, C. & Tector, A. J. (2010). *Severe hypernatremia in deceased liver donors does not impact early transplant outcome*, Transplantation, Vol. 90, No. 4, (Aug 27 2010), pp. 438-43

Markin, R. S., Wisecarver, J. L., Radio, S. J., Stratta, R. J., Langnas, A. N., Hirst, K. & Shaw, B. W., Jr. (1993). *Frozen section evaluation of donor livers before transplantation*, Transplantation, Vol. 56, No. 6, (Dec 1993), pp. 1403-9

McCormack, L., Petrowsky, H., Jochum, W., Mullhaupt, B., Weber, M. & Clavien, P. A. (2007). *Use of severely steatotic grafts in liver transplantation: a matched case-control study*, Ann Surg, Vol. 246, No. 6, (Dec 2007), pp. 940-6; discussion 946-8

Nakanuma, Y. (1990). *Nodular regenerative hyperplasia of the liver: retrospective survey in autopsy series*, J Clin Gastroenterol, Vol. 12, No. 4, (Aug 1990), pp. 460-5

Nocito, A., El-Badry, A. M. & Clavien, P. A. (2006). *When is steatosis too much for transplantation?*, J Hepatol, Vol. 45, No. 4, (Oct 2006), pp. 494-9

Nonomura, A., Mizukami, Y., Muraoka, K., Yajima, M. & Oda, K. (1994). *Angiomyolipoma of the liver with pleomorphic histological features*, Histopathology, Vol. 24, No. 3, (Mar 1994), pp. 279-81

Noujaim, H. M., de Ville de Goyet, J., Montero, E. F., Ribeiro, C. M., Capellozzi, V. L., Crescentini, F., Casagrande, M., Santos, R. G., Curvello, L., de Miranda, M. P. & Genzini, T. (2009). *Expanding postmortem donor pool using steatotic liver grafts: a new look*, Transplantation, Vol. 87, No. 6, (Mar 27 2009), pp. 919-25

Palmiero, H. O., Kajikawa, P., Boin, I. F., Coria, S. & Pereira, L. A. (2010). *Liver recipient survival rate before and after model for end-stage liver disease implementation and use of donor risk index*, Transplant Proc, Vol. 42, No. 10, (Dec 2010), pp. 4113-5

Patkowski, W., Zieniewicz, K., Skalski, M. & Krawczyk, M. (2009). *Correlation between selected prognostic factors and postoperative course in liver transplant recipients*, Transplant Proc, Vol. 41, No. 8, (Oct 2009), pp. 3091-102

Peters, R. L., Edmondson, H. A., Mikkelsen, W. P. & Tatter, D. (1967). *Tetracycline-induced fatty liver in nonpregnant patients. A report of six cases*, Am J Surg, Vol. 113, No. 5, (May 1967), pp. 622-32

Picciotto, A., Ciravegna, G., Lapertosa, G. & Celle, G. (1983). *One or two liver biopsies during laparoscopy?*, Hepatogastroenterology, Vol. 30, No. 5, (Oct 1983), pp. 192-3

Rey, J. W., Wirges, U., Dienes, H. P. & Fries, J. W. (2009). *Hepatic steatosis in organ donors: disparity between surgery and histology?*, Transplant Proc, Vol. 41, No. 6, (Jul-Aug 2009), pp. 2557-60

Rosenthal, J. T., Shaw, B. W., Jr., Hardesty, R. L., Griffith, B. P., Starzl, T. E. & Hakala, T. R. (1983). *Principles of multiple organ procurement from cadaver donors*, Ann Surg, Vol. 198, No. 5, (Nov 1983), pp. 617-21

Schaefer, B., Meyer, G., Arnholdt, H. & Hohlbach, G. (1989). *[Heterotopic pancreatic pseudocyst of the liver]*, Chirurg, Vol. 60, No. 8, (Aug 1989), pp. 556-8

Schlitt, H. J., Loss, M., Scherer, M. N., Becker, T., Jauch, K. W., Nashan, B., Schmidt, H., Settmacher, U., Rogiers, X., Neuhaus, P. & Strassburg, C. (2011). *[Current developments in liver transplantation in Germany: MELD-based organ allocation and incentives for transplant centres]*, Z Gastroenterol, Vol. 49, No. 1, (Jan 2011), pp. 30-8

Schon, M. R., Kollmar, O., Akkoc, N., Matthes, M., Wolf, S., Schrem, H., Tominaga, M., Keech, G. & Neuhaus, P. (1998). *Cold ischemia affects sinusoidal endothelial cells while warm ischemia affects hepatocytes in liver transplantation*, Transplant Proc, Vol. 30, No. 5, (Aug 1998), pp. 2318-20

Shah, V. R. (2008). *Aggressive management of multiorgan donor*, Transplant Proc, Vol. 40, No. 4, (May 2008), pp. 1087-90

Smith, M. (2004). *Physiologic changes during brain stem death--lessons for management of the organ donor*, J Heart Lung Transplant, Vol. 23, No. 9 Suppl, (Sep 2004), pp. S217-22

Spitzer, A. L., Lao, O. B., Dick, A. A., Bakthavatsalam, R., Halldorson, J. B., Yeh, M. M., Upton, M. P., Reyes, J. D. & Perkins, J. D. (2010). *The biopsied donor liver: incorporating macrosteatosis into high-risk donor assessment*, Liver Transpl, Vol. 16, No. 7, (Jul 2010), pp. 874-84

Van Steenbergen, W., Joosten, E., Marchal, G., Baert, A., Vanstapel, M. J., Desmet, V., Wijnants, P. & De Groote, J. (1985). *Hepatic lymphangiomatosis. Report of a case and review of the literature*, Gastroenterology, Vol. 88, No. 6, (Jun 1985), pp. 1968-72

Weismuller, T. J., Fikatas, P., Schmidt, J., Barreiros, A. P., Otto, G., Beckebaum, S., Paul, A., Scherer, M. N., Schmidt, H. H., Schlitt, H. J., Neuhaus, P., Klempnauer, J., Pratschke, J., Manns, M. P. & Strassburg, C. P. (2011). *Multicentric evaluation of model for end-stage liver disease-based allocation and survival after liver transplantation in Germany--limitations of the 'sickest first'-concept*, Transpl Int, Vol. 24, No. 1, (Jan 2011), pp. 91-9

Wood, K. E., Becker, B. N., McCartney, J. G., D'Alessandro, A. M. & Coursin, D. B. (2004). *Care of the potential organ donor*, N Engl J Med, Vol. 351, No. 26, (Dec 23 2004), pp. 2730-9

Woolf, G. M. & Vierling, J. M. (1993). *Disappearing intrahepatic bile ducts: the syndromes and their mechanisms*, Semin Liver Dis, Vol. 13, No. 3, (Aug 1993), pp. 261-75

Yanoff, M. & Rawson, A. J. (1964). *Peliosis Hepatis. An Anatomic Study with Demonstration of Two Varieties*, Arch Pathol, Vol. 77, No. (Feb 1964), pp. 159-65

Zak, F. G. (1950). *Peliosis hepatis*, Am J Pathol, Vol. 26, No. 1, (Jan 1950), pp. 1-15, incl 2 pl

12

Initial Poor Graft Dysfunction and Primary Graft Non-Function After Orthotopic Liver Transplantation

Chen Hao, Xie Junjie, Shen Baiyong, Deng Xiaxing,
Tao Ran, Peng Chenghong and Li Hongwei
*Center of Organ Transplantation, Ruijin Hospital,
Shanghai Jiao Tong University School of Medicine,
P.R.China*

1. Introduction

Orthotopic liver transplantation (OLT) has become the effective treatment for end-stage liver diseases. Since the 1980s, the successful rate of liver transplantation has increased with the improvement of operative methods and the use of University of Wisconsin (UW) solution. Nevertheless, liver procurement and implantation are inevitably associated with allograft damage. Lack of donor liver hinders OLT and leads to an increase in the number of deaths on the waiting list and as a consequence the transplant community has greatly expanded the use of non-ideal donors to improve the rate of transplant (Delmonico et al., 2005). Donor pool expansion strategies such as the use of living donors, cadaveric split livers, and "extended criteria donors" (ECD)/marginal donors are being pursued. These may predispose recipients to graft dysfunction and increase long-term risk and survival in recipients.
Primary graft non-function (PGNF) is the most severe type of graft damage after OLT, followed by initial poor graft function (IPGF) (Chui et al., 2000). Emergency hepatic retransplantation is necessary because of the extreme high mortality of PGNF. Evaluation of IPGF is determined by a high level of alanine aminotransferase (ALT) and/or aspartate aminotransferase (AST). IPGF directly influences the survival in the hepatic graft. Ultimately, some grafts recover completely while others need to be retransplanted (Pokorny et al., 2000). IPGF and PGNF are associated with many factors, such as status of donor, quality of hepatic graft, long-term warm ischemia, cold ischemia, primary liver disease, status of liver function of recipients and operative techniques (Brokelman et al., 1999). For evaluation of the donor hepatic allograft with regard to pre-existing diseases, in particular macrovesicular steatosis and post-transplant evaluation of hepatic graft function, liver biopsy is the most challenging and valuable clinical practice. Recently, some progress has been made in the prevention and treatment of early hepatic graft dysfunction. The present review provides broad discussion in the relevant sections.

2. The definitions and clinical features

2.1 Definitions of IPGF and PGNF

The concept of primary graft dysfunction is not clear. In clinical liver transplantation, primary dysfunction is defined as IPGF or PGNF. The difference between IPGF and PGNF

considers the degree of dysfunction, the timing and length after liver transplantation and the need for urgent retransplantation.
The diagnostic standard for IPGF has not been set yet, and there are different opinions among some reported definitions (Table 1). The criteria of Ploeg et al (Ploeg et al., 1993) and Gonzalez et al (Gonzalez et al., 1994) are adopted by some earlier studies. The introduction of Nanashima et al's criteria (Nanashima et al., 2002), which is simpler, more convenient and dependable, for an ALT and/or AST level above 1500 IU/L within 72 hours after OLT means poor hepatic allograft function as early as possible and also puts us on guard to prevent PGNF.

Definitions of IPGF	References
Graded initial liver function	(Gonzalez et al., 1994)
Severe: sum of score 7-9	
Moderate: 5 or 6	
Mild: 3 or 4	
AST > 2000 IU/L and prothrombin time >16 s	(Ploeg et al., 1994)
on days 2-7	
ALT > 2500 IU/L within 3 days	(Ardite et al., 1999)
AST or ALT > 2500 IU/L within 24 hours	(Chui et al., 2000)
ALT or AST > 1500 IU/L within the first 3 days	(Nanashima et al., 2002)

Table 1. Diagnostic definitions of IPGF

PGNF is manifested by hepatic cytolysis and rapidly rising transaminases, absence of bile production, severe liver-related coagulation deficit, hypoglycemia, high lactate levels, and hepatic hemodynamic instability (Uemura et al., 2007). According to the United Network for Organ Sharing (UNOS), PGNF is defined as irreversible graft function requiring emergency liver replacement during the first 10 days after liver transplantation. It is characterized by an AST ≥ 5000 UI/L, an international normalized ratio of prothrombin (INR) ≥ 3.0, and acidosis (pH ≤ 7.3 and/or lactate concentration ≥ 2× normal).
Silberhumer et al (Silberhumer et al., 2007) proposed four grades of initial graft function over the first postoperative 5 days as: (1) good function, AST maximal 1000 UI/L and spontaneous prothrombin time > 50%; (2) fair function, AST 1000-2500 UI/L, clotting factor support < 2 days; (3) IPGF, AST > 2500 UI/L, clotting factor support > 2 days; and (4) PGNF, retransplantation required within 7 days.

2.2 Clinical features

IPGF is a severe clinical complication after OLT, with elevation of serum aminotransferase. Some patients may further develop PGNF (Mor et al., 1992), which is manifested by hepatocellular necrosis, rapidly rising transaminases, absence of bile production, severe liver-related coagulation deficit, high lactate levels, systemic hemodynamic instability and acute renal failure (Pokorny et al., 2000).
Nevertheless, it is inconvenient to make the diagnosis of IPGF or PGNF due to the lack of precise to objective criteria in clinical practice. The great variability in the incidences reported in different series, which ranges from 2% and 23%. Ploeg et al reported the rates of IPGF and PGNF for 22% and 6%, respectively (Ploeg et al., 1993). Ardite et al's study showed the rates of IPGF and PGNF for 19% and 0% (Ardite et al., 1999) in contrast to 29.5%

and 0.93%, respectively in Chui et al's investigation (Chui et al., 2000). In the study by Chen et al, the rates of IPGF and PGNF were 36.25% and 1.3%, respectively (Chen et al., 2007). In The Scientific Registry for Transplant Recipients (SRTR) analysis enrolling 10545 deceased donors, adult first transplants, 613 (5.8%) cases of PNGF occurred (Johnson et al., 2007). In another single-center analysis of donors after cardiac death (DCD), PGNF occurred in 6.4% of brain dead donors (DBD) vs. 11.8% of DCD (Abt et al., 2004).

In partial liver transplantation, the biochemical profile of small for-size syndrome (SFSS) includes cholestasis with elevated conjugated bilirubin, mild to moderate elevation of transaminases, and prolonged prothrombin time. Approximately 50% of recipients with SFSS will die of sepsis within 4 - 6 weeks after septicemia (Heaton, 2003).

3. The impact of donor, recipient and factors associated with IPGF and PGNF

Graft dysfunction can be a result of various factors including status of donor, quality of hepatic graft, organ harvesting, ischemia-reperfusion injury, SFSS, primary liver disease, status of liver function of recipients and operative techniques, etc. Although ECD from older donors or steatotic grafts provide a solution for the shortage of allografts, donor factors could still predispose recipients to IPGF and/or PGNF. With extended application of living donor liver transplantation (LDLT), SFSS has become the main problem. The occurrence of SFSS depends on a number of recipient, graft and technical factors.

3.1 Recipient' factors

3.1.1 Child-Pugh classification and Model for End Stage Liver Disease (MELD) score

In a retrospective study (Chen et al., 2007), Child-Pugh classification had no influence on the occurrence of IPGF, yet the ratio of Child-Pugh C in the IPGF group was higher than in the non-IPGF group. Their data suggested that Child-Pugh C of recipients was one possible risk factor leading to IPGF.

The MELD score, which combines the serum creatinine, bilirubin, and INR of recipient to predict waitlist mortality, has been considered to be controversial in evaluating the occurrence of PGNF. In the SRTR analysis by Johnson et al, MELD score as a compound of risk factors was not included in models to predict PGNF (Johnson et al., 2007).

Although MELD score at the time of transplantation showed only a trend of an association with recipient survival, it had no significant impact on initial graft function (Silberhumer et al., 2007).

3.1.2 Other factors before transplantation

Elderly recipient and urgent recipient status with the use of ECD graft were associated with an increased risk of death by 50% (Cameron et al., 2006). Although the recipient's age and clinical status before OLT were related to IPGF (Moreno Sanz et al., 1999), it was not confirmed in a recent study (Chen et al., 2007). In addition, the incidence of PGNF was more in male recipients receiving grafts from female donors than in patients with male donors (Marino et al., 1995).

Avolio et al considered that hyperbilirubinemia before OLT was associated with PGNF (Avolio et al., 1999). In the STRT anslysis by Johnson et al, it was showed that by life support, mechanical ventilation, use of inotropes, hemodialysis, initial status 1 and use of a shared transplant were risk factors for PGNF by univariate analysis on recipients (Johnson et al., 2007). In the multivariate model, only recipient serum creatinine, bilirubin, on life support and status 1 at transplant were significant risk factors for PGNF. For pediatric recipients, diagnosis of tumor, dialysis prior to transplant, recipient body weight ≤ 6 kg increased the risk of graft failure (Lee et al., 2008).

Controversies exist regarding the morbidity and mortality of patients undergoing OLT at the extremes of the body mass index (BMI). An extremely BMI is defined as a BMI < 18.5 kg/m^2 or a BMI > 40 kg/m^2. In a study of the UNOS database, which reviewed 73,538 adult liver transplants, there was no significant impact of underweight or very severely obese on the occurrence of PGNF though these patients experienced significantly higher rates of morbidity and mortality compared with recipients with intermediate BMI range (Dick et al., 2009).

3.2 Donor's factors

3.2.1 Extended criteria donors and marginal donors

The use of ECDs is associated with increased graft loss and decreased survival. At present, no consensus has been reached for the definition of ECD graft. However, several risk factors associated with an increased rate of IPGF or PGNF have been identified. These risk factors include donor's factors (age, gender, obesity, weight, height, BMI, elevated liver functions, hypotension/increased administration of vasopressor and hypernatremia, cause of donor death and graft steatosis) and transplant factors such as type of graft and cold ischemia time (CIT) (Müllhaupt et al., 2008).

Definition for ECD by the suggestion of Chung et al includes age > 65 years, macrovesicular steatosis > 40%, serum sodium > 155 mmol/L, positive serological data, carcinoma outside the liver, DCD, and split-graft liver transplantation (Chung et al., 2010). In a large retrospective cohort study of 1153 OLT (Cameron et al., 2006), the ECD included donor age over 55 years, donor hospital stay >5 days, CIT >10 hours and warm ischemia time (WIT) > 40 minutes.

Marginal donors were considered by Pokorny et al as follows (Pokorny et al., 2005): older than 60 years, a prolonged intensive care unit (ICU) stay > 4 days with ventilatory support, a prolonged CIT >10 hours, a high vasopressor support (high-dose dopamine or any other vasoactive amines), a donor peak serum sodium > 155 mEq/L, a donor serum creatinine > 1.2 mg/100 mL and BMI > 30. When patients had more than three cumulative marginal donor criteria, the rate of PGNF was 36% (Pokorny et al., 2005).

3.2.2 Age

Hepatic graft from old donor may increase susceptibility to cold ischemia-induced endothelial injury with impaired adenosine triphosphate (ATP) synthesis post reperfusion and result in decreased regenerative capacity and synthetic function (Gordon Burroughs & Busuttil, 2009).

Donor age has been a well-recognized factor affecting PGNF. In the study by Feng et al, donor age over 40 years was associated significantly with the relative risk of graft failure (Feng et al., 2006). In the multivariate analysis by Lake et al, donor age over 40 was related with a 1.67 increased risk of graft failure in HCV-infected recipients and with 2.21 increased risk of graft failure when donor age was more than 60 years (Lake et al., 2005). In the SRTR analysis by Johnson et al, donor age more than 40 years was an independent factor for the prediction of PGNF (Johnson et al., 2007). Inversely, in other studies, donor age was not confirmed to increase the incidence of PGNF (Busquets et al.,2001; Grande et al.,1998; Washburn et al.,1996). However, these studies were based on a much smaller scale.

3.2.3 Steatosis

Hepatic steatosis is more common in donors of advanced age, as well as in those with a history of obesity, dyslipidemia, metabolic disorders, or diabetes.

The decreased allograft survival rate after using fatty livers is seen in the early post-transplant period (Verran et al., 2003). In contrast to macrovesicular steatosis, livers with predominantly microvesicular steatosis show less injury and allograft survival rates are similar to those in nonsteatotic grafts (Fishbein et al., 1997). So, adoption of an allograft with microvesicular steatosis is safe and the pool of donors has expanded. However, macrovesicular steatosis is one of the important risk factors leading to IPGF (Selzner & Clavien, 2001). Macrovesicular steatosis may impaire mitochondrial oxidation of fatty acids, increase synthesis and delivery of fatty acids to hepatocytes, reduce the removal of hepatocyte triglycerides, and microcirculatory disruption with narrowing of the hepatic sinusoids by enlarged, fat-laden hepatocytes (Reddy & Rao, 2006). Further more, macrovesicular steatosis may increase the oxidative injury of endothelial cell and hepatocyte and the vulnerability to secondary insults, including the cytokine surge associated with brain death as well as cold ischemic injury (Gordon Burroughs & Busuttil, 2009). In addition, the occurrence of IPGF or PGNF may be due to the release of free lipids from fatty hepatocytes, probably as a consequence of cold ischemia. Free lipids result in the production of reactive oxygen species after reperfusion initiating a cascade, which finally leads to sinusoidal endothelial cell damage (Selzner & Clavien, 2001; Kupiec-Weglinski & Busuttil, 2005). Severe fatty livers are more susceptible to warm and cold ischemia reperfusion injury than normal ones (Kukan & Haddad, 2001). The type of damage is not through the pathway of cellular apoptosis, but necrosis (Selzner & Clavien, 2000). Overexpression of the mitochondrial uncoupling protein 2 in fatty livers may contribute to decreased cellular ATP levels (Serviddio et al., 2008), which reduces the capacity for hepatic regeneration (Selzner et al., 2000). There are some other factors which may play a role in fatty livers after reperfusion, like the down-regulation of peroxisome proliferator-activated receptor-α, an important regulator of the hepatic inflammatory response to ischemia reperfusion, and overexpression of adiponectin, a fat cell-secreted hormone with antidiabetic and antiinflammatory activities (Massip-Salcedo et al., 2008).

Ureña et al considered that hepatic allografts with moderate macrovesicular steatosis (30% - 60%) can be used selectively in critical situations; mild macrovesicular steatosis (< 30%) is relatively safe, and severe cases (> 60%) enhance the rate of PGNF (Ureña et al., 1998; D'Alessandro et al., 1991). Canelo et al reported that PGNF can occur with donors having moderate macrovesicular steatosis. In this study, mild macrovesicular steatosis was 27.1% in the non-IPGF group and 13.8% in the IPGF group (Canelo et al., 2000). There was no significant difference between those groups.

In the study by Verran et al, 6% of patients receiving grafts with severe macrovesicular fat required retransplantation within 3 months versus 1.4% of those receiving mildly steatotic grafts (Verran et al., 2003). In another multivariate analysis by Salizzoni et al, cumulative adverse factors on the incidence of PGNF included donor age, recipient HCV viremia, and prolonged CIT by use of grafts with over 15% macrovesicular steatosis (Salizzoni et al., 2003).

3.3 Small-for-size syndrome (SFSS)

SFSS is a well-recognized complication that occurs primarily in living donor or reduced size liver transplantation. The principal pathogenesis of SFSS is the unbalance between the accelerated liver regeneration and the increased demand of liver function, leading to severe graft dysfunction with prolonged hyperbilirubinemia and increased ascites (Ikegami et al., 2008). SFSS is caused by multiple factors including graft quality, recipient conditions and technique problems. SFSS is seen most frequently when the graft volume/standard liver volume ratio (GV/SLV) is less than 30% or partial liver grafts with graft weight/recipient weight ratios (GW/RW) less than 0.8%. Another important factor leading to SFSS is portal venous hypertension (Shimamura et al., 2001). In recent study by Hill et al, GW/RW did not appear to be the only determinant of outcome after partial liver transplantation and the occurrence of SFSS was influenced not only by the graft size but also by other factors such as the degree of portal hypertension as well (Hill et al., 2009). For adult patient receiving right lobe graft, low intraoperative body temperature, graft size of < 35% of the estimated standard graft weight, and middle hepatic vein occlusion were significantly independent factors in determining hospital mortality (Fan et al., 2003). Other factors may impact the occurrence of SFSS (Emond et al., 1996; Yoshizumi et al., 2008): donor-related factors including advanced donor age and steatotic graft and recipient-related factors including higher MELD scores, septic complications, rejection and biliary complications. Donor age over 50 years is associated with reduced regenerative capacity, increased susceptibility to prolonged cold ischemia, increased rates of IPGF/PGNF and prolonged cholestasis. Fatty infiltration of 30% or more in grafts in splitting or auxiliary liver transplantation may increase incidence of SFSS (Heaton & Rela, 2001).

3.4 Ischemia reperfusion injury

Hepatic ischemia reperfusion injury is an important factor related to IPGF (Mueller et al., 1997). During the course of clinical liver transplantation, warm ischemia, cold ischemia, rewarming ischemia, and reperfusion occur sequentially in the allograft. Severe ischemia reperfusion injury leads to immediate graft non-function and triggers irreversible ischemic biliary lesions.

3.4.1 Warm ischemia

Hepatic warm ischemia occurs when the liver is maintained at body temperature but is inadequately perfused with blood. Although grafts from DCD increase the number of organs abailable, longer non-heart beating time and hypotension lead to warm ischemia, which may cause cell necrosis in the hepatic parenchyma after reperfusion and more easily result in IPGF or PGNF.

The process of warm ischemia reperfusion injury involves activation of immune pathways and is dominated by hepatocellular injury. There are 2 distinct phases: the early phase (less than 2 hours after reperfusion) is marked by activation of immune cells (CD4+T cells and Kupffer cells) and production of oxidant stress; the later injury (6 to 48 hours after reperfusion) is characterized by neutrophil-mediated inflammation and hepatocellular injury (Klune & Tsung, 2010). In addition, warm ischemia also damages endothelial cells (Selzner et al., 2003; Teoh & Farrell, 2003).

As prolonged WIT is common with uncontrolled DCD, standardized criteria in donor selection have not been established and limited data concerning its use have been reported. D'Alessandro et al reported that the average WIT was 16.4 minutes in 19 cases of OLT using a DCD and the rate of PGNF was 10.5% (D'Alessandro et al., 2000). Gomez et al also reported that with 5-15 minutes average WIT, IPGF occurred in 6 of 8 cases and PGNF in the other two cases (Gomez et al., 1997). In a matched-pair analysis, PGNF was occurred 5.1% in livers of DCD versus 0% in those of DBD (Pine et al., 2009). In another retrospective study, PGNF was presented 3.7% in livers of DCD versus 1.4% in those of DBD (Grewal et al, 2009). In the study of 141 patients by de Vera et al, the incidence of PGNF was 12% in livers of DCD versus 3% in livers of DBD. WIT over 20 minutes was associated with poorer DCD outcomes (de Vera et al., 2009). In the study by Chen et al, the average WIT was significantly longer in the IPGF group than in the non-IPGF (Chen et al., 2007). Changes after warm ischemia were seen in liver biopsies before OLT. Furthermore, WIT was 7 minutes in only one case who suffered from PGNF. From logistic regression analysis, the possibility of IPGF was enhanced significantly when WIT exceeded 3 minutes. These results suggested that extension of WIT is a direct risk factor in bringing on IPGF. Recently, an analysis of OPTN/UNOS data demonstrates donor age > 60 years, WIT > 30 minutes, CIT > 10 hours, retransplantation, and recipient cardiopulmonary support pre-OLT to be the most important predictors of significantly PGNF and patient survival after transplantation of a DCD graft (Mateo et al., 2006). Similarily, the University of California, Los Angeles (UCLA) reported with controlled DCD that PGNF occurred only in 2.6% of the recipients with about 30 minutes of mean WIT (Gordon Burroughs & Busuttil, 2009).

3.4.2 Cold ischemia

Although the cold preservation time of the allograft is extended greatly by the use of UW solution in clinical liver transplantation, cold ischemia is an important factor for IPGF and PGNF.

Some investigations showed that sinusoidal endothelial cells are damaged first in cold ischemia reperfusion, then hepatocellular cells, because of activation of Kupffer cells and neutrophilic leukocytes, and the release of inflammatory mediators, which leads to impairment of hepatic allografts (Jaeschke, 2006). During the phase of cold ischemia, loss of mitochondrial respiration and ATP depletion occur consequently though hypothermia reduces the metabolic rate and prolongs the time that anoxic cells can retain essential metabolic functions (Selzner et al., 2003). Energy-dependent metabolic pathways and transport processes deteriorate and proteinases and metalloproteinases are activated. These changes lead to the sinusoidal endothelial cells to be lifted away from the underlying matrix. Loss of sinusoidal microvascular integrity and function that occurs during cold preservation is attributable to the reperfusion phase. The degree of endothelial damage has been correlated with functional impairment of the liver following reperfusion.

Piratvisuth et al retrospectively summarized 230 cases of liver transplantation where the rate of IPGF was significantly higher when CIT was more than 720 minutes (Piratvisuth et al., 1995). In the study by Janny et al, AST level increased significantly after OLT if cold ischemia time was above 600 minutes (Janny et al., 1997). Adam et al thought that the possibility of hepatic allograft loss was significantly enhanced when cold ischemia time was over 720 minutes (Adam et al., 1992). De Vera et al suggested that CIT over 8 hours was significantly related to the occurence of PGNF (de Vera et al., 2009). In the study by Chen et al, the cold preservation time in all cases was within 1000 minutes, averaging 622 minutes in the IPGF group and 515 minutes in the non-IPGF group (Chen et al., 2007). A significant difference was shown by univariate analysis and not by multi-regression analysis. The results above suggested that extension of CIT is a potential risk factor for IPGF and PGNF.

3.4.3 Rewarm ischemia

The anhepatic phase was defined as the time from the physical removal of the liver from the recipient to the time of graft recirculation. During the anhepatic period, rewarming ischemia injury occurs because of the rise of allograft temperature. Strasberg et al considered that rewarming ischemia injury as the most important risk factor for IPGF can lead to increased AST level and decreased rate of allograft survival (Strasberg et al., 1994). The tolerance limits of allografts to rewarm ischemia time are not clear. In the study by Chen et al, although rewarming ischemia time was significantly longer in the IPGF group than in the non-IPGF group, shown by univariate ayalysis, multiregression analysis showed no significant difference between the two groups when rewarming ischemia time was above 45 minutes (Chen et al., 2007). In Nanashima et al's investigation, average rewarming ischemia time was about 110 minutes in both IPGF group and non-IPGF group (Nanashima et al., 2002). Platz et al reported that serum levels of ALT, AST, E-selectin and hyaluronic acid increased significantly if the anhepatic period was above 90 minutes (Platz et al., 1997). Delva et al thought that rewarm ischemia time should not exceed 60 minutes (Delva et al., 1989). Recently, in a logistic regression analysis by Ijtsma et al, the anhepatic phase over 100 minutes [odds ratio (OR), 4.28] was an independent predictive factor for graft dysfunction (Ijtsma et al., 2009). These results suggested that extended rewarming ischemia time is an important risk factor for IPGF.

4. Histopathological characteristics

For evaluation of the donor hepatic allograft with regard to pre-existing diseases, in particular macrovesicular steatosis and post-transplant evaluation of hepatic graft function, liver biopsy is the most challenging and valuable clinical practice.

4.1 Steatosis of donors

Excessively fatty liver, specifically macrovesicular (large droplet) fatty liver, is associated closely with risk for IPGF or PGNF. Microvesicular (small droplet) fat in the donor liver is not a contraindication for transplantation (Fishbein et al., 1997). As macroscopy is unreliable in the appraisal of the severity of steatosis, bioptical evaluation before transplantation is recommended in cases where significant steatosis is suspected. The percentage of steatosis should be determined by liver biopsy before transplantation.

4.2 Ischemia reperfusion injury

According to the experiences of Demetris et al, it is electron microscopy, not light microscopic examination, before transplantation which can be used to accurately assess the cold ischemia injury and post-transplant allograft function (Demetris et al., 2009). However, after reperfusion, light microscopic examination is more informative. Reperfusion biopsies show the damage, with reasonable accuracy, can predict IPGF or PGNF during the first few weeks post operation.

Severe cold preservation reperfusion damage is one of the major reasons for PGNF. Histologically, it is characterized by massive necrosis, which becomes evident within the first 48 hours after transplantation (Chazouillères et al., 1993). The hepatic microenvironment involving in the pathogenesis of preservation injury includes lymphocytes, hepatocytes, bile duct epithelium, sinusoidal cells, Kupffer cells, neutrophilic leukocytes and platelets. Sinusoidal endothelial cells are the first affected then hepatic parenchymal cells (Clavien, 1998) and finally hepatic allograft function is impaired.

Most biopsy specimens were essentially normal before transplantation except for focal mild spotty acidophilic necrosis, a slight increase in sinusoidal inflammatory cells and mild hepatocellular swelling. It is important that the integrity of the sinusoidal lining cells could not be evaluated reliably with immersion fixed, paraffin-embedded and hematoxylin and eosin-stained slides of biopsy specimens before transplantation. By contrast to biopsy specimens before transplantation, various pathological findings after reperfusion are demonstrated. In severe cold ischemia reperfusion injury under the examination of light microscopy (Kakizoe et al., 1990), larger areas of necrosis appeared, which were classified as focal or zonal with periportal or bridging necrosis, and severe neutrophilic exudation. The focal or zonal necrosis was either centrilobular, periportal, or both in its distribution. In general, the degree of inflammation increased after revascularization and paralleled the degree of necrosis. For hepatocytes, microvesicular steatosis, focal hepatocellular cytoaggregation and mild hydropic cell swelling were detected. In more severe injury, if hepatocellular necrosis was mainly in zone 3, centrilobular hepatocyte dropout is seen. The adjacent viable zone 2 hepatocytes proliferate to restore the liver parenchyma, and mitoses are seen. If periportal necrosis and bridging necrosis are present, the parenchymal collapse triggers ductular reaction that can link adjacent portal tracts and distort the architecture. More severe injury is also usually accompanied by centrilobular hepatocellular swelling, and canalicular and cholangiolar cholestasis (Demetris et al., 1987).

Ultrastructural analysis by Kakizoe et al revealed that the sinusoidal microvasculature was more sensitive to organ procurement and cold preservation than the endothelium of larger vessels or hepatocytes (Kakizoe et al., 1990). These changes at the end of cold ischemia before transplantation included endothelial cell vacuolization and a partial or complete detachment of individual cells, resulting in denudation with loss of the space of Disse. The sinusoids contained cellular debris, presumably fragments of hepatocytes, detached endothelial cells and occasional inflammatory cells. The hepatocellular changes detected were relatively mild and included cytoplasmic fat vacuolization, a decrease in the mitochondrial matrix, formation of hepatocellular cytoplasmic blebs protruding into the sinusoids and occasional loss of hepatocyte microvilli on the sinusoidal surface. After reperfusion, increased sinusoidal cellular debris, focal sinusoidal endothelial cell denudation and occasional active appearing Kupffer cells that contained cytoplasmic vacuoles and electron-dense material are observed. Inflammatory cells were often clustered in areas of microarchitectural distortion and sinusoidal lining cell denudation. They were also seen near Kupffer cells and directly adherent to hepatocytes or amidst cellular debris. Hepatocyte alterations were relatively mild. The changes included an increase in lipid vacuolization, detachment of cytoplasmic blebs and, in some areas, formation of electrondense material in the cytoplasm. The mitochondria in some cases showed mild

swelling, and the rough endoplasmic reticulum showed focal mild fusiform dilatation when compared with samples taken before transplantation.
In some circumstances, the histological findings showed minimal alterations in some patients who experienced IPGF or PGNF. Biopsies after reperfusion may be performed too soon after reperfusion to detect morphological changes of irreversible ischemic injury.

4.3 SFSS

The histopathologic features of SFSS had been summarized by Demetris et al (Demetris et al., 2006). The portal vein and sinusoidal injury could be divided into early, intermediate, and late changes. Early changes include focal endothelial denudation that is accompanied by hemorrhage into the portal connective tissue that occasionally dissects deeper into the hepatic parenchyma when it is severe. Denudation of portal vein and periportal sinusoidal endothelium, severe congestion with frank rupture and thrombosis of the periportal sinusoids may occur as early as 5 minutes after transplantation in grafts of less than 30% expected liver volume (Kelly et al., 2004). Intermediate and late portal venous changes are associated with repair of the early changes. Endothelial cell hypertrophy, subendothelial edema accompanied by an in-growth of myofibroblasts and endothelial cells resulting in focal fibrosis, and luminal obliteration or recanalization of thrombi may be present.
In addition, functional dearterialization could be observed because of arterial vasospasm and/or arterial thrombosis. The arterial lesions are invariably accompanied by large perihilar bile duct necrosis, cholangitic abscesses, leakage of bile in the surrounding connective tissue, and scattered parenchymal infarcts. The most characteristic triad of histopathologic findings present include centrilobular hepatocanalicular cholestasis, centrilobular hepatocyte microvesicular steatosis, and a low-grade ductular reaction at the interface zone. The ductular reaction consisted of portal tract expansion because of an increase of ductal profiles at the interface zone accompanied by acute neutrophilic periductular inflammation.
Based on the above pathological manifestations, Demetris et al proposed the following sequence of SFSS (Demetris et al., 2006). First, portal venous hyperperfusion causes portal vein and sinusoidal endothelial cell injury which leads to intraparenchymal dissecting hemorrhage in severe cases. Second, portal hyperperfusion triggers the arterial buffer response (Marcos et al., 2000), hepatic arterial vasospasm, and decreased hepatic artery perfusion. Decreased hepatic arterial blood flow can also be presented in most reduced-size liver allografts (Marcos et al., 2000). Third, centrilobular microvesicular steatosis and infarcts in the periphery are caused by poor arterial flow and ischemia. In the hilum, it manifests as ischemic cholangitis in severe cases (Ludwig et al., 1992). Last, remnants of portal vein pathology often cause organizing mural thrombi or thickening in large branches portal vein branches and partial or complete luminal obliteration or recanalization in small portal vein branches.
However, the histopathologic and pathophysiologic manifestations of SFSS have not been depended completely on peripheral core needle biopsies (Demetris et al., 2006). Under the examination of peripheral core needle biopsies, affected grafts most commonly show the following triad: centrilobular hepatocanalicular cholestasis, centrilobular hepatocyte microvesicular steatosis, and a ductular reaction at the interface zone. Venous pathology could not be detected by peripheral core needle biopsies in failed allograft though the presentation of venous changes is particularly helpful for the diagnosis of SFSS. In addition, it should be kept in mind that the changes in zone 3 and ductular reaction are not specific for SFSS. The detection should include suboptimal arterial flow as hepatic artery thrombosis

or bile duct stricturing are not related to the SFSS, and systemic causes such as sepsis with or without systemic hypotension.

5. The strategy for prevention and treatment

As PGNF is the most severe type of IPGF and a life threatening condition, there is growing need for early identification of IPGF and PGNF. This may help to determine further therapeutic interventions, changes in therapeutic protocols or additional diagnostic procedures aiming at preventing IPGF and PGNF.

5.1 Early diagnosis

At present, confirmation of IPGF and PGNF still depends on daily monitoring of liver function, renal function, blood coagulation function, hemodynamic and respiratory parameters, as well as liver biopsy. In order to reach a quick and accurate diagnosis, it requires careful interpretation of allograft biopsy and correlation of hepatic histopathological characteristics with clinical and laboratory findings. As laboratory tests may reflect later results of IPGF or PGNF, early biomarkers should be searched.

Recently, Dahaba et al assessed Bispectral index (BIS) monitoring as an early intraoperative indicator of living-donor or DCD graft function (Dahaba et al., 2009). BIS monitoring, an electroencephalographic (EEG)-derived parameter, is a useful measure for grading and monitoring the degree of central nervous system involvement in patients with chronic liver disease. BIS increase was associated significantly with non-IPGF but not with the occurrence of IPGF, which indicates predictive power of BIS monitoring as an indicator of the return of cerebral activity with the restoration of graft hepatic function.

In animal model of liver transplantation by using non-heart beating donor, the levels of serum β-galactosidase, IL-6, hyaluronic acid and redox-activate iron are closely associated with early confirmation of IPGF and PGNF (Monbaliu et al., 2007).

5.2 Donor-recipient matching models

As various donor and recipient risk factors influence graft function and survival after OLT (see Table 2), identifying the right set of donor and recipient matching characteristics may be very important, especially in the face of increasing use of DCD.

From the data of SRTR, Feng et al identified seven donor characteristics that be independently used to predict significantly increased risk of graft failure and developed a quantitative donor risk index (DRI) using Cox regression models (Feng et al., 2006). By using DRI, the risk of donor liver graft could be assessed quantitatively. In another large analysis by using the data from the UNOS of 20,301 recipients, a comprehensive model that predicts survival after liver transplantation was developed and validated based on donor and recipient characteristics (Ioannou, 2006). These models could adequately predict survival after OLT in patients with or without hepatitis C virus and have a large effect on post-transplant survival.

By using the OPTN/SRTR data base on 21673 liver transplant recipients, Rana et al identified 13 recipient factors, 4 donor factors and 2 operative factors (warm and cold ischemia) as significant predictors of recipient mortality (Rana et al., 2008). The multivariate analysis in this study included all of the variables considered in the SRTR risk-adjusted model. The Survival Outcomes Following Liver Transplant (SOFT) score was evaluated by utilizing 18 risk factors to successfully predict 3-month recipient survival following liver transplantation. Furthermore, the proposed SOFT risk score can be used to predict outcomes for a particular recipient and donor allograft prior to transplantation comparing against waitlist mortality predicted by the MELD score. However, the SOFT score addresses only 3-month mortality comparing other studies which look at longerterm outcome.

Study	Markmann	Cuende	Busuttil	Feng	Ioannou	Rana
References	(Markmann et al., 2001)	(Cuende et al., 2005)	(Busuttil et al., 2005)	(Feng et al., 2006)	(Ioannou et al., 2006)	(Rana et al., 2008)
Number in study	1393	5150	3200	20023	38811	21673
Year range of data	1992 - 1998	1994 - 2110	1984 - 2001	1998 - 2002	1994 - 2003	2002 - 2006
Data source	UCLA	Spain	UCLA	SRTR	UNOS	UNOS
Donor factors						
Age	•	•	•	•	•	•
Race				•	•	•
Gender					•	
Height				•		
Hypertension		•				
Cause of donor death				•		•
DCD				•		•
Length of donor hospital/ICU stay		•	•			
Serum sodium level	•					
Serum bicarbonate level		•				
Serum creatinine level						•
Recipient factors						
Age	•		•		•	•
Recipient urgency			•		•	•
Preoperative mechanical ventilation	•					
Serum creatinine level	•					
Serum albumin level					•	
Cause of recipient's liver disease			•		•	
Retransplantation			•			•
BMI					•	•
MELD score					•	•
Transplant factors						
Warm ischemia time			•			•
Cold ischemia time			•		•	•
Partial- or split-liver graft				•		

Table 2. Factors effecting graft function or graft survival

Given the importance of advanced donor age and graft quality, Halldorson et al developed a statistic, D-MELD, the product of donor age and preoperative MELD, calculated from laboratory values (Halldorson et al., 2009). Using a cutoff D-MELD score of 1600, they defined a subgroup of donor-recipient matches with significantly poorer short- and long-term outcomes as measured by survival and length of stay. It can be used to accurately estimate the risk for various donor/recipient combinations and predicte worse outcome in recipients after OLT if D-MELD ≥ 1600. In an observational cohort study that prospectively enrolled liver transplantations performed at 20 out of 21 Italian Transplant Centres, it was demonstrated that the liver donor population used for transplantation in Italy has a higher risk profile mainly because of older donor age (Angelico et al., 2011).

The models above are aimed to help clinicians balance waitlist mortality with posttransplant outcome and make right decisions on a particular allograft. Freeman (Freeman, 2008) suggested that the differences between statistical calculations and decision made for individual patients with various treatment options should be emphasized though these models have some useful information for donor-recipient matching.

5.3 Prevention and treatment

5.3.1 General consideration

Recently, some progress has been made in the prevention and treatment of early hepatic graft dysfunction. In the clinical practice, limitation of the use of liver grafts from patients older than 50 years should be complied. For steatotic donor grafts, restricting the use of steatotic livers to those with less than 40% macrovesicular steatosis is recommended. Livers with large droplet fat in excess of 60% are at increased risk for primary graft dysfunction/nonfunction and are therefore typically excluded from transplantation (Trevisani et al., 1996/Ploeg et al., 1993). As with other ECD grafts, recipient matching should be based on the number and extent of recipient risk factors and the absence of other negative donor variables, such as advanced donor age and prolonged CIT, to minimize the negative impact on graft and patient's outcome. Determination of the BMI seems to be a helpful and non-invasive method to estimate the degree of liver steatosis, particularly in living donors (Rinella et al., 2001; Trotter, 2001). Individuals with normal BMI usually do not have steatosis (Rinella et al., 2001).

5.3.2 Surgical strategies

For reduction of severe ischemia reperfusion injury of graft, surgical strategies have been undertaken. It is recommended that the time from pronouncement of cardiac death until liver perfusion with preservation solution and CIT should be between 20 minutes to 12 hours. For the use of uncontrolled non-heart-beating donors, normothermic extracorporeal membrane oxygenation (NECMO) were adopted in a prospective case-control study on adult patients undergoing OLT, and the results are encouraging (Jiménez-Galanes et al., 2009). Prior to major hepatectomy, ischemic preconditioning (IP) of the liver has been successfully employed to protect against subsequent prolonged periods of ischemia (Clavien et al., 2000). The aim of IP is to induce resistance to a subsequent longer episode of ischemia by a short episode of ischemia reperfusion. The development of hepatic preconditioning can be differentiated into 2 phases. An early phase of protection occurs immediately after IP. The subsequent phase (late preconditioning) begins 12-24 hours after the stimulus and the induction of cytoprotective genes, including HSP70, HSP27, and HSP32/heme oxygenase 1. Hepatic preconditioning is not limited to parenchymal cells but also ameliorates sinusoidal perfusion, prevents postischemic Kupffer cell activation, neutrophil infiltration, and decreases the production of proinflammatory cytokines, oxidative injury and apoptosis (Carini & Albano, 2003). In a prospective randomized study on 100 patients undergoing major liver resection to the impact of ischemic preconditioning was evaluated (Clavien et al.,

2003). Postoperative serum transaminase levels were significantly lower in preconditioned group than in control group, with even more benefits in younger patients, longer duration of inflow occlusion, where resected volume <50%, and in the presence of steatosis (Clavien et al., 2003). Recently in experimental settings, graft preservation by normothermic machine perfusion has proven superiority over static cold storage. Normothermic perfusion could preserve extended criteria grafts for long periods, assess the viability of these grafts during perfusion and improve the condition of the grafts (Vogel et al., 2010). However, the feasibility and the device of the normothermic machine perfusion should be introduced and evaluated in human livers.

5.3.3 Pharmacological strategies

Pharmacological treatments include (Bahde & Spiegel, 2010): first, antioxidant therapy aiming at supporting endogenous antioxidants and inhibiting ROS generation; second, vasoactive mediators, such as ET, angiotensin II, thromboxane A2, NO, carbon monoxide, prostaglandin E1 and prostacyclin, can ameliorate the hepatic microcirculation; third, anti-inflammatory drugs in order to reduce ischemia reperfusion injury via selectin, cyclo-oxygenase 2 and protease inhibition, cytokines (including TNF-α and IL-1) and chemokine blockade; fourth, antiapoptotic strategies, including mitochondrial permeability transition inhibitors (ciclosporin A, trifluoperazine), anti-Fas or anti-Fas ligand antibodies, antiapoptotic proteins, caspase inhibitors and others; fifth, pharmacological preconditioning imitating the protective mechanisms induced by IP; finally, glucose infusion, by supplying glucose for ATP generation. A total of 14 RCTs were identified for evaluating these pharmacological measurements. Although some pharmacological strategies showed promising results with improved hepatic function and clinical outcome, but there is still not solid evidence to recommend its application in clinical. However, methylprednisolone (Aldrighetti et al., 2006; Pulitanò et al., 2007) and sevoflurane (Beck-Schimmer et al., 2008) are the most promising drugs for reduction of ischemia reperfusion injury.

5.3.4 SPSS

For prevention of SFSS in partial liver transplantation, several interventions should be considered. First, selection of grafts from healthy donors without advanced age. Second, graft steatosis of 30% or more should preclude. Third, sufficient graft volume should be guaranteed. In the pediatric population, the recipient receives an adult lateral left segment or left lobe. In adult-to-adult LDLT, an extended right lobe graft with or without middle hepatic vein can increase graft volume though the donor is relatively small (Lo et al., 2004; Cattral et al., 2004). Finally, ischemic preconditioning may also be of benefit in partial liver transplantation to protect SFSS grafts, as it has been shown to maintain the hepatic microcirculation and decrease the activation of Kupffer cells (Franco-Gou et al., 2004; Vajdová et al., 2004).

5.3.5 Retransplantation

Early retransplantation is the only choice of treatment in patients with PGNF. It was reported by Grande et al that the third postoperative day is a crucial time in making the decision of retransplantation in patients with IPGF (Grande et al., 1992). It is because that the improvement of liver function began on the third day in almost all patients whose graft dysfunction spontaneously ameliorated. Upon the diagnosis of PGNF, rescue hepatectomy of the non-functioning liver can achieve a dramatic temporary clinical improvement as failing graft causes the pathophysiology of this disorder and extrahepatic sequelae. Retransplant after PGNF in the initial transplant can achieve relatively good long-term survival (Uemura et al., 2007). However, a second or third transplant after PGNF did not demonstrate long-term survival, and hospital mortality was 57% (Uemura et al., 2007). In addition, the patient's and graft's survival were lower in recipients with hepatitis C virus infection who received retransplantation when compared with those without HCV infection as HCV was an independent predictor of mortality after retransplantation (Yoo et al., 2003).

6. Conclusion

IPGF is a severe complication after OLT while PGNF is a life-threatening event. The factors of donor, recipient and operation contribute to the occurrences of IPGF or PGNF. For evaluation of the donor hepatic allograft and post-transplant evaluation of hepatic graft function, liver biopsy as well as with clinical and laboratory findings are important for early diagnosis in clinical practice. For prevention of IPGF or PGNF, it is necessary for careful consideration of donor and recipient factors before OLT. Surgical and pharmacological interventions should be undertaken cautiously.

7. Acknowledgment

The author would like to thank Dr. Lu Hui for his help in revising the manuscript and support of all doctors and nurses of the Center for Organ Transplantation in Ruijin Hospital.

8. References

Abt, PL.; Desai, NM.; Crawford, MD.; Forman, LM.; Markmann, JW.; Olthoff, KM. & Markmann, JF. (2004) Survival following liver transplantation from non-heart-beating donors. *Annals of Surgery*, Vol.239, No.1, (January 2004), pp. 87-92, ISSN: 1528-1140

Adam, R.; Bismuth, H.; Diamond, T.; Ducot, B.; Morino, M.; Astarcioglu, I.; Johann, M.; Azoulay, D.; Chiche, L. & Bao, YM. (1992) Effect of extended cold ischaemia with UW solution on graft function after liver transplantation. *Lancet*, Vol.340, No.8832, (December 1992), pp. 1373-1376, ISSN: 0140-6736

Aldrighetti, L.; Pulitanò, C.; Arru, M.; Finazzi, R.; Catena, M.; Soldini, L.; Comotti, L. & Ferla, G. (2006) Impact of preoperative steroids administration on ischemia-reperfusion injury and systemic responses in liver surgery: a prospective randomized study. *Liver Transplantation*, Vol.12, No.6, (June 2006), pp. 941-949, ISSN: 1527-6473

Angelico, M.; Cillo, U.; Fagiuoli, S.; Gasbarrini, A.; Gavrila, C.; Marianelli, T.; Costa, AN.; Nardi, A.; Strazzabosco, M.; Burra, P.; Agnes, S.; Baccarani, U.; Calise, F.; Colledan, M.; Cuomo, O.; De Carlis, L.; Donataccio, M.; Ettorre, GM.; Gerunda, GE.; Gridelli, B.; Lupo, L.; Mazzaferro, V.; Pinna, A.; Risaliti, A.; Salizzoni, M.; Tisone, G.; Valente, U.; Rossi, G.; Rossi, M.; Zamboni, F. & Liver Match Investigators. (2011) Liver Match, a prospective observational cohort study on liver transplantation in Italy: study design and current practice of donor-recipient matching. *Digestive and Liver Disease*, Vol.43, No.2, (February 2011), pp. 155-164, ISSN: 1590-8658

Ardite, E.; Ramos, C.; Rimola, A.; Grande, L.; Fernandez-Checa, JC. (1999) Hepatocellular oxidative stress and initial graft injury in human liver transplantation. Journal of *Hepatology*, Vol.31, No.5, (November 1999), pp. 921-927, ISSN: 0168-8278

Avolio, AW.; Agnes, S.; Chirico, AS. & Castagneto, M. (1999) Primary dysfunction after liver transplantation: donor or recipient fault? *Transplantation Proceedings*, Vol.31, No.1-2, (February-March 1999), pp. 434-436, ISSN: 0041-1345

Bahde, R. & Spiegel, HU. (2010) Hepatic ischaemia-reperfusion injury from bench to bedside. *Br J Surg*, Vol.97, No.10, (October 2010), pp. 1461-1475, ISSN: 1365-2168

Beck-Schimmer, B.; Breitenstein, S.; Urech, S.; De Conno, E.; Wittlinger, M.; Puhan, M.; Jochum, W.; Spahn, DR.; Graf, R. & Clavien, PA. (2008) A randomized controlled trial on pharmacological preconditioning in liver surgery using a volatile anesthetic. *Annals of Surgery*, Vol.248, No.6, (December 2008), pp. 909-918, ISSN: 1528-1140

Brokelman, W.; Stel, AL. & Ploeg, RJ. (1999) Risk factors for primary dysfunction after liver transplantation in the University of Wisconsin Solution era. *Transplantation Proceedings*, Vol.31, No.5, (August 1999), pp. 2087-2090, ISSN: 0041-1345

Busquets, J.; Xiol, X.; Figueras, J.; Jaurrieta, E.; Torras, J.; Ramos, E.; Rafecas, A.; Fabregat, J.; Lama, C.; Ibañez, L.; Llado, L. & Ramon, JM. (2001) The impact of donor age on liver transplantation: influence of donor age on early liver function and on subsequent patient and graft survival. *Transplantation*, Vol.71, No.12, (June 2001), pp. 1765-1771, ISSN: 1534-0608

Busuttil, RW.; Farmer, DG.; Yersiz, H.; Hiatt, JR.; McDiarmid, SV.; Goldstein, LI.; Saab, S.; Han, S.; Durazo, F.; Weaver, M.; Cao, C.; Chen, T.; Lipshutz, GS.; Holt, C.; Gordon, S.; Gornbein, J.; Amersi, F. & Ghobrial, RM. (2005) Analysis of long-term outcomes of 3200 liver transplantations over two decades: a single-center experience. *Annals of Surgery*, Vol.241, No.6, (December 2005), pp. 905-916, ISSN: 1528-1140

Canelo, R.; Braun, F.; Dopkens, K.; Ramadori, G. & Ringe, B. (2000) Characterization and influence of risk factors on initial liver function after transplantation. *Transplantation Proceedings*, Vol.32, No.1, (February 2000), pp. 60-61, ISSN: 0041-1345

Cameron, AM.; Ghobrial, RM.; Yersiz, H.; Farmer, DG.; Lipshutz, GS.; Gordon, SA.; Zimmerman, M.; Hong, J.; Collins, TE.; Gornbein, J.; Amersi, F.; Weaver, M.; Cao, C.; Chen, T.; Hiatt, JR. & Busuttil, RW. (2006) Optimal utilization of donor grafts with extended criteria: a single-center experience in over 1000 liver transplants. *Annals of Surgery*, Vol.243, No.6, (June 2006), pp. 748-753, ISSN: 1528-1140

Carini, R. & Albano, E. (2003) Recent insights on the mechanisms of liver preconditioning. *Gastroenterology*, Vol.125, No.5, (November 2003), pp. 1480-1491, ISSN: 0016-5085

Cattral, MS.; Molinari, M.; Vollmer, CM Jr.; McGilvray, I.; Wei, A.; Walsh, M.; Adcock, L.; Marks, N.; Lilly, L.; Girgrah, N.; Levy, G.; Greig, PD. & Grant, DR. (2004) Living-donor right hepatectomy with or without inclusion of middle hepatic vein: comparison of morbidity and outcome in 56 patients. *American Journal of Transplantation*, Vol.4, No.5, (May 2004), pp. 751-757, ISSN: 1600-6143

Chazouillères, O.; Calmus, Y.; Vaubourdolle, M. & Ballet, F. (1993) Preservation-induced liver injury. Clinical aspects: mechanisms and therapeutic approaches. *Journal of Hepatology*, Vol.18, No.1, (April 1993), pp. 123-134, ISSN: 0168-8278

Chen, H., Peng, CH., Shen, BY., Deng, XX., Shen, C., Xie, JJ., Dong, W. & Li, HW. (2007) Multi-factor analysis of initial poor graft function after orthotopic liver transplantation. *Hepatobiliary & Pancreatic Diseases International*, Vol.6, No.2, (April 2007), pp. 141-146, ISSN: 1499-3872

Chui, AK.; Shi, LW.; Rao, AR.; Anasuya, A.; Hagl, C.; Pillay, P.; Verran, D.; McCaughan, GW. & Sheil, AG. (2000) Primary graft dysfunction after liver transplantation. *Transplantation Proceedings*, Vol.32, No.7, (November 2000), pp. 2219-2220, ISSN: 0041-1345

Chung, HY.; Chan, SC.; Lo, CM. & Fan, ST. (2010) Strategies for widening liver donor pool. *Asian Journal of Surgery*, Vol.33, No.2, (April 2010), pp. 63-69, ISSN: 1015-9584

Clavien, PA. (1998) Sinusoidal endothelial cell injury during hepatic preservation and reperfusion. *Hepatology*, Vol.28, No.2, (August 1998), pp. 281-285, ISSN: 1665-2681

Clavien, PA.; Yadav, S.; Sindram, D. & Bentley, RC. (2000) Protective effects of ischemic preconditioning for liver resection performed under inflow occlusion in humans. *Annals of Surgery*, Vol.232, No.2, (August 2000), pp. 155-162, ISSN: 1528-1140

Clavien, PA.; Selzner, M.; Rüdiger, HA.; Graf, R.; Kadry, Z.; Rousson, V. & Jochum, W. (2003) A prospective randomized study in 100 consecutive patients undergoing major liver resection with versus without ischemic preconditioning. *Annals of Surgery*, Vol.238, No.6, (December 2003), pp. 843-850, ISSN: 1528-1140

Cuende, N.; Miranda, B.; Cañón, JF.; Garrido, G. & Matesanz, R. (2005) Donor characteristics associated with liver graft survival. *Transplantation*, Vol.79, No.10, (May 2005), pp. 1445-1452, ISSN: 1534-0608

D'Alessandro, AM.; Kalayoglu, M.; Sollinger, HW.; Hoffmann, RM.; Reed, A.; Knechtle, SJ.; Pirsch, JD.; Hafez, GR.; Lorentzen, D. & Belzer, FO. (1991) The predictive value of donor liver biopsies for the development of primary nonfunction after orthotopic liver transplantation. *Transplantation*, Vol.51, No.1, (January 1991), pp. 157-163, ISSN: 1534-0608

D'Alessandro, AM.; Hoffmann, RM.; Knechtle, SJ.; Odorico, JS.; Becker, YT.; Musat, A.; Pirsch, JD.; Sollinger, HW. & Kalayoglu, M. (2000) Liver transplantation from controlled non-heart-beating donors. *Surgery*, Vol.128, No.4, (October 2000), pp. 579-588, ISSN: 1530-0358

Dahaba, AA.; Feng, ZY.; Zhu, SM.; Bornemann, H.; Rehak, PH. & Metzler, H. (2009) The utility of using bispectral index monitoring as an early intraoperative indicator of initial poor graft function after orthotopic or split-graft liver transplantation. *Gut*, Vol.58, No.4, (April 2009), pp. 605-606, ISSN: 1468-3288

de Vera, ME.; Lopez-Solis, R.; Dvorchik, I.; Campos, S.; Morris, W.; Demetris, AJ.; Fontes, P. & Marsh, JW. (2009) Liver transplantation using donation after cardiac death donors: long-term follow-up from a single center. *American Journal of Transplantation*, Vol.9, No.4, (April 2009), pp. 773-781, ISSN: 1600-6143

Delmonico, FL.; Sheehy, E.; Marks, WH.; Baliga, P.; McGowan, JJ. & Magee, JC. (2005) Organ donation and utilization in the United States, 2004. *American Journal of Transplantation*, Vol.5, No.4 Pt 2, (April 2005), pp. 862-873, ISSN: 1600-6143

Delva, E.; Camus, Y.; Nordlinger, B.; Hannoun, L.; Parc, R.; Deriaz, H.; Lienhart, A. & Huguet, C. (1989) Vascular occlusions for liver resections. Operative management and tolerance to hepatic ischemia: 142 cases. *Annals of Surgery*, Vol.209, No.2, (February 1989), pp. 211-218, ISSN: 1528-1140

Demetris, AJ.; Jaffe, R. & Starzl, TE. (1987) A review of adult and pediatric post-transplant liver pathology. *Pathology Annual*, Vol.22, No.Pt 2, (1987), pp. 347-386, ISSN: 0079-0184

Demetris, AJ.; Kelly, DM.; Eghtesad, B.; Fontes, P.; Wallis, Marsh, J.; Tom, K.; Tan, HP.; Shaw-Stiffel, T.; Boig, L.; Novelli, P.; Planinsic, R.; Fung, JJ. & Marcos, A. (2006) Pathophysiologic observations and histopathologic recognition of the portal hyperperfusion or small-for-size syndrome. *American Journal of Surgical Pathology*, Vol.30, No.8, (Augest 2006), pp. 986-993, ISSN: 1532-0979

Demetris, AJ.; Crawford, JM.; Minervini, MI.; Nalesnik, M.; Ochoa, E.; Randhawa, P.; Sasatomi, E. & Wu, T. (2009) Transplantation pathology of the liver. In: *Surgical pathology of the GI tract: liver, biliary tract and pancreas*, Odze, RD. & Goldblum, JR., eds, pp. 1169-1229, Saunders/Elsevier, ISBN 978-14160-4059-0, Philadelphia

Dick, AA.; Spitzer, AL.; Seifert, CF.; Deckert, A.; Carithers, RL Jr.; Reyes, JD. & Perkins, JD. (2009) Liver transplantation at the extremes of the body mass index. *Liver Transplantation*, Vol.15, No.8, (August 2009), pp. 968-977, ISSN: 1527-6473

Emond, JC.; Renz, JF.; Ferrell, LD.; Rosenthal, P.; Lim, RC.; Roberts, JP.; Lake, JR. & Ascher, NL. (1996) Functional analysis of grafts from living donors. Implications for the treatment of older recipients. *Annals of Surgery*, Vol.224, No.4, (October 1996), pp. 544-552, ISSN: 1528-1140

Fan, ST.; Lo, CM.; Liu, CL.; Yong, BH. & Wong, J. (2003) Determinants of hospital mortality of adult recipients of right lobe live donor liver transplantation. *Annals of Surgery*, Vol.238, No.6, (December 2003), pp. 864-869, ISSN: 1528-1140

Feng, S.; Goodrich, NP.; Bragg-Gresham, JL.; Dykstra, DM.; Punch, JD.; DebRoy, MA.; Greenstein, SM. & Merion, RM. (2006) Characteristics associated with liver graft failure: the concept of a donor risk index. *American Journal of Transplantation*, Vol.6, No.4, (April 2006), pp. 783-790, ISSN: 1600-6143

Fishbein, TM.; Fiel, MI.; Emre, S.; Cubukcu, O.; Guy, SR.; Schwartz, ME.; Miller, CM. & Sheiner, PA. (1997) Use of livers with microvesicular fat safely expands the donor pool. *Transplantation*, Vol.64, No.2, (September 1997), pp. 248-251, ISSN: 1534-0608

Franco-Gou, R.; Peralta, C.; Massip-Salcedo, M.; Xaus, C.; Serafín, A. & Roselló-Catafau, J. (2004) Protection of reduced-size liver for transplantation. *American Journal of Transplantation*, Vol.4, No.9, (September 2004), pp. 1408-1420, ISSN: 1600-6143

Freeman, RB Jr. (2008) SOFT endpoints in liver transplantation. *American Journal of Transplantation*, Vol.8, No.12, (December 2008), pp. 2483-2484, ISSN: 1600-6143

Gómez, M.; Garcia-Buitrón, JM.; Fernandez-Garcia, A.; Vilela, D.; Fernández-Selles, C.; Corbal, R.; Fraguela, J.; Suárez, F.; Otero, A.; Alvarez, J. & Mánez, R. (1997) Liver transplantation with organs from non-heart-beating donors. *Transplantation Proceedings*, Vol.29, No.8, (December 1997), pp. 3478-3479, ISSN: 0041-1345

Gonzalez, FX.; Rimola, A.; Grande, L.; Antolin, M.; Garcia-Valdecasas, JC.; Fuster, J.; Lacy, AM., Cugat, E., Visa, J. & Rodés, J. (1994) Predictive factors of early postoperative graft function in human liver transplantation. *Hepatology*, Vol.20, No.3, (September 1994), pp. 565-573, ISSN: 1665-2681

Gordon Burroughs, S. & Busuttil, RW. (2009) Optimal utilization of extended hepatic grafts. *Surgery Today*, Vol.39, No.9, (September 2009), pp. 746-751, ISSN: 0941-1291

Grande, L.; Rimola, A.; García-Valdecasas, JC.; Mas, A.; Fuster, J.; Navasa, M.; Lacy, AM.; Llach, J.; Gonzalex, FX.; Robusté, J. & Visa, J. (1992) Recovery of liver graft after initial poor function. *Transplantation*, Vol.53, No.1, (January 1992), pp. 228-230, ISSN: 1534-0608

Grande, L.; Matus, D.; Rimola, A.; Manyalic, M.; Cabrer, C.; García-Valdecasas, JC. & Visa, J. (1998) Expanded liver donor age over 60 years for hepatic transplantation. *Clinical Transplantation*, (1998) pp.297-301, ISSN: 0902-0063

Grewal, HP.; Willingham, DL.; Nguyen, J.; Hewitt, WR.; Taner, BC.; Cornell, D.; Rosser, BG.; Keaveny, AP.; Aranda-Michel, J.; Satyanarayana, R.; Harnois, D.; Dickson, RC.; Kramer, DJ. & Hughes, CB. (2009) Liver transplantation using controlled donation after cardiac death donors: an analysis of a large single-center experience. *Liver Transplantation*, Vol.15, No.9, (September 2009), pp. 1028-1035, ISSN: 1527-6473

Halldorson, JB.; Bakthavatsalam, R.; Fix, O.; Reyes, JD. & Perkins, JD. (2009) D-MELD: a simple predictor of post liver transplant mortality for optimization of donor/recipient matching. *American Journal of Transplantation*, Vol.9, No.2, (February 2009), pp. 318-326, ISSN: 1600-6143

Heaton, N. & Rela, M. (2001) Auxiliary liver transplantation. In: *Transplantation of the liver*, Maddrey, WC., Schiff, ER. & Sorrell, MF. eds, Lipincott Williams and Wilkins, pp. 121, ISBN-10 0781720397, ISBN-13 978-0781720397, Philadelphia

Heaton, N. (2003) Small-for-size liver syndrome after auxiliary and split liver transplantation: donor selection. *Liver Transplantation*, Vol.9, No.9, (September 2003), pp. S26-28, ISSN: 1527-6473

Hill, MJ.; Hughes, M.; Jie, T.; Cohen, M.; Lake, J.; Payne, WD. & Humar, A. (2009) Graft weight/recipient weight ratio: how well does it predict outcome after partial liver transplants? *Liver Transplantation*, Vol.15, No.9, (September 2009), pp. 1056-1062, ISSN: 1527-6473

Ijtsma, AJ.; van der Hilst, CS.; de Boer, MT.; de Jong, KP.; Peeters, PM.; Porte, RJ. & Slooff, MJ. (2009) The clinical relevance of the anhepatic phase during liver transplantation. *Liver Transplantation*, Vol.15, No.9, (September), pp. 1050-1055, ISSN: 1527-6473

Ikegami, T.; Shimada, M.; Imura, S.; Arakawa, Y.; Nii, A.; Morine, Y. & Kanemura, H. (2008) Current concept of small-for-size grafts in living donor liver transplantation. *Surgery Today*, Vol.38, No.11, (October 2008), pp. 971-982, ISSN: 0941-1291

Ioannou, GN. (2006) Development and validation of a model predicting graft survival after liver transplantation. *Liver Transplantation*, Vol.12, No.11, (November 2006), pp. 1594-1606, ISSN: 1527-6473

Jaeschke, H. (2006) Mechanisms of Liver Injury. II. Mechanisms of neutrophil-induced liver cell injury during hepatic ischemia-reperfusion and other acute inflammatory conditions. *American Journal of Physiology-Gastrointestinal and Liver Physiology*, Vol.290, No.6, (June 2006), pp. G1083-1088, ISSN: 1522-1547

Janny, S.; Sauvanet, A.; Farges, O.; LeMée, J.; Maillochaud, JH.; Marty, J. & Belghiti, J. (1997) Outcome of liver grafts with more than 10 hours of cold ischemia. *Transplantation Proceedings*, Vol.29, No.5, (August 1997), pp. 2346-2347, ISSN: 0041-1345

Jiménez-Galanes, S.; Meneu-Diaz, MJ.; Elola-Olaso, AM.; Pérez-Saborido, B.; Yiliam, FS.; Calvo, AG.; Usera, MA.; González, MC.; González, JC. & González, EM. (2009) Liver transplantation using uncontrolled non-heart-beating donors under normothermic extracorporeal membrane oxygenation. *Liver Transplantation*, Vol.15, No.9, (September 2009), pp. 1110-1118, ISSN: 1527-6473

Johnson, SR.; Alexopoulos, S.; Curry, M. & Hanto, DW. (2007) Primary nonfunction (PNF) in the MELD Era: An SRTR database analysis. *American Journal of Transplantation*, Vol.7, No.4, (April 2007), pp. 1003-1009, ISSN: 1600-6143

Kakizoe, S.; Yanaga, K.; Starzl, TE. & Demetris, AJ. (1990) Evaluation of protocol before transplantation and after reperfusion biopsies from human orthotopic liver allografts: considerations of preservation and early immunological injury. *Hepatology*, Vol.11, No.6, (June 1990), pp. 932-941, ISSN: 0168-8278

Kelly, DM.; Demetris, AJ.; Fung, JJ.; Marcos, A.; Zhu, Y.; Subbotin, V.; Yin, L.; Totsuka, E.; Ishii, T.; Lee, MC.; Gutierrez, J.; Costa, G.; Venkataraman, R. & Madariaga, JR. (2004) Porcine partial liver transplantation: a novel model of the "small-for-size" liver graft. *Liver Transplantation*, Vol.10, No.2, (February 2004), pp. 253-263, ISSN: 1527-6473

Klune, JR. & Tsung, A. (2010) Molecular biology of liver ischemia/reperfusion injury: established mechanisms and recent advancements. *Surgery Clinics of North America*, Vol.90, No.4, (August 2010), pp. 665-677, ISSN: 1042-3699

Kukan, M. & Haddad, PS. (2001) Role of hepatocytes and bile duct cells in preservation-reperfusion injury of liver grafts. *Liver Transplantation*, Vol.7, No.5, (May 2001), pp. 381-400, ISSN: 1527-6473

Kupiec-Weglinski, JW. & Busuttil, RW. (2005) Ischemia and reperfusion injury in liver transplantation. *Transplantation Proceedings*, Vol.37, No.4, (May 2005), pp. 1653-1656, ISSN: 0041-1345

Lake, JR.; Shorr, JS.; Steffen, BJ.; Chu, AH.; Gordon, RD. & Wiesner, RH. (2005) Differential effects of donor age in liver transplant recipients infected with hepatitis B.; hepatitis C and without viral hepatitis. *American Journal of Transplantation*, Vol.5, No.3, (March 2005), pp. 549-557, ISSN: 1600-6143

Lee, KW.; Cameron, AM.; Maley, WR.; Segev, DL. & Montgomery, RA. (2008) Factors affecting graft survival after adult/child split-liver transplantation: analysis of the UNOS/OPTN data base. *American Journal of Transplantation*, Vol.8, No.6, (June 2008), pp. 1186-1196, ISSN: 1600-6143

Lo, CM.; Fan, ST.; Liu, CL.; Yong, BH.; Wong, Y.; Lau, GK.; Lai, CL.; Ng, IO. & Wong, J. (2004) Lessons learned from one hundred right lobe living donor liver transplants. *Annals of Surgery*, Vol.240, No.1, (July 2004), pp. 151-158, ISSN: 1528-1140

Ludwig, J.; Batts, KP. & MacCarty, RL. (1992) Ischemic cholangitis in hepatic allografts. *Mayo Clinic Proceedings*, Vol.67, No.6, (June 1992), pp. 519-526, ISSN: 1942-5546

Marcos, A.; Olzinski, AT.; Ham, JM.; Fisher, RA. & Posner, MP. (2000) The interrelationship between portal and arterial blood flow after adult to adult living donor liver transplantation. *Transplantation*, Vol.70, No.12, (December 2000), pp. 1697-1703, ISSN: 1534-0608

Marino, IR.; Doyle, HR.; Aldrighetti, L.; Doria, C.; McMichael, J.; Gayowski, T.; Fung, JJ.; Tzakis, AG. & Starzl, TE. (1995) Effect of donor age and sex on the outcome of liver transplantation. *Hepatology*, Vol.22, No.6, (December 1995), pp. 175417-175462, ISSN: 0168-8278

Markmann, JF.; Markmann, JW.; Markmann, DA.; Bacquerizo, A.; Singer, J.; Holt, CD.; Gornbein, J.; Yersiz, H.; Morrissey, M.; Lerner, SM.; McDiarmid, SV. & Busuttil, RW. (2001) Preoperative factors associated with outcome and their impact on resource use in 1148 consecutive primary liver transplants. *Transplantation*, Vol.72, No.6, (September 2001), pp. 1113-1122, ISSN: 1534-0608

Massip-Salcedo, M.; Zaouali, MA.; Padrissa-Altés, S.; Casillas-Ramirez, A.; Rodés, J.; Roselló-Catafau, J. & Peralta, C. (2008) Activation of peroxisome proliferator-activated receptor-alpha inhibits the injurious effects of adiponectin in rat steatotic liver undergoing ischemia-reperfusion. *Hepatology*, Vol.47, No.2, (February 2008), pp. 461-472, ISSN: 0168-8278

Mateo, R.; Cho, Y.; Singh, G.; Stapfer, M.; Donovan, J.; Kahn, J.; Fong, TL.; Sher, L.; Jabbour, N.; Aswad, S.; Selby, RR. & Genyk, Y. (2006) Risk factors for graft survival after liver transplantation from donation after cardiac death donors: an analysis of OPTN/UNOS data. *American Journal of Transplantation*, Vol.6, No.4, (April 2006), pp. 791-796, ISSN: 1600-6143

Monbaliu, D.; van Pelt, J.; De Vos, R.; Greenwood, J.; Parkkinen, J.; Crabbé, T.; Zeegers, M.; Vekemans, K.; Pincemail, J.; Defraigne, JO.; Fevery, J. & Pirenne, J. (2007) Primary graft nonfunction and Kupffer cell activation after liver transplantation from non-heart-beating donors in pigs. *Liver Transplantation*, Vol.13, No.2, (February 2007), pp. 239-247, ISSN: 1527-6473

Mor, E.; Klintmalm, GB.; Gonwa, TA.; Solomon, H.; Holman, MJ.; Gibbs, JF.; Watemberg, I.; Goldstein, RM. & Husberg, BS. (1992) The use of marginal donors for liver transplantation. A retrospective study of 365 liver donors. *Transplantation*, Vol.53, No.2, (February 1992), pp. 383-386, ISSN: 1534-0608

Moreno Sanz, C.; Jiménez Romero, C.; Moreno González, E.; García García, I.; Seoane González, I.; Loinaz Segurola, C.; García Ureña, MA. & González Chamorro, A. (1999) Primary dysfunction after liver transplantation. Is it possible to predict this complication? *Revista Española de Enfermedades Digestivas*, Vol.91, No.6, (June 1999), pp. 401-419, ISSN: 1130-0108

Mueller, AR.; Platz, KP.; Schumacher, G.; Riger, J.; Gebauer, B.; Neumann, U. & Neuhaus, P. (1997) Mechanisms of preservation and reperfusion injury in human liver transplantation. *Transplantation Proceedings*, Vol.29, No.8, (December 1997), pp. 3455-3457, ISSN: 0041-1345

Müllhaupt, B.; Dimitroulis, D.; Gerlach, JT. & Clavien, PA. (2008) Hot topics in liver transplantation: organ allocation--extended criteria donor--living donor liver transplantation. *Journal of Hepatology*, Vol.48, No.Suppl 1, (February 2008), pp.S58-67, ISSN: 0168-8278

Nanashima, A.; Pillay, P.; Verran, DJ.; Painter, D.; Nakasuji, M.; Crawford, M.; Shi, L. & Ross, AG. (2002) Analysis of initial poor graft function after orthotopic liver transplantation: experience of an australian single liver transplantation center. *Transplantation Proceedings*, Vol.34, No.4, (June 2002), pp. 1231-1235, ISSN: 0041-1345

Pine, JK.; Aldouri, A.; Young, AL.; Davies, MH.; Attia, M.; Toogood, GJ.; Pollard, SG.; Lodge, JP. & Prasad, KR. (2009) Liver transplantation following donation after cardiac death: an analysis using matched pairs. *Liver Transplantation*, Vol.15, No.9, (September 2009), pp. 1072-1082, ISSN: 1527-6473

Piratvisuth, T.; Tredger, JM.; Hayllar, KA. & Williams, R. (1995) Contribution of true cold and rewarming ischemia times to factors determining outcome after orthotopic liver transplantation. *Liver Transplantation & Surgery*, Vol.1, No.5, (September 1995), pp. 296-301, ISSN: 1074-3022

Platz KP.; Mueller AR.; Schäfer C.; Jahns S.; Guckelberger O. & Neuhaus P. (1997) Influence of warm ischemia time on initial graft function in human liver transplantation. *Transplantation Proceedings*, Vol.29, No.8, (December 1997), pp. 3458-3459, ISSN: 0041-1345

Ploeg, RJ.; D'Alessandro, AM.; Knechtle, SJ.; Stegall, MD.; Pirsch, JD.; Hoffmann, RM.; Sasaki, T.; Sollinger, HW.; Belzer, FO. & Kalayoglu, M. (1993) Risk factors for primary dysfunction after liver transplantation--a multivariate analysis. *Transplantation*, Vol.55, No.4, (April 1993), pp. 807-813, ISSN: 1534-0608

Pokorny, H.; Gruenberger, T.; Soliman, T.; Rockenschaub, S.; Langle, F. & Steininger, R. (2000) Organ survival after primary dysfunction of liver grafts in clinical orthotopic liver transplantation. *Transplant International*, Vol.13, No.Suppl 1, (2000), pp. S154-157, ISSN: 1432-2277

Pokorny, H.; Langer, F.; Herkner, H.; Schernberger, R.; Plöchl, W.; Soliman, T.; Steininger, R. & Muehlbacher, F. (2005) Influence of cumulative number of marginal donor criteria on primary organ dysfunction in liver recipients. *Clinical Transplantation*, Vol.19, No.4, (August 2005), pp. 532-536, ISSN: 0902-0063

Pulitanò, C.; Aldrighetti, L.; Arru, M.; Finazzi, R.; Soldini, L.; Catena, M. & Ferla, G. (2007) Prospective randomized study of the benefits of preoperative corticosteroid administration on hepatic ischemia-reperfusion injury and cytokine response in patients undergoing hepatic resection. *HPB (Oxford)*, Vol.9, No.3, (2007), pp. 183-189, ISSN:1365-182X

Rana, A.; Hardy, MA.; Halazun, KJ.; Woodland, DC.; Ratner, LE.; Samstein, B.; Guarrera, JV.; Brown, RS Jr. & Emond, JC. (2008) Survival outcomes following liver transplantation (SOFT) score: a novel method to predict patient survival following liver transplantation. *American Journal of Transplantation*, Vol.8, No.12, (December 2008), pp. 2537-2546, ISSN: 1600-6143

Reddy, JK. & Rao, MS. (2006) Lipid metabolism and liver inflammation. II. Fatty liver disease and fatty acid oxidation. *American Journal of Physiology-Gastrointestinal and Liver Physiology*, Vol.290, No.5, (May 2006), pp. G852-858, ISSN: 1522-1547

Rinella, ME.; Alonso, E.; Rao, S.; Whitington, P.; Fryer, J.; Abecassis, M.; Superina, R.; Flamm, SL. & Blei, AT. (2001) Body mass index as a predictor of hepatic steatosis in living liver donors. *Liver Transplantation*, Vol.7, No.5, (May 2001), pp. 409-414, ISSN: 1527-6473

Salizzoni, M.; Franchello, A.; Zamboni, F.; Ricchiuti, A.; Cocchis, D.; Fop, F.; Brunati, A. & Cerutti, E. (2003) Marginal grafts: finding the correct treatment for fatty livers. *Transplant International*, Vol.16, No.7, (July 2003), pp. 486-493, ISSN: 1432-2277

Selzner, M. & Clavien, PA. (2000) Failure of regeneration of the steatotic rat liver: disruption at two different levels in the regeneration pathway. *Hepatology*, Vol.31, No.1, (January 2000), pp. 35-42, ISSN: 0168-8278

Selzner, M.; Rudiger, HA.; Sindram, D.; Madden, J. & Clavien, PA. (2000) Mechanisms of ischemic injury are different in the steatotic and normal rat liver. *Hepatology*, Vol.32, No.6, (December 2000), pp. 1280-1288, ISSN: 0168-8278

Selzner, M. & Clavien, PA. (2001) Fatty liver in liver transplantation and surgery. *Seminars in Liver Disease*, Vol.21, No.1, (2001), pp. 105-113, ISSN: 0272-8087

Selzner, N.; Rudiger, H.; Graf, R. & Clavien, PA. (2003) Protective strategies against ischemic injury of the liver. *Gastroenterology*, Vol.125, No.3, (September 2003), pp. 917-936, ISSN: 0016-5085

Serviddio, G.; Bellanti, F.; Tamborra, R.; Rollo, T.; Capitanio, N.; Romano, AD.; Sastre, J.; Vendemiale, G. & Altomare, E. (2008) Uncoupling protein-2 (UCP2) induces mitochondrial proton leak and increases susceptibility of non-alcoholic steatohepatitis (NASH) liver to ischaemia-reperfusion injury. *Gut*, Vol.57, No.7, (July 2008), pp. 957-965, ISSN: 1468-3288

Shimamura, T.; Taniguchi, M.; Jin, MB.; Suzuki, T.; Matsushita, M.; Furukawa, H. & Todo, S. (2001) Excessive portal venous inflow as a cause of allograft dysfunction in small-for-size living donor liver transplantation. *Transplantation Proceedings*, Vol.33, No.1-2, (February-March 2001), pp. 1331, ISSN: 0041-1345

Silberhumer, GR.; Pokorny, H.; Hetz, H.; Herkner, H.; Rasoul-Rockenschaub, S.; Soliman, T.; Wekerle, T.; Berlakovich, GA.; Steininger, R. & Muehlbacher, F. (2007) Combination of extended donor criteria and changes in the Model for End-Stage Liver Disease score predict patient survival and primary dysfunction in liver transplantation: a retrospective analysis. *Transplantation*, Vol.83, No.5, (May 2007), pp. 588-592, ISSN: 1534-0608

Strasberg, SM.; Howard, TK.; Molmenti, EP. & Hertl, M. (1994) Selecting the donor liver: risk factors for poor function after orthotopic liver transplantation. *Hepatology*, Vol.20, No.4Pt1, (October 1994), pp. 829-838, ISSN: 0168-8278

Teoh, NC. & Farrell, GC. (2003) Hepatic ischemia reperfusion injury: Pathogenic mechanisms and basis for hepatoprotection. Journal of Gastroenterology and *Hepatology*, Vol.18, No.8, (August 2003), pp. 891-902, ISSN: 1440-1746

Trevisani, F.; Colantoni, A.; Caraceni, P. & Van Thiel, DH. (1996) The use of donor fatty liver for liver transplantation: a challenge or a quagmire? *Journal of Hepatology*, Vol.24, No.1, (January 1996), pp. 114-121, ISSN: 0168-8278

Trotter, JF. (2001) Thin chance for fat people (to become living donors). *Liver Transplantation*, Vol.7, No.5, (May 2001), pp. 415-417, ISSN: 1527-6473

Uemura, T.; Randall, HB.; Sanchez, EQ.; Ikegami, T.; Narasimhan, G.; McKenna, GJ.; Chinnakotla, S.; Levy, MF.; Goldstein, RM. & Klintmalm, GB. (2007) Liver retransplantation for primary nonfunction: analysis of a 20-year single-center experience. *Liver Transplantation*, Vol.13, No.2, (February 2007), pp. 227-233, ISSN: 1527-6473

Ureña, MA.; Ruiz-Delgado, FC.; González, EM.; Segurola, CL.; Romero, CJ.; García, IG.; González-Pinto, I. & Gómez Sanz, R. (1998) Assessing risk of the use of livers with macro and microsteatosis in a liver transplant program. *Transplantation Proceedings*, Vol.30, No.7, (November 1998), pp. 3288-3291, ISSN: 0041-1345

Vajdová, K.; Heinrich, S.; Tian, Y.; Graf, R. & Clavien, PA. (2004) Ischemic preconditioning and intermittent clamping improve murine hepatic microcirculation and Kupffer cell function after ischemic injury. *Liver Transplantation*, Vol.10, No.4, (April 2004), pp. 520-528, ISSN: 1527-6473

Verran, D.; Kusyk, T.; Painter, D.; Fisher, J.; Koorey, D.; Strasser, S.; Stewart, G. & McCaughan, G. (2003) Clinical experience gained from the use of 120 steatotic donor livers for orthotopic liver transplantation. *Liver Transplantation*, Vol.9, No.5, (May 2003), pp. 500-505, ISSN: 1527-6473

Vogel, T.; Brockmann, JG. & Friend, PJ. (2010) Ex-vivo normothermic liver perfusion: an update. *Current Opinion in Organ Transplantation*, Vol.15, No.2, (April 2010), pp. 167-172, ISSN: 1531-7048

Washburn. WK.; Johnson. LB.; Lewis. WD. & Jenkins. RL. (1996) Graft function and outcome of older (> or = 60 years) donor livers. *Transplantation*, Vol.61, No.7, (April 1996), pp. 1062-1066, ISSN: 1534-0608

Yoo, HY.; Maheshwari, A. & Thuluvath, PJ. (2003) Retransplantation of liver: primary graft nonfunction and hepatitis C virus are associated with worse outcome. *Liver Transplantation*, Vol.9, No.9, (September 2003), pp. 897-904, ISSN: 1527-6473

Yoshizumi, T.; Taketomi, A.; Soejima, Y.; Uchiyama, H.; Ikegami, T.; Harada, N.; Kayashima, H.; Yamashita, Y.; Shimada, M. & Maehara, Y. (2008) Impact of donor age and recipient status on left-lobe graft for living donor adult liver transplantation. *Transplant International*, Vol.21, No.1, (January 2008), pp. 81-88, ISSN: 1432-2277

13

Role of Liver Biopsy After Liver Transplantation

Marco Carbone and James Neuberger
Liver Unit, Queen Elizabeth Hospital,
United Kingdom

1. Introduction

Assessment of liver histology following orthotopic liver transplantation is an essential component of management in the transplant recipient. Most programs recommend liver biopsies when there are changes in the patient's status or biochemical tests. The use of protocol allograft biopsies, that is in asymptomatic recipients with normal or near-normal liver tests, is controversial. Considerations such as potential morbidity and mortality, cost, inconvenience, use of resources, and potential impact of unexplained histopathological findings should be weighed against potential individual and societal benefits. More than one insult can contribute to late posttransplantation dysfunction and immunosuppression can influence the histological findings and the severity of many disease such as recurrent viral hepatitis, autoimmune hepatitis (AIH), and rejection. Histological analysis can help to determine the main component of injury, but careful clinicopathological correlation is needed. Biopsy interpretation should include an assessment of adequacy of the sample, and more than 6 portal tracts are considered adequate, a systematic examination, and a correlation with clinical aspects such as the original disease, immunosuppression, liver tests, viral serology, immunology and radiologic findings. Many transplant units follow center-specific criteria; however, a wide use of the standardized criteria (Anonymous, 1997; Demetris 2000) would enable centers to compare and pool results, improve management, and better understand the pathophysiology of disease mechanisms.

2. Early post-transplant period

Of the many causes of graft dysfunction in the early posttransplantation period, acute allograft rejection, preservation or reperfusion injury, drug-induced liver injury, viral infection and bile duct injury are the most common, and a liver biopsy may be required for their specific diagnosis and optimal management. The histological changes of preservation/reperfusion injury are uncommonly severe and typically resolve during the immediate and early posttransplant period. Acute cellular rejection (ACR) normally occurs within the first month of transplantation and liver biopsy represents a valuable tool for its diagnosis and guiding treatment. Though the histological diagnosis is often straightforward, several clinical situations can pose diagnostic challenges, such as patients with co-exiting viral hepatitis and other forms of tissue injury. In the early postoperative period, transplant recipients receive many drugs that are potentially hepatotoxic, such as antibiotics, analgesics, immunosuppressive agents and total parenteral nutrition. Although the histological features of drug-induced liver injury are rarely diagnostic, recognition of drug-induced graft damage will allow prompt withdrawal. While bacterial and fungal infection are often systemic, many viral infections directly affect the graft and usually require histology to differentiate infection from rejection and, as the two often co-exist, the histological findings will usually guide the need for any change in immunosuppression. The two opportunistic viral infections most frequently observed in liver allograft biopsies are cytomegalovirus (CMV) and Epstein-Barr virus (EBV) (Hubscher, 2006). Other opportunistic viral infections that can involve the liver allograft include adenovirus (mainly in pediatric liver transplant recipients), herpes simplex virus, varicella zoster virus, and human herpesvirus 6 (Kusne, 2006; Ohashi 2008). Most complications of the biliary tree are diagnosed radiologically, therefore liver biopsy has a limited role in this setting. Several reports have clearly indicated that serum liver tests have poor sensitivity and specificity in the diagnosis of graft disfunction. We have found that the extent of changes seen on liver histology, evaluated by protocol liver biopsy on the 7th postoperative day and assessed using the Banff criteria, has only a weak correlation with the liver tests. Furthermore, the change in the liver test is unreliable in predicting the histological severity of graft rejection (Neuberger et al., 1998). There is no evidence that patient outcome is improved with use of early protocol biopsies. A systematic review of 15 studies including 1566 liver transplant recipients showed that 32% of the patients had histologic acute cellular rejection (ACR) on protocol biopsy without associated biochemical graft dysfunction; without additional treatment, only 14% of these patients subsequently developed biochemical graft dysfunction. The authors, therefore, advised against the early protocol biopsy, after considering the small but definite risk associated with this procedure, and suggested that liver biopsy should be delayed until patients develop biochemical graft dysfunction, unexplained fever, or other surrogate markers of rejection or other early graft harmful event (Bartlett et al., 2002).

3. Late post-transplant period

Allograft biopsies in the late post-transplant period may be done on a protocol basis or as part of the diagnostic work-up of patients who are experiencing biochemical or clinical graft dysfunction, for monitoring recurrence of disease and response to therapy (e.g. recurrent hepatitis C infection). A wide spectrum of histological changes has been reported in the late posttransplant period. General classification is difficult as changes may reflect a variety of factors including the indications for liver transplant, the center's policy regarding protocol liver biopsies, the consequences of differing regimens of immunosuppression and differences in describing changes. Most of the main complications that occur during the early post-transplant period can also be seen in the later period. Changes seen in late post-transplant biopsies are often complex and may reflect more than one pathological process; histology may help to identify the dominant cause of graft damage in such cases.

Protocol liver biopsies are defined as those biopsies done according to agreed-on guidelines and not in response to changes in clinical status or biochemical tests. An informal survey of 35 transplant units located in North America, Europe, and Australasia, carried out in our unit in 2007, showed that whereas 65% of units undertake protocol biopsies for patients grafted for hepatitis C virus infection, only 25% do so for patients grafted for other indications (Mells, 2008). Furthermore, protocol biopsies are done less frequently than in the past. The lack of consensus regarding the use of protocol liver biopsies is due, in part, to the risks associated with the procedure, uncertainty about the usefulness of these biopsies in patients with normal liver function tests, costs. Part of the rationale for protocol biopsies was the need to understand the range of histological findings in the 'normal' allograft and the histological and clinical correlations; it is believed that these changes are now understood (Table 1).

Pros	Cons
Liver tests are associated with poor sensitivity and specificity in the diagnosis of graft dysfunction and provide little information on the severity of graft damage	Risk of morbidity and mortality associated with the procedure
Protocol liver biopsies are able to detect the early stage of many diseases occurring late after transplant and allow a early treatment that may avoid or delay graft injury and graft loss	The information provided by protocol biopsies can be obtained by other means
Knowledge of the histological changes may improve the understanding of the post-transplant diseases that could improve post-transplant care	Histologic findings often do not influence management when liver tests are normal and the patient is well
	High costs
	Interpretation of the biopsy may be jeopardized by differences in interpretation between observers
	Sampling variability

Table 1. Pros and Cons of a Protocol Biopsy

Percutaneous liver biopsies carry a risk of morbidity and mortality, that is relatively low, however this risk needs to be outweighed by benefits. Early studies reported a rate of major complications, represented mostly by bleeding and infection, between 0.2% and 1.79%, with a mortality rate up to 0.2% (Bubak, 1991; Chezmar, 1991; Lang, 1999; Larson, 1997; Perez Roldan, 1995; Van Thiel, 1993). The main factors associated with morbidity and mortality after a liver biopsy in the immunocompetent patient, such as the presence of a gallbladder or an unsuspected abnormal vascular anatomy or dilated bile ducts, generally do not apply to a liver transplant recipient; therefore, a lower rate of complication may be anticipated in these patients. Whether the presence of a Roux-en-Y choledochojejunostomy is associated with an increased risk of septic complication compared with duct-to-duct anastomosis (Ben-Ari, 1996; Galati, 1994) is controversial; in our center, as with many other units, a single prophylactic dose of antibiotic is given before a percutaneous liver biopsy is performed in recipients with Roux loop bilary anastomosis. Liver biopsies are relatively expensive, with a cost estimated at USD$1,032 in those without complications and USD$2,745 with complications (Poynard, 2004), and where resources are limited, this represents an important argument against a controversial diagnostic tool. Furthermore, the reliability of liver histology in making a specific diagnosis; this should be evaluated in terms of differences in interpretation between observers, evidenced in the assessment of hepatitis C and rejection in allograft biopsies (Demetris, 1991; Netto, 2006), and in terms of sampling variability (Maharaj, 1986; Poniachik, 1996; Ratziu, 2005; Regev, 2002); although studies of sampling variability in liver allograft biopsies have not been reported; however this is likely to be similar to that in the native liver.

The justification for doing protocol biopsies is based on many arguments:

- Liver tests (LFTs) are associated with poor sensitivity and specificity in the diagnosis of graft dysfunction and provide little information on the severity of graft damage;

- graft function is better preserved if liver damage is diagnosed and treated early;
- knowledge of the histological changes in the allograft in different clinical situations may result in better understanding of the post-transplant diseases that could improve post-transplant care.

There is a poor correlation between liver tests and histological findings in the late post-transplant setting. Thus, Berenguer reported that 11 (11.5%) of 97 recipient who were found to have abnormal histology at 1-year protocol biopsy had normal liver tests (Berenguer, 2001). Similar findings were reported with a longer follow-up of 10 years. Duclos-Valee et al, who documented recurrent autoimmune hepatitis in 7 (41%) of 17 patients and reported that in 4 (23%) of these patients the histologic findings of disease recurrence on protocol allograft biopsies preceded biochemical abnormalities by 1 to 5 years (Duclos-Valla, 2003). Sebagh et al evaluated 10-year post-OLT protocol biopsies of 134 patients and calculated that the sensitivity and specificity of normal liver tests for the detection of histologic abnormalities was only 75% and 54%, respectively. More recently, Abraham et al. evaluated 165 protocol allograft biopsies taken from 100 liver transplant patients at the time of normal LFTs and normal clinical function and evidenced as a significant fraction of protocol allograft biopsies harbor histologic (27%) and clinically significant (11.5%) abnormalities, most commonly fatty liver disease, low-grade/low-stage recurrent hepatitis C and primary biliary cirrhosis, and central venulitis, including some cases with subsequent fibrosis progression (Abraham, 2008) (Table 2).

Study	Years post-LT	Sample size	Patients with abnormal histology [n(%)]	Patients with normal LFTs and abnormal histology [n(%)]	Histologic findings
Berenguer	1	231	97 (42%)	11 (11.5%)	-
Duclos-Vallée	10	17	7 (41%)	4 (57%)	Autoimmune hepatitis
Sebagh	10	143	115 (80%)	53 (46%)	PBC, viral, CH, AIH, CR, undetermined
Abraham*	3 to 8 months (21.8%) 1 year (31.5%) 2 to 3 years (32.7%) 4 to 5 years (13.9%)	165	44 (27%)	44 (27%)	Fatty liver disease, recurrent disease (PBC, hepatitis C, sarcoidosis), Ito cell hyperplasia, central venulitis, mild acute portal rejection

* protocol allograft biopsies were taken at the time of normal LFTs.
Abbreviations: PBC, primary biliary cirrhosis; CH, chronic hepatitis; AIH, autoimmune hepatitis; CR, chronic rejection.

Table 2. Association between liver tests and histological findings

3.1 Hepatitis C

Another potential indication for protocol liver allograft biopsies is represented by recurrence of hepatitis C (rHCV), that is almost universal following liver transplantation (Everhart, 1999). In addition to confirming a diagnosis of rHCV (and excluding other causes of graft dysfunction), sequentially liver biopsies are used to assess the need for treatment, disease severity and progression. The majority of studies assessing the usefulness of long-term liver biopsies have been performed in centers with a low prevalence of viral infection, and this has led to an underestimation of the clinical importance of this tool. Histological abnormalities are often present in protocol biopsies from HCV-positive patients who are clinically well with apparently normal graft function (Berenguer, 2001; Sebagh, 2003) and these changes may have implications for prognosis and treatment (Roche, 2010). The posttransplant course of hepatitis C is associated with a more rapid progression of fibrosis than in the native liver, with the development of cirrhosis after 5 years in 28% of cases (Samuel, 2006). Early recognition and intervention of recipients with rapidly evolving recurrent hepatitis C following orthotopic liver transplantation (OLT) is the only practical approach to improve outcome of these patients (Gane, 2008).

Histologic changes at 1 year, such as fibrosis stage of >2 or an hepatitis activity index score>4, predict the subsequent course of recurrent hepatitis C and provide not only an early indication of which patients should receive antiviral treatment (Firpi, 2004) but are also used to monitor treatment responses (Bahra, 2007). Moreover, diagnosis of HCV-related graft cirrhosis before clinical decompensation may facilitate an early referral for liver retransplantation at a stage when the probabilities of a favorable outcome are greater. Combinations of laboratory test with or without clinical parameters, direct biochemical markers of hepatic extracellular matrix turnover, and more complex assays such as FibroTest, Fibrometer, and Hepascore, have been evaluated in the non-transplant setting for the assessement of progression of fibrosis (Lok, 2005; Leroy, 2004; Imbert-Bismut, 2001; Cales, 2005; Adams, 2005) and have also more recently been used in a similar manner in liver allograft recipients (Carrion, 2010; Cholongitas, 2010). Some authors have recently developed a model, the FibroTransplant score, based on the presence/absence of HCV infection, time since transplant, alpha 2-macroglobulin, AP, total protein, INR, and glucose - *1/(1+EXP{- [-20.5+(0.99 x presence of HCV infection)+(0.008 x time since LT) + (0.096 x total protein) + (6.36 x international normalized ratio [INR]) x (0.277 x glucose) + (0.007 x alkaline phosphatase [AP]) + (0.97 x alpha 2-macroglobulin)]})* - which accurately distinguished patients with mild to moderate fibrosis from those with advanced fibrosis (Beckebaum, 2010). As fibrosis progresses, total protein decreases, whereas INR and the concentration of the protease inhibitor alpha 2-macroglobulin increase; moreover, elevated alkaline phosphatase, HCVinfection and diabetes have been described as risk factors for progression to severe fibrosis (Berenguer, 2000; Syn, 2007). The optimal cutoff value for diagnosis of F>3 was 0.55, with a specificity of 90.2%, a sensitivity of 61.8%, a positive predictive value (PPV) of 77.2% and a negative predictive value (NPV) of 81.4%. Recently, Berres et al have shown as early serum levels of chemokines CXCL10 (interferon-inducible protein 10) independently predict the progression of liver fibrosis after LT for HCV infection (Berres, 2011). The most promising tool for non-invasive assessement of fibrosis progression in recurrent hepatitis C is the transient elastography; this is a reproducible technique that assesses liver stiffness, has been validated in patients with chronic hepatitis C for the assessment of hepatic fibrosis and can identify patients with rapidly progressive hepatitis C in the first year following OLT, differentiating them from patients with slowly progressive hepatitis C (Carrion, 2010);

however liver stiffness measurement (LSM) seems to be less reliable in the intermediate stages of fibrosis (Beckebaum, 2010), as already reported in the non-transplant setting (Foucher, 2006; Ganne-Carrie, 2006). These noninvasive methods, however, should be interpreted with caution in the transplant population as there are other possible causes of graft fibrosis, there may be atypical features, some related to the effects of immunosuppression such as fibrosing cholestatic hepatitis (FCH), and there may be a combination of hepatitis C recurrence and graft rejection, that cannot be detected unless a liver biopsy is performed. It is likely that non invasive methods will lead to a changing role for liver biopsy in the assessment of allograft damage in HCV-positive patients. These are not expected to replace liver biopsy in the immediate future, however currently they represent an additional tool capable to reduce the frequencies of biopsies for monitoring fibrotic changes during follow-up in selected populations, such as patients under anticoagulative therapy, with coagulopathy, or those declining a biopsy.

Patients undergoing liver transplantation for reasons other than HCV have not a strict need to undergo protocol liver biopsies. However, abnormal histological findings among non-HCV+ve recipients with normal aminotransferase levels are not uncommon (Ayata, 2000; Mells, 2009; Pappo, 1995; Slapak, 1997); the histological assessment of the graft using protocol biopsies in this setting may be helpful in improving the management of these patients. The more important histologic abnormalities other than HCV recurrence that may be revealed by protocol liver allograft biopsy are reported below.

3.2 Chronic rejection

Chronic rejection (CR) is a rare condition that affects the liver graft with a prevalence of 1-2% but it can lead to graft loss within the first 12 months of transplantation (Hubscher, 2007; Sebagh, 2003). It is characterized by obliterative arteriopathy leading to loss of medium-sized arteries, ischemic cholangiopathy, and progressive loss of interlobular and septal bile ducts extent to more than 50% of portal tracts (Demetris, 1998). However, duct loss can be patchy in distribution and the assessment of bile duct numbers should be interpreted with caution, particularly in small biopsies with fewer than 10 portal tracts. Improvements in immunosuppression have resulted, not only in a reduced prevalence of graft failure from CR , but also in a different pattern of presentation. More cases now occur later (> 12 months post transplant) with a more insidious presentation and an indolent course, in some cases running for a period of several years without progressing to graft failure (Nakazawa, 2000; Sebagh, 2003). In the early stage of chronic rejection there is a loss of bile ducts in less than 50% of portal tracts; this is characterized by inflammatory and degenerative changes in bile ducts, which have an atrophic or 'dysplastic-like' appearance associated with features of replicative senescence (Demetris, 2000). Early-stage CR is associated with normal or slightly abnormal LFTs and so is detected only by using protocol biopsies; this may be reversible simply by altering immunosuppression (IMS) (Wiesner, 1999). However whether the early recognition of chronic rejection and a prompt change in IMS have some impact on graft survival is an open question.

3.3 Hepatitis B

Allograft histology is not as useful in patients transplanted for HBV cirrhosis, as with HCV because the virological and serological markers highly reliable for monitoring recurrent hepatitis B. However, protocol biopsies may be useful to detect other causes of late allograft dysfunction in patients who received a liver transplant for HBV-related cirrhosis, like chronic hepatitis (CH) despite normal liver tests and negative virological markers (Targhetta, 2006).

3.4 Autoimmune hepatitis

Autoimmune hepatitis (AIH) recurs in up to 30% to 40% of patients after liver transplantation (Ayata, 2000; Reich 2000; Vogel 2004;), and if untreated may lead to loss of the graft. Protocol biopsies allow early detection of AIH in the allograft because histologic changes may precede biochemical disturbance, even by several years (Duclos-Vallee, 2003) and therefore a prompt addition or increase in corticosteroid therapy may prevent significant injury to the allograft.

3.5 Cholestatic liver disease

Primary biliary cirrhosis (PBC) and Primary sclerosing cholangitis (PSC) may recur after liver transplantation (Lerut, 1988; Neuberger, 1982), although the impact of recurrent disease on long-term survival is controversial. Unlike PSC, liver biopsy represent the gold standard for the diagnosis of recurrent PBC with the histological findings of granulomatous cholangitis or florid duct lesions, since LFTs and serum AMA after transplant are not reliable and it is also important to differentiate recurrent disease from other causes of bile-duct damage. Protocol biopsies may provide early signs of recurrence of primary disease, and a early use of ursodeoxycholic acid treatment may be beneficial in the long-term, although there are no strong evidences supporting this.

3.6 Chronic hepatitis

A common histological finding in late allograft liver graft is an unspecified chronic hepatitis (CH), defined as a mononuclear portal and lobular infiltrate without features of acute or chronic rejection or any other identifiable causes of graft injury (Neuberger, 2005). CH is a common finding in late allograft biopsies, occurring in up to 30% to 70% of biopsies taken after 12 months and is poorly correlated with the clinical and serologic findings (Hubscher, 1990; Mells 2009). CH is clinically important because it may be associated with progressive fibrosis which may lead to graft cirrhosis (Evans, 2006). In most of the transplant recipients CH may be related to identifiable factors such as viral infections, recurrent autoimmune diseases, de novo autoimmune hepatitis, fatty liver disease and drug toxicity (Banff Working Group, 2006; Brunt, 1999; Haydon, 2002; Hubscher, 2001; Nakhleh, 2005; Pappo, 1995; Slapak, 1997). However, many patients with CH still do not have any clear cause of graft damage. Idiopathic CH may represent a late cellular rejection from suboptimal immunosuppression, as suggested by limited evidences (Evans, 2006; Syn, 2007); this may justify changes in the IMS and a closer follow-up of these patients.

3.7 Withdrawal of immunosuppression

Protocol biopsy may be a useful tool to drive the reduction of immunosuppression after transplantation. Some of the major causes of late mortality, such as renal impairment, vascular disease, and some de novo malignancies, are clearly related to immunosuppression; the absence of significant inflammation or fibrosis in a late protocol biopsy may help to identify patients in whom immunosuppression can be safely reduced or even withdrawn completely in the hope of achieving "operational tolerance" , with a long-term benefits for the patient.

4. Timing of protocol liver biopsy

In HCV recipients, fibrosis of the graft progresses since the first year after transplantation with a rate of 0.2-0.3 of fibrosis units (FU)/year; the progression seems not to be linear during a 10-year follow-up, and may be accelerated in the second half. Therefore, in order to monitor the aggressiveness of recurrent disease protocol liver biopsies should be performed in those transplanted for HCV-related cirrhosis since the first year from transplant and then annually.

For non-HCV-related transplants, the usual schedule in many centers that undertake protocol biopsies is a biopsy at 1, 2 or 3, 5, 10, and 15 years (Mells, 2008); however, there are no strong evidences supporting this and the right timing remains to be assessed.

5. Conclusion

Protocol allograft liver biopsies represent a useful tool in HCV-recipients for detection and follow-up of HCV recurrence.

The usefulness of long-term protocol liver biopsies in non-HCV liver transplant recipients is controversial. They may be useful to detect the early stage of many diseases occurring late after transplant, such as chronic rejection or PBC recurrence, and so allow a early treatment that may avoid or delay graft injury and graft loss. They may also represent an important tool to optimize immunosuppression management and identify recipients that might be successfully weaned. Last but not least, protocol biopsies may offer a better understanding of the allograft structure and function. However, clear evidence that these are cost-effective and improve patient and graft outcomes is lacking. Further studies are required to devise optimal algorithms for the use of liver biopsy in the assessment of the long-term liver allograft.

6. References

Adams LA, Bulsara M, Rossi E, et al. (2005) Hepascore: An accurate validated predictor of liver fibrosis in chronic hepatitis C infection. *Clin Chem,* Vol. 51, (2005), pp.(1867).

Anonymous. (1997). Banff schema for grading liver allograft rejection: an international consensus document. *Hepatology,* Vol. 25, (1997), pp. (658-663).

Ayata G, Gordon FD, Lewis WD, et al. (2000).Liver transplantation for autoimmune hepatitis: A long-term pathologic study. *Hepatology.* Vol. 32, (2000), pp. (185-92).

Bahra M, Neumann UP, Jacob D, Langrehr JM, Berg T, Neuhaus R, & Neuhaus P. (2007). Fibrosis progression in hepatitis C positive liver recipients after sustained virologic response to antiviral combination therapy (interferon-ribavirin therapy). *Transplantation,* Vol. 83, (2007), pp. (351-353).

Bartlett AS, Ramadas R, Furness S, Gane E, & McCall JL. The natural history of acute histologic rejection without biochemical graft dysfunction in orthotopic liver transplantation: a systematic review. (2002). *Liver Transpl.* Vol. 8, No12, (Dec 2002), pp. (1147-53).

Beckebaum S, Iacob S, Klein CG, Dechêne A, Varghese J, Baba HA, Sotiropoulos GC, Paul A, Gerken G, & Cicinnati VR. (2010). Assessment of allograft fibrosis by transient elastography and noninvasive biomarker scoring systems in liver transplant patients. *Transplantation.* Vol 27, No 89, (Apr 2010), pp. (983-93).

Ben-Ari Z, Neville L, Rolles K, et al. (1996).Liver biopsy in liver transplantation: No additional risk of infections in patients with choledochojejunostomy. *J Hepatol,* Vol 24, (1996), pp.(324).

Berenguer M, Ferrell L, Watson J, et al. (2000) HCV-related fibrosis progression following liver transplantation: Increase in recent years. *J Hepatol,*Vol. 32, (2000), pp.(673).

Berenguer M, Rayon JM, Prieto M, et al. (2001). Are posttransplantation protocol liver biopsies useful in the long term? *Liver Transpl.* Vol. 7, (2001), pp. (790–796).

Berres ML, Trautwein C, Schmeding M, Eurich D, Tacke F, Bahra M, Neuhaus P, Neumann UP, & Wasmuth HE. (2011). Serum chemokine CXC ligand 10 (CXCL10) predicts fibrosis progression after liver transplantation for hepatitis C infection. Hepatology. Vol 53, No 2, (Feb 2011), pp. (596-603).

Brunt EM, Janney CG, Di Bisceglie AM, Neuschwander- Tetri BA, & Bacon BR. (1999). Nonalcoholic steatohepatitis: a proposal for grading and staging of histological lesions. *Am J Gastroenterol,* Vol. 94, (1999), pp.(2467-2474).

Brunt EM. (2001). Nonalcoholic steatohepatitis: definition and pathology. Semin Liver Dis, Vol. 21, (2001), pp. (3-16).

Bubak ME, Porayko MK, Krom RA, et al. (1991). Complications of liver biopsy in liver transplant patients: Increased sepsis associated with choledochojejunostomy. *Hepatology* Vol. 14, (1991), pp. (1063).

Cales P, Oberti F, Michalak S, et al. (2005). A novel panel of blood markers to assess the degree of liver fibrosis. *Hepatology* ,Vol. 42 (2005), pp. (1373).

Carrion JA, Fernandez-Varo G, Bruguera M, Garcia-Pagan JC, Garcia-Valdecasas JC, Perez-Del-Pulgar S, Forns X, Jimenez W, & Navasa M. (2010). Serum fibrosis markers identify patients with mild and progressive hepatitis C recurrence after liver transplantation. Gastroenterology, Vol. 138, (2010), pp. (147-58).

Carrion JA, Torres F, Crespo G, Miquel R, Garcı`a-Valdecasas JC, Navasa M, et al. (2010). Liver stiffness identifies two different patterns of fibrosis progression in patients with hepatitis C virus recurrence after liver transplantation. *Hepatology,* Vol 51, (2010), pp. (23-34).

Chezmar JL, Keith LL, Nelson RC, et al. (1991). Liver transplant biopsies with a biopsy gun. *Radiology,* Vol. 179, (1991), pp. (447).

Cholongitas E, Tsochatzis E, Goulis J, & Burroughs AK. (2010). Noninvasive tests for evaluation of fibrosis in HCV recurrence after liver transplantation: a systematic review. *Transpl Int,* Vol 23, (2010), pp. (861-70).

Demetris AJ, Belle SH, Hart J, et al. (1991). Intraobserver and interobserver variation in the histopathological assessment of liver allograft rejection. The Liver Transplantation Database (LTD) Investigators. *Hepatology,* Vol. 14, (1991), pp. (751).

Demetris AJ, Seaberg EC, Batts KP, et al. (1998). Chronic allograft rejection. *Am J Surg Pathol,* Vol. 22, (1998), pp. 28.

Demetris A, Adams D, Bellamy C, et al. (2000). Update of the International Banff Schema for Liver Allograft Rejection: working recommendations for the histopathologic staging and reporting of chronic rejection. An International Panel. *Hepatology* Vol 31, (2000), pp.(792).

Duclos-Vallee JC, Sebagh M, Rifai K, et al. (2003). A 10 year follow up study of patients transplanted for autoimmune hepatitis: histological recurrence precedes clinical and biochemical recurrence. *Gut.* Vol. 52, (2003), pp. (893–897).

Evans HM, Kelly DA, McKiernan PJ, et al. (2006). Progressive histological damage in liver allografts following paediatric liver transplantation. *Hepatology,* Vol. 43, (2006), pp. (1109).

Everhart JE, Wei Y, Eng H, et al. (1999). Recurrent and new hepatitis C virus infection after liver transplantation. *Hepatology,*Vol. 29, (1999), pp.(1220).

Fabrega E, Castro B, Crespo J, et al. (2000). Different time course of circulating adhesion molecules and hyaluran during hepatic allograft rejection. *Transplantation,*Vol. 69, (2000), pp. (569).

Firpi RJ, Abdelmalek MF, Soldevila-Pico C, et al. (2004). One-year protocol liver biopsy can stratify fibrosis progression in liver transplant recipients with recurrent hepatitis C infection. *Liver Transpl,* Vol. 10, (2004), pp. (1240).

Foucher J, Chanteloup E, Vergniol J, et al. (2006). Diagnosis of cirrhosis by transient elastography (FibroScan): A prospective study. *Gut,*Vol. 55, (2006), pp. (403).

Galati JS, Monsour HP, Donovan JP, et al. (1994). The nature of complications following liver biopsy in transplant patients with Roux-en-Y choledochojejunostomy. *Hepatology Vol.* 20, (1994), pp. (651).

Gane EJ. (2008). The natural history of recurrent hepatitis C and what influences this. Liver Transpl Vol. 14, Suppl 2, (2008), pp. (36-44).

Ganne-Carrie N, Ziol M, de Ledinghen V, et al. (2006).Accuracy of liver stiffness measurement for the diagnosis of cirrhosis in patients with chronic liver diseases. *Hepatology* Vol. 44, (2006), pp. (1511).

Haydon G, Lalor PF, Hubscher SG, & Adams DH. (2002). Lymphocyte recruitment to the liver in alcoholic liver disease. *Alcohol,* Vol. 27, (2002), pp. (29-36).

Hubscher SG. (1990).Chronic hepatitis in liver allografts. *Hepatology,* Vol. 12, (1990), pp. (1257).

Hubscher SG. (2001). Recurrent autoimmune hepatitis after liver transplantation: diagnostic criteria, risk factors, and outcome. Liver Transpl Vol. 7, (2001), pp. (285-291).

Hubscher SG. (2006). Recurrent and de-novo disease in the liver allograft. *Current Opinion in Organ Transplantation* Vol. 11, (2006), pp. (283-288).

Hubscher SG, Portmann BC. (2007). Transplantation pathology. In: *MacSween's Pathology of the Liver*. 5th ed. Edinburgh: Churchill Livingstone, (2007), pp. (815–879).

Imbert-Bismut F, Ratziu V, Pieroni L, et al. (2001). Biochemical markers of liver fibrosis in patients with hepatitis C virus infection: A prospective study. *Lancet,* Vol. 357, (2001), pp. (1069).

Kusne S, & Blair JE. (2006). Viral and fungal infections after liver transplantation–part II. *Liver Transpl,* Vol. 12, No. 1, (2006), pp. (2–11).

Lang M, Neumann UP, Muller AR, et al. (1999). Complications of percutaneous liver biopsy in patients after liver transplantation. *Z Gastroenterol* 1999, Vol. 37, (1999), pp. (205).

Larson AM, Chan GC, Wartelle CF, et al. (1997). Infection complicating percutaneous liver biopsy in liver transplant recipients. *Hepatology,* Vol. 26, (1997), pp. (1406).

Leroy V, Monier F, Bottari S, et al. (2004). Circulating matrix metalloproteinases 1, 2, 9 and their inhibitors TIMP-1 and TIMP-2 as serum markers of liver fibrosis in patients with chronic hepatitis C: Comparison with PIIINP and hyaluronic acid. *Am J Gastroenterol,* Vol. 99, (2004), pp. (271).

Lerut J, Demetris AJ, Stieber AC, Marsh JW, Gordon RD, Esquivel CO, et al. (1988). Intrahepatic bile duct strictures after human orthotopic liver transplantation.

Recurrence of primary sclerosing cholangitis or unusual presentation of allograft rejection? *Transpl Int*, Vol. 1, (1988), pp. (127-30).

Lok AS, Ghany MG, Goodman ZD, et al. Predicting cirrhosis in patients with hepatitis C based on standard laboratory tests: Results of the HALT-C cohort. *Hepatology*, Vol. 42, (2005), 282.

Maharaj B, Maharaj RJ, Leary WP, et al. (1986). Sampling variability and its influence on the diagnostic yield of percutaneous needle biopsy of the liver. *Lancet*, Vol. 1, (1986), pp. (523).

Mells G, & Neuberger J. (2008). Protocol liver allograft biopsies. Transplantation. Vol. 85, No. 12, (Jun 2008) pp.(1686-92).

Mells, Neuberger J. (2009). Late Protocol Liver Biopsies in the Liver Allograft: A Neglected Investigation?. *Liver Transplantation*, Vol15, (2009), pp. (931-938).

Nakazawa Y, Jonsson JR, Walker NI, Kerlin P, Steadman C, Lynch SV, Strong RW, Clouston AD. (2000). Fibrous obliterative lesions of veins contribute to progressive fibrosis in chronic liver allograft rejection. *Hepatology*, Vol. 32, (2000), pp. (1240-1247).

Nakhleh RE, Krishna M, Keaveny AP, Dickson RC, Rosser B, Nguyen JH, Steers JL. (2005). Review of 31 cases of morphologic hepatitis in liver transplant patients not related to disease recurrence. *Transplant Proc*, Vol 37, (2005), pp. (1240-1242).

Netto GJ, Watkins DL, Williams JW, et al. (2006). The hepatitis C 3 trial group. interobserver agreement in hepatitis C grading and staging and in the Banff grading schema for acute cellular rejection: the "hepatitis C 3" multi-institutional trial experience. *Arch Pathol Lab Med*,Vol. 130, (2006), pp. (1157).

Neuberger J, Portmann B, Macdougall BR, Calne RY, Williams R. (1982). Recurrence of primary biliary cirrhosis after liver transplantation. *N Engl J Med*, Vol. 306, (1982), pp. (1-4).

Neuberger J., Wilson P., & Adams D. (1998) Protocol liver biopsies: the case in favour. *Transplant Proceeding*, Vol. 30, No. 4, (Jun 1998), pp. (1497-9).

Neuberger J. (2003). Recurrent primary biliary cirrhosis. *Liver Transpl* 2003;Vol. 9, (2003), pp. (539).

Neuberger J. (2005). Chronic allograft dysfunction: diagnosis and management. Is it always progressive? *Liver Transpl* , Vol. 11, (2005), pp. (63).

Ohashi M, Sugata K, Ihira M, et al. (2008). Human herpesvirus 6 infection in adult living related liver transplant recipients. *Liver Transpl*, Vol.14, No.1, (2008), pp. (100–109).

Pappo O, Ramos H, Starzl TE, et al. (1995). Structural integrity and identification of causes of liver allograft dysfunction occurring more than 5 years after transplantation. *Am J Surg Pathol* , Vol. 19, (1995), pp. (192).

Perez Roldan F, Banares R, Clemente G, et al. (1995). Severe complications of percutaneous hepatic biopsy in patients with orthotopic liver transplantation. *Gastroenterol Hepatol* 1995; Vol. 18, (1995), pp (410).

Perkins JD, Nelson DL, Rakela J, et al. (1989). Soluble interleukin 2 receptor level in liver allograft recipients: an indicator of rejection. *Transplant Proc* 1989;Vol. 21, (1989), pp. (2275).

Piccinino F, Sagnelli E, Pasquale G, et al. (1986). Complications following percutaneous liver biopsy. A multi-centre retrospective study on 67,276 biopsies. *J Hepatol* 1986; Vol. 2, (1986), pp. (165).

Poniachik J, Bernstein DE, Reddy KR, et al. (1996). The role of laparoscopy in the diagnosis of cirrhosis. *Gastrointest Endosc* ,Vol. 43, (1996), pp.(568).

Poynard T, Imbert-Bismut F, Ratziu V (2004). "Serum markers of liver fibrosis". *Hepatology Reviews*, Vol 1, (2004), pp. (23–31).

Ratziu V, Charlotte F, Heurtier A, et al. (2005). Sampling variability of liver biopsy in nonalcoholic fatty liver disease. *Gastroenterology,* Vol. 128, (2005), pp. (1898).

Regev A, Berho M, Jeffers LJ, et al. (2002). Sampling error and intraobserver variation in liver biopsy in patients with chronic HCV infection. *Am J Gastroenterol,* Vol. 97, (2002), pp. (2614).

Reich DJ, Fiel I, Guarrera JV, et al. (2000). Liver transplantation for autoimmune hepatitis. *Hepatology* 2000; Vol. 32, (2000), pp. (693).

Roche B, Samuel D. (2010). Hepatitis C virus: up to the minute. *Liver Transpl,* Vol. 16, (2010), pp. (S26-S35).

Samuel D, Forns X, Berenguer M, Trautwein C, BurroughsA, Rizzetto M, et al. (2006). Report of the monothematic EASL conference on liver transplantation for viral hepatitis (Paris, France, January 12-14, 2006). *J Hepatol* Vol. 45, (2006), pp. (127-143).

Sebagh M, Rifai K, Feray C, Yilmaz F, Falissard B, Roche B, Bismuth H, Samuel D, & Reynes M. (2003). All liver recipients benefit from the protocol 10-year liver biopsies. Hepatology Vol. 37, (2003), pp. (1293-1301).

Slapak GI, Saxena R, Portmann B, Gane E, Devlin J, Calne R, Williams R. (1997). Graft and systemic disease in long-term survivors of liver transplantation. Hepatology, Vol 25, (1997), pp. (195-202).

Syn W-K, Nightingale P, Gunsen B, et al. (2007). Natural history of unexplained chronic hepatitis after liver transplantation. *Liver Transpl,*Vol. 13, (2007), pp. (984).

Targhetta S, Villamil F, Inturri P, et al. (1997). Protocol liver biopsies in longterm management of patients transplanted for hepatitis B-related liver transplantation. *Hepatology*, Vol. 5, (1997), pp. (195-202).

Trull AK, Facey SP, Rees GW, et al. (1994). Serum alpha-glutathione Stransferase–a sensitive marker of hepatocellular damage associated with acute liver allograft rejection. *Transplantation,* Vol. 58, (1994), pp. (1345).

Van Thiel DH, Gavaler JS, Wright H, et al. (1993). Liver biopsy. Its safely and complications seen at a liver transplant center. *Transplantation,*Vol. 55, (1993), pp.(1087).

Vogel A, Heinrich E, Bahr MJ, et al. (2004). Long-term outcome of liver transplantation for autoimmune hepatitis. *Clin Transplant,*Vol.18, (2004), pp. (62).

Weisner RH, Batts KP, Krom RAF. Evolving concepts in the diagnosis, pathogenesis, and treatment of chronic hepatic allograft rejection. *Liver Transpl Surg,* Vol. 5, (1999), pp. (388).

14

The Present Role of Liver Biopsy in Kidney Transplant Candidates in the Management of Hepatitis B and C Patients

Teresa Casanovas, Carme Baliellas and Maria Carmen Peña Cala
Hospital Universitari de Bellvitge, Institut Català de la Salut, IDIBELLL, Hospitalet de Llobregat-Barcelona, Spain

1. Introduction

This chapter will deal with the present role of Liver Biopsy in determining liver disease prognosis in hepatitis B and C patients on haemodialysis and its role in establishing treatment strategies and in the decision-making process prior to kidney transplant. In recent years, progress has been made in determining the natural history of this disease in renal patients (Espinosa et al., 2004; Jadoul et al., 2004).

Chronic hepatitis due to HCV is frequent in renal transplant recipients and in dialysis patients and has a significant impact on their survival (Hanafusa et al., 1998; Orloff et al., 1995; Pouteil-Noble et al., 1995). Mathurin et al., (1999) demonstrated in a case-control study that anti-HCV and HBsAg positive were independently associated with patient and graft survival. This was the first time that a 10 year follow-up was carried out; previous publications are based on shorter follow-ups and fewer patients.

It is known that the prevalence of chronic infection with the hepatitis C virus (HCV) in patients with chronic kidney disease is higher than in the general population (Lavanchy, 2009). The estimated prevalence of chronic infection in haemodialysis patients is 13%, ranging from 10 to 65 %, depending on the geographical zone (Hmaied et al., 2006; Huraib et al., 1995; Santos & Souto, 2007; Shamshiraz et al., 2004).

When considering patients candidates to kidney transplantation we have to take into account that immunosuppressive therapy after renal transplantation predisposes a reactivation of chronic viral hepatitis B or C, which is usually a mild disease for patients remaining under haemodialysis.

It should be noted that HBV and HCV may induce de novo glomerulonephritis and chronic allograft nephropathy which can lead to graft failure (Aouifi & Garcia, 2001). In such cases, patients have to undergo dialysis again and therefore it is beneficial to eradicate HCV RNA before transplantation and to control and maintain HBV DNA negative (Huskey & Wiseman, 2011).

A routine liver histological analysis could improve a patient's chance of being selected for renal transplantation. Liver biopsy has been considered the "gold standard" for many years, because it provides us with information that was otherwise unobtainable (Ghany et al., 2010). Nowadays however, due to progress in non-invasive methods, liver biopsy is only necessary in selected cases or in patients with a lack of correlation between clinical and analytical data (Alric et al., 2009; Stasi et al., 2009).

In solid organ transplant patients, who are HBV or HCV carriers under immunosuppressives, an increasing frequency of fibrosing cholestatic hepatitis has been described. This type of hepatitis evolves rapidly to liver cirrhosis, significantly increases morbidity and mortality and leads to the need for a liver transplantation in selected cases (Boletis et al., 2000; Delladetsima et al., 1999; Vallet-Pichard et al., 2011). (Table 1).

Typical viral hepatitis	Fibrosing cholestatic hepatitis
- Portal lymphocytic infiltrates are observed, with various degrees of periportal interface inflammatory activity. - Lobular necroinflammatory change is present, the inflammatory component chiefly lymphocytic. Granulomatous hepatitis, have been reported in chronic HCV infection. - Different morphologic changes are specifically seen in particular hepatotropic virus: a. HCV: Portal lymphoid aggregates and follicles, focal duct damage, and mild fatty change often occur. b. HBV: "Ground glass" cells and sometimes mild fatty change may be seen.	- Described in patients under immunosuppressors and related to a direct viral cytopathic effect on the liver cells and although fibrosing cholestatic hepatitis is seen in both HBV and HCV infection, it is more common in the former. - Portal expansion with periportal and intrasinusoidal collagen deposition, bile ductular proliferation, but with minimal portal inflammation are seen. - Prominent ballooning change of liver cells occurs, with associated cholestasis but mild lobular inflammation. - Variable but sometimes prominent fatty change (steatoviral) may occur. In severe cases, bridging and multiacinar necrosis can be seen, leading to the graft failure.

Table 1. Chronic Hepatitis major morphologic features. Typical viral hepatitis vs Fibrosing cholestatic hepatitis. (Adapt., Kanel, G. C. & Korula, J. *(2011) Atlas of Liver Pathology,* Elsevier Saunders, ISBN: 978-1-4377-0765-6)

2. General approach

2.1 Preliminary considerations

Active HCV infection in dialysis patients, namely HCV-RNA positive by PCR, requires evaluation of liver fibrosis preferentially by liver biopsy. New tools for assessing fibrosis by non-invasive methods have been developed, and although they have yet to be validated for chronic kidney patients they will be discussed in this chapter.

General management of chronic viral hepatitis and in particular the indication of liver biopsy, in a practical clinical approach, has the objective to avoid liver-related mortality and to promote allograft survival in kidney transplanted patients (Sezer et al., 2004).

2.2 Historical background

Over the past few decades, medical progress has been made and new specialities have emerged in areas such as solid organ transplants and chronic viral hepatitis treatments. Nephrology and hepatology specialities have to plan an interdisciplinary care approach for

patients candidates for transplantation and for those receiving immunosuppressors especially in hepatitis virus carriers (Fabrizi et al., 2010a, Carriero et al., 2008).
One quarter of HCV positive patients evaluated for a kidney transplant have advanced fibrosis or cirrhosis in the liver biopsy. In the past they should require a combined liver and kidney transplant. Currently, this concept is not fully accepted, for the following two reasons:

1. Due to the scarcity of donors some patients with cirrhosis or advanced liver fibrosis, but never decompensated, are being accepted for renal transplantation only .
2. Liver biopsies, which were mandatory several years ago, are being replaced by non-invasive methods in mild or severe hepatitis. However, patients diagnosed inconclusively must undergo a liver biopsy to confirm the diagnosis (Sebastiani & Alberti, 2006).

2.3 Our experience

In 1991 we initiated a prospective, non-randomized study to assess the tolerability and efficacy of Interferon (IFN) alfa for treating chronic hepatitis C in kidney transplant candidates undergoing haemodialysis. The aims were to evaluate the efficacy and safety of IFN alfa in this setting. We studied HCV RNA status at the end of treatment and during follow-up and the complications related to haemodialysis, to primary renal disease, and to the use of IFN during treatment. We also studied the evolution of the kidney graft in transplanted patients and the evolution of hepatitis after transplantation to investigate the risk of accelerated liver disease. It should be noted that although we now evaluate the results of the anti-virals with viral kinetics, at the begining of the study PCR qualitative of RNA-HCV was the only available method.
This study was published in 2001, and the results showed that 64% had Sustained Viral Response (SVR) and HCV-RNA was repeatedly negative during the follow-up (Casanovas-Taltavull et al., 2001). Moreover a lesser development of de novo glomerulonephritis was observed in patients to whom IFN alfa had been administered (Cruzado et al., 2003).
We have to take into account that in those days our dialyzed patients had a higher prevalence of viral hepatitis. The prevalence of HBV and HCV infections has markedly decreased in patients who are candidates for transplantation since the introduction of screening, hygiene and prevention measures, including systematic vaccination against HBV, screening of blood and organ donations, use of erythropoietin, compliance with universal hygiene rules, and isolation of HBV-infected and HCV positive patients from non-infected patients (Fabrizi et al., 2004).
Blood transfusions were common in the past because they were thought to improve graft tolerance and erithropoietin had yet to be approved for this indication (Light et al., 1982).
While an anti-Hepatitis B vaccine is indicated in these patients, an anti-HCV vaccine has yet to be developped. Preventive and general measures are therefore crucial for stopping viral transmission (Sauné et al., 2010).

3. Clinical spectrum and natural history of the disease

3.1 Epidemiology and prevalence of liver diseases in patients under substitutive renal treatment

Reports on the natural history of hepatitis C infection in the dialysis population vary and consequently is not completely understood. The slow progression of the HCV-associated liver disease may mask the consequences of HCV infection in the dialysis population (Okoh et al., 2008). Previous studies that focused on liver disease demonstrated a low proportion of HCV-positive dialysis patients with bridging hepatic fibrosis or cirrhosis (Gane & Pilmore, 2002).

The possible explanation for such a distinct difference is a reduction of the viral load via adsorption of viral particles with their subsequent destruction (Kaiser et al., 2008). In the same way, alanine aminotransferase (ALT) may be filtered through the dialyser membrane and ALT levels may be normal in patients with otherwise advanced liver disease (Lopes et al., 2006).

Because of the persisting contradictions reported, there is an urgent need for better communication between specialists to establish clear guidelines for the management of chronic viral hepatitis in ESRD patients. Phase 3 trials of new antivirals, in combination with pegIFN and ribavirin in the general population, which have a primary end point of SVR efficacy, are expected to be performed. Before administering these new drugs to patients under hemodialysis it will be necessary to perform PK studies and to obtain a toxicological profile of these new drugs in this setting.

3.2 Risk factors (Table 2) some concerns

Studies on viral isolates have suggested a nosocomial patient-to-patient transmission of HCV infection among dialysis patients in some centers despite dialysis centers having routine protocols to prevent hepatitis transmission and to control the infection (McLaughlin et al., 1997). Several dilemmas regarding the management of these patients have yet to be resolved:

1. Should HCV-RNA testing and complete HBV serologies be included in the routine screening of HD population for chronic hepatitis infection, considering the fact that anti-HCV remains positive even in cured patients and that in some RNA-HCV positive cases, antibodies may be negative ("occult-hepatitis") (Angelico et al., 2000).
2. Does periodic serum ALT testing have a role in HD patients for hepatitis infection although it is known that ALT may be normal in this population?
3. Should HCV or HBV-infected subjects be isolated and dialyzed by segregated machines? This situation is not totally resolved and can lead to misunderstandings among medical teams and cured patients.

Intravenous drug use
Number of blood transfusions received before 1999
Duration of hemodialysis
Mode of dialysis
Prevalence of HCV infection in the dialysis unit
Previous organ transplantation
Male gender / Older age
Intravenous drug use
Previous HBV infection
General risk of nosocomial transmission of HCV

Table 2. Risk Factors for HCV infection in dialysis patients (Alavian, S. M., 2009).

3.3 Impact of transplantation on the natural history of hepatitis

Renal Transplantation is recognized as the treatment of choice in most patients with end stage renal disease but the decision-making process for kidney transplant in hepatitis cases is complex. Recently, however, it has been shown that clinical evolution is better in patients who have received a kidney transpant, even in those who are non responders to antivirals, than in patients who have to remain under haemodialysis. (Sezer et al., 2004).

3.4 Hepatitis B virus (HBV) in renal patients

Although the prevalence of hepatitis B virus (HBV) infection has declined in haemodialysis patients and in renal transplant recipients, it remains high within countries with endemic HBV infection (especially Asia-Pacific and Africa). Renal transplantation is associated with reduced survival in HBsAg+ hemodialysis patients (Aroldi et al., 2005).

Treatment of hepatitis B is indicated among kidney transplanted patients and haemodialysis patients with HBV in replicative phase, (same indications as the general population) but the anti-HBV treatment has to be pursued as a preventive measure once the patient has received the transplant in order to avoid progression of the liver disease which could affect the liver and also the graft (Daudé et al., 2011).

Lamivudine used to be the only option for such cases but severe forms of exacerbation were described due to resistant mutants. Present anti-HBV therapy based on nucleos(t)ide analogues, such as tenofovir or entecavir, are now recommended. They are more potent, have a higher genetic barrier than lamivudine and are well tolerated. The dosing and administration depends on the creatinine clearance (Vigano et al., 2005).

Treatment with entecavir or tenofovir is indicated in all HBsAg-positive candidates for transplantation and after transplantation in order to maintain HBV DNA negative. Better graft survival has been described in HBsAg negative patients in comparison with patients with HBV infection (HBsAg positive or only anti-HBc positive) undergoing immunosuppressor treatment (Gane & Pilmore, 2002).

A liver biopsy in HBV positive patients has to be considered when image test results, such as ultrasound echography or fibroscan, are unclear or misleading and if there is no correlation between clinical and analytical data. A three phase liver CAT (Computed Axial Tomography) scan with injection of contrast medium is indicated when an ultrasound echography detects signs of a possible tumour.

Whatever the baseline histological evaluation, with the new anti-HBV anti-virals, sustained suppression of necro-inflammation may result in regression of fibrosis or cirrhosis, which in turn may lead to decreased disease-related morbidity and improved survival (Vallet-Pichard et al., 2011). Regular monitoring with liver function tests and HBV DNA measurements should enable early detection and rescue in case of appearance of demonstrated virus resistance.

3.5 Hepatitis C virus (HCV) in renal patients

We consider that haemodialysis patients (presenting no severe co-morbidities or contra-indications) are candidates to anti-HCV treatment only if they are being evaluated for the waiting list for kidney transplant and as long as they have no contraindications to interferon therapy, because the evolution of hepatitis C is generally mild for patients remaining on dialysis (Kidney Disease Improving Global Outcomes [KDIGO], 2008).

Although anti-HCV treatment must be proposed to all candidates for renal transplantation who had no contraindications to interferon, whatever their baseline histopathology, in HCV-infected patients undergoing chronic dialysis who are non-candidates for renal transplantation, the indication for antiviral therapy has to be individualized and is usually limited to patients with significant fibrosis (Gordon et al., 2009).

After transplantation, interferon- α is contraindicated but may be used in patients for whom the benefits of antiviral treatment clearly outweigh the risks, especially that of allograft rejection. Due to this risk, dialysis patients recieving anti-viral treatment are taken off the waiting list.

Questions about efficacy and safety of HCV treatment have yet to be resolved because practice and guidelines accepted for the general population cannot be applied to dialysed cases. These patients are considered as a special population and the treatment is only indicated for selected cases after weighing the pros and cons. Sustained viral response rates as high as 50 to 60% have been demonstrated with interferon monotherapy in dialysis (Fabrizi et al., 2008; Fabrizi et al., 2010a).

The therapeutical anti-viral option with pegylated interferon was incorporated in 2000 to the protocols for HCV treatment and adopted for the management of dialyzed patients due to its positive results and because it requires only one injection a week. Previously, standard interferon was administered three times weekly after every dialysis session. Currently, the question of whether results with pegylated interferon are better than those observed in the past with standard interferon remains unanswered. Ribavirine was totally contraindicated in uremic patients, but due with a better sustained response to anti-HCV treatment obtained with the combination of pegilated interferon and ribavirine in the general population, it now has a role in the HCV treatment in patients undergoing dialysis (Fabrizi et al., 2010b).

Concerns about its use are present due to the risk of severe anemia in this setting. Combining ribavirine in uremic cases has only been accepted with extreme caution regarding doses, recommending only 200 mg, 1 pill a week. In the event of good tolerance the dose may be increased to 2-3 pills weekly, always combined with erythropoietin (Carriero et al., 2008).

Treatment of chronic HCV infection with pegylated interferon and ribavirin in kidney transplant recipients is associated with a risk of acute or chronic cellular rejection of 30% or more, resulting in graft loss and reduced patient survival. Therefore, indications for treatment must be tailored accordingly. The indication should be assessed on a case-by-case basis, if HCV infection is life-threatening.

Hepatitis C virus (HCV) infection influences glomerular pathologic findings in renal allografts and affects the graft outcome. In diagnostic renal allograft biopsies, after kidney transplant, the presence of de novo immune-mediated glomerulonephritis has been observed, especially type I membrano prolipherative glomerulonephritis (MPGN), which is strongly associated with HCV infection and results in accelerated loss of the graft. Cruzado et al., (2003) proved that patients previously treated with interferon were less at risk of developing MPGN.

4. Diagnostic procedures

4.1 Serological assays and blood liver tests

The assessment of liver disease should include biochemical markers, such as alanine aminotransferase (ALT) and aspartate aminotransferase (AST), gamma-glutamyl transpeptidase (GGT), alkaline phosphatase, bilirubin, prothrombin time or INR (International Normalized Ratio); albumin; gammaglobulins and full blood counts. Abdominal ultrasound should be obtained as basic hepato-biliary imaging (Kidney Disease Improving Global Outcomes [KDIGO], 2008).

Various serological assays are available for the diagnosis and follow-up of HCV infection. Third generation serological tests for determining the presence of HCV antibodies are highly sensitive and specific. In case of positive serology, viral load should be determined by HCV RNA. In addition, quantitative real time PCR should be determined at least once in each patient in order to diagnose cases that have 'escaped' lower-sensitivity tests (Angelico et al., 2000).

ALT, as mentioned previously, is a helpful, although non-specific, marker of the presence of HCV infection in the dialysis population. Serial determinations of ALT are vague when reflecting the severity of liver disease and do not correlate with the liver histology or viral load (Lopes et al., 2006).

According to our experience, all patients with end-stage renal disease should undergo serological tests to screen for HCV and HBV and have their status confirmed by PCR before starting renal replacement therapy (hemo-dialysis, peritoneal dialysis).

4.2 Non-invasive imaging techniques

The ideal non-invasive test has to be simple and reproducible, readily available, easy to perform, less expensive than biopsy, and able to predict the full spectrum of fibrosis and to reflect changes occurring over time (Gaiani et al., 1997; Lackner et al., 2005).

The majority of studies have focused on HCV cases, the most prevalent liver disease in the general population, but there are few studies addressing chronic kidney patients under dialysis treatment (Alric et al., 2009).

Non-invasive methods include blood/serum markers and imaging/scanning techniques. Ultrasonography and Elastography (Fibroscan) combined with blood indexes, are the most reliable for detecting liver cirrhosis. However, in kidney patients their clinical use is limited because they have not been totally validated. This is a developing field and in the future a combination of data will probably be available in order to establish prognosis and diagnosis of cirrhosis.

4.2.1 Blood tests to diagnose chronic liver disease

Fibrosis assessment in research is done with serum fibrosis markers which can be divided into direct and indirect markers, with a preference for indirect markers.

a) Direct markers are involved in the formation of an extracellular matrix during fibrosis, and indirect markers reflect hepatic dysfunction. Several studies on the diagnosis of liver cirrhosis using direct fibrosis markers, such as collagen and hyaluronic acid, had a low sensitivity and specificity (approximately 80%). Fibrosis markers are expensive and not available for clinical practice.

b) Indirect fibrosis markers include the AST-to-ALT ratio (AAR), the AST-to-platelet ratio index (APRI), and Forns's index (Forns et al., 2002) which is the most popular as it enables the required data to be obtained easily.

Sebastian et al. (2009) have published results showing that combining the results of fibroscan and blood tests may reduce the indication of liver biopsy. In clinical practice diagnosis of compensated cirrhosis is based on ultrasonography and routine blood tests.

4.2.2 Ultrasonographic (US) imaging

Ultrasonographic (US) imaging with Doppler analysis is being widely used for the diagnosis of chronic hepatitis and compensated and decompensated cirrhosis.

US is safe, inexpensive, and routinely used within hospitals, it is also available in individual doctor's practices and in mobile settings. It offers real-time capability without the need for much data processing and analysis. However, it is recognized that the US technique needs a skilled operator, which is an important drawback.

The combination of gray scale US and Doppler US improves diagnostic accuracy and is essential for diagnosis of cirrhosis or fibrosis. It is known that liver fibrosis and steatosis can have similar appearances and can be present at the same time in a "fatty-fibrotic pattern" (Borrioni et al., 2006). US can show a small, nodular liver in advanced cirrhosis, but surface nodularity or increased echogenicity can be seen in hepatic steatosis as well as in cirrhosis (Hirche et al., 2007).

	ADVANTAGES	DISADVANTAGES
Liver biopsy	• Great experience • Evaluates other parameters in addition to fibrosis • Accurately differenciates varying stages of fibrosis	• Sampling errors • Varies depending on the observer's interpretation • Invasive method (morbidity and mortality) • Hospitalization required • Expensive
Hepatic Elastography (Fibroscan)	• Good reproductibility • More comprehensive assessment of liver tissue • Non-invasive method • Does not require admission • Inexpensive	• No experience in dialysis patients • Less applicable if obesity, ascites, or/and small intercostal spaces • Unreliable fibrosis results if cholestasis, cytolysis or liver edema • Only evaluates fibrosis • Does not discriminate between intermediate stages of fibrosis

Table 3. Theoretical advantages and disadvantages of liver biopsy and hepatic transient elastography of the liver in patients on dialysis, providing the lack of validation studies.

Gaiani et al., (1997) investigated the accuracy of an ultrasonographic score derived from liver, spleen, and portal vein features in predicting the final diagnosis in patients with compensated chronic liver disease. After comparing results obtained by ultrasonography to those obtained by percutaneous liver biopsy, they identified liver surface nodularity and portal flow velocity as factors independently associated with cirrhosis. Enlargement of the caudate lobe and spleen size besides the specific echogenicity pattern have been found to be associated with cirrhosis in other studies. Spleen size was assessed longitudinally and considered normal up to 12 cm.

A model consisting of liver surface nodularity obtained by echography, may be useful for the identification of compensated cirrhosis with a high degree of accuracy in daily practice, when a platelet count of less than 100,000/mm^3, an albumin level of less than 3.5 g/dL, and a prothrombin time or an INR of more than 1.3, is observed.

Albumin and prothrombin time or INR indicate the synthetic activity of the liver and platelet count reflects the degree of portal hypertension. As these variables, excepting the platelet count, are used in the Child-Pugh scoring system, the most used classification for cirrhosis prognosis, the specificity of the items appears to be high.

The albumin level and INR has more than 95% specificity in identifying cirrhosis, but sensitivity is low. A platelet count of less than 100,000/ mm^3 has been widely accepted as the cut-off level of portal hypertension.

With strengths and limitations, the usual blood tests and ultrasonographic variables are the basis for the diagnosis of compensated liver cirrhosis (Fontana & Lok., 2002; Sebastiani et al., 2006).

4.2.3 Hepatic elastography (fibroscan)

The fibrogenic evolution of chronic viral hepatitis B and C towards cirrhosis represents a key issue in clinical hepatology. Traditionally, liver fibrosis has been assessed by liver biopsy. One of the most important reasons for which a liver biopsy has been indicated in many situations including patients with chronic renal failure and viral hepatitis is fibrosis assessment. The liver biopsy has a low although non-negligible morbidity and mortality rate.

The fragment of liver tissue studied is small and represents only 1/50.000 of the liver. Liver biopsy obtains a semiquantitative result leading to a possible inaccurate fibrosis assessment, because fibrosis is heterogeneously distributed. Furthermore, the evaluation of the specimen requires an experimented pathologist to give his/her diagnostic opinion. There may therefore be cases of inter or intra-observer variations. Some studies show that there can be differences of up to 35% variability and of up to 20% interobservational, which can lead to errors when studying the hepatic fibrosis of a particular patient (Standish et al., 2006).

In the past ten years, non-invasive methodologies have been proposed to predict the presence of fibrosis in chronic liver disease, especially the introduction of transient elastography or FibroScan ® (Castera et al., 2005; Ziol et al., 2005) which represents a further advancement.

This technique is based on the estimate of liver tissue elasticity by ultrasound. This is done by measuring the speed of propagation of a mechanical wave within the liver parenchyma. Results, expressed in kilo Pascals, are obtained from the speed of the recorded wave (meters / second). Hepatic elastography provides a number of advantages compared to liver biopsy (Table 3).

The evaluated tissue volume is about 100 times bigger than the biopsy which is therefore likely to be much more representative of the total liver tissue. As it is non-invasive, this method can be repeated in the same patient. It has also shown good reproducibility between observers. Nevertheless, this technique also has its limitations. In 5-15% of patients it is impossible to use because of its inability to pass the mechanical wave and to reach the liver in obese patients and in patients with small intercostal spaces or due to the presence of ascites. Furthermore, some situations or comorbidities of the patient may produce unreliable results of this test. This can occur if there is liver stasis, marked elevation of transaminases or a presence of significant cholestasis. Hepatic elastography has demonstrated a high sensitivity and specificity enabling a correct diagnosis of fibrosis even when cirrhosis is already present, but this method is not as efficient for classifying intermediate fibrosis stages. Establishing the exact stage of fibrosis can be improved by using hepatic elastography in conjunction with fibrosis serum markers or the fibrotests mentioned above. Fibroscan has proved its utility in diverse liver diseases (chronic HCV or HBV, NASH, sclerosing cholangitis....) in immunocompetent patients but also in immunosuppressed patients such as in recurrent chronic hepatitis C after liver transplantation. There are no specific studies comparing liver biopsy to transient elastography for assessing liver fibrosis in patients with chronic renal failure on dialysis. Probably, and by analogy with other populations, this could be useful. We must bear in mind that it is more important to establish the fibrosis stage and disregard cirrhosis in such patients, which consequently entails a different management of the patient, even though anti-viral treatment is always indicated, in order to protect the renal graft after transplantation. In addition, liver biopsy in patients on dialysis has a higher morbidity and higher risk of bleeding in comparison to the general population. Specific studies well designed to assess the usefulness of elastography versus liver biopsy in patients undergoing dialysis would be justified.

4.2.3.1 Combination of blood test and fibroscan

Fibroscan can only evaluate tissue elasticity, however when it is combined with blood tests and new algorithms it can be indicated in different liver diseases. In the future, new formulas combining Fibroscan and diagnostic characteristics will be available for more reliable prognosis in different etiologies. A summary of current methods for assessing fibrosis are exposed in Table 4.

CURRENT METHODS FOR ASSESSING FIBROSIS				
INVASIVE	LIVER BIOPSY	Needs specific preparation and nowadays is only indicated in selected patients		
NON-INVASIVE			Blood/Serum markers	Settings in which validation exists
		APRI	AST to platelets ratio	Hepatitis B and C
		Fib-4	Age,AST,ALT, platelets	Hepatitis C
		Fibro-Test,	Alpha2-macroglobulin, GGT, haptoglobin, apolipoprotein A1, total bilirubin	Hepatitis B and C, alcoholic hepatitis, non-alcoholic fatty liver
		Forns' Index	Combination of GGT, cholesterol, BMI age	Hepatitis B and C
IMAGING/SCANNING TECHNIQUES				
Ultrasonography with Doppler analysis		Identification of portal hypertension. Doppler measures velocity of blood flow and hemodynamic variations		
Elastography (Fibroscan),		Liver stiffness. Not possible if: presence of ascites, narrow intercostal spaces, obesity		
Computed Tomography		Identifies microvascular changes, but can not be performed in renal failure or in patients who are contrast allergic		
Magnetic Resonance		Observes changes in liver parenchyma. Useful studying tumours. High cost		

Table 4. Current methods for assessing fibrosis

4.3 Liver biopsy

At present, cases with an inconclusive diagnosis can only be resolved by liver biopsy. Liver biopsy is considered the "gold standard" for obtaining information concerning the extent of

HCV-associated liver disease and further non-suspected diagnosis such as hemosiderosis, steatosis, non-alcoholic fatty liver disease etc. Liver biopsy should be carried out in the initial study of all patients except in cases of contraindications or clinical and/or ultrasonographic established cirrhosis. Desmet et al. (2003a)

Liver biopsy is an invasive procedure which is associated with an increased risk of bleeding in dialysis patients. A liver biopsy may be obtained percutaneously or via the transjugular route which is associated with a lower risk. In addition, the transjugular approach can be used to measure the hepatic venous pressure gradient and confirm the existence of portal hypertension.

Nowadays, liver biopsy only seems to be mandatory in the evaluation of non-conclusive cases. In such cases an assessment of the severity of the liver disease is needed for choosing the most suitable treatment. There is an urgent need for non-invasive validated markers of hepatic fibrosis in this setting.

4.3.1 Liver biopsy procedure

Before the liver biopsy procedure, imaging studies and a detailed coagulation analysis have to be performed to investigate hepatobiliary disease. Because of the high risk of bleeding in uremic patients, in our unit, liver biopsy is obtained after a dialysis session without heparin. An hematocrit at least, of 30% is mandatory; patients whose hematocrit levels are below this value receive a blood transfusion. To improve platelet function, a dose of 0.3 mg/kg of body weight of Minurin (Ferring SA, Madrid, Spain) is administered intravenously 30 minutes before the biopsy when indicated by hemostatic studies. Transjugular liver biopsy is used in patients with platelet levels of less than 100,000/mm3, and a percutaneous approach using a needle which is guided by Computed Tomography or Ultrasonography, and not blindly as in the past, is indicated in patients with normal coagulation analysis and in those in whom it is not necessary to measure portal pression. A better specimen is obtained using this last approach.

4.3.2 Histological assessment

The primary objective of histologic assessment is to evaluate disease progression in all forms of compensated liver disease independently of etiology (viral, toxic, metabolic etc.) and to evaluate the extent and type of hepatic fibrosis. Biopsies have to be evaluated by experienced pathologists.

Thus staging of liver fibrosis represents the most useful data for prognosis. Specimens are processed with routine stains, hematoxylin and eosin, and connective tissue stains (reticulin and trichrome method staining) used for accurate assessment of liver architecture and hepatic fibrosis. Specimens are stained by the periodic acid-Schiff method, and the presence of hemosiderin in macrophages and Kupffer cells is investigated by Perl's iron stain method. The presence of hepatitis B surface and core antigen is searched for in the cytoplasm and nucleus respectively, by immunohistochemistry. If a positive staining for either antigen is found, it is indicative of a replicative phase of HBV chronic infection.

Fat accumulation in hepatocytes ("steatosis") appears as clearly defined transparent spaces within the cytoplasm and can be both macro and microvesicular in nature. Moreover many of the liver diseases that contain fat have associated inflammation (e.g. neutrophils in alcoholic hepatitis, lymphocytes in chronic viral hepatitis due to HCV infection).

Pathologists have developed scores for reading and interpreting liver biopsies by sharing and correlationing their results with clinical data. Histologic staging (degree of fibrosis) and grading (degree of necroinflammatory activity) has become a very useful tool for the clinician when deciding the prognosis and therapeutic options. It is recommended to begin the histologic description with the etiology of hepatitis (e. g., chronic hepatitis C) followed by the degree of fibrosis, and the degree of activity, with appropriate numerical codes using one classification and scoring system. Various scoring systems have been validated for use in chronic hepatitis C. Desmet et al. (2003b)

The most widely used in Europe are METAVIR, Scheuer, Ishak, and Knodell's Hepatitis Activity Index. Metavir and Scheuer's scores are more reproducible and less prone to observer variation, but less discriminant both for fibrosis and for necroinflammation than Ishak and Knodell (Table 5).

FIBROSIS STAGE	DESCRIPTION	CRITERIA
0	No fibrosis	Normal connective tissue
1	Portal fibrosis	Fibrous portal expansion
2	Periportal fibrosis	Periportal or rare portal-portal septa
3	Septal fibrosis	Fibrous septa with architectural distortion; no obvious cirrhosis
4	Cirrhosis	Cirrhosis

INFLAMMATORY GRADE	DESCRIPTION	LYMPHOCYTIC PIECEMEAL NECROSIS	LOBULAR INFLAMMATION AND NECROSIS
0	Portal inflammation only; no activity	None	None
1	Minimal	Minimal, patchy	Minimal, occasional spotty necrosis
2	Mild	Mild, involving some or all portal tracts	Mild, little hepatocellular change
3	Moderate	Moderate, involving all portal tracts	Moderate, with noticeable hepatocellular change
4	Severe	Severe, may have bridging fibrosis	Severe, with prominent diffuse hepatocellular damage

Table 5. The liver biopsy interpretation in chronic hepatitis: Staging and Grading Systems (Batts, 1995, as cited in Kanel, G. C. & Korula, J. (2011) Atlas of Liver Pathology)

In our unit, biopsies are scored according to the classical system proposed by Scheuer, in which necroinflammatory activity (portal/periportal hepatitis and lobular activity) and fibrosis are evaluated separately, and are classified on a scale of a 0-4, as follows: F0, no fibrosis; F1, portal fibrosis; F2, periportal fibrosis; F3, septal fibrosis; and F4, cirrhosis based on the recommended criteria. Bile duct and cholangiolar proliferation may be present but are not prominent, except in instances of severe liver cell injury. Other findings such as iron deposits are studied in Kupffer and liver cells and are classified as mild, moderate, or severe. But over the years, steatosis, non-alcoholic fatty liver, has become more important.

Liver biopsy provides information regarding the presence or absence of cirrhosis especially if a study of portal pression is incorporated to the procedure. In the cirrhotic stage, the regenerative nodules are often "macronodular", more than 3 mm. If they are less than 3 mm, they are micronodular. Sometimes a mixed pattern with both macro and micronodules can be detected.

Recently, the great advances in radiological imaging techniques have focused attention on hepatic premalignant nodular lesions. The histological differential diagnosis of these nodules can often be difficult, especially in needle biopsy specimens with limited material. Diagnostic considerations differ significantly between livers with and without cirrhosis: In the noncirrhotic liver, the differential diagnosis includes liver cell adenoma, nodular regenerative hyperplasia, and hepatocellular carcinoma. In cirrhosis, dysplastic nodules (low and high grade), dysplasia (large and small cell) as well as hepatocellular carcinoma may occur. The standardization and the uniform use of the nomenclature of these entities are necessary for a better understanding of the biological nature and etiopathology of these lesions. Only a commonly accepted nomenclature makes a comparison of different therapeutic treatment regimens feasible.

Liver biopsy also assesses the disease severity by evaluating the parenchyma structure and other possible tissue damage related to non-suspected lesions. It helps to determine the degree of disease progression, the need for anti-viral treatment, patient motivation and the indication of a combined liver and kidney transplant.

4.3.3 Diagnosis of hepatic fibrosis and cirrhosis

Cirrhosis can be defined as the end stage consequence of fibrosis of the hepatic parenchyma resulting in nodule formation and altered hepatic function.

Up to 40% of patients with cirrhosis are asymptomatic and may remain so for more than a decade, but progressive deterioration is inevitable once complications develop, including ascites, variceal hemorrhage or encephalopathy. Early diagnosis of liver cirrhosis in chronic hepatitis patients is critical in its management. All cirrhotic patients, notably after solid organ transplantation, should be screened for hepatocellular carcinoma. Liver biopsy increases costs and has potential risks, however, diagnosis of compensated liver cirrhosis usually requires doing a liver biopsy and assessment of portal hypertension (fibrosgastroscopy and direct measurement). Liver biopsy is the most accurate diagnostic method in the diagnosis of compensated liver cirrhosis, but a liver biopsy is performed in few patients in clinical practice.

Complications in the general population are very low (1/4000–10,000), but the risk of hemorrhage in uremics has to be taken into account, false negative probability due to sampling error is reported to be of 20 to 30%. A liver specimen obtained to be evaluated has to be more than 1 cm in length.

For these reasons, nowadays it is necessary to establish non-invasive diagnostic methods, validated predominantly for chronic HCV, to allow for an easier diagnosis of liver cirrhosis in different populations.

4.3.4 Liver biopsy data in dialysis patients

A few researchers have evaluated histologic severity of liver disease in HCV-positive patients with end stage renal disease. Martin et al., (2000) reported 37 anti-HCV positive patients, who were referred for renal transplant, most of whom were already dialysis dependent and had undergone liver biopsy. Mild or moderate necroinflammatory activity occurred in all patients; bridging fibrosis was present in 3 of 37 (8%), and frank cirrhosis in 9 (24%). No relationship between severity of histologic changes and HCV viral load or genotype or ALT activity was reported. In this study, a history of alcohol abuse was elicited in 38% of patients, perhaps accounting in part for the frequency of advanced fibrosis. Sterling et al., (1999) evaluated liver histology in 50 consecutive patients with chronic HCV awaiting renal transplantation. Bridging fibrosis or cirrhosis was present in 22%, which was not significantly different from a control group of HCV-positive patients with intact renal function and normal ALT, although there was a trend toward more fibrosis in the dialysis group.

The impact of renal transplantation on the natural history of HCV infection has been shown by Zylberberg et al. In a case-control study including 28 kidney transplanted HCV-infected patients compared with 28 matched immunocompetent controls, they observed histopathological deterioration in 70% of the transplanted patients compared to 19% of the controls. The median time elapsed between kidney transplantation and the final liver biopsy in the study was 13.6 years (range 2.6–23.9 years). The progressive nature of liver disease in HCV-infected renal transplanted recipients is probably related to numerous factors. There is evidence that acute HCV acquired perioperatively acts more aggressively in such patients, perhaps reflecting an acute infection at the time the patient is receiving maximum immunosuppression. It appears that therapeutic immunosuppression following renal transplant may accelerate the course of HCV infection leading to hepatocellular failure. On the other hand, the overall survival advantage conferred by transplant may outweigh the potential negative effects of immunosuppression for many renal transplant patients.

5. Impact of viral eradication on mortality related to hepatitis

Despite the fact that HCV and HBV infections adversely affect the survival of dialysis and renal transplant patients and its high prevalence in these groups of patients, large clinical trials are rare.

5.1 Hemodialysis patients

Due to the negative long-term impact of HCV infection after transplantation and to the current lack of treatment options for HCV after kidney transplantation, treatment of haemodialysis patients should be attempted when possible.

Careful patient selection and side effect management are important. Combination treatment with pegylated interferon and ribavirin might be considered by experienced physicians, with individualized ribavirin dosing and substantial hematopoietic support, as suggested by few preliminary studies.

The optimal treatment of HCV in dialysis patients and a more in depth profile of patients has not been determined. We perform Electroencephalography, and echocardiography in order to be aware of unexpected risks and therefore be able to prevent them.

5.2 Therapeutic options after kidney transplant

Although treatment of kidney transplants recipients who have hepatitis C is not routinely recommended because of the potential risk for precipitating rejection, some clinical presentations warrant consideration of interferon-based therapy. The most pressing reasons to consider HCV therapy are recurrent and progressive HCV-associated glomerulopathy in the transplanted kidney, severe cholestatic hepatitis, and advanced histologic stages of liver disease.

5.3 HCV-mediated glomerulonephritis

HCV-mediated glomerulonephritis may be effectively managed with interferon-based therapy. The current "best therapy" for these situations is combination therapy with interferon and ribavirin, because combination therapy is the most likely to achieve a sustained viral response.

6. Algorithms and new perspectives

Although practices regarding whether patients with cirrhosis should be referred for combined liver and kidney transplantation or whether they should be considered for kidney transplantation alone vary by center, an algorithm for assessment of the fibrosis stage or presence of cirrhosis and evaluation for anti- hepatitis C treatment may be suggested.

By adding non invasive methods such as Fibroscan to the routine tests (abdominal ultrasonography with Doppler and blood analysis) liver biopsy may be avoided in the majority of cases and it could be indicated only when there is a discrepancy between clinical and analytical data.

Patients with liver cirrhosis with portal hypertension, and who had some liver decompensation do not need liver biopsy and have to be considered candidates to combined liver and kidney transplant while patients with cirrhosis or advanced fibrosis should undergo more in depth studies.

7. Conclusion

- At present, Hepatitis C and B infection represent a major medical and epidemiologic challenge both in patients on renal replacement therapy and patients undergoing kidney transplantation. The major concern, however, is the lack of safe and effective drugs to treat HCV-infected patients with chronic kidney disease.
- Unfortunately, there have not been any large scale clinical trials performed on this population, therefore the evidence for treatment recommendations is scant and the role of liver biopsy in selected cases is vigent.
- Assessment of the severity of liver fibrosis is important in decision making in patients with chronic hepatitis C under dialysis which is why liver biopsy is still regarded as the reference method to assess the grade of inflammation and the stage of fibrosis. Patients on dialysis, even those diagnosed with chronic hepatitis, have the possibility to receive a kidney transplant, which may have a more favourable evolution if prior to transplant viral eradication is achieved. Another concern in patients also suffering from chronic liver disease is deciding whether they will only need a kidney transplant or whether a combined kidney and liver transplantation is necessary.
- Until recently, a combined transplant was always recommended for patients with advanced fibrosis or cirrhosis. However, nowadays due to a lack of donors, in some centers, patients are only being referred for a kidney transplant, providing that the patient has never suffered from decompensated liver disease.
- Furthermore, in recent years transient elastography (Fibroscan) has been progressively introduced in order to resolve diagnosis uncertainty regarding the fibrosis stage in different clinical settings, especially in patients with chronic hepatitis C due to its high prevalence worldwide, but it has not been validated for kidney patients yet.

- In kidney transplant recipients, HCV infection is associated with an increased risk of de novo glomerulonephritis and liver-related mortality, both HCV related.
- In conclusion, as cirrhosis is an important predictor of poor post-kidney transplant survival after kidney transplantation, it is advisable to obtain a liver biopsy from selected HCV-positive kidney transplant candidates, considering that the combination of common blood tests, abdominal echography and Fibroscan can improve accuracy and reduce the necessity of using liver biopsy.

8. References

Print Book

Kanel, G. C. & Korula, J. (2011) *Atlas of Liver Pathology,* (3rd Edition) Elsevier Saunders, ISBN 978-1-4377-0765-6, Philadelphia, PA 19103-2899

Papers in journals

Ahmed, M.S., Wong, C.F., Shawki, H., et al., (2008) Rapidly deteriorating renal function with membranoproliferative glomerulonephritis Type 1 associated with hepatitis C treated successfully with steroids and antiviral therapy: a case report and review of literature. *Clin Nephrol.* Vol 69, No issue 4, pp. (298-301), ISSN 1555-9041

Alavian, S. M. (2009) A shield against a monster: Hepatitis C in hemodialysis patients. *World J Gastroenterol,* Vol 15, No issue 6, pp. (641-646), ISSN 1007-9327

Alric, L., Kamar, N. Bonnet, D. et al., (2009) Comparison of liver stiffness, fibrotest and liver biopsy for assessment of liver fibrosis in kidney-transplant patients with chronic viral hepatitis. *Transpl Int,* Vol 22, No issue 5, pp (568-573), ISSN 0934-0874

Angelico, M. Morosetti, M. Passalacqua, S. et al., (2000) Low levels of hepatitis C virus RNA in blood of infected patients under maintenance haemodialysis with high-biocompatibility, high-permeability filters. *Dig Liver Dis,* Vol 32, No issue 8, pp. (724-728), ISSN 1590-8658

Aoufi Rabih, S., & García Agudo, R. (2011) Management of HCV infection in chronic kidney disease. *Nefrología.* (Official Publication of the Spanish Nephrology Society), Vol 31, No issue 3, pp. (260-267), ISSN 0211-6995

Aroldi, A. Lampertico, P. Montagnino, G. et al., (2005) Natural history of hepatitis B and C in renal allograft recipients. *Transplantation,* Vol 79, No issue 9, pp. (1132-1136), ISSN 1534-0608.

Bedossa, P., Dargère, D., Paradis, V. (2003) Sampling variability of liver fibrosis in chronic hepatitis C. *Hepatology,* Vol 38, No issue 6, pp. (1449-1457), ISSN 1665-2681

Bedossa, P., Poynard, T. (1996) An algorithm for the grading of activity in chronic hepatitis C. The METAVIR Cooperative Study Group. *Hepatolog,* Vol 24, No issue 2, pp. (289-293), ISSN 1665-2681

Bejarano, P.A, Koehler, A. & Sherman, K.E. (2001) Second opinion pathology in liver biopsy interpretation. *Am J Gastroenterol,* Vol 96, No issue11, pp.(3158-3164), ISSN 0002-9270

Borroni, G. Ceriani, R., Cazzaniga, M. et al., (2006) Comparison of simple tests for the non-invasive diagnosis of clinically silent cirrhosis in chronic hepatitis C *Aliment Pharmacol & Therap,* Vol 24, No issue 5, pp.(797–804), ISSN0269-2813, 1365-2036

Bravo, A.A., Sheth, S.G., Chopra, S. (2001) Liver biopsy. *N Engl J Med,* Vol 34, No issue 7, pp. (495-500), ISSN 0028-4793

Carriero, D., Fabrizi, F., Uriel, A.J., et al., (2008) Treatment of dialysis patients with chronic hepatitis C using pegylated interferon and low-dose ribavirin. *Int J Artif Organs,* Vol 31, No issue 4, pp. (295-302), ISSN 0391-3988

Carrión, J.A., Navasa, M., Bosch, J., et al., (2006) Transient elastography for diagnosis of advanced fibrosis and portal hypertension in patients with C recurrence after liver transplantation. *Liver Transplantation,* Vol.12, No.12, pp. (1791-1798), ISSN1527-6465

Casanovas-Taltavull, T., Baliellas, C., Benasco, C., et al., (2001) Efficacy of interferon for chronic hepatitis C virus-related hepatitis in kidney transplant candidates on hemodialysis: results after transplantation. *Am J Gastroenterol,* Vol 96, No issue 4 , pp. (1170-1177), ISSN 0002-9270

Castéra, L., Faucher, J., Bernard, P.H., et al., (2010) Pitfalls of liver stiffness measurement: A 5-year prospective study of 13,369 examinations. *Hepatology,* Vol.51, No.3, pp. (828-835), ISSN 1665-2681

Cholongitas, E., Quaglia, A., Samonakis, D., et al., (2006) Transjugular liver biopsy: how good is it for accurate histological interpretation?. *Gut,* Vol 55, No issue 12, pp. (1789-1794), ISSN 0017-5749

Colloredo, G., Guido, M., Sonzogni, A., Leandro, G. (2003) Impact of liver biopsy size on histological evaluation of chronic viral hepatitis: the smaller the sample, the milder the disease. *J Hepatol,* Vol 39, No issue 2, pp. (239-244), ISSN 0168-8278

Cruzado, J.M., Casanovas-Taltavull, T., Torras, J., et al., (2003) Pretransplant interferon prevents hepatitis C virus-associated glomerulonephritis in renal allografts by HCV-RNA clearance. *Am J Transplant,* Vol 3, No issue 3, pp. (357-360), ISSN 1600-6143

Daudé, M., Rostaing, L., Sauné, K., et al., (2011) Tenofovir therapy in hepatitis B virus-positive solid-organ transplant recipients. *Transplantation,* Vol 91, No issue 8, pp. (916-920), ISSN 1534-0608

Delladetsima, J.K., Boletis, J.N., Makris, F., et al., (1999) Fibrosing cholestatic hepatitis in renal transplant recipients with hepatitis C virus infection. *Liver Transpl Surg,* Vol 5, No issue 4, pp. (294-300), ISSN 1074-3022

Desmet, V. (1997) Histological classification of chronic hepatitis. *Acta Gastroenterol Belg,* Vol 60, No issue 4, pp. (259-2567), ISSN 0001-5644

Desmet, V. (2003a) Liver tissue examination. *J Hepatol,* Vol 39, Suppl 1, pp. (S43-S49), ISSN 0168-8278

Desmet, V. (2003b) a "Knodell RG, Ishak KG, et al., Formulation and application of a numerical scoring system for assessing histological activity in asymptomatic chronic active hepatitis. [*Hepatology,* 1981; Vol 1, pp. 431–435]". *Journal of Hepatology,* Vol 38, No issue 4, pp. (382-386), ISSN 0168-8278

Espinosa, M., Martn-Malo, A., Ojeda, R., et al., (2004) Marked reduction in the prevalence of hepatitis C virus infection in hemodialysis patients: causes and consequences. *Am J Kidney Dis,* Vol 43, No issue 4, pp. (685-689), ISSN 0272-6386

Fabrizi, F, Martin P, Dixit V, Bunnapradist S (2004) Meta-analysis: Effect of hepatitis C virus infection on mortality in dialysis. *Aliment Pharmacol Ther,* Vol 20, No issues 11-12, pp. (1271-1277), ISSN 0269-2813, 1365-2036

Fabrizi, F., Takkouche, B., Lunghi, G., et al., (2007) The impact of hepatitis C virus infection on survival in dialysis patients: meta-analysis of observational studies. *J Viral Hepat,* Vol 14, No issue 10, pp. (697-703), ISSN 1352-0504

Fabrizi, F., Dixit, V., Messa, P., Martin, P. (2008) Interferon monotherapy of chronic hepatitis C in dialysis patients: meta-analysis of clinical trials. *J Viral Hep,* Vol 15, No issue 2, pp. (79-88), ISSN 1352-0504

Fabrizi, F., Dixit, V., Messa, P., Martin, P. (2010b) Pegylated interferon monotherapy of chronic hepatitis C in dialysis patients: Meta-analysis of clinical trials. *J Med Virol,* Vol 82, No issue 5, pp. (768-775), ISSN 0146-6615

Fabrizi, F., Martin, P. & Messa, P. (2010a) Hepatitis B and hepatitis C virus and chronic kidney disease. *Acta Gastroenterol Belg,* Vol 73, No issue 4, pp. (465-471), ISSN 0001-5644

Fontana, R.J. & Lok, A.S.F. (2002) Noninvasive Monitoring of Patients With Hepatitis C *Hepatology,* Vol 36, No issue 5, Suppl 1, pp. (S57-S64), ISSN 1665-2681

Forns, X., Ampurdanès, S., Llove,t J.M., et al., (2002) Identification of chronic hepatitis C patients without hepatic fibrosis by a simple predictive model. *Hepatology,* Vol 36, No issue 4, Pt 1, pp. (986-992), ISSN 1665-2681

Gaiani, S., Gramantieri, L., Venturoli, N., et al., (1997) What is the criterion for differentiating chronic hepatitis from compensated cirrhosis? A prospective study comparing ultrasonography and percutaneous liver biopsy. *J Hepatol,* Vol 27, No issue 6, pp. (979-985), ISSN 0168-8278

Gane, E. & Pilmore, H., (2002) Management of chronic viral hepatitis before and after renal transplantation. *Transplantation,* Vol 74, No issue 4, pp. (427-437), ISSN 1534-0608

Ghany, M.G., Lok, A.S., Everhart, J.E., et al. (2010) HALT-C Trial Group. Predicting clinical and histologic outcomes based on standard laboratory tests in advanced chronic hepatitis C. *Gastroenterology,* Vol 138, No issue 1, pp. (136-146), ISSN 0002-9270

Gordon, C.E., Uhlig, K., Lau, J., et al., (2009) Interferon for hepatitis C virus in hemodialysis--an individual patient meta-analysis of factors associated with sustained virological response. *Clin J Am Soc Nephrol,* Vol 4, No issue 9, pp. (1449-1458), ISSN: 1555-9041

Hanafusa, T., Ichikawa, Y., Kishikawa, H., et al., (1998) Retrospective study on the impact of hepatitis C virus infection on kidney transplant patients over 20 years. *Transplantation,* Vol 66, No issue 4 , pp. (471-476), ISSN 1534-0608

Hinrichsen, H., Leimenstoll, G., Stegen, G., et al., (2002) PHV Study Group. Prevalence and risk factors of hepatitis C virus infection in haemodialysis patients: a multicentre study in 2796 patients. *Gut,* Vol 51, No issue 3, pp. (429-433), ISSN 0017-574

Hirche, T.O., Ignee, A., Hirche, H., et al., (2007) Evaluation of hepatic steatosis by ultrasound in patients with chronic hepatitis C virus infection. *Liver Int,* Vol 27, No issue 6, pp. (748-757), ISSN 1478-322

Hmaied, F., Ben Mamou, M., Saune-Sandres, K., et al., (2006) Hepatitis C virus infection among dialysis patients in Tunisia: incidence and molecular evidence for nosocomial transmission. *J Med Viro,* Vol 78, No issue 2, pp. (185-191), ISSN 1096-9071

Huraib, S., al-Rashed, R., Aldrees, A., et al., (1995) High prevalence of and risk factors for hepatitis C in haemodialysis patients in Saudi Arabia: a need for new dialysis strategies. *Nephrol Dial Transplant* , Vol 10, No issue 4, pp. (470-474),. ISSN 0932-0509

Huskey J, Wiseman AC. (2011) Chronic viral hepatitis in kidney transplantation. *Nat Rev Nephro,* Vol 7, No issue 3, pp. (156-165) , ISSN 1759-5061

Jadoul, M., Poignet, J.L., Geddes, C., et al., (2004) HCV Collaborative Group. The changing epidemiology of hepatitis C virus (HCV) infection in haemodialysis: European multicentre study. *Nephrol Dial Transplant* , Vol 19 , No issue 4, pp. (904-909), ISSN 0931-0509

Kaiser, T., Damerow, H.C., Tenckhoff, S., et al., (2008) Kinetics of hepatitis C viral RNA and HCV-antigen during dialysis sessions: evidence for differential viral load reduction on dialysis. *J Med Virol.,* Vol 80, No issue 7, pp. (1195-1201), ISSN 0146-6615

Kalambokis, G., Christou, L., Stefanou, D., et al., (2007) Association of liver cirrhosis related IgA nephropathy with portal hypertension. *World J Gastroenterol,* Vol 13, No issue 43, pp. (5783-5786), ISSN 1007-9327

Kidney Disease: Improving Global Outcomes (KDIGO). (2008) KDIGO clinical practice guidelines for the prevention, diagnosis, evaluation, and treatment of hepatitis C in chronic kidney disease. *Kidney Int,* Vol 73, Suppl 109s, pp.(S1-S99), ISSN 0098-6577

Lackner, C., Struber, G., Liegl, B., et al., (2005) Comparison and validation of simple noninvasive tests for prediction of fibrosis in chronic hepatitis C. *Hepatology,* Vol 41, No issue 6, pp. (1376-1382), ISSN: 1665-2681

Lavanchy, D. (2009) The global burden of hepatitis C. *Liver Int,* Vol 29, Suppl 1, pp. (74-81), ISSN 1478-3223

Light, J.A., Metz, S., Oddenino, K., et al., (1982) Donor-specific transfusion with diminished sensitization. *Transplantation,* Vol 34, No issue 6, pp. (352-355), ISSN 1534-0608

Lopes, E.P., Gouveia, E.C., Albuquerque, A.C., et al., (2006) Determination of the cut-off value of serum alanine aminotransferase in patients undergoing hemodialysis, to identify biochemical activity in patients with hepatitis C viremia. *J Clin Virol,* Vol 35, No issue 3, pp. (298-302), ISSN 1386-6532

Martin, P., Carter, D., Fabrizi, F., et al., (2000) Histopathological features of hepatitis C in renal transplant candidates. *Transplantation,* Vol 69, no Issue 7, pp. (1479-1484), ISSN 1534-0608

Martin, P. & Fabrizi, F. (2008) Kidney Disease in Patients with Chronic Hepatitis C. *J Hepatol,* Vol 49, No issue 4, pp. (613-624), ISSN 0168-8278

Martínez, S.M., Crespo, G., Navasa, M., & Forns X. (2011) Noninvasive assessment of liver fibrosis. *Hepatology,* Vol 53, No issue 1, pp. (325-335), ISSN 1665-2681

Mathurin, P., Mouquet, C., Poynard, T. et al., (1999) Impact of hepatitis B and C virus on kidney transplantation outcome. *Hepatology,* Vol 29, No issue 2, pp. (257–263), ISSN 1665-2681

McLaughlin, K.J., Cameron, S.O., Good, T., et al., (1997) Nosocomial transmission of hepatitis C virus within a British dialysis centre. *Nephrol Dial Transplant,* Vol 12, No issue 2, pp. (304-309), ISSN 1460-2385

Morales, J.M., Marcén, R., Andres, A., et al. (2010) Renal transplantation in patients with hepatitis C virus antibody. A long national experience. *NDT Plus,* Vol 3, (Suppl- 2), ii41-ii46, ISSN 1753-0792 ISSN 1753-0784

Noureddin, M. & Ghany, M.G. (2010) Pharmacokinetics and pharmacodynamics of peginterferon and ribavirin: implications for clinical efficacy in the treatment of chronic hepatitis C. *Gastroenterol Clin North Am,* Vol 39, No issue 3, pp. (649-658), ISSN 1558-1942

Okoh, E.J., Bucci, J.R., Simon, J.F. & Harrison, S.A. (2008) HCV in patients with end-stage renal disease. *Am J Gastroenterol,* Vol 103, No issue 8, pp. (2123-2134), ISSN 0002-9270

Orloff, S.L., Stempel, C.A., Wright, T.L., et al., (1995) Long-term outcome in kidney transplant patients with hepatitis C (HCV) infection. *Clin Transplant,* Vol 9, No issue 2, pp. (119-124), ISSN 0902-0063

Persico, M., Palmentieri, B., Vecchione, R., et al., (2002a) Diagnosis of chronic liver disease: reproducibility and validation of liver biopsy. *Am J Gastroenterol,* Vol 97, No issue 2, pp. (491-492), ISSN 0002-9270

Persico, M., Palmentieri, B., Coppola, L., et al., (2002b) Occurrence of HCC in asymptomatic HCV-related chronic hepatitis. *Dig Dis Sci, Vol* 47, No issue 11, pp. (2407-2410), ISSN: 1590-8658

Pouteil-Noble, C., Tardy, J.C., Chossegros, P., et al., (1995) Co-infection by hepatitis B virus and hepatitis C virus in renal transplantation: morbidity and mortality in 1098 patients. *Nephrol Dial Transplant,* Vol 10, Suppl 6, pp. (122-124), ISSN 0931-0509

Rousselet, M.C., Michalak, S., Dupré, F., et al. (2005) Sources of variability in histological scoring of chronic viral hepatitis. *Hepatology,* Vol 41, No issue 2, pp. (257-264), ISSN 1665-2681

Salama, G., Rostaing, L., Sandres, K. & Izopet, J. (2000) Hepatitis C virus infection in French hemodialysis units: a multicenter study. *J Med Virol,* Vol 61, No issue 1, pp. (44-51), ISSN 1096-9071

Santos, M.A. & Souto, F.J. (2007) Infection by the hepatitis C virus in chronic renal failure patients undergoing hemodialysis in Mato Grosso state, central Brazil: a cohort study. *BMC Public Health,* Vol 7, pp. (32-40), ISSN 1471-2478

Scott, D.R., Wong, J.K., Spicer, T.S., et al., (2010) Adverse impact of hepatitis C virus infection on renal replacement therapy and renal transplant patients in Australia and New Zealand.*Transplantation,* Vol 90, No issue 11, pp. (1165-1171), ISSN 1534-0608

Sebastiani, G. & Alberti, A. (2006) Non invasive fibrosis biomarkers reduce but not substitute the need for liver biopsy. *World J Gastroenterol, Vol* 12, No issue 23, pp. (3682-3694), ISSN 1007-9327

Sebastiani, G., Halfon, P., Castera, L., et al., (2009) SAFE biopsy: a validated method for large-scale staging of liver fibrosis in chronic hepatitis C. *Hepatology, Vol* 49, No issue 6, pp. (1821-1827), ISSN 1665-2681

Sebastiani, G., Vario, A., Guido, M., et al., (2006) Stepwise combination algorithms of non-invasive markers to diagnose significant fibrosis in chronic hepatitis C. *J Hepatol*, Vol 44, No issue 4, pp. (686-693), ISSN 0168-8278

Seeff, L.B., Everson, G.T., Morgan, T.R., et al., (2010) HALT–C Trial Group. Complication rate of percutaneous liver biopsies among persons with advanced chronic liver disease in the HALT-C trial. *Clin Gastroenterol Hepatol*, Vol 8, No issue 10, pp.(877-883), ISSN 1542-3565

Sezer, S., Ozdemir, F.N., Akcay, A., et al., (2004) Renal transplantation offers a better survival in HCV-infected ESRD patients. *Clin Transplant*, Vol 18, No issue 5, pp. (619-623), ISSN 1399-0012

Shaheen, A.A., Wan, A.F., Myers, R.P. (2007) FibroTest and FibroScan for the prediction of hepatitis C-related fibrosis: a systematic review of diagnostic test accuracy. *Am J Gastroenterol* , Vol 102, No issue 11, pp. (2589-600), ISSN 0002-9270

Shamshirsaz, A.A., Kamgar, M., Bekheirnia, M. R. et al., (2004) The role of hemodialysis machines dedication in reducing Hepatitis C transmission in the dialysis setting in Iran: A multicenter prospective interventional study. *BMC Nephrol*, Vol 5, Oct 7, pp. (13-17), ISSN 1471-2369

Siddique, I., El-Naga, H.A., Madda, J.P., et al., (2003) Sampling variability on percutaneous liver biopsy in patients with chronic hepatitis C virus infection. *Scand J Gastroenterol*, Vol 38, No issue 4, pp. (427-432), ISSN 0036-5521

Standish, R.A., Cholongitas, E., Dhillon, A., et al., (2006) An appraisal of the histopathological assessment of liver fibrosis. *Gut*, Vol.55, No 4, pp. (569-578), ISSN 0017-5749

Stasi, C., Arena, U., Vizzutti, F., et al., (2009) Transient elastography for the assessment of liver fibrosis in patients with chronic viral hepatitis: the missing tool?. *Dig Liver Dis, Vol* 41, No issue 12, pp. (863-866), ISSN 1590-8658

Sterling, R.K., Sanyal, A.J., Luketic, V.A., et al., (1999) Chronic hepatitis C infection in patients with end stage renal disease: characterization of liver histology and viral load in patients awaiting renal transplantation. *Am J Gastroenterol,* Vol 94, No issue 12, pp. (3576-3582), ISSN: 0002-9270

Tannapfel, A. & Wittekind, C. (2001) Preneoplasia of the liver. Definition—differential diagnosis-clinical consequences. *Pathologe,* Vol 22, No issue 6, pp. (399-406), ISSN 0172-8113

Tobkes, A.I. & Nord, H.J. (1995) Liver biopsy: review of methodology and complications. *Dig Dis. Sci* , Vol13, No issue 5, pp: (267-74), ISSN 1573-2568

Vallet-Pichard, A., Fontaine, H., Mallet, V. & Pol, S. (2011a) Viral hepatitis in solid organ transplantation other than liver. *J Hepatol,* Vol 55, No issue 2, pp (472-478) PMID: 21241754. ISSN 0168-8278

Vallet-Pichard, A., Pol, S., Mallet, V., (2011b) Assessment and reversibility of liver fibrosis in viral hepatitis. *Rev Prat.*,Vol 61 No issue 1 pp. (39-43), ISSN:0035-2640

Viganò, M., Colombo, M., Aroldi, A., et al., (2005) Long-term lamivudine monotherapy in renal-transplant recipients with hepatitis-B-related cirrhosis. *Antivir Ther* Vol10 No issue 6 pp. (709-713), ISSN 1359-6535

Vizzutti, F., Arena, U., Marra, F. & Pinzani, M, (2009) Elastography for the non-invasive assessment of liver disease: limitations and future developments. *Gut*, Vol.58, No.2, pp. (157-160), ISSN 0017-5749

Zeman, M., Campbell, P. & Bain, V.G. (2006) Hepatitis C eradication and improvement of cryoglobulinemia-associated rash and membranoproliferative glomerulonephritis with interferon and ribavirin after kidney transplantation. *Can J Gastroenterol,* Vol 20 No issue 6 pp. (427-431), ISSN 0835-7900

Ziol, M., Handra-Luca, A., Kettaneh, A., et al., (2005) Noninvasive asessment of liver fibrosis by measuremcnt of stiffnss in patients with chronic hepatitis C. *Hepatology,* Vol.41, No. 1, pp: (48-54), ISSN 1665-2681

Zylberberg, H., Nalpas, B., Carnot, F., et al., (2002) Severe evolution of chronic hepatitis C in renal transplantation: a case control study. *Nephrol Dial Transplant,* Vol 17, No issue 1 , pp. (129-133, ISSN 0931-0509)

15

Immunohistochemical Staining of Liver Grafts for Recurrent Hepatitis C After Liver transplantation

Hiroshi Sadamori[1], Tetsuya Ogino[2], Takahito Yagi[1] and Toshiyosi Fujiwara[1]
[1]*Departments of Gastroenterological Surgery,*
[2]*Departments of Pathology,*
Okayama University Graduate School of Medicine, Dentistry and Pharmaceutical Sciences,
Japan

1. Introduction

Chronic hepatitis C virus (HCV) infection is the leading reason for liver transplantation in both the USA and Europe. Also, with increasing numbers of adult recipients, HCV associated liver disease is now becoming the leading indication for liver transplantation in Japan as well. The recurrence of HCV infection in the grafted liver is inevitable and HCV re-infection precedes acute hepatitis, which is usually detected between 1 and 3 months post-transplantation. Acute HCV is characterized by a rising serum alanine transaminase level and sometimes by a moderate elevation in bilirubin levels, resulting in varying degrees of liver graft damage. Acute HCV usually evolves to chronic hepatitis, which impairs both the graft and patient survival because the progression to liver cirrhosis is faster after liver transplantation than in nontransplant patients. A biopsy of the transplanted graft is helpful in establishing a diagnosis of recurrent HCV, in aiding the decision to undertake antiviral treatment, and in assessing the treatment response. The biopsy is assessed for grade (degree of necro-inflammation) and stage (extent of fibrosis) which help predict the likelihood of disease progression.

There are still several problems with the diagnosis and treatment of recurrent HCV after liver transplantations. Especially during the first 6 months following transplantation, recurrent HCV infection frequently causes severe liver graft dysfunction. Also during this period, recurrent HCV is sometimes difficult to differentiate from other complications such as acute cellular rejection (ACR) and biliary complications because the histopathological changes of a grafted liver with recurrent HCV infection are often atypical. Thus, a definite histopathological diagnosis of recurrent HCV sometimes cannot be made solely based on the findings of hematoxylin-eosin (H&E) stained liver biopsies. The diagnosis of recurrent HCV and the decision to launch antiviral treatment is often difficult and stressful for clinicians.

The detection of HCV replicative intermediates or antigens in liver biopsies may be helpful in the diagnosis and medical management of patients with recurrent HCV. In the following section, previous reports about the immunohistochemical detection of HCV antigens in liver grafts are reviewed and our data about immunohistochemical staining using IG222 monoclonal antibody (mAb) against the HCV-envelope 2 (E2) protein are described.

2. Immunohistochemical analysis of liver grafts for recurrent HCV after liver transplantation

2.1 Immunohistochemical detection of HCV antigens in patients with chronic HCV infection

The identification of HCV antigens in the liver was first reported in 1990 (Krawczynski et al., 1990). Several antibodies have been induced for the detection of HCV in liver biopsies. HCV antigens were detected exclusively in the cytoplasm of hepatocytes in specimens obtained from the livers of patients with chronic HCV infection, with a detection rate of 23-100% (Roskams, 2002; Scheuer et al., 1997). According to these reports, the number of positive hepatocytes and the intensity of staining were relatively low in most of the liver specimens. Clinically, the indication and management of antiviral therapy for HCV infection is decided according to liver biochemical tests, HCV genotype, and serum HCV-RNA levels. Thus, histopathological findings from liver biopsy are not necessarily essential for managing patients with chronic HCV infection. In addition, the histopathological features of chronic HCV infection are typical and are easily assessed for the disease diagnosis and progression from H&E stained liver biopsy specimens. Therefore, immunohistochemical detection of HCV antigens doesn't necessarily seem to be valuable for the medical management of patients with chronic HCV infection.

2.2 Immunohistochemical detection of HCV antigens for liver transplantation

2.2.1 Problems of diagnosing and managing recurrent HCV

In recurrent HCV infection in grafted livers, histopathological changes often exhibit from acute lobular hepatitis to chronic hepatitis in the majority of patients after transplantation. The severity of these changes, including necro-inflammatory activity and fibrosis progression, may vary depending on each case and the time after transplantation. Especially during the first 6 months following transplantation, recurrent HCV infection may cause severe liver graft dysfunction. During this period, the histopathological changes of a grafted liver with recurrent HCV infection are often atypical and difficult to differentiate from other complications, such as ACR and biliary complications. A definite histopathological diagnosis of recurrent HCV can be made when H&E stained liver biopsies show findings characteristic of recurrent HCV such as a variable degree of mononuclear portal inflammation, interface activity, lobular disarray, and spotty hepatocyte necrosis. However, in practice, the examination of H&E-stained liver biopsy is often done before a definite diagnosis of recurrent HCV hepatitis can be established. The clinical situations associated with the diagnosis and management of recurrent HCV are often stressful for clinicians.

Antiviral treatment can be initiated in the early weeks after liver transplantation, irrespective of biochemically or histologically proven recurrent HCV hepatitis. However, according to preliminary studies, the response rate is not higher than in treatment initiated after a definite diagnosis and the tolerability of treatment in these early transplant periods is limited. This pre-emptive antiviral therapy soon after liver transplantation is still under evaluation. At present, antiviral treatment after a definite diagnosis of recurrent HCV is accepted as a standard therapy. Since early recurrent HCV often causes severe liver graft dysfunction, an early definite histopathological diagnosis is essential for the early commencement of antiviral therapy. Therefore, the detection of HCV replicative intermediates or antigens in liver biopsies may be helpful for the early diagnosis and optimal medical management of patients with recurrent HCV after liver transplantation.

2.2.2 Immunohistochemical detection of HCV antigens for recurrent HCV after liver transplantation

The post-transplant HCV-RNA serum levels usually reach 10-20 times the pre-transplantation levels, presumably because of immunosuppression. Although it is easy to show systemic HCV infection through serum HCV-RNA levels, it is more difficult to evaluate the actual state of HCV infection in the grafted liver. The presence of HCV-RNA in liver biopsy specimens has been shown by *in situ* hybridization (Agnello et al., 1998) or by reverse-transcriptase *in situ* polymerase chain reaction (Fragulidis et al., 1998). However, these methods have technical difficulties and have not been widely used. In contrast, the detection of HCV antigens in liver grafts is easy and sensitive enough for clinical use in the management of patients after liver transplantation. Thus, considering the above-mentioned problems of diagnosing recurrent HCV, immunohistochemical detection of HCV antigens in liver grafts could provide potentially important pathological information, making possible a correlation between viral replication in liver grafts and recurrent HCV after liver transplantation. Several studies suggested that the immunohistochemical staining of HCV antigens in liver grafts correlated with the severity of recurrent HCV after liver transplantation (Gane et al., 1996; Pessoa et al., 2008; Vargas et al., 1998; Verslype et al., 2003).

2.3 Immunohistochemical staining of liver grafts using IG222 mAb against HCV-Envelope 2

Several monoclonal and polyclonal antibodies against HCV antigens have been used for the immunohistochemical analysis of HCV antigens in liver biopsy specimens of hepatitis C patients. Of these antibodies, IG222 is reported to have a strong immunoreactivity to the HCV-E2 protein in both fresh-frozen tissue and paraffin-embedded tissue (Verslype et al., 2003). Verslype et al. reported that immunohistochemical staining using IG222 mAb had a sensitivity of 96%, a specificity of 91% and an overall accuracy of 94.8% in their 253 patients with chronic hepatitis C. Based on those findings, we decided to use IG222 for the immunohistochemical analysis of liver grafts. In this section, we describe our data (Sadamori et al., 2009) about the immunohistochemical staining of liver grafts using IG222 mAb in patients who underwent liver transplantation for HCV associated liver failure.

2.3.1 Longitudinal immunohistochemical analysis of a case of recurrent HCV

Figure 1 summarizes the clinical course of a patient with early recurrent HCV after living donor liver transplantation (LDLT). Immunoreactivity to IG222 mAb was weakly positive on a liver biopsy specimen on postoperative day (POD) 31 showing moderate ACR (Fig. 2A and 3A). After the improvement of liver function tests by steroid pulse therapy, the liver function tests increased again around POD 55. A H&E stained liver biopsy on POD 59 showed mild portal inflammation, endothelial inflammation of portal venules, and an intra-acinar acidophilic body, leading to the diagnosis of probable recurrent HCV (Fig. 2B). At that stage, the immunoreactivity to IG222 mAb was already moderate (Fig. 3B). With further deterioration shown in liver function tests, another liver biopsy on POD 80 confirmed a definite diagnosis of recurrent HCV (Fig. 2C) accompanied by marked immunoreactivity to IG222 mAb (Fig. 3C). The findings in this case show the diagnostic usefulness of the immunohistochemical staining of liver grafts using IG222 mAb.

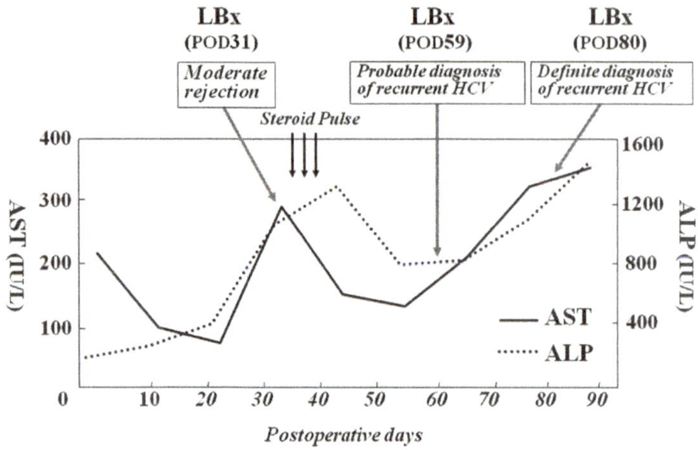

Fig. 1. Clinical course of a representative patient with post-LDLT early recurrent HCV.

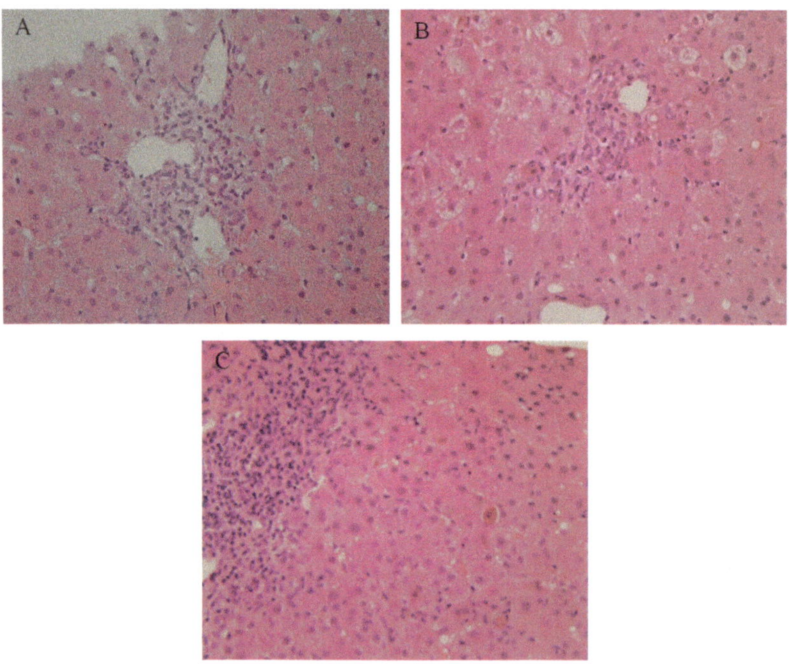

Fig. 2. Findings of H&E stained liver biopsy specimens (A) Liver biopsy specimen obtained on POD 31 showed moderate acute cellular rejection. (Original magnification x160) (B) Liver biopsy specimen obtained on POD 59 showed mild portal inflammation and an intra-acinar acidophilic body, leading to the diagnosis of probable recurrent HCV. (Original magnification x160) (C) Liver biopsy specimen obtained on POD 80 showed marked portal inflammation, intra-acinar inflammatory cell infiltration and intra-acinar spotty necrosis, leading to the diagnosis of definite recurrent HCV. (Original magnification x160)

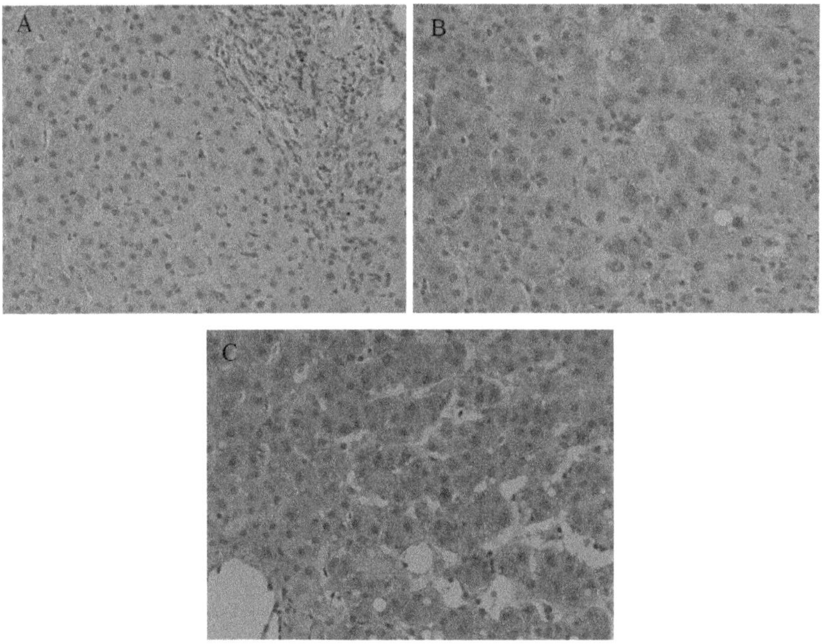

Fig. 3. Immunohistochemistry for HCV-E2 in liver biopsy specimens
(A) Immunohistochemistry for HCV-E2 in a liver biopsy obtained on POD 41 based on a suspected acute rejection episode. Note the weakly positive immunoreactivity to IG222. (Original magnification x200) (B) Immunohistochemistry for HCV-E2 in liver biopsy obtained on POD 59 of a case with probable diagnosis of recurrent HCV based on the examination of H&E-stained sections. Note the moderate immunoreactivity to IG222. (Original magnification x200) (C) Immunohistochemistry for HCV-E2 in a liver biopsy obtained on POD 80, of a case with definite diagnosis of recurrent HCV based on the examination of H&E-stained sections. Note the marked immunoreactivity to IG222. (Original magnification x200).

2.3.2 Serial changes in immunoreactivity to IG222 mAb after LDLT

Previous study reported that HCV antigen expression in transplanted liver grafts was detected as early as 10 days post-transplantation in 25% of liver biopsy specimens and within 3 weeks in 50% of specimens (Ballardini et al., 2002). By the time histological recurrent HCV is clinically overt, HCV antigens can be detected in more than 90% of liver biopsy specimens (Ballardini et al., 2002; Gane et al., 1996; Guerrero et al., 2000). We performed immunohistochemical staining using IG222 mAb on 84 liver biopsy specimens obtained from 28 patients who underwent LDLT for HCV associated liver failure. Immunohistochemistry using IG222 mAb was performed on paraffin sections of all liver biopsies by a two-step indirect EnVision technique. To investigate serial changes of HCV antigen expression in liver grafts, the 84 liver biopsy specimens were divided into three groups according to the time elapsed from LDLT: Group $POD_{1\text{-}30}$ (28 specimens), Group $POD_{31\text{-}179}$ (34 specimens), and Group $POD_{\geq 180}$. (22 specimens). Table 1 lists the grade of immunoreactivity to IG222 mAb in the above-mentioned three groups classified according to the time after LDLT. Immunoreactivity to IG222 for HCV-E2 was detected in 78.6% of the liver biopsy specimens obtained during the first month after LDLT, and there were no significant differences in the grades of immunohistochemical staining between the three groups classified according to the time elapsed from LDLT. Our data shows that constant HCV antigen expression in liver grafts is observed relatively early after liver transplantation and is not associated with the time elapsed from the transplantation.

Group	No.of liver specimens	No.of patients	Grade of Anti-HCV-E2 immunoreactivity	Serum HCV-RNA level (KIU/ml)
POD_{1-30}	28	22	0+ :6 1+ :11 2+ :8 3+ :3	2124 ± 354
POD_{31-179}	34	24	0+ :4 1+ :19 2+ :9 3+ :2	3196 ± 295
$POD_{>180}$	22	19	0+ :1 1+ :17 2+ :4 3+ :0	2778 ± 381

IHS: Immunohistochemical staining HCV-E2: HCV-envelope 2 POD: Postoperative days

NOTE. Comparison of IHS grades (Mann-Whitney *U* test): There were no significant comparisons among three groups.
Comparison of serum HCV-RNA levels (Mann-Whitney *U* test): There were no significant comparisons among three groups.
*The grade of IHS from 0+ to 3+ scale (0+ : neg, 1+: <5%, 2+: 5-20%, 3+: >20% positive hepatocytes).

Table 1. The grades of IHS and serum HCV-RNA levels among three groups classified according to the time after LDLT

2.3.3 Immunohistochemical staining with IG222 mAb for differentiating recurrent HCV from other complications

Based on our histological evaluation of H&E stained specimens, 34 liver biopsy specimens obtained from LDLT recipients were diagnosed as follows: definite recurrent HCV in 12, probable recurrent HCV in 7, definite ACR in 7 and other complications in 8. The other complications comprised of drug-induced liver injury in 1, cytomegalovirus hepatitis in 1, cholestasis due to biliary stricture in 3 and non-specific cholestasis in 3. Figure 4 shows the grade of immunohistochemical staining with IG222 mAb in the above-mentioned four different post-transplant conditions. In our study, the grade of HCV-E2 expression was significantly higher in liver grafts with definite and probable recurrent HCV compared with those with ACR and other complications (mainly biliary complications). These data suggested that strong HCV-E2 expression in liver grafts is associated with recurrent HCV after LDLT when IG222 mAb is used for the immunohistochemical staining of the liver grafts. Therefore, immunohistochemical staining of liver grafts using IG222 mAb can be an innovative approach for differentiating recurrent HCV from other complications including ACR and for aiding the decision to commence antiviral treatment.

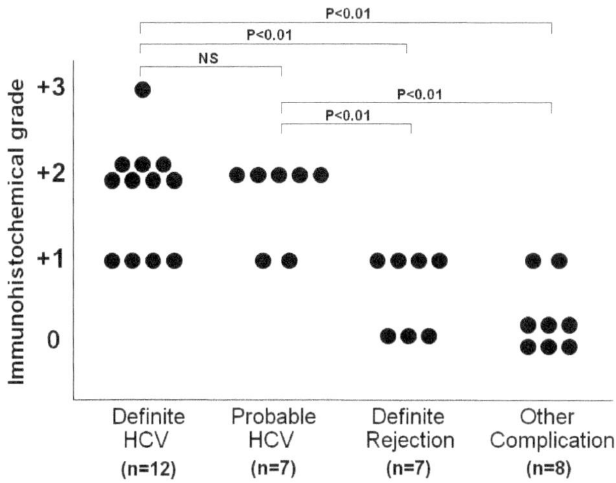

Fig. 4. IG222 immunohistochemical grading in four different post-transplant conditions.

2.3.4 Correlation between immunohistochemical grading and serum HCV-RNA levels

Previous reports investigated the relationship between serum HCV-RNA levels and recurrent HCV after liver transplantation. Some of these studies showed a close correlation between serum HCV-RNA levels and the presence and severity of recurrent HCV (Di Martino et al., 1997; Feray et al., 1994; Gottschlich et al., 2001). However, others groups

Histological assessment	No.of liver specimens	Grade of Anti-HCV-E2 immunoreactivity *	Serum HCV-RNA level (KIU/ml)
Definite HCV	12	0+ :0 1+ :4 2+ :7 3+ :1	3368 ± 525
Probable HCV	7	0+ :0 1+ :2 2+ :5 3+ :0	3671 ± 840
Definite rejection	7	0+ :3 1+ :4 2+ :0 3+ :0	2925 ± 639
Other complications	8	0+ :5 1+ :3 2+ :0 3+ :0	4211 ± 408

IHS: Immunohistochemical staining HCV-E2: HCV-envelope 2

NOTE. Comparison of IHS grades (Mann-Whitney *U* test): Definite HCV *v* Probable HCV, P = NS; Definite HCV *v* Definite rejection, P = .002; Definite HCV *v* Other complications, P = .0001; Probable HCV *v* Definite rejection, P = .009; Probable HCV *v* Other complications, P = .002; Definite rejection *v* Other complications, P = NS.

Comparison of serum HCV-RNA levels (Mann-Whitney *U* test): There were no significant comparisons among four post-transplant conditions.

*The grade of IHS from 0+ to 3+ scale (0+: neg, 1+: <5%, 2+: 5-20%, 3+: >20% positive hepatocytes).

Table 2. The grades of IHS and serum HCV-RNA levels in four different post-transplant conditions.

found no such correlation (Chazouilleres et al., 1994; Freeman et al., 1996; Zhou et al., 1996). In our study, the serum HCV-RNA levels in the specimens with definite and probable recurrent HCV were comparable with those with definite ACR and other complications (Table 2). In addition, the expression of HCV-E2 in liver grafts did not correlate with serum HCV-RNA levels when our data of 84 liver biopsy specimens was analyzed. Previous studies indicated that HCV can replicate efficiently in extrahepatic tissues and cell types, including peripheral blood mononuclear cells, lymph nodes, and bone marrow, particularly in immunosuppressed patients (Blackard et al., 2006; Laskus et al., 1998; Radkowski et al., 1998). Extrahepatic replication of HCV may help explain the lack of correlation between serum HCV-RNA levels and HCV-E2 staining in liver grafts.

2.3.5 Assessment of antiviral treatment response after liver transplantation

The course of HCV recurrence after liver transplantation progresses more rapidly and more aggressively than in the immunocompetent non-transplant HCV-infected population. Chronic HCV is observed in almost 70 % of patients 3 years after transplantation (Feray et al., 1994). Moreover, as the progression rate of fibrosis is faster after transplantation, the rate of cirrhosis reaches about 20% at 5 years (Berenguer et al., 2000; Gane et al., 1996). Several attempts have been made to prevent a poor prognosis due to HCV recurrence. Antiviral therapy for patients on the waiting list is attractive, but many patients do not meet the inclusion criteria and cannot receive antiviral treatment. Even if antiviral treatment is initiated despite poor hepatic reserve, many patients will withdraw due to frequent serious adverse events.

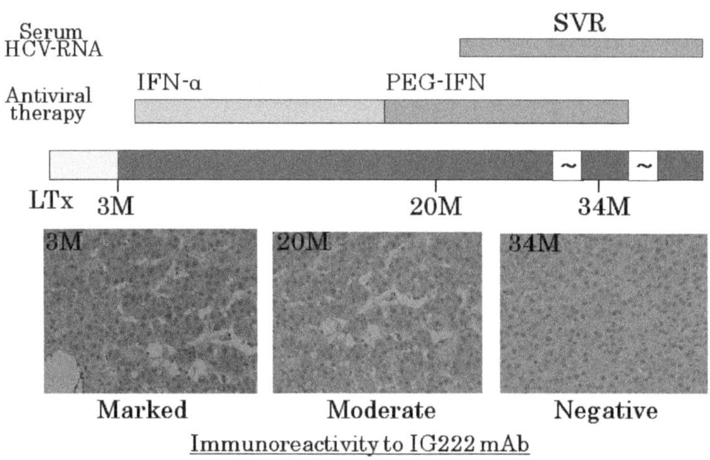

Fig. 5. Clinical course and immunohistochemical staining of liver grafts using IG222 mAb of a patient with recurrent HCV, who achieved sustained virological response (SVR) by antiviral therapy.

Antiviral therapy after transplantation can contribute to the improvement of HCV disease progression in a minority of the overall HCV liver transplant population. In studies using combination therapy with interferon (IFN)-alpha and ribavirin or, more recently, pegylated interferon-alpha (PEG-IFN) plus ribavirin, a sustained virological response (SVR) was achieved in 20-30% of patients (Carrion et al., 2007; Samuel et al., 2003). Figure 5 shows the clinical course and immunohistochemical staining of liver grafts using IG222 mAb of a patient with recurrent HCV, who achieved SVR by antiviral therapy. The grade of HCV-E2 expression on the liver grafts decreased according to the continuation of antiviral therapy and became almost negative when SVR was achieved.

At present, there is no effective therapy for those that don't respond to antiviral therapy or patients who experience a viral relapse after antiviral therapy. For those patients, new innovative strategies to improve therapeutic efficacy and tolerability are needed for the medical management of recurrent HCV after liver transplantation. In addition, immunohistochemical staining of liver grafts with IG222 mAb, directed against HCV-E2, may be useful for the actual evaluation of new medical treatment responses especially for those that don't respond to antiviral therapy.

3. Conclusion

Through the immunohistochemical staining of HCV antigens using reliable antibodies we can assess the actual HCV re-infection and replication in transplanted liver grafts. According to previous studies and our data, the immunohistochemical staining of HCV antigens on liver grafts can contribute to the early and prompt diagnosis of recurrent HCV after liver transplantation. Based on our study, immunohistochemical staining of liver grafts using IG222 mAb is sensitive enough for clinical use and can be useful for differentiating recurrent HCV from other complications, including ACR, and for aiding in the decision to commence antiviral treatment. In the future, the immunohistochemical staining of HCV antigens on liver grafts should be able to contribute toward identifying patients suitable for early antiviral therapy and assessing the antiviral treatment response for recurrent HCV after liver transplantation.

4. Acknowledgement

This project was supported by an unrestricted research grant from Novartis Japan Inc.

5. References

Agnello V, Abel G, Knight GB, et al. (1998). Detection of widespread hepatocyte infection in chronic hepatitis C. *Hepatology*, 28, pp.573-84.

Ballardini G, De Raffele E, Groff P, et al. (2002). Timing of reinfection and mechanisms of hepatocellular damage in transplanted hepatitis C virus-reinfected liver. *Liver Transpl*, 8, pp.10-20.

Blackard JT, Kemmer N, Sherman KE. (2006). Extrahepatic replication of HCV: Insight into clinical manifestation and biological consequences. *Hepatology*, 44, pp.15-22.

Berenguer M, Ferrell L, Watson J, et al. (2000). HCV-related fibrosis progression following liver transplantation: increase in recent years. J *Hepatol*, 32, pp.673-84.

Carrion JA, Navasa M, Garcia-Retortillo M, *et al.* (2007). Efficacy of antiviral therapy on hepatitis C recurrence after liver transplantation: a randomized controlled study. *Gastroenterology*, 132, pp.1746-56.

Chazouilleres O, Kim M, Combs C, *et al.* (1994). Quantitation of hepatitis C virus RNA in liver transplant recipients. *Gastroenterology*, 106, pp.994-9.

Di Martino V, Saurini F, Samuel D, *et al.* (1997). Long-term longitudinal study of intrahepatic hepatitis C virus replication after liver transplantation. *Hepatology*, 26, pp.1343-50.

Feray C, Gigou M, Samuel D, *et al.* (1994). The course of hepatitis C virus infection after liver transplantation. *Hepatology*, 20, pp.1137-43.
Fragulidis GP, Citrocco RE, Weppler D, et al. (1998). In situ enzymatic oligonucleotide amplification of hepatitis C virus-RNA in liver biopsy specimens (reverse transcriptase in situ polymerase chain reaction) after orthotopic liver transplantation for hepatitis C-related liver disease. *Transplantation*, 66, pp.1472-6.
Freeman RB, Tran S, Lee YM, et al. (1996). Serum hepatitis C RNA titers after liver transplantation are not correlated with immunosuppression or hepatitis. *Transplantation*, 61, pp.542-6.
Gane EJ, Naoumov NV, Qian KP, et al. (1996). A longitudinal analysis of hepatitis C virus replication following liver transplantation. *Gastroenterology*, 110, pp. 167-77.
Gane EJ, Portmann BC, Naoumov NV, et al. (1996). Long-term outcome of hepatitis C infection after liver transplantation. *N Eng J Med*, 334, pp. 815-20.
Gottschlich MJ, Aardema KL, Burd EM, *et al.* (2001). The use of hepatitis C viral RNA levels in liver tissue to distinguish rejection from recurrent hepatitis C. *Liver Transpl*, 7, pp.436-41.
Guerrero RB, Batts KP, Burgart LJ, *et al.* (2000). Early detection of hepatitis C allograft reinfection after orthotopic liver transplantation: a molecular and histologic study. *Mod Pathol*, 13, pp.229-37.
Krawczynski K, Beach M, Di Bisceglie A, et al. (1990). Hepatocellular HCV-associated antigen and antibody: viral specificity and relation to natural history of infection. *Hepatology*, 12, pp. 905-10.
Laskus T, Radkowski M, Wang L, et al. (1998). Search for hepatitis C virus extrahepatic replication sites in patients with acquired immunodeficiency syndrome: specific detection of negative-strand viral RNA in various tissues. *Hepatology*, 28, pp.1398-401.
Pessoa MG, Alves V, Wakamatsu A, et al. (2008). Post-transplant recurrent hepatitis C: immunohistochemical detection of hepatitis C virus core antigen and possible pathogenic implications. *Liver Int*, 28, pp.807-13.
Radkowski M, Wang L, Vargas H, et al. (1998). Detection of hepatitis C virus replication in peripheral blood mononuclear cells after orthotopic liver transplantation. *Transplantation*, 66, pp.664-6.
Roskams T. (2002). The role of immunohistochemistry in diagnosis. *Clin Liver Dis*, 6, pp.571-89.
Sadamori H, Yagi T, Iwagaki H, et al. (2009). Immunohistochemical staining of liver grafts with a monoclonal antibody against HCV-Envelope 2 for recurrent hepatitis C after living donor liver transplantation. J Gastroenterol Hepatol, 24, pp. 574-580.
Samuel D, Bizollon T, Feray C, et al. (2003). Interferon-alpha 2b plus ribavirin in patients with chronic hepatitis C after liver transplantation: a randomized study. *Gastroenterology*, 124, pp. 642-50.
Scheuer PJ, Krawczynski K, Dhillon AP, et al. (1997). Histopathology and detection of hepatitis C virus in liver. *Springer Immunopathols*, 19, pp. 27-45.
Vargas V, Krawczynski K, Castells L, et al. (1998). Recurrent hepatitis C virus infection after liver transplantation: Immunohistochemical assessment of the viral antigen. *Liver Transpl*, 4, pp. 320-7.
Verslype C, Nevens F, Sinelli N, et al. (2003). Hepatic immunohistochemical staining with a monoclonal antibody against HCV-E2 to evaluate antiviral therapy and reinfection of liver grafts in hepatitis C viral infection. *J Hepatol*, 38, pp.208-14.
Zhou S, Terrault NA, Ferrell L, *et al.* (1996). Severity of liver disease in liver transplantation recipients with hepatitis C virus infection: Relationship to genotype and level of viremia. *Hepatology*, 4, pp.1041-6.

Part 3

Liver Biopsy in Children

16

Liver Biopsy as a Useful Tool in the Management of Autoimmune Liver Diseases in Childhood

Giuseppe Maggiore, Marco Sciveres and Aurelio Sonzogni
Department of Pediatrics University of Pisa,
Pediatric Hepatology and Liver Transplant Unit and Pathology Unit,
UPMC-Ismett,
Italy

1. Introduction

Autoimmune diseases of the liver and biliary tract are inflammatory diseases of unknown origin that progress spontaneously, in most cases, to severe fibrosis and cirrhosis (Maggiore et al, 2009). They are characterized by an inflammatory infiltrate in the liver tissue involving the lobule and the portal tract and, most frequently, by the presence of non-organ and liver-specific autoantibody reactivity (Mieli Vergani & Vergani, 2009). There are at least three principal disorders in humans, in which the liver damage is thought to be caused by an autoimmune mechanism: autoimmune hepatitis (AIH), where the target of the autoimmune attack is the hepatocyte, and two other conditions, autoimmune cholangitis (AIC) and primary biliary cirrhosis (PBC), where the target is the cholangiocyte. Between these three disorders exists a range of overlap of liver damage both at diagnosis and/or during the follow-up, recognized as "overlap syndrome" (Alvarez, 2006). Any autoimmune disorder may overlap with the other two. Autoimmune cholangitis may be limited, at diagnosis and during the follow-up, to the smallest intrahepatic (forth order) bile ducts in case of the so-called "small duct sclerosing cholangitis" (Chapman, 2002), or may be diffuse affecting also larger bile duct and giving the typical radiological or MRI imaging of "sclerosing cholangitis"). In children, primary biliary cirrhosis is exceptionally described, particularly before adolescence. Moreover, a rare and peculiar form of autoimmune hepatitis, typical of infancy exists, and is characterized by the unique association of Coombs positive autoimmune hemolytic anemia with the peculiar histopathological finding of diffuse giant cell transformation of the hepatocytes at a very unusual age even for infants (Maggiore et al, 2011).

Immunosuppressive treatment is usually efficacious in most cases of AIH, but it is less effective in autoimmune cholangitis, particularly in case of delayed diagnosis at the stage of diffuse sclerosing cholangitis (Maggiore et al, 2009). Immunosuppressive treatment is also the only life-saving treatment recognized in "infantile giant cell hepatitis associated with autoimmune hemolytic anemia" (Maggiore et al, 2011).

Liver biopsy is of paramount importance in the diagnostic work-up of autoimmune diseases of the liver and biliary tract as recognized by the major guidelines. Histological examination of liver tissue allow to confirm the diagnosis through the presence of suggestive features; to evaluate the degree of biliary tract damage; to establish the severity of architectural injury and the eventual presence of cirrhosis and when necessary, to confirm the diagnosis of relapse in case of discontinuation of treatment.

2. Autoimmune hepatitis

Autoimmune hepatitis is a severe liver disease carrying a high mortality rate if untreated. All ages and genders are affected, with a peak of incidence in prepubertal girls, even if the disease has been diagnosed as early as age six months. The disease often presents acutely or can follow a chronic but fluctuating course, usually progressing to cirrhosis and liver failure, even though the rapidity of progression to end-stage liver diseases is highly variable (Lohse AW & Mieli-Vergani, 2011).

Waldenström first described this disease entity in 1950 in a young woman with a chronic inflammatory liver disease, rapidly evolving to cirrhosis, elevated gamma globulins and amenorrhea. The disease was defined as "lupoid hepatitis" because of the presence of antinuclear antibodies (ANA) and of lupus erythematosus cells. Further progress in the identification and characterization of the autoantibodies typically present in AIH patients, led to a consensus on the definition and classification of this disease.

Autoimmune hepatitis is a rare disease, occurring in all races and in all geographic areas, but with a wide range of prevalence in different populations. Studies in adults have reported, in Europe, a prevalence of 1: 10.000 (Boberg, 2002); however the insidious character of the disease in some patients suggests a considerable higher frequency. In childhood, the incidence of AIH is unknown, but it is apparently increasing in the last 20 years, representing today about 10% of all chronic liver diseases in patients referred to a tertiary pediatric liver centre, in Europe (Mieli Vergani & Vergani, 2008). Female gender is mostly involved, with an F/M ratio from 3:1 up to 9:1. Even though all ages are affected, AIH is mainly a pediatric disease since about 40% of diagnoses of AIH-1 and 80% of AIH-2 are made during childhood and adolescence (Alvarez, 2009).

2.1 Pathogenesis

The mechanisms leading to autoimmune attack of the hepatocytes are unknown, but several observations suggest that AIH is a multifactorial disease (Longhi et al, 2009). The histological pictures of interface hepatitis and immunohistochemical studies have identified, among the immune-reactive inflammatory cells, a large predominance of activated T lymphocytes positive for the CD4+ helper/inducer phenotype. The CD4+ T lymphocytes are believed to recognize one or more self antigens on the cell surface of the hepatocytes, thus triggering the autoimmune response.

2.1.1 Autoantigen presentation

The first step in an immune reaction is the presentation of the antigen to naive CD4+ T lymphocytes. The antigenic peptide is carried by professional antigen-presenting cells (APC) on their membrane within the binding groove of class II human leukocyte antigen (HLA) molecules. These HLA class II molecules are encoded in close proximity to HLA I and HLA III genes, configuring a number of ancestral haplotypes due to strong linkage disequilibrium among the HLA *loci*. The HLA class II molecules expressed on the membrane of APC are able to hold only short peptides of 13-23 amino acid residues, which are the final product of the internalization and partial digestion by the APC of extracellular proteins. The recognition of the complex "HLA II-exogenous peptide" is restricted by the specificity of the T-cell receptor and hampered by ligand to ligand co-stimulation. Consequently, HLA class II plays a central role in regulating CD4+ T helper activity. The functional site of HLA class II, the peptide binding groove, is hosted within the DRα and DRβ polypeptidic chain, which composes together the DR heterodimers. Alleles of the DRβ *locus* are highly polymorphous and present three hypervariable regions encoding amino acid motifs. The consequence of this polymorphism is that each individual carries different DR molecules with different binding properties and affinities. Consequently, the nature and the structure of HLA class II polypeptidic chains, and especially of the DR molecules, critically affect both the nature and the alignment of the antigenic peptide and the affinity and avidity of the linkage between the antigen major histocompatibility complex (MHC) II and the T-cell receptor. Thus, the suitability of certain autoantigens to trigger an immune response is genetically determined and depends strictly on the genotypic asset of HLA class II.

2.1.2 Genetic background

In the Caucasian population, the HLA A1-B8-DR3 haplotype is associated to AIH-1 as well as with several autoimmune disorders. The HLA DR3 and DR4 haplotypes were identified as independent risk factors for AIH-1, whereas HLA DR2 was accounted to have a protective role. With the availability of high-resolution HLA-typing methods, the molecular basis of this association became investigable and the principal susceptibility allele for AIH-1 was recognized in *DRB1*0301* (Czaja, 2000). This allele not only confers an increased risk to develop AIH-1, but also influences some features of the disease. Patients bearing *DRB1*0301* in fact present at younger age, respond less favorably to corticosteroid treatment, carry a higher risk of relapse, and require liver transplantation more frequently for end-stage liver failure. Genetic predisposition to AIH-1 has, however, a relevant regional variation, and studies outside Europe and North America have found different susceptibility alleles at the DRB1 *locus*. In Japan, the prevalence of DR3 haplotype in the general population is very low and DR4 is the principal risk factor for AIH type. In an adult Brazilian mixed population with different percentages of whites, blacks, and Amerindians, a weak association with *DRB1*1301* (DR6) was found, while in Mexicans of mixed ancestry, the primary HLA association is with *DRB1*0404* as a part of the DR4 serologic subset.

Data concerning HLA typing in children with AIH-1 are scant. European children show the typical pattern for AIH-1 in Caucasoid patients, with a significant prevalence of DR3 (*DRB1*0301*) and DR52a (*DRB3*0101*) and with a low prevalence of DR4. In a large Argentinean series, DR6 (*DRB1*1301*) was the primary susceptibility allele, with a secondary association with *DRB1*0301*, while HLA *DRB1*1302*, which differs by only one amino acid, showed a weak protective role. A study concerning a mixed Brazilian population with a prevalence of patients older than 16 years reported comparable results: *DRB1*1301* was observed more frequently in children than in adults. A secondary association with *DRB1*0301* was recorded in all age groups, but *DRB1*1301* patients were significantly younger than the *DRB*0301* counterpart. More recently, in an array of 50 families from France and Quebec, once more, the *DRB1*1301* allele resulted as the primary genetic risk factor for AIH-1 in children.

Genetic background of AIH-2 has been poorly investigated to date because of the low prevalence of this form in adults. Two reports from Europe focused on the *DRB1*03* and *DQB1*02* alleles, whereas another study conducted in a German population reported an increased frequency of *DRB1*07*, *DRB4*01*, and *DQB1*06*. In a population from Brazil, composed for the large part by pediatric patients, a significant increase of *DRB1*07*, *DRB4*, and *DQB1*02* was observed when compared with healthy controls. The last two alleles were in strong linkage disequilibrium with *DRB1*07*. Speculating on this data in comparison with the patterns of susceptibility showed in adult patients, we can argue that *DRB1*1301* is a relevant risk factor peculiar to pediatric age and, interestingly, among adult patients it is associated with younger age.
The DR4 family of alleles seems not to be implicated in children, whereas in adults they have been described as a marker of a mild, late-onset disease. This might explain the peculiar epidemiology of AIH-1 in Japan, where HLA DR3 has a very low prevalence in the general population and pediatric cases of AIH are rare.

2.1.3 Autoantigens

The autoimmune response, independently of the trigger, develops against one or more autoantigens (Bogdanos, 2009). Recognition of these autoantigens might be the key factor in developing an etiologic-based therapy. Unfortunately, most of the antigens recognized by autoantibodies detected in AIH are either nonspecific or intracellular molecules and unlikely to be involved in breaking self-tolerance and provoking the emergence of liver-infiltrating immunocytes. The most likely candidate autoantigens seem to be the asialoglycoprotein receptor (ASGP-R) for AIH-1 and CYP2D6 for AIH-2. The ASGP-R is an organ-specific molecule located in the membrane and with a prevalent periportal expression. Both peripheral and infiltrating lymphocytes taken from adults and children with AIH show a proliferative response to purified human ASGP-R and can induce autologous B-lymphocytes to produce anti-ASGP-R autoantibodies *in vitro*. A lack of T suppressing function specific for ASGP-R has been also reported both in patients and in their healthy relatives. This defect seems to reside in a subpopulation of CD4+ T-cells and it is inherited as an autosomal, non HLA-linked trait and it is corrigible by immunosuppressive therapy. Unfortunately, auto-reactivity against ASGP-R is not AIH-specific and its pathogenetic role is far from being defined.
Seven isoforms of cytochrome P450 are highly expressed in human liver: two major isoforms, CYP2C and CYP3A that account for 50% of total CYP expression and five minor isoforms, including CYP2D6. All these isoforms have been identified as LKM targets in different types of liver diseases such as autoimmune, viral, and drug-induced liver diseases. The likely molecular target of AIH-2, CYP2D6, is an intracellular enzyme active in phase I detoxification of several drugs. The CYP2D6 was extensively studied to map the most frequent epitopes in LKM-1. Several short sequences were identified and each of them was labeled, *via* gene bank searches, as cross-reacting with viral proteins, or human proteins involved in other autoimmune disorders. The sequence 193-212 of CYP2D6 is recognized by 93% of the AIH-2 sera and 50% of the LKM-1/HCV-positive sera, and presents extensive cross-reaction with HCV and cytomegalovirus peptides. Furthermore, inhibition studies of the CYP2D6 enzymatic activity showed clearly that conformational epitopes exist and are functionally prevalent. By the effect of some cytokines, CYP2D6 can be expressed on hepatocyte surfaces, becoming a potential target for auto reactive T-cells. Several viruses

had been proposed as triggering factors in the pathogenesis of AIH such as measles virus, Epstein-Barr virus, hepatitis A virus, or herpes simplex virus. Molecular mimicry had been equally invoked between CYP2D6 and the IE 175 protein of herpes simplex virus, but presently none of these viruses is considered as a specific cause of AIH in genetically susceptible individuals.

2.1.4 Autoimmune reaction as a defect of immune regulation

High titers of antibodies against different microbial antigens are present in patients with AIH; this non antigen-specific defect, also present in first-degree relatives, is correctable both *in vivo* and *in vitro* by pharmacologic doses of corticosteroids and is related to a generic impairment of "T-cell suppression". Children with this condition have low level of CD8-expressing T-cells, which segregate with the possession of HLA haplotype B8 DR3. Furthermore, patients with AIH have been reported to have a specific defect in a subpopulation of T lymphocytes controlling the immune response to liver-specific antigens expressed on the hepatocyte membrane. More recently, a CD4+ T-cell subset expressing the interleukin 2 (IL-2) receptor, known as CD25 regulatory T-cells, have been found to be reduced in number at diagnosis of AIH. This CD4+ T-cell subset regulates the proliferation of auto-reactive T-cells through the release of immunoregulatory cytokines such as IL-10.

2.2 Clinical features

Autoimmune hepatitis is heterogeneous in nature and it is usually classified in two types according to the pattern of the autoantibody panel detected at the time of diagnosis (Odièvre, 1983). Type 1 AIH is characterized by the presence of anti-smooth muscle antibody and/or antinuclear antibody and AIH-2 by the presence of anti-liver-kidney microsomal antibody type 1 and/or anti-liver cytosol type 1 antibody. The ratio of incidence of the two types in Europe is 2:1, while it is 7:1 or greater in America and in Japan. In Europe, AIH-2 represents about 20% of new diagnoses of AIH, while in the USA AIH-2 represents only 5%. Differences between the two types consist in the epidemiologic distribution, genetic markers, and clinical presentation (table 1), which might underlie the different pathogenetic mechanism and include (Mieli Vergani & Vergani, 2009):

- AIH-1 affects children and adults, while AIH-2 is almost exclusively a childhood disease;
- Patients with AIH-2 are younger and have a higher tendency to present as an acute liver failure;
- Hypergammaglobulinemia, which is quite typical of AIH-1, is moderate and occasionally absent in AIH-2;
- AIH-2 progresses through "flares" of necrosis usually spontaneously regressing and this can explain why AIH-2 can be characterized by transitory phases of mild histological activity;
- AIH-2 is almost never associated to evidence of bile duct lesions, dissimilar to AIH- 1 where different degrees of bile duct lesion are common;
- Extrahepatic autoimmune disorders are reported in patients with both types of AIH and in first-degree relatives with a higher prevalence of autoimmune thyroid (Grave's and Hashimoto diseases) and skin (vitiligo and alopecia) disorders in AIH-2.

	AIH type 1	AIH type 2	Small ducts autoimmune sclerosing cholangitis	Autoimmune diffuse sclerosing cholangitis
Age of onset	infancy and early childhood	infancy and early childhood	all ages	usually adolescence
Symptoms at onset	Symptomatic acute hepatitis	Symptomatic acute hepatitis	Often related to the associated inflammatory bowel disease	Often related to the associated inflammatory bowel disease
Cirrhosis at onset	not frequent	not frequent	not frequent	possible
Hypergammaglobulinemia	possible	possible	possible	possible
Biliary lesions	absent	absent	constant	constant
Autoantibodies	LKM1, LC1	LKM1, LC1	ANA, SMA, p/cANCA, SLA	ANA, SMA, p/cANCA, SLA
Extrahepatic disorders except IBD	Frequent	Frequent	possible	possible
Associated IBD	Unusual	Unusual	frequent	almost constant
Response to immunosuppressive treatment	usually good	usually good	possible	uncertain

Table 1. Main clinical features of autoimmune hepatitis in children.

Despite this heterogeneity, available data suggest a similar outcome and a similar response to treatment.

Beside these two main clinical-serological subtypes, in about 10% of patients AIH may present as a cryptogenic chronic hepatitis with the same demographic, biochemical, histological features and the same response to immunosuppressive therapy of both subtypes of AIH, but in absence of any recognizable autoantibody reactivity pattern. This entity recently described in adults as seronegative autoimmune hepatitis it has been also recognized in children. Recognition and treatment of SAIH are necessary to prevent progression to end-stage liver disease and liver biopsy in such patients play a pivotal role.

Overall, there are three clinical patterns of disease onset:

- The most frequent is indistinguishable from that of an acute viral hepatitis, with malaise, anorexia, nausea, vomiting, and abdominal pain followed by jaundice, dark urine, and pale stools. Some patients, particularly anti-LKM-1 positive, may develop acute liver failure with encephalopathy (Maggiore et al, 1990). Identifying autoimmune hepatitis as the etiology of acute liver failure is potentially important, because administering appropriate immunosuppressive therapy might avoid the need for liver transplantation. Even clinical and histological criteria of autoimmune acute liver failure have not been fully defined; liver histology may be particularly helpful in suggesting the diagnosis.
- About 30% of patients, with a higher frequency for AIH type 1, have an insidious onset with an illness characterized by progressive fatigue, anorexia, weight loss, or a relapsing course with jaundice eventually followed by a spontaneous partial recovery, sometimes even a complete normalization of liver function tests, even if acute exacerbation is usually experienced within a few months (Maggiore et al 1993). Patients may progress with a fluctuating course lasting for several months/years before diagnosis (Maggiore et al 1984). Firm hepatomegaly, splenomegaly and signs of liver function impairment are, however, frequent and cirrhosis or severe fibrosis is often present at diagnosis.
- Between 10-15% of patients may be completely asymptomatic when the underlying disease is accidentally discovered by the finding of hepatomegaly or by an increase of aminotransferase activity.
- Rarely, AIH may present with bleeding from esophageal varices as a complication of portal hypertension, or with symptoms related to an associated extrahepatic autoimmune disorder such as chronic diarrhea, weight loss, and goiter.

Autoimmune extrahepatic disorders are reported in about 30% of patients and include autoimmune thrombocytopenia, autoimmune hemolytic anemia, type 1 insulin-dependent, diabetes, autoimmune thyroiditis, vitiligo, cutaneous vasculitis, uveitis, glomerulonephritis, juvenile chronic arthritis, systemic lupus erythematosus, and Sjögren's disease. Celiac disease, in particular, may be associated with all types of autoimmune liver disorders with a particular high frequency (Caprai et al, 2008).

A form of AIH akin to AIH-2 affect some 20% of patients with autoimmune polyendocrinopathy-candidiasis-ectodermal dystrophy (APECED). APECED is an autosomal-recessive disorder caused by mutations in the autoimmune regulator (AIRE1) gene, and is characterized by a variety of autoimmune diseases accompanied by chronic muco-cutaneous candidiasis. These disorders include hypoparathyroidism and autoimmune adrenalitis. The AIRE1 gene is highly expressed in the thymus and the protein encoded by the gene is involved in clonal deletion of self-reactive T-cells. AIRE1 monoallelic mutations have been reported also in a few children with severe AIH-2 and extrahepatic autoimmune disorders.

2.3 Laboratory findings

Besides the presence of specific autoantibodies that characterize the two types of AIH, abnormal laboratory findings exploring evidence of liver injury and/or abnormal liver function are frequent in AIH. Serum aminotransferase activity, which is the most sensitive test of ongoing liver injury, is increased in all untreated patients, sometimes markedly, up to or more than 50-times the upper normal limit. Gamma glutamyltransferase (GGT) activity commonly exploring evidence of bile duct injury, may be normal or slightly elevated. A significant increase of GGT should lead to suspect relevant bile duct damage as in the case of autoimmune cholangitis or overlap syndrome. Total serum gamma globulins are elevated in about 80% of patients, sometimes markedly; the increase concerns particularly immunoglobulin G class. This feature is typical of AIH-1, but may be absent in young patients with AIH-2 presenting with acute onset. Partial or complete serum immunoglobulin class A deficiency and genetically determined low levels of C4 can be found and are more common in AIH-2. Serum albumin may be normal in the early phases of the disease, but it may be reduced in case of cirrhosis with liver insufficiency. Reduction of protrombin activity reflects the severity of liver function impairment together with the level of total bilirubin, in case of acute presentation with severe liver dysfunction.

2.3.1 Autoantibodies

Determination of traditional autoantibodies (ANA, SMA and LKM-1) is very helpful when diagnosing AIH (Krawitt, 2011). Their assessment is performed by indirect immunofluorescence (IF), a diagnostic technique, somewhat out of fashion because it is time-consuming and requires experienced technicians and laboratory physicians (Vergani et al, 2004). However, IF testing on murine tissue sections remains the gold standard for the detection ANA, SMA and LKM-1 reactivity. ANA fluorescence pattern, which in AIH is usually homogeneous, can be further characterized using Hep2 cells which are less specific when used as a screening. Both ANA and SMA are hallmarks of AIH-1, and they are usually present at high (≥ 1:100) titer and their presence is usually mutually exclusive.
Rat stomach is commonly used as substrate to detect SMA: uniform staining of the *muscolaris mucosae* as well as staining of the blood vessels walls (V) and of the parietal cell is characteristic. In rat kidney tissue, a faint staining of the mesangial area of glomeruli (G) and of the brush border of proximal renal tubular cells (T) is also present. The "VG" and "VGT" are the most frequent IF staining pattern detected in AIH. Smooth muscle antigen is directed against structural components of the cytoskeleton such as actin, desmin, and troponin. The SMA reactivity in AIH is mostly directed against filamentous (F) actin, present in the hepatocytes as a part of the cytoskeleton in close proximity to the plasma membrane. Anti-F-actin reactivity, which corresponds to the "VGT" IF pattern, is present in the majority of patients with AIH, especially children, even if its absence does not exclude the diagnosis of AIH (Maggiore et al, 1993). Antinuclear antibodies have various patterns of IF: homogeneous, the most common (60%), speckled (15-25%), and mixed homogeneous/speckled. Several nuclear antigens with a wide range of molecular weight were identified as a target of ANA reactivity. There is no evidence in ANA-positive AIH

patients of an association of a particular nuclear antigen with specific clinical manifestations of AIH or with treatment outcome. The IF ANA pattern is not counted on to have clinical importance and it could vary in the same patient during follow-up. The cut-off titer for the positivity of ANA is commonly indicated to be 1:40 in children. Our experience, however, suggests in clinical practice to raise the cut-off point to 1:100 to avoid over diagnosis due to low specificity of such autoantibody.

Anti-LKM-1 serum reactivity defines AIH-2 (Maggiore et al, 1986). Anti-microsomal antibodies are a heterogeneous group, associated to a number of immune-mediated hepatic diseases such as drug-induced hepatitis, chronic viral hepatitis (HCV and HDV) and APECED. The distinctive IF pattern of LKM-1 on rodent liver and kidney sections is a diffuse cytoplasmic staining of microsome of hepatocytes and of the proximal renal tubular cells (P3 portion). A weak staining of the distal tubules is occasionally present and this can generate confusion with anti-mitochondrial antibody (AMA). Positivity for AMA in childhood patients should therefore be considered with caution since AMA-positive AIH or primary biliary cirrhosis are entities extremely rare in this age group. The LKM-1 target a 50 kDa antigen identified as cytochrome P450 2D6 (CYP2D6) (Gueguen et al, 1988) and inhibits *in vitro* but not *in vivo* CYP2D6 activity. Also, LKM-1 can be present in a small proportion (5-10%) of HCV-related hepatitis, even if the target epitopes are different. The role of LKM-1 antibody in the pathogenesis of liver cell injury is debated. The recent demonstration that CYP2D6 can be expressed on liver cell surface and the finding that immunization in mice with human CYP2D6 can induce liver damage suggests that LKM-1 might play a role in inducing liver cell damage in AIH (Muratori et al, 2000).

Anti-liver cell cytosol antibody 1 is an organ-specific autoantibody and its presence also characterizes AIH-2. It was identified by IF, immunodiffusion, and immunoblotting techniques and characteristically stains the cytoplasm of the rat hepatocytes in a homogeneous pattern, sparing the cellular layer around lobular central veins without staining of the proximal renal tubules (Martini et al, 1988). Liver cytosol-1 antibodies recognize a 58-62 kDa liver-specific antigen identified as formiminotransferase cyclodeaminase (Lapierre et al, 1999). Liver cytosol-1 can be present on its own as a sole autoantibody (Bridoux-Henno et al, 2004), can be found associated with LKM-1 reactivity in about 50% of AIH-2, and occasionally it has also been described associated with anti-SMA at low titer and in adults with HCV-related chronic hepatitis.

In 20-30% of adult patients lacking ANA, SMA, or LKM-1, the diagnosis of AIH can be suggested by the finding of other, less common autoantibodies such as anti-soluble liver antigen (SLA/LP) or anti-neutrophil cytoplasmic antibody (ANCA). None of these autoantibodies except SLA is specific for AIH since they are found either in several systemic autoimmune diseases, or in liver diseases of infectious etiology such as HCV infection. Anti-soluble liver antigen is a non specie-specific, non organ-specific antibody currently assessed by immuno-enzymatic or radio immunological assays. The target antigen is likely to be a 50 kDa 422-amino acid protein, identical to previous liver pancreas antigen. Soluble liver antigens are present in patients with AIH-1, AIH-2. Antibodies to SLA/LP are of a major diagnostic value for AIH-1, including overlap syndromes but are not found in association with anti-liver/kidney/microsome type 1 or antibodies to liver cytosol type 1. They are rarely present in other liver diseases such as hepatitis C and drug-induced hepatitis.

Antineutrophil cytoplasmic antibodies have a heterogeneous pattern of target antigens and are commonly distinguished as cytoplasmic (cANCA), perinuclear (pANCA) and atypical perinuclear (apANCA). They have been described in AIH-1 and in ASC patients with all types of pattern, while they are virtually absent in AIH-2.

Once diagnosis is made, autoantibody reactivity fluctuates during treatment, reducing in titer in case of remission, but also independently. Autoantibody status is not predictive of laboratory and histological features; moreover, high serum titers at presentation do not identify patients with more aggressive disease or different treatment outcomes. Finally, the disappearance of autoantibodies is not predictive of low risk of relapse during treatment or of sustained remission in case of stopping the treatment.

2.4 Histology

The histological hallmark of AIH is "interface hepatitis", defined as a dense, inflammatory infiltrate of mononuclear cells, lymphocytes (mainly T helper and natural killer), plasma cells and activated macrophages infiltrating the portal tract, invading the adjacent parenchyma and surrounding apoptotic hepatocytes with erosion of the limiting plate (Figure 1). Interface hepatitis may be present in other inflammatory liver diseases of different etiologies (viral, drug-induced, etc.) and this peculiar histological picture is to be properly integrated in clinical and biochemical setting.

Plasmacells are considered another significant histopathological hallmark of autoimmune disease; they may be diffusely evident in interface and lobular hepatitis areas, but in about one third of the cases plasmacells are patchy localized within liver parenchyma.

A considerable amount of eosinophilic granulocytes is often present within the portal infiltrate, especially in patients with co-existent celiac disease (Caprai et al, 2008). Most patients with autoimmune hepatitis have parenchymal complications of chronic inflammation such as severe fibrosis and about a third of them are already cirrhotic at presentation. In children, this proportion seems to be even higher. Only patients with very acute presentation may lack features of chronic hepatitis and fibrosis. Cirrhosis in autoimmune hepatitis is often macronodular, and may easily be overlooked by percutaneous liver biopsy. Anyway a confident histological diagnosis of cirrhosis should be proposed only in case of well-defined nodular fibrotic transformation, mainly in cases with severe features of activity, as massive necrosis with parenchymal collapse may lead to a nodular appearance of the liver. Laparoscopy, a minimally invasive technique with the currently available very small diameter endoscopes, is helpful in making a diagnosis of cirrhosis in autoimmune hepatitis, as cirrhosis maybe overlooked in up to 50% of cases without macroscopic assessment of the liver. Diagnosis of cirrhosis may influence the choice and dose of the immunosuppressive agents prescribed, has prognostic implications, and forms the basis for regular screening for complications of cirrhosis, such as esophageal varices bleeding.

Liver histology plays a major role in two particularly challenging diagnostic conditions: the AIH with very acute onset and the seronegative AIH. In case of very acute onset, the inflammatory liver injury, in contrast to classical autoimmune hepatitis, predominates in the centrilobular zone and it is often associated with reticular collapse. In such cases four features may suggest an autoimmune pathogenesis: the presence of massive/submassive hepatic necrosis (Figure 2), the presence of lymphoid follicles within portal tracts (Figure 3), a plasma cell-enriched inflammatory infiltrate and central perivenulitis. Ductular (intermediate) hepatocytes are considered a reactive/regenerative response to injury and more commonly present in case of massive/submassive necrosis serving as hepatic progenitor cells, and could be seen as cytokeratin 7 (CK7)-positive hepatocytes in immunohistochemistry. In case of seronegative autoimmune hepatitis the liver histology represent an invaluable diagnostic tool showing features suggesting an autoimmune pathogenesis. Centrilobular changes are prominent due to the high frequency of acute icteric onset.

Bile duct inflammatory changes are not considered a typical lesion of autoimmune hepatitis. They can be found in limited proportion (about 25% of patients with AIH-1) in form of destructive or not destructive cholangitis and ductopenia. Patients with and without bile duct changes had similar laboratory findings but diagnostic scores for AIH are lower in case of bile duct damage. Patients with destructive cholangitis and/or ductopenia respond as well to therapy as patients with nondestructive cholangitis, and outcome is similar to those of patients without biliary changes.

2.5 Diagnosis

The diagnosis of AIH in children can be easy when all the typical hallmarks of the disease are present, such as the presence of another autoimmune disease in the same patient, hypergammaglobulinemia of IgG type with the demonstration of specific autoantibodies and a suggestive histology. However, in some patients the diagnosis be challenging, and in this case it is usually made by a combination of clinical, serologic, and histologic criteria and by the exclusion of other possible known causes of severe hepatic disease, such as chronic hepatotropic virus infections and Wilson's disease, by appropriate tests.

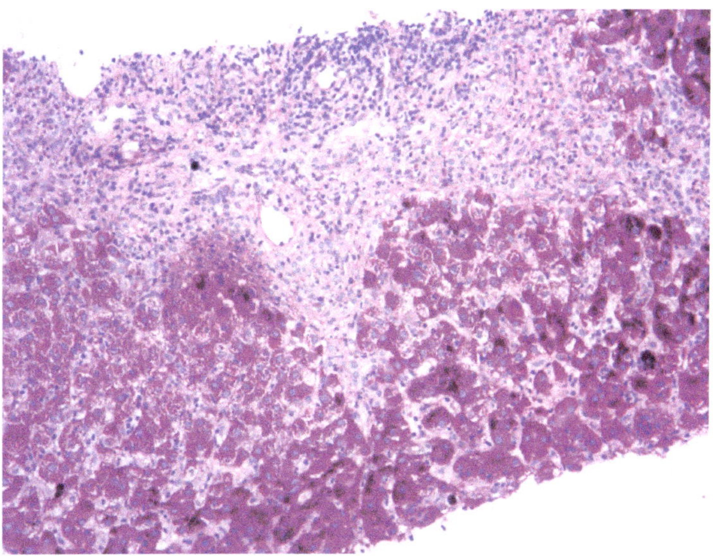

Fig. 1. Presence of dense portal and periportal inflammatory infiltrate with lymphocytes, histiocytes, neutrophilic and eosinophilic granulocytes and plasma cells with interface activity.

Even if histopathology features pathognomonic of autoimmune hepatitis are lacking, liver histology should be always performed at diagnosis if hemostasis allows it. The characteristic lesion of "interface hepatitis", characterized by a predominantly lymphoplasmacytic, necroinflammatory, and periportal infiltrate with or without lobular involvement should suggest the diagnosis. Other suggestive features include the presence of portal-portal or central-portal bridging necrosis, formation of liver cell rosettes and the presence of nodular regeneration, even in the early stages, in the most severe cases. Storage of metals like iron, copper, or intracellular proteins have to be excluded by appropriate histochemical techniques.

Features of biliary damage are usually absent or limited. In case of absence of typical serum autoantibodies, it is mandatory to send a serum sample to a reference laboratory to investigate the presence of autoantibodies not routinely assessed such as ANCA or LC-1. If doubt persists, in case of severe cryptogenetic inflammatory disease, once Wilson's disease is excluded, it is advisable to attempt an immunosuppressive treatment for at least six weeks to evaluate the sensitivity of the disease to immunosuppressive therapy.

To help the diagnosis of autoimmune hepatitis, a panel of physicians and pathologists has published a descriptive set of criteria to classify patients as having either "definite" or "probable" autoimmune hepatitis. This scoring system has been used in a large number of studies and it has shown a good sensibility (89.9%) but a low specificity (60.8%), particularly in cases of immune-mediated biliary diseases like autoimmune cholangitis or primary biliary cirrhosis, which often score as a "probable" autoimmune hepatitis. In 1999 the score was reviewed; however, this scoring system still remains more adapted to adulthood than to childhood since some items, for example, concerning the use of the alkaline phosphatase/aminotransferase ratio due to the low discriminating role of this enzyme in childhood in exploring bile duct damage or alcohol consumption.

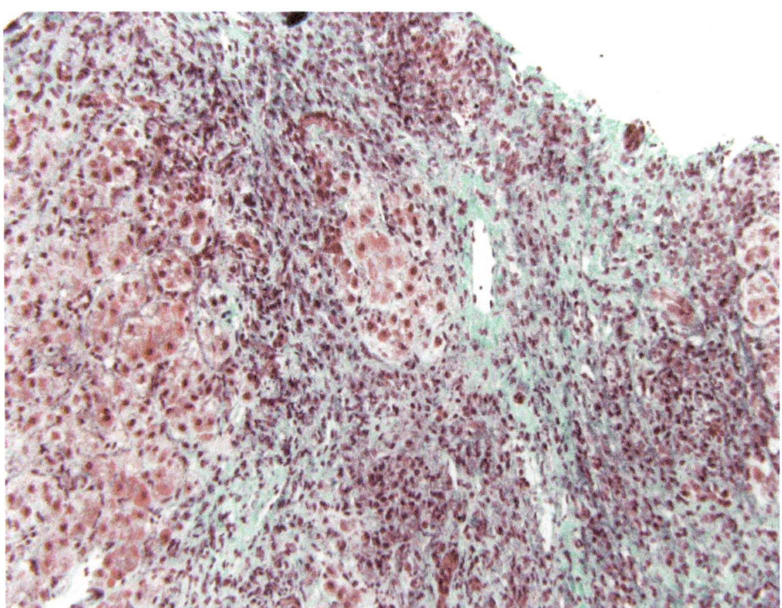

Fig. 2. Submassive necrosis with panlobular and portal inflammatory infiltrate with CD3 and CD20 positive lymphocyte plasmacells and polymorphonuclear eosinophils and neutrophils in a girl with AIH-1 with marked hypergammaglobulinemia and acute onset.

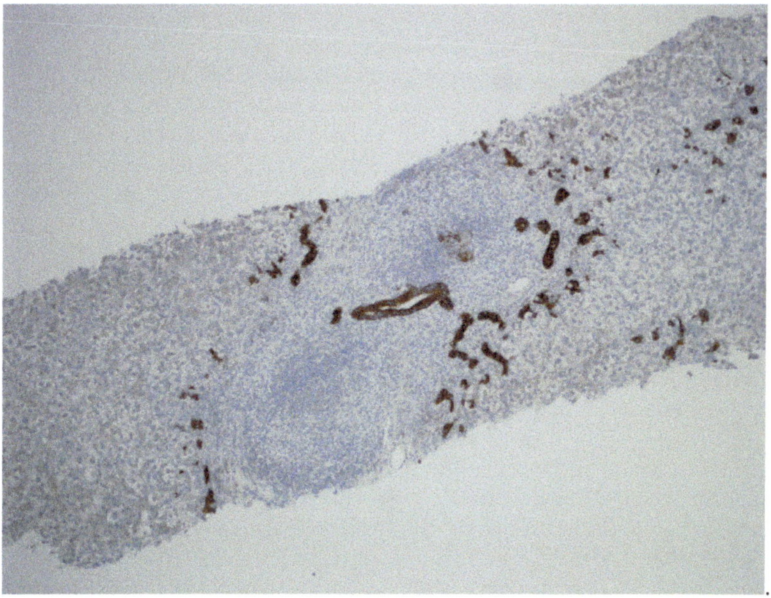

Fig. 3. Lymphocytic infiltrate shaped as lymphoid follicles surrounding two biliary structures with features of destructive cholangitis and marked ductular proliferation (CK7 immunostaining).

2.6 Management

Currently, the most effective therapy for AIH is immunosuppression. The degree of response to treatment depends on the severity of the disease at presentation. Standard treatment includes prednisolone as monotherapy or a combination of prednisone and azathioprine. Prednisone or prednisolone is used at a dose of 2 mg/kg/day (maximum daily dose of 60 mg in adolescents), and azathioprine is prescribed starting from 1 mg/kg/day up to a maximum 2.5 mg/kg/day. Combination therapy from the start of treatment is generally preferred because of the "steroid-sparring" effect of azathioprine that allows reducing the steroid dose more rapidly, avoiding the severe side effects related to their prolonged use at high doses (Maggiore et al, 1984).

2.6.1 Efficacy of the treatment

The first goal of the treatment in AIH is to induce a complete remission of the clinical signs (jaundice, hepatomegaly, and/or splenomegaly) and of the biochemical "activity" of the disease (aminotransferases, gamma globulins). Treatment generally is associated with a measurable clinical and laboratory response within 6-10 weeks that is usually followed by restoration of liver function, when impaired at onset, as demonstrated by the normalization of protrombin activity (Maggiore et al, 1984). Once the response to treatment is established, prednisone doses are gradually decreased, being aware, however, that complete normalization of biochemical parameters takes a longer period of from 6-9 months. Different therapeutic schedules of treatment discontinuation exist; however, discontinuation of therapy should be tailored for individual patients in relation to their characteristics. The shift to alternate-day use of corticosteroids is very suitable as soon as possible because it is associated with a lower incidence of side effects, particularly concerning growth, without increasing the risk of relapse (Maggiore et al, 1984). About 10% of cases, with severe liver function impairment at onset, however, deteriorate despite compliance to therapy. In these cases a "rescue" immunosuppressive therapy, with 2 mg/kg/day of steroids or 1 mg/kg day plus cyclosporine to a target blood level of 200 ± 50 ng/mL has been proven successful in 90% of patients in a mean period of 3 weeks (Cuarterolo et al, 2011). Eventually, the adjunction of cyclosporin as a third immunosuppressant agent or the substitution of azathioprine with mycophenolate mofetil should be assayed (Schramm C & Lohse AW, 2011). Treatment failure should lead to promptly discuss of the opportunity of an early liver transplantation.

2.6.2 Sustained response

Once complete remission is achieved, the goal of treatment becomes to maintain remission and to prevent relapses. The dose of prednisone is to be reduced further to the lowest dose compatible with a clinical and biochemical remission (strictly normal aminotransferases and gamma globulins levels). Small doses of prednisone on alternate-day schedule combined with azathioprine are in fact effective in maintaining remission. Once remission is achieved, a relapse can occur and in most cases it is related to inappropriate patient compliance to the prescribed treatment. To demonstrate histologic remission by a liver biopsy in a patient with long-standing, complete biochemical remission is a question of debate since histologic remission is not absolutely predictive of no risk of relapse. Hepatic fibrosis progresses only in a minority of patients who are compliant to treatment and who maintain a persistent remission. In some cases, fibrosis can even diminish during treatment.

2.6.3 Duration of treatment

No evidence-based data exist on the optimal duration of immunosuppressive treatment. Relapse is frequent if treatment is withdrawn within the first two years. Current experience suggests that sustained remission should be maintained for at least five years, then, in the case of treatment combining prednisone and azathioprine, prednisone should be stopped during the sixth year, maintaining a sustained remission on azathioprine monotherapy for at least another year. Azathioprine monotherapy, as in adults, reduces the likelihood of relapse and maintains sustained remission in most patients with AIH, independent of its serological type. Absence of serum autoantibodies is not predictive of an absence of relapse; however, a sharp increase of the titer of autoantibodies prompts caution in reducing the immunosuppression.

2.6.4 Side effects of treatment

Combination therapy is associated with side effects, mostly caused by prednisone that produces increased appetite, moderate weight increase, sometimes marked and a transitory reduction of height growth. Severe side effects are less frequent in specialized centers, but frequent in less experienced centers and include obesity, growth failure, severe cosmetic changes, cutaneous *striae*, vertebral collapse, hyperglycemia, cataracts responsible for visual impairment, and psychosis. Azathioprine is rarely responsible for severe side effects such as cytopenia necessitating a dosage reduction. Teratogenicity and oncogenicity issues of azathioprine in humans have not been conclusively demonstrated. However, pregnancy should be ruled out in adolescent girls before starting treatment since azathioprine therapy during pregnancy cannot be recommended.

2.6.5 Alternative treatments

Failure to respond to conventional treatment or severe side effects of corticosteroids are clear indications for the use of cyclosporine A. Cyclosporine therapy is effective in inducing remission in patients with AIH at a median dose of 5 mg/kg/day to obtain serum cyclosporine initial concentration in the range of 200-250 ng/ml even if lower levels are often equally effective. Side effects of cyclosporine treatment are few, well tolerated, and disappear after reduction of the dose (Sciveres et al 2004). Once remission is achieved, treatment may be continued at lower doses or patients may be shifted to conventional treatment. Mycophenolate mofetil (MMF, 20 mg/kg twice a day) has been successfully employed in addition to steroids in patients who either did not tolerate azathioprine or did not respond to standard therapy, suggesting that it may represent another alternative strategy of treatment. Side effects of MMF include headache, diarrhea, dizziness, hair loss, and neutropenia.

Liver transplantation is the treatment option of choice in end-stage AIH or in patients with acute severe/fulminant onset who do not respond to rescue immunosuppression. The 5-year posttransplant survival for these AIH-patients is 86% and patient and graft survival, infectious and metabolic complications, and retransplantation rates did not differ between AIH and non-AIH patients (Martin et al 2011). The higher risk for late acute rejection and the greater degree of immunosuppression needed does not compromise outcomes of liver transplantation for AIH.

2.6.6 Long-term prognosis

The long-term prognosis of children with AIH remains uncertain. A sustained remission can be maintained in most patients, without notable side effects, with low-dose immunosuppression. A limited number of patients maintain a sustained remission once the treatment is stopped. Some patients with cirrhosis, in the absence of an evident relapse of the disease, may develop progressive liver insufficiency and need liver transplantation.

3. Autoimmune bile duct disorders

Autoimmune bile duct damage includes primary biliary cirrhosis in adults, autoimmune cholangitis and autoimmune overlap syndrome in adults and children. Since this chapter is devoted to autoimmune disorders in childhood PBC will not be examined.

3.1 Autoimmune cholangitis (AIC)

Autoimmune cholangitis is a chronic, immune-mediated, cholestatic disease of uncertain etiology, characterized by progressive inflammatory damage of intra and extrahepatic bile ducts resulting in obliterative fibrosis and destruction of small bile ducts and fibrosclerotic lesions of large bile ducts. Autoimmune cholangitis (AIC) may be distinguished in two main entities: the more traditional form, the so-called Primary Sclerosing Cholangitis (PSC), a chronic and diffuse inflammatory cholangiopathy potentially involving all orders of intra and extrahepatic bile ducts, characterized by radiographically visible biliary stricture and dilations of large and medium size bile ducts and a variant form with a damage at least initially limited to small bile ducts, the so- called small duct sclerosing cholangitis, (SDSC).

In this form, biliary imaging explored both endoscopic cholangiography or magnetic resonance is normal or present only minor abnormalities. PSC is more common and typical of adulthood, usually progresses to cirrhosis and liver failure and carries an increased risk of cholangiocarcinoma. SDSC is more typical of childhood, and diagnosis may be suspected only on clinical, biochemical, and histologic features showing evidence of biliary inflammatory injury.

3.1.2 Autoimmune (primary) sclerosing cholangitis (PSC)

Autoimmune sclerosing cholangitis is also defined as primary sclerosing cholangitis (PSC) to be distinguished by secondary forms where a wide range of insults may produce similar cholangiographic imaging pattern. Secondary sclerosing cholangitis (SSC) is thought to develop as a consequence of known injuries or secondary to pathological processes of the biliary tree. The most frequently described causes of SSC are longstanding biliary obstruction, surgical or blunt abdominal trauma to the bile duct, ischemic injury to the biliary tree, intra-arterial chemotherapy, portal biliopathy, eosinophilic and/or mast cell cholangitis, recurrent pyogenic cholangitis, primary immune deficiency, and AIDS-related cholangiopathy. PSC can usually be differentiated on the basis of patient's history and the strong association of PSC with inflammatory bowel disease (IBD).

PSC is a rare disease, the true incidence and prevalence of PSC in children is grossly underestimated: recent studies suggest a mean annual incidence rate of 0.23/100,000 compared to 0.77 cases per 100,000 person-year in adults. The incidence of PSC is similar in North American and European countries, but it continues to increase over time, this disease being diagnosed more frequently also in children and adolescents because of increased awareness of this condition and of the widespread use of noninvasive biliary imaging.

3.1.2.1 Pathogenesis

The etiology and pathogenesis of PSC remain very poorly understood. As the disease is associated with autoantibodies and peculiar HLA haplotypes as well as being closely related to IBD, it would appear to be immune mediated. An autoimmune mediated destructive process is also suggested by lymphocytic infiltration into areas of portal damage. PSC is not however a classical autoimmune disease, as it occurs with a slight male predominance compared with the typical female predominance found in classical autoimmune liver diseases such as PBC and AIH. Moreover, PSC does not have the characteristic response to immunosuppressive treatment as seen in classical autoimmune diseases. Circumstantial evidence that PSC may be immune mediated comes from the independent association of PSC with a number of autoimmune diseases. Simultaneous or sequential occurrence of PSC and AIH has been described in both adult and pediatric populations. In general, PSC in children is characterized by more pronounced autoimmune features with a possible overlap with AIH. Serum autoantibodies and in particular, anti-neutrophil cytoplasmic antibodies (ANCA) are largely present in the serum of patients with PSC. They are however not specific for PSC and are also found in AIH. These ANCA may have atypical features distinct from perinuclear-staining anti-neutrophil cytoplasmic antibody (p-ANCA) and by cytoplasmic-staining anti-neutrophil cytoplasmic antibody (c-ANCA). The target antigen for these atypical ANCA is probably a neutrophil nuclear envelope protein. Some authors have suggested that the term p-ANNA is therefore more appropriate as the recognized antigen is not cytoplasmic but originating in the nuclear membrane. The importance of these autoantibodies in the development of PSC is unknown, but current evidence suggests that they are unlikely to play a role in the pathogenesis of PSC. A high proportion of non-specific autoantibodies in addition to p-ANNA are found in patients with PSC, they are of unclear relevance and unhelpful in diagnosis. They include anti-nuclear antibodies anti-smooth muscle antibody, and anti-cardiolipin antibodies without however a demonstrated association with thrombotic disease.

Association studies have identified various HLA molecules and other immunoregulatory genes as determinants of disease susceptibility and progression in PSC. There is an increased frequency of *HLA B8* and *DR3* (*HLA DRB1*0301*) in PSC. *HLA B8* and *DR3* are in linkage disequilibrium and this haplotype is also associated with several organ specific autoimmune diseases including AIH-1, diabetes mellitus, myasthenia gravis and thyrotoxicosis.

There is a T cell predominant portal infiltrate in PSC although the relative proportions and importance of the CD4 and CD8 cells are not known. CD4 cells are seen more commonly in the portal tracts and CD8 cells predominate in areas of interface hepatitis, when present. The cell infiltrate may change as the disease progresses. These cells are functional and are likely to be involved in the pathogenesis of disease.

PSC is strongly linked to IBD but it also runs a course independent from the bowel disease since the disease can develop many years after colectomy. It has been suggested that T lymphocytes generated in the gut during active inflammation persist as long-lived memory cells and undergo enterohepatic circulation and can then trigger an inflammatory response in the liver when activated by an appropriate stimulus. The nature of the stimulus remains unclear; possibilities include hepatic expression of the original priming antigen or possibly mediation solely by the aberrant expression of gut specific adhesion molecules and chemokines. Bacterial antigens may act as molecular mimics in genetically susceptible individuals and cause an immune reaction responsible for initiating PSC. The bacteria are able to get through gut walls made permeable by colonic inflammation; chemokines and cytokines are then released from Kupffer cells in the liver attracting macrophages, monocytes, lymphocytes, activated neutrophils and fibroblasts to the portal tracts.

Finally, defects in the hepatobiliary transport system and in particular, in knockout mice for the *Mdr2* (*Abcb4*) gene, which corresponds to human *MDR3/ABCB4* gene defects, spontaneously develop sclerosing cholangitis with features similar to human PSC. A non-functional ABCB4 protein leads to the formation of a "toxic" bile with increased concentration of free, non-micellar bile acids which cause cholangiocyte injury, pericholangitis, periductal fibrosis and, eventually, sclerosing cholangitis. Studies in PSC patients, however, did not find ABCB4 mutations.

In summary, immune mechanisms play an important role in the pathogenesis of PSC, although it remains unclear whether it is a classical autoimmune disease. There are strong major histocompatibility complex genetic associations including HLA molecules. HLA haplotypes however do not account for all the genetic susceptibility in the development of PSC and there is uncertainty about the importance of genes outside this region. Bacterial antigens may act as molecular mimics in hosts who are genetically susceptible and therefore cause an immune reaction leading to PSC initiation. Lymphocytes may move from the inflamed gut in IBD *via* the enterohepatic circulation and cause inflammation of the liver when activated by a specific stimulus such as bacterially derived antigens.

3.1.2.2 Clinical features

The mean age at diagnosis of PSC in the pediatric population is approximately 13 years with a slight (2:1) predominance in males, but there are an increased number of earlier diagnoses in the first decade of life (Feldstein , 2003). PSC is strictly associated with an inflammatory bowel disease (IBD) reaching more than 80% of cases, while, only 2 -7.5% of children or adolescents affected by IBD develop sclerosing cholangitis (Miloh 2009). This form of IBD predominantly has the features of an ulcerative colitis and in a minority of a Crohn's colitis. A distinctive IBD phenotype, consisting of a prevalence of diffuse colonic involvement (pancolitis), with however a less active disease and even asymptomatic in about 10% of cases; with eventual rectal sparing and backwash ileitis, but with an increased risk in the long term of colonic adenocarcinoma has been suggested (Loftus, 2005). The diagnosis of IBD may precede or closely follow the onset of PSC. A prior history of abdominal pain, diarrhea, and eventually blood in stools is frequently reported by patients or their parents. Two thirds of children who have PSC are symptomatic at the time of diagnosis and the most frequent initial symptoms are related to the IBD or to a generalized inflammatory process. The abdominal pain is fluctuant, whereas fatigue is progressive and usually followed by anorexia and weight loss. Signs or symptoms directly related to the liver disease are rare, particularly in younger patients, and include hepatomegaly, splenomegaly, jaundice, and pruritus. Frequently the disease is discovered because of an occasional finding of increased aminotransferase level without any sign or symptom. The association with other extrahepatic autoimmune disorders, such as autoimmune hemolytic anemia, autoimmune thrombocytopenic purpura, Sjögren's syndrome, and celiac disease, is less frequent than in AIH, but is reported in up to 25% of cases.

3.1.2.3 Laboratory findings

Although there are no specific laboratory features specific of PSC, elevated serum GGT activity is almost always present in these children and reflects the presence of ongoing bile duct injury (Feldstein, 2003). Serum aminotransferase activity is generally elevated in most patients, but the increase of these enzymes is not specific. Serum alkaline phosphatase levels are not as helpful in childhood because of the wide range of normal values for this enzyme during pediatric age, resulting from the increase of bone formation related to growth. Total bilirubin concentration is usually within a normal range in most patients, and signs of hepatic failure are unusual at diagnosis. An increased direct bilirubin level usually characterizes more severe, long-lasting forms with evident macroscopic fibrosclerotic lesions of bile ducts and cirrhosis. On the other hand, jaundice may be transient, secondary to bacterial cholangitis, which can be recurrent and could even finally represent an indication for liver transplantation. Thrombocytopenia and diminished white blood cell count secondary to portal hypertension due to hypersplenism can found in children with splenomegaly. Elevated IgG levels are found in 70% of children with PSC, and circulating autoantibodies that usually characterize AIH-1, such as ANA and/or SMA, are detected in serum of more than 80% of patients. Antineutrophil cytoplasmic antibody, with staining mainly but not exclusively in the periphery of the nucleus, is usually found by indirect IF. Anti-LKM-1 is practically never detected in these patients.

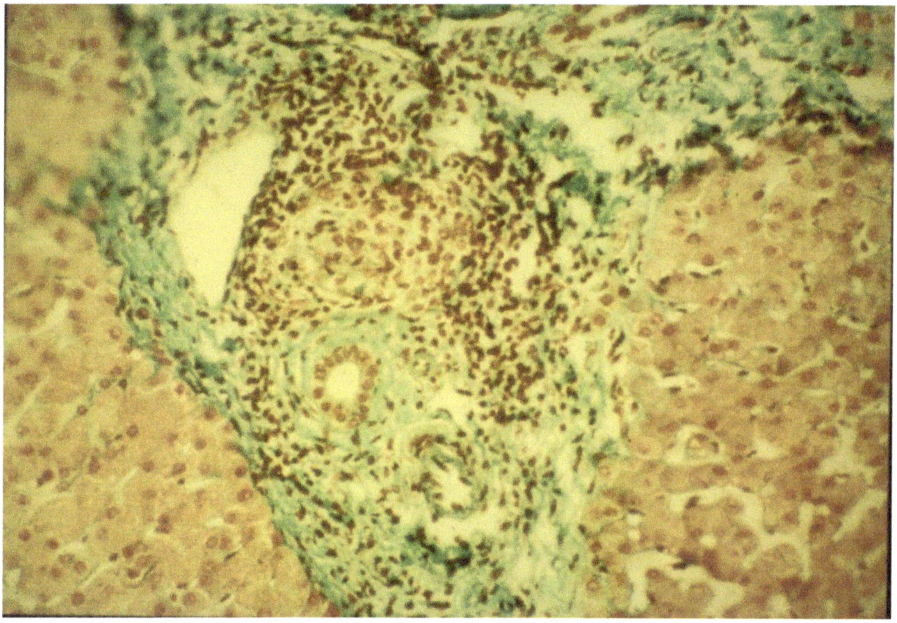

Fig. 4. Autoimmune cholangitis. An intrahepatic bile duct surrounded by an inflammatory infiltrate and ductal and periductal fibrosis.

3.1.2.4 Histology

In patients with PSC, percutaneous liver biopsy documents the presence of an inflammatory and/or fibrotic cholangiopathy (Figure 4) with progressive damage, atrophy and ultimately loss of small size bile ducts (ductopenia) (Figure 5). Edema and fibrosis around the interlobular bile ducts progressing to concentric periductal fibrosis ('onion-skinning') (Figure 6), narrowing , obliteration of the small bile ducts, leaving a bile duct scar may be considered the main histologic feature of PSC, although may be missed in the liver sample as it is a focal histological feature. However, often only lesions of acute cholangitis are present, such as infiltration and destruction of biliary epithelium (Figure 6 B) with the finding of lymphoid folliculi or even granuloma, usually encompassing a bile duct. Inflammatory infiltrate around the bile duct is polymorphous mainly with lymphocytes, histiocytes; however a significant number of eosinophils can be present around bile duct and in the colonic cryptae in case of associated IBD (figure 7).

Bridging fibrosis is frequent at diagnosis while typical lesions are present only in a limited number of patients with advanced fibrosis and more frequently findings are those of an aspecific cholangiopathy with ductular proliferation and loss of very small bile ducts. Septal fibrosis or cirrhosis is found in the initial liver biopsy of more than half of newly diagnosed children with PSC. An inflammatory infiltrate ranging from a mixture of lymphocytes and polymorphonuclear cells to a lymphoplasmacytic infiltrate with the features of interface hepatitis can be observed in about a third of patients. These features characterize the overlap syndrome. In advance disease, liver parenchyma show features of long standing cholestasis, i.e positive immunostaining to biliary-type citocheratin 7 and feathery degeneration of liver cells cytoplasm.

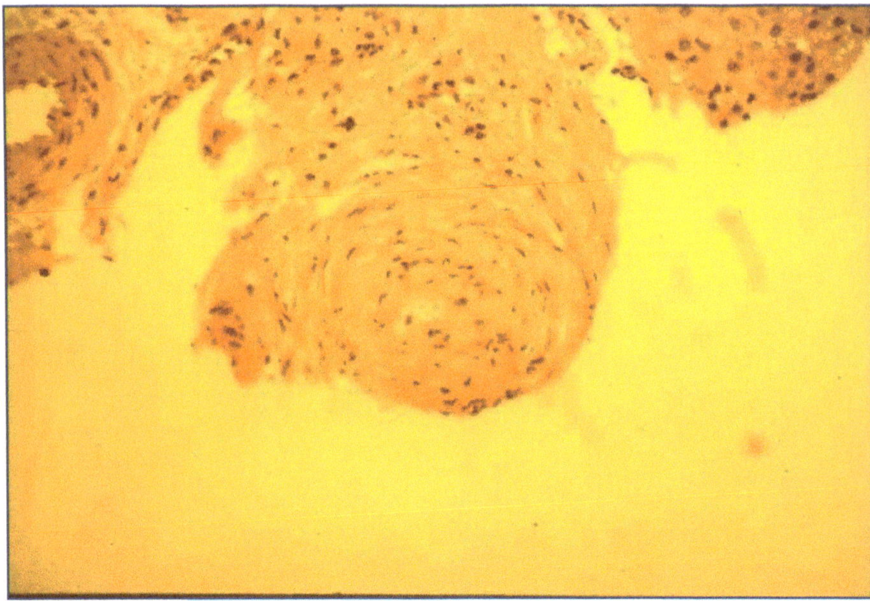

Fig. 5. Autoimmune cholangitis. A concentric fibrotic scar obliterating an intrahepatic bile duct.

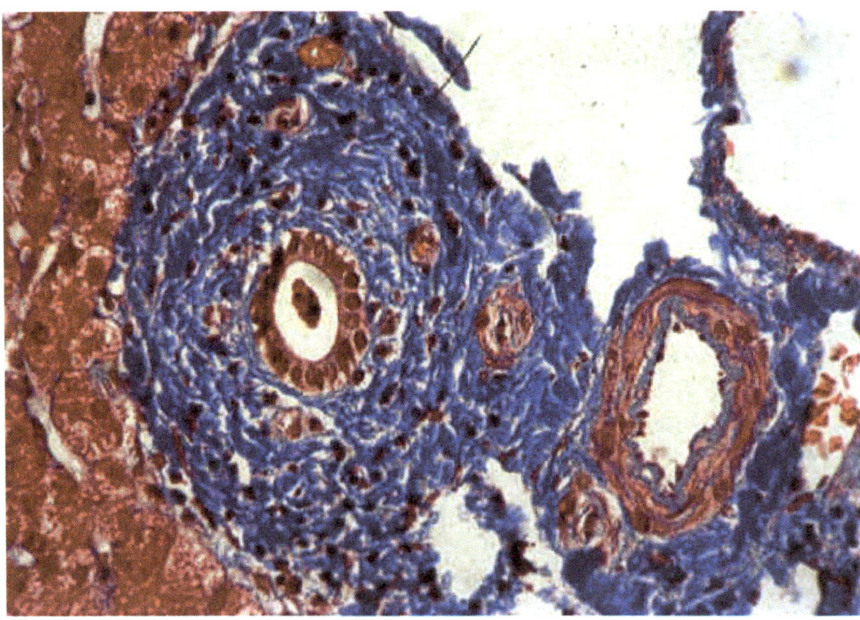

Fig. 6. Autoimmune cholangitis. An intrahepatic bile duct surrounded by concentric periductal fibrosis ('onion-skinning').

3.1.2.5 Biliary imaging

Visualization of intra and extrahepatic bile ducts by direct opacification of the biliary tree or by magnetic resonance (MR) cholangiopancreatography is an essential part of the diagnostic workup. Until recently, endoscopic retrograde cholangiography or transhepatic, transcholecystic, percutaneous cholangiography were used to visualize the biliary tree.

Currently, MRI cholangiopancreatography provides an excellent quality of resolution for imaging intrahepatic and extrahepatic bile ducts in older children. Abnormal features observed include duct wall irregularities, strictures, irregular dilations, and beading resulting in the characteristic "bead-on-a-string" appearance (Figures 7 and 8). Lesions restricted to the intrahepatic branches are found in 30-40% of patients, whereas abnormalities limited exclusively to the extrahepatic ducts are rare. Cholelithiasis may be present, with the majority of patients being asymptomatic.

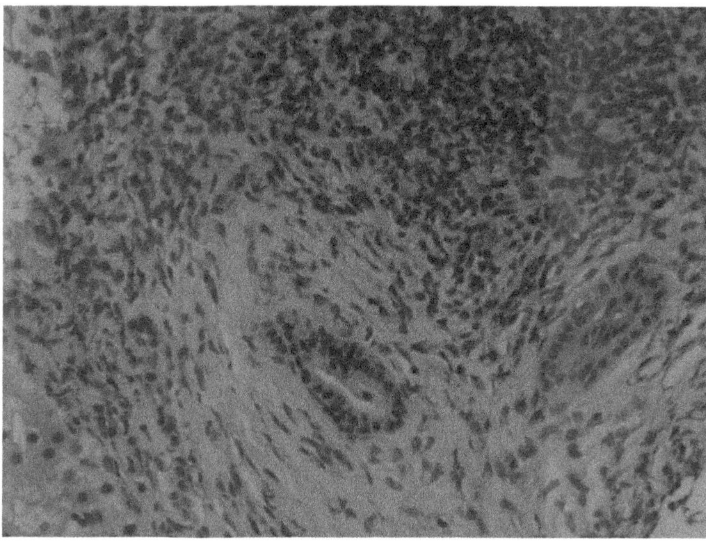

Fig. 7. Autoimmune cholangitis. Inflammatory portal fibrosis with destructive ductular lesions and biliary proliferation without ductopenia

3.1.2.6 Diagnosis

Suspicion of PSC should arise when a patient presents with signs or symptoms of chronic liver disease, such as hepatomegaly, splenomegaly, stellar angiomas, palmar erythema, fatigue (more frequent in adolescents), anorexia, pruritus, or jaundice. The most common laboratory finding is an increase of the serum GGT activity. The possibility of PSC should be considered in any patient who has IBD and an increased liver enzyme serum activity, particularly if laboratory features suggesting cholestasis or symptoms or signs of chronic liver disease are present. Definitive diagnosis requires a liver biopsy and a biliary imaging. The diagnosis may be challenging in patients asymptomatic who do not have autoantibodies and hypergammaglobulinemia. In these patients, liver histology and the presence of an associated IBD may suggest the diagnosis. The differential diagnosis of PSC should include other causes of liver injury reported in patients who have IBD, including those such as drug-induced liver damage.

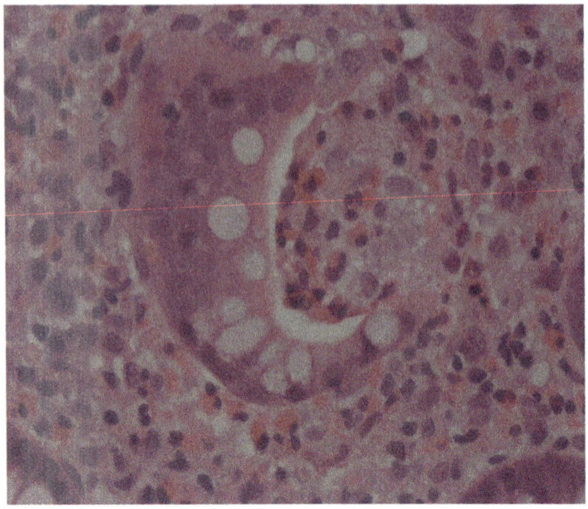

Fig. 8. Inflammatory bowel disease associated with Autoimmune cholangitis. Eosinophilic cryptitis

In children who have ulcerative colitis and who have abnormal liver laboratory tests, a liver biopsy and a biliary imaging are usually indicated. Moreover, distinction between PSC and AIH-1 is not always easy. Traditionally, AIH and PSC are regarded as separate disease entities, but recently it was hypothesized that both diseases are part of the same process.

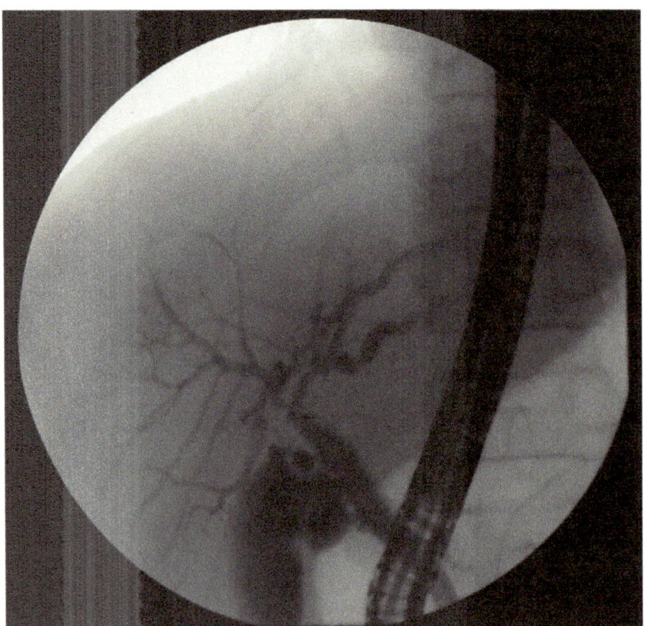

Fig. 9. Endoscopic cholangiopancreatography showing irregular intrahepatic bile ducts with stenosis and dilation prevalent in left liver sections.

This condition corresponding to the overlap syndrome, which would encompass both PSC and AIH, may respond satisfactorily to immunosuppressive therapy. In fact, approximately 50% of children with features of autoimmune liver disease present cholangiographic features typical of sclerosing cholangitis, though generally less advanced than those observed in adult patients with sclerosing cholangitis. All these patients present with the clinical features of typical AIH, many do not have typical histologic evidence of fibro-obliterative bile duct damage on liver biopsy, and virtually all have the autoantibody pattern of AIH-1

3.1.2.7 Management and prognosis

Children with PSC have a significantly shorter survival than the expected for age-matched general population. Many children with PSC progress to end-stage liver disease with the consequent need for liver transplantation. Currently, no specific therapy is clearly standardized for PSC. Patients with PSC seem to have a more severe prognosis than those who have bile duct lesion limited to fourth order bile ducts (small duct sclerosing cholangitis, SDSC). Lesions of the large bile ducts and the consequent obstruction of bile flow contribute to the rapid progression of liver injury.

Treatment with ursodeoxycholic acid leads to improvement of biochemical tests in most patients, but does not seem to affect survival in children or adults. One third of newly diagnosed patients have biochemical signs of inflammation as well as interface hepatitis at liver biopsy. Immunosuppressive therapy is not effective in adults with PSC, even if there is increasing evidences of some benefit in adults and children with SDSC. However, in these cases corticosteroids and azathioprine are frequently administered. No impact on long term outcome has been reported with these drugs in small pediatric series or in larger adult series. This lack of improvement in outcome occurs despite a good control of the inflammatory process. Stabilization or even regression of the cholangiographic lesions has been however observed, however, in half of patients treated after a median follow-up of four years. Immunosuppressant drugs are indicated in the frequent occurrence of overlap syndrome and it should be considered that anti-inflammatory and immunosuppressive drugs administered to maintain remission of associated IBD might interfere with the natural history of PSC, particularly in children. It can be speculated that the duration of the inflammatory process and development of fibrosis in the bile ducts before diagnosis influence the outcome. The overall median survival rate without liver transplantation is approximately 12 years in children who have PSC. A younger age at onset and significant portal hypertension are clinical variables associated with shorter survival in children.

Surgical, endoscopic, or radiologic dilatation of bile duct strictures has been attempted in some patients who have PSC. Although transitory good results have been reported with this intervention, there seems to be no effect on long-term outcome. Any invasive procedure in these children can be complicated by bacterial cholangitis that would be difficult to treat, given the abnormal bile flow. Complications caused by chronic decrease in bile flow could be prevented with adequate nutritional support, including administration of liposoluble vitamins. Dominant strictures in PSC with significant cholestasis should be treated with balloon dilatation. Some patients also appear to benefit from short-term stenting. No randomized, prospective controlled trials have been performed to assess the efficacy of endoscopic treatment in PSC, and the application is presently performed based on individual assessment of each patient. Complications secondary to portal hypertension or recurrent bacterial cholangitis can be considered possible indications for liver transplantation even if liver function is somewhat preserved

Liver transplantation is the only therapeutic option for a child who has PSC, cirrhosis, and signs of liver failure. However, retransplantation rates are higher for patients with PSC than other diagnoses with a 25% recurrence rate in transplanted liver. An increased risk of acute cellular rejection in PSC has been demonstrated in several series, it is not clear whether PSC patients are particularly at risk or whether the risk is related to autoimmune liver disease in general. Furthermore, there is an increased risk of acute rejection in patients with pre-transplant IBD as compared with patients without IBD and the risk of chronic rejection also seems to be higher in PSC patients with IBD.

Recently prolonged treatment with oral vancomycin has been shown may be beneficial in difficult-to-treat PSC associated with inflammatory bowel disease.

An increased incidence of colorectal neoplasia has been described in adult patients who have PSC-related IBD. This complication is the most frequent cause of death after liver transplantation in patients who have ASC. Cholangiocarcinoma may complicate PSC in adults, and is significantly more common in patients who have colorectal neoplasia.

3.1.3 Autoimmune overlap syndrome

Overlap syndrome in children and adolescents concerns only autoimmune hepatitis and autoimmune cholangitis features and includes patients within the spectrum of autoimmune liver diseases presenting with the characteristics of both PSC or SDSC and AIH. AIH and AIC are not homogeneous disorders and patients within each diagnosis may present with a range of clinical, biochemical, serological, and histological findings. However, the diagnosis of overlap syndrome should not be overlooked; certainly AIH should not be diagnosed in presence of definite bile duct pathology, but some coincidental biliary injury may be observed. The presence of some degree of biliary involvement in AIH should therefore not necessarily lead to a change in diagnosis but an adequate biliary imaging study should be considered in such patients. Several types of relationship between the autoimmune liver disorders in the same patient have been described: 1. sequential presentation of two disorders: 2. concomitant presence of two distinct disorders; autoimmune diseases are often associated with one another and it can be argued that an individual who has developed one autoimmune liver disease is predisposed to develop another one as well; 3. existence of a continuum of pathological changes between two disorders, without strict boundaries and with "overlaps" localized in the center; 4. "overlap syndromes" are distinct entities on their own, with a variety of autoimmune manifestations presenting in a susceptible individual; 5. the presence of one primary disorder that also has one or more characteristics of another: this contention has been supported by a majority. The diagnosis of AIH-AIC overlap syndrome could be established in a patient with inflammatory colangiopathy diffuse or limited to intrahepatic bile duct on the presence of: 1. significant biochemical disease activity (moderate to severe increase of aminotransferases, hypergammaglobulinemia); 2. ANA or ASMA antibodies present in a titer at least ≥1:40; 3. a liver histology with interface hepatitis, moderate to severe lobular necrosis, moderate to severe periportal or periseptal inflammation. The major guidelines suggest that patients with AIH-AIC overlap syndrome should be treated with immunosuppressive regimen associated with ursodeoxycholic acid (UDCA) even if this recommendation is not evidence-based. Ursodeoxycholic acid (UDCA) is widely used in autoimmune cholangitis due to its beneficial effects on serum liver tests, histological features, prognostic surrogate markers, and development of colonic dysplasia associated with accompanying ulcerative colitis, although long-term efficacy of UDCA still remains unproven. UDCA at higher doses (> 20 mg/kg daily) may be superior to standard doses and has also been used in the treatment of AIH-PSC overlap syndrome. Use of UDCA in combination with immunosuppressive drugs in AIH-AIC overlap syndrome, and the long-term course has been considered favorable in the long term. The response to immunosuppressive therapy appears to be better in children with AIH-AIC overlap than in adults.

3.1.4 Autoimmune small duct sclerosing cholangitis (SDSC)

A minority of patients with sclerosing cholangitis of unknown etiology with similar cholestatic and histologic features as those with classic PSC has normal biliary imaging, and they have been referred to as SDSC (Chapman, 2002). Patients with SDSC: 1. Are generally younger than patients with PSC and presents with more active disease, with overlap features; 2. may however progress to PSC and to end-stage liver disease with the consequent need of liver transplantation; 3. may progress to end-stage liver disease even without evidence of development of large-duct disease; 4. may suffer from recurrence of SDSC in the allograft in case of liver transplant; 5. do not seem to develop cholangiocarcinoma; 6. generally seem to have a significantly better long-term prognosis as compared with patients with large-duct PSC.

3.1.5 IgG4-related sclerosing cholangitis (IgG4-SC)

Biliary stricture, mimicking bile duct carcinoma and primary sclerosing cholangitis are frequently seen in IgG4-related systemic diseases. IgG4-related sclerosing cholangitis is almost constantly associated with autoimmune sclerosing pancreatitis (AIP). This syndrome affects predominantly middle-aged and elderly patients, with male predominance. The patients present with symptoms referable to the involvement of one or more sites, usually in the form of mass lesions. also defined as type 1, most commonly presenting as painless obstructive jaundice with or without a pancreatic mass. Other common sites of involvement are the hepatobiliary tract, salivary gland, orbit, and lymph node, but practically any organ-site can be affected, such as retroperitoneum, aorta, mediastinum, soft tissue, skin, central nervous system, breast, kidney, prostate, upper aerodigestive tract, and lung. Some patients have low titers of autoantibodies such as antinuclear antibodies and rheumatoid factor. The natural history is characterized by the development of multiple sites of involvement with time, sometimes after many years. However, the disease can remain localized to one site in occasional patients. The patients usually have a good general condition, with no fever or constitutional symptoms. The disease often shows excellent response to steroid therapy with however relapse after steroid withdrawal. The main pathologic findings in various extranodal sites include lymphoplasmacytic infiltration, lymphoid follicle formation, sclerosis and obliterative phlebitis, accompanied by atrophy and loss of the specialized structures of the involved tissue (such as secretory acini in pancreas, salivary gland, or lacrimal gland). Immunostaining shows increased IgG4+ cells in the involved tissues (>50 per high-power field, with IgG4/IgG ratio >40%). The lymph nodes show an increase in IgG4+ plasma cells on immunostaining. The nature and pathogenesis of IgG4-related sclerosing disease are still elusive. Very few pediatric reports of AIP exist.

4. Giant cell hepatitis combined with autoimmune hemolytic anemia

Transformation of hepatocytes into giant multinucleated cells is mostly observed in the neonatal period, when it is considered a nonspecific reaction of the immature liver cell to various forms of aggression. In older children and adults, giant cell transformation is rare and has been described sporadically in cases of viral, toxic, autoimmune, and genetic disease, as well as in diseases of unknown origin. When present, it is considered to carry a severe prognosis, with a risk of recurrence after liver transplantation.

In 1981, four young children were reported associating a giant cell hepatitis and Coombs-positive hemolytic anemia of the immunoglobulin G-positive (IgG+) C type: three of them died of liver failure, but for the remaining child, immunosuppressive treatment with prednisone and azathioprine was beneficial. Because of the association with a positive Coombs test and a positive response to immunosuppressive treatment, it was postulated that this entity might be of autoimmune origin. Since this original description, a total of 18 children with giant cell hepatitis and Coombs-positive hemolytic anemia have been reported confirming the onset of this condition in early childhood after the neonatal period, the severity of the liver condition that can progress to liver failure, and in many instances, the response to immunosuppressive treatment, but with less favorable initial control than in conventional autoimmune hepatitis, which occurs later in childhood. In the studies reported, mortality or the need for liver transplantation were 39% of reported cases and were due to liver cell failure and/or bacterial infection as well as relapse after liver transplantation.

The diagnosis of giant cell hepatitis combined with autoimmune hemolytic anemia should be considered in any child between ages 1 month and 2 years presenting with autoimmune hemolytic anemia, acute liver disease of unknown cause, or both. Assay for serum aminotransferase activities should be part of the investigation in young children with autoimmune hemolytic anemia, both at the onset of the disease and during follow-up.

Unexplained elevated aminotransferase activity should lead to liver biopsy in a search for signs of giant cell hepatitis (Figure. 7). In such cases, any reduction of the dose of steroids initially given to treat hemolytic anemia should be gradual, because the liver condition may degenerate to liver cell failure if the dose is lowered too fast. Conversely, a direct Coombs test should be part of the search for acute hepatitis of unknown origin in early childhood. If the test is positive of the IgG+ C type, liver biopsy should be performed as soon as possible; if giant cell hepatitis is found, immunosuppressive therapy should be rapidly started.

Except in cases of acute refractory liver cell failure, which would require liver transplantation, immunosuppressive therapy with prednisone and azathioprine is the first-line treatment. This is similar to that used in the treatment of older children with the most common type of autoimmune hepatitis. If appropriately administered, this treatment may control the liver disease. Here again, extreme caution should be exercised when reducing steroid doses. Thus, the high initial dose should be maintained for as long as possible until serum aminotransferase activity has returned to normal, because early relapse may occur. Hepatitis relapses are difficult to manage: in some cases they may be controlled by increasing the steroid dosage or adding cyclosporine to the initial regimen. Sometimes, however, hepatitis is refractory to drug therapy and rescue treatment with other drugs or biological agent such as Rituximab can be attempted. Liver transplantation must be considered when signs of liver failure occur early or during a relapse and are refractory to immunosuppressive treatment even if a relapse of the initial liver disease can be observed.

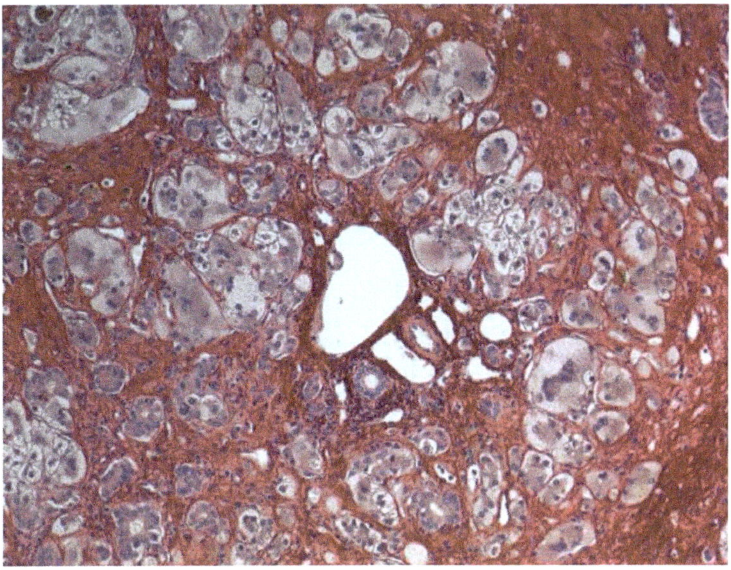

Fig. 10. Liver biopsy showing diffuse giant cell transformation in a child with autoimmune hemolytic anemia.

The evolution of anemia may be independent of the evolution of hepatitis: anemia can be extremely severe and require repeated erythrocyte transfusions and may be refractory to all kinds of drug therapy. In such cases, Rituximab should be considered. Before Rituximab became available, splenectomy was used with success. Once the disease has been under control for 5 years of management with immunosuppressive therapy, treatment can be stopped in most patients without relapse of the hepatitis.

5. Conclusions

In conclusion, in the pediatric population two predominant forms of autoimmune diseases of the liver, AIH and AIC, have been clearly identified, although the distinction between the two diagnoses is not always easy. The diagnosis of AIH must be considered in patients who have symptoms and signs of acute or chronic hepatitis, particularly when an extrahepatic autoimmune disorder is present. Hypergammaglobulinemia and circulating antibodies are of great help in supporting diagnosis of AIH. The fluctuating course of the disease can be responsible for alternating periods of remission and relapse. Therefore, a low-intensity inflammatory syndrome at onset does not preclude instituting immunosuppressive treatment. Rapid, complete, and sustained control of liver inflammation improves the short- and long-term outcome. Because it has been shown that liver fibrosis can regress in patients responding to treatment, an aggressive approach to confirm the diagnosis of AIH is justified.

The diagnosis of AIC must be evoked in patients who have IBD and clinical and laboratory features of cholestasis and/or bile duct injury. Liver biopsy and bile duct imaging are essential for the diagnosis and in distinguishing diffuse (PSC) from limited (SDSC) entities. Even if effective treatment has yet been described to control the progression of this disease, patient with features overlapping with AIH may be efficaciously treated with conventional immunosuppressive treatment. Liver transplantation is the only definitive therapy, for patients with acute AIH unresponsive to rescue immunosuppressive treatment and for patients with end stage liver failure. Liver transplantation is also the treatment of choice for patient with sclerosing cholangitis and end stage liver disease. In both condition however the risk of relapse of the disease in the graft is not negligible.

6. References

Alvarez, F. (2006). Autoimmune hepatitis and primary sclerosing cholangitis. *Clinics in Liver Disease,* Vol. 10, No. 1, (February 2006), pp. 89-107, ISSN 1089-3261

Boberg, KM. (2002). Prevalence and epidemiology of autoimmune hepatitis. *Clinics in Liver Disease,* Vol. 6, No. 3, (August 2002), pp. 347-355, ISSN 1089-3261

Bogdanos DP., Mieli-Vergani G., & Vergani D. (2009). Autoantibodies and their antigens in autoimmune hepatitis. *Seminars in Liver Disease,* Vol. 29, No. 3, (August 2009), pp. 241-253, ISSN 0272-8087

Bridoux-Henno L., Maggiore G., Joahnet C., Fabre M., Vajro P., Dommergues JP., Reinert P., & Bernard O. (2004). Features and outcome of AIH type 2 presenting with isolated positivity for anti-liver cytosol antibody. *Clinical Gastroenterology and Hepatology,* Vol. 2, No. 9, (September 2004), pp. 825-830, ISSN 1542-3565.

Caprai S., Vajro P., Ventura A., Sciveres M., & Maggiore G, SIGENP Study Group for Autoimmune Liver Disorders in Celiac Disease (2008). Autoimmune Liver disease associated with celiac disease in childhood: a multicenter study. *Clinical Gastroenterology and Hepatology,* Vol. 6, No. 7, (July 2008), pp. 803-806, ISSN 1542-3565

Chapman RW. (2002). Small duct primary sclerosing cholangitis. *Journal of Hepatology,* Vol. 36, No. 5, (May 2002), pp. 692-694, ISSN 0168-8278

Cuarterolo ML., Ciocca ME., López SI., de Dávila MT., & Alvarez F. (2011). Immunosuppressive therapy allows recovery from liver failure in children with autoimmune hepatitis. *Clinical Gastroenterology and Hepatology,* Vol. 9, No. 2, (February 2011), pp. 145-149, ISSN 1542-3565

Czaja AJ., & Donaldson PT. (2000). Genetic susceptibility for immune expression and liver cell injury in autoimmune hepatitis. *Immunological Review,* Vol. 174, (April 2000), pp. 250-259, ISSN 1600-065X

Debray D., Maggiore G., Girardet JP., Mallet E., & Bernard O. (1999). Efficacy of cyclosporin A in children with type 2 autoimmune hepatitis. *The Journal of Pediatrics,* Vol. 135, No. 1, (July 1999), pp. 111-114, ISSN 0022-3476

Feldstein AE., Perrault J., El-Youssif M., Lindor K., Freese D., & Angulo P. (2003). Primary sclerosing cholangitis in children: a long-term follow-up study. *Hepatology,* Vol. 38, No. 1, (July 2003), pp 210-217, ISSN 1527-3350

Gueguen M., Meunier-Rotival M., Bernard O., & Alvarez F. (1988). Anti-liver kidney microsome antibody recognize CYP450 from the IID subfamily. *Journal of Experimental Medicine,* Vol. 168, No. 1, (August 1988), pp. 801-816, ISSN 0022-1007

Gregorio GV., Portmann B., Reid F., Donaldson PT., Doherty DG., McCartney M., Mowat AP., Vergani D., & Mieli-Vergani G. (1997). Autoimmune hepatitis in childhood: a

20-year experience. *Hepatology,* Vol. 25, No. 3, (March 1997), pp. 541-547, ISBN 1527-3350

Gregorio GV., Portmann B., Karani J., Harrison P., Donaldson PT., Vergani D., & Mieli-Vergani G. (2001). Autoimmune hepatitis/sclerosing cholangitis overlap syndrome in childhood: a 16-year prospective study. *Hepatology,* Vol. 33, No. 3, (March 2001), pp. 544-553, ISBN 1527-3350

Lapierre P., Hajoui O., Homberg JC. & Alvarez F. (1999). Formiminotransferase cyclodeaminase is an organ-specific autoantigen recognized by sera of patients with AIH. *Gastroenterology,* Vol. 116, No 3 (March 1999), pp. 643-649, ISSN 0016-5085

Lohse AW., & Mieli-Vergani G. (2010). Autoimmune hepatitis. *Journal of Hepatology,* Vol. 55, No. 1, (July 2011), pp. 171-182, ISBN 0168-8278

Loftus EV. Jr, Harewood GC., Loftus CG., Tremaine WJ., Harmsen WS., Zinsmeister AR., Jewell DA., & Sandborn WJ. (2005) PSC-IBD: a unique form of inflammatory bowel disease associated with primary sclerosing cholangitis. *Gut,* Vol. 54, No 1, (January 2005), pp. 91-96, ISSN 0017-5749

Longhi MS., Ma Y., Mieli Vergani G., & Vergani D. (2010). Aetiopathogenesis of autoimmune hepatitis. *Journal of Immunology,* Vol. 34, No 1, (February 2010), ISSN 0022-1767

Krawitt EL. (2011). Discrimination of autoimmune hepatitis: autoantibody typing and beyond. *Journal ofGastroenterology,* Vol. 46, Suppl. 1, (January 2011), pp. 39-41, ISSN 0944-1174

Maggiore G., Bernard O., Hadchouel M., Hadchouel P., Odièvre M., & Alagille D. (1984). Treatment of autoimmune chronic active hepatitis in childhood. *The Journal of Pediatrics,* Vol. 104, No. 6, (June 1984), pp. 839-844, ISBN 0022-3476

Maggiore G., Bernard O., Homberg JC., Hadchouel M., Alvarez F., Hadchouel P., Odièvre M., & Alagille D. (1986). Liver disease associated with anti-liver-kidney microsome antibody in children. *The Journal of Pediatrics, Vol.* 108, No. 3, (March 1986), pp. 399-401, ISSN 0022-3476.

Maggiore G., Porta G., Bernard O., Hadchouel M., Alvarez F., Homberg JC., & Alagille D. (1990). Autoimmune hepatitis with initial presentation as acute hepatic failure in young children. *The Journal of Pediatrics,* Vol. 116, No. 2, (February 1990), pp. 280-282, ISSN 0022-3476

Maggiore G., Veber F., Bernard O., Hadchouel M., Homberg JC., Alvarez F., Hadchouel P. & Alagille D. (1993). Autoimmune hepatitis associated with anti-actin antibodies in children. *Journal of Pediatric Gastroenterology and Nutrition,* Vol. 17, No. 4, (November 1993), pp. 376-381, ISSN 0277-2116

Maggiore G., Riva S., & Sciveres M. (2009). Autoimmune diseases of the liver and biliary tract and overlap syndromes in childhood. *Minerva Gastroenterologica e Dietolologica,* Vol. 55, No. 1, (March 2009), pp. 53-70, ISSN 1121-421X

Maggiore G., Sciveres M., Fabre M., Gori L., Pacifico L., Resti M., Choulot JJ., Jacquemin E., & Bernard O. (2011). Giant Cell Hepatitis with Autoimmune Hemolytic Anemia in Early Childhood: Long-Term Outcome in 16 Children. *The Journal of Pediatrics,* Vol. 159, No. 1 (July 2011), pp. 127-132, ISSN 0022-3476

Martin SR., Alvarez F., Anand R., Song C., & Yin W. (2011). Outcomes in children who underwent transplantation for autoimmune hepatitis. *Liver Transplantation*, Vol. 17, No. 4, (April 2011), pp. 393-401, ISSN 1527-6465

Martini E., Abuaf N., Cavalli F., Durand V., Johanet C., & Homberg JC. (1988). Antibody to liver cytosol (anti-LC1) in patients with autoimmune chronic active hepatitis type 2. *Hepatology*, Vol. 8, No. 6, (November-December 1988), pp. 1662-1666, ISSN 1527-3350

Mieli Vergani G., & Vergani D. (2008) .Autoimmune pediatric liver disease. *World Journal of Gastroenterology*, Vol. 14, No. 21, (June 2008), pp. 3360-3367, ISSN 1007-9327

Mieli Vergani G., & Vergani D. (2009). Autoimmune hepatitis in children: what is different from adult AIH? *Seminars in Liver Disease*, Vol. 29, No. 3 (August 2009), pp. 297-306, ISSN 0272-8087

Miloh T., Arnon R., Shneider B., Suchy F., & Kerkar N. (2009). A retrospective single-center review of primary sclerosing cholangitis in children. *Clinical Gastroenterology and Hepatology*, Vol. 7, No. 2, (February 2009), pp. 239-245, ISSN 1542-3565

Muratori L., Parola M., Ripalti A., Robino G., Muratori P., Bellomo G., Carini R., Lenzi M., Landini MP., Albano E., & Bianchi FB. (2000). Liver/kidney microsomal antibody type 1 targets CYP2D6 on hepatocyte plasma membrane. *Gut*, Vol. 46, No. 4, (April 2000), pp. 553-561, ISSN 0017-5749

Odièvre M., Maggiore G., Homberg JC., Saadoun F., Courouсé AM., Yvart J., Hadchouel M., & Alagille D. (1983). Seroimmunologic classification of chronic hepatitis in 57 children. *Hepatology*, Vol. 3, No. 3, (May-June 1983), pp. 407-409, ISBN 1527-+3350

Schramm C., & Lohse AW. (2011). Role of mycophenolate mofetil in the treatment of autoimmune hepatitis. *Journal of Hepatology*, in press, (Jan 28,. Epub ahead of print) ISBN 0168-8278

Sciveres M., Caprai S., Palla G., Ughi C., & Maggiore G. (2004). Effectiveness and safety of cyclosporine as therapy for autoimmune diseases of the liver in children and adolescents. *Alimentary Pharmacology and Therapeutics*, Vol. 19, No. 2, (January 2004), pp. 209-17, ISSN 1365-2036

Vergani D., Alvarez F., Bianchi FB., Cançado EL., Mackay IR., Manns MP., Nishioka M. & Penner E; International Autoimmune Hepatitis Group (2004). Liver autoimmune serology: a consensus statement from the committee for autoimmune serology of the International Autoimmune Hepatitis Group. *Journal of Hepatology*, Vol. 41, No. 4, (October 2004), pp. 677-683, ISBN 0168-8278

17

Needle Biopsy in Children With Liver Diseases

A. Pietrobattista[1], A. Alterio[1], G. Natali[2], R. Fruhwirth[2], D. Comparcola[1], M. R. Sartorelli[1] and V. Nobili[1]
[1]*Department of Hepatogastroenterology and Nutrition, Pediatric Hospital Bambino Gesù,*
[2]*Radiology Interventional Unit, Pediatric Hospital Bambino Gesù, Italy*

1. Introduction

The diagnosis of most liver diseases in children requires histological confirmation, thus liver biopsies are routine procedures in specialist centre. Although sensitive and relatively accurate blood tests used to detect and diagnose liver disease have now become widely available, percutaneous needle biopsy provides the histopathological examination and assessment of liver disease and remains the cornerstone in the evaluation and management of parenchymal liver diseases [1–5]. Paul Ehrlich is credited with performing the first percutaneous liver biopsy in 1883 in Germany. However, the technique required up to a 15-minute intrahepatic phase, making it impractical and probably unsafe. In 1958, Menghini reported a new technique, which became more widely used [5, 6]. Historically liver biopsy was used exclusively for adult patients, just in the last 50 years, following the developing knowledge in pediatric hepatology, it has taken on an important role in the clinical practice. In the past and even today many authors, discuss about when liver biopsy is recommended, regarding indications and timing.

2. Indications for liver biopsy in children overview

Actually numerous studies strongly suggest that due to the limitations and risks of biopsy, as well as the improvement of the diagnostic accuracy of new noninvasive biomarkers (Fibroscan, FibroTest, ELF) (7-14), liver biopsy should no longer be considered mandatory as a first line estimate of fibrosis in the most frequent chronic liver diseases. In reality even if the development of non-invasive markers of liver injury must be encouraged especially for the assessment of liver fibrosis, the consensus in many conference statements recommend liver biopsy for the diagnosis and the management of almost all patients with liver diseases (15-18).

To date liver biopsy has three major roles: for diagnosis, for assessment of prognosis (disease staging), and/or to assist in making therapeutic management decisions.

As said, when to order a liver biopsy is a subject of contention in the medical community especially whether deciding to recommend a liver biopsy in a child.

Nearly all doctors agree that a liver biopsy should routinely ordered when tests reveal raised liver enzyme over several months. The liver enzyme elevation that merits a histological evaluation can range from 1.5 times to twice the normal range for a child of that weight and age. Considering the chronic trend of altered liver enzymes (almost 6 months) as one of the major indication, instead the acute flares of elevated enzymesin children often end to find a spontaneously resolution being related to some infections, fever or medical treatments.Diseases and situations in which liver biopsy may be indicated are listed in Tables 1. It is essential to have information about liver size and consistency and the presence of cyst or dilatated bile ducts from ultrasound, and if necessary to have a "spot"marked on the abdomento ensure an accurate biopsy. Correct information about coagulation parameters is crucial. Prothrombin time should be within 3 s of control values; platelets > 80.000/L. The patient's blood group should be known, and it is prudent to cross-match a unit of blood prior to the procedure.However even when present an indication, liver biopsy could be difficult to perform because of clinical conditions of the patient. Abnormal coagulationis the main contraindications while in presence of ascitis different techniques other than the needle aspiration should be considered (table 2). In these cases when liver biopsy is strictly necessary alternative techniques will be used, such as transjugular biopsy and the procedure should be performed in high experienced centre (19-20).

2.1 Use of liver biopsy in specific disease

Neonatal cholestasis is a relevant condition in which liver biopsy play a pivotal role and has to be considered as soon as possible to provide specific treatment. In case of biliary atresia early diagnosis in vital, as the Kasai portoenterostomy is less likely to be successful the later is performed. Biliary atresia is the cause of liver disease in approximately 25% on infants presenting with neonatal cholestasis and percutaneous liver biopsy is essential and has high diagnostic specificity. Features of bile duct obstruction (duct reaction, previously known as ductular proliferation; bile plugs; portal tract edema) are usually obvious along with variable fibrosis and giant cell transformation (Figure 1). However the earlier the liver biopsy is performed, the more difficult it may be to interpret. Particularly in the setting of abnormal liver tests of unclear etiology, the risks and benefits of a liver biopsy should be carefully weighed, and the decision to perform a liver biopsy must be individualized. The liver biopsy plays a pivotal role in the follow-up of liver transplant (OLT). Pediatric liver transplant recipients often need to undergo liver biopsies for the detection and specification of complications such as acute or chronic graft rejection, infection, or drug toxicity. It is always necessary to have an histological confirmation (mixed inflammatory infiltrate in the portal tract with subendothelial lymphoid infiltration) (Figure 2). Some liver transplant programs perform liver biopsy on a protocol basis after transplantation (e.g., annually), even in those patients with normal liver tests, although compelling evidence to support this approach is lacking. In contrast, there is good evidence suggesting that fibrosis progression may be predicted by using liver histology in patients following transplantation (21-23).Nevertheless when the medical history, physical examination, biochemical, serological, or imaging investigation have shown the presence of specific markers liver biopsy should be brought forward to ruled out liver diseases that need to be treated such as Wilson disease or autoimmune hepatitis (figure 3) or to make a diagnosis of non alcoholic steatohepatitis (figure 4).

Neonatal cholestatic jaundice
Abnormal liver tests of unknown etiology
Focal of diffuse abnormalities on imaging studies
Need of liver tissue to further analisys (Wilson disease, metabolic disorders)
Prognosis—Staging of known parenchymal liver disease
Management—Developing treatment plans based on histologic analysis
Suspicion of inherited metabolic liver disease
Suspicion of autoimmune liver disease
Liver transplant follow up

Table 1. Indications for liver biopsy in children

Absolute
Severe coagulopathy (INR > 1,5, PLT < 50.000 mm^3)*
Possible vascular lesion
Treatment with FANS in the last week
Impossibility of blood transfusion, if necessary
Relative
Ascites
Obesity
Hemophilia*

* possible in some cases with blood products transfusion

Table 2. Contraindications to percutaneousliver biopsy in children

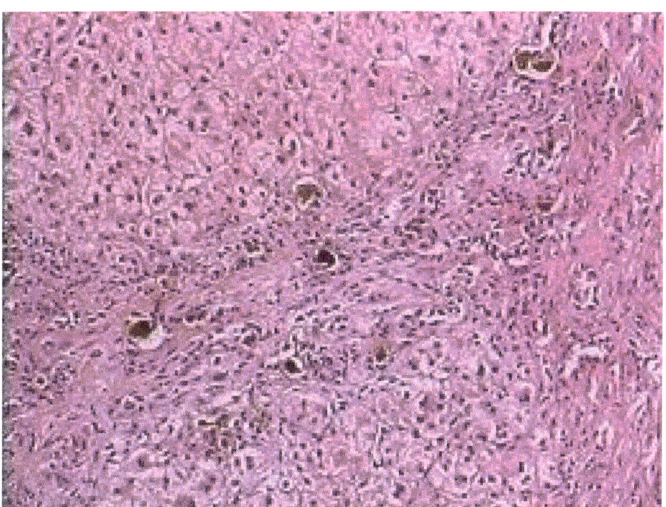

Fig. 1. Liver histology of a patient with biliary atresia

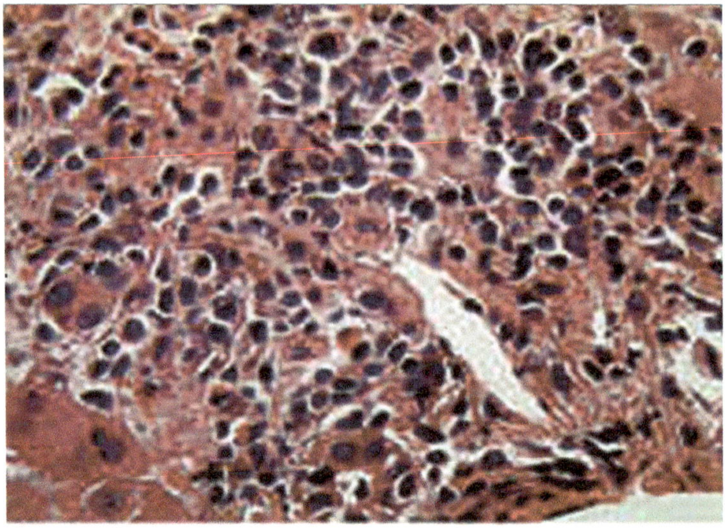

Fig. 2. Liver transplant histology showing acute showing expansion of portal spaces, due to ductular rejection proliferation, bile plugging in bile ductules and giant cells

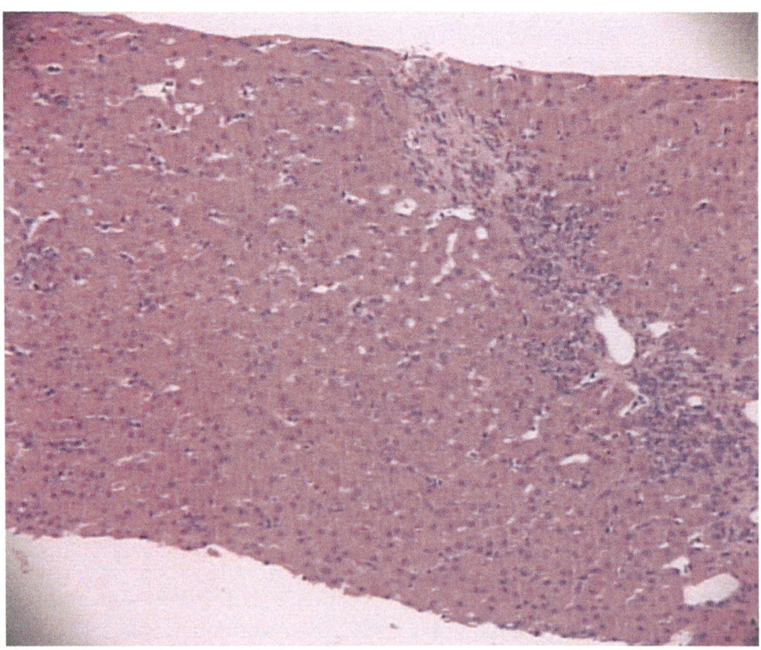

Fig. 3. Histology of an autoimmune hepatitis, portal

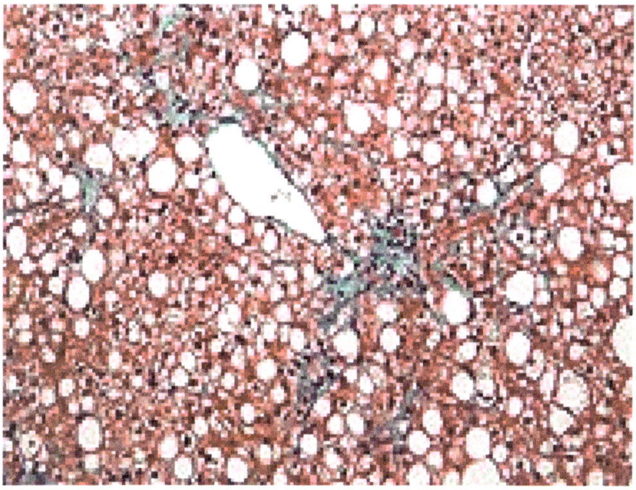

Fig. 4. Liver histology in a children with non alcoholic and peryportal lymphoplasmocityc infiltrate steatohepatitis

2.2 Risks and complications

Liver biopsy is generally regarded as a safe procedure, but an aspiration technique using a Menghini needle has a complication risk 1: 1000, while mortality rates up to 1:10,000 have been reported (24). The risks related to any procedure should always be balanced against potential benefits, and this is particularly pertinent in relation to children. Paediatric studies suggest an overall complication rate for percutaneous biopsy of 0.- 6.83% (2.4 - 4.5% major complications) (25-28). The data is difficult to compare between series as authors vary in their definition of major and minor complications, and in the exclusion criteria they employ. Complications include intraperitoneal haemorrhage, biliary peritonitis, haemobilia and injury to the duodenum, colon or lung. The risk of significant bleeding after an image-guided percutaneous liver biopsy, as measured by a decrease in haematocrit, is reported to be up to 3%. Paediatric studies have shown that the risk of complications is greater in patients with malignant disease, cirrhosis or recent bone marrow. It may be that these children should always be considered for a transjugular biopsy approach. Tumour seeding along the biopsy track remains a significant concern but unlike in hepatocellular carcinoma in the adult population, is rare in the commoner paediatric lesions such as hepatoblastoma. Smaller risks include lack of an adequate sample. With good operative technique, post-operative pain should be minimal, and post-operative infection rare. It is important to remember that sick children may deteriorate for clinical reasons unrelated to the liver biopsy itself. In table 3 are listed the rates of complications after needle biopsy as reported by D'Antiga and Mieli Vergani (29). The majority of complications occur in the first 3 hours after liver biopsy (30-35).

The complications of this potentially dangerous procedures are much reduced if performed in experts hands in specialized units under controlled conditions. Especially for children is crucial a well established post procedure observation to early recognize possible complications. (tab 4)

Complications	Rate %
Pain	0.056-22
Intraperitoneal haemorrhage	0.03-0.7
Intrahepatic bleeding	0.059-23
biliary peritonitis	0.03-0.22
haemobilia	0.059-0.2
Lung injury	0.08-0.28
Anhestetic reaction	0.029
Death	0.0083-0.03

Table 3. Rate of complications after liver biopsy. From D'antiga L and Mi Vergani G in Training and Educational corner, Bollettino Sigemp, 2010.

Blood pressure, pulse, respiration and temperature
15 min for 2h
30 min for 2h
Hourly for 2h
4 hourly as required
Chest X-rat/abdominal ultrasound may be required if bleeding if suspected

Table 4. Post liver biopsy observation

3. Liver biopsy procedure

Several techniques may be used to obtain liver tissue; a table including/defining specific terms has been provided in an effort to standardize terminology (Table 5).

The liver biopsy should be performed in a dedicated area, with adequate space for the operator, assistants, emergency equipment if necessary, or for family members during recovery.

All liver biopsy techniques require specific training so as to ensure appropriate-sized specimen retrieval and the lowest rate of complications. The main techniques are listed below:

- Percutaneous or needle biopsy
- Laparoscopic or open biopsy
- Transjugular biopsy

Percutanous Biopsy. This method may be undertaken in three different ways, namely palpation/percussionguided, image-guided, and real-time image-guided. A palpation/percussion-guided transthoracic approach, after infiltration of local anesthesia, is the classic percutaneous method. An aspiration technique with Menghini needle (or disposable variant) has a complication risk of 1 in 1000 biopsies. In fibrotic or chirrotic liver a Tru-Cut needle, which removes a larger core, may be necessary (Fig 5). The entry site is marked on the skin surface and the area is prepared and draped in sterile fashion. Local anesthetic is injected on the entry site.

Term	Definition
Liver biopsy	Any type of liver biopsy
Transthoracic palpation/percussion guided	The most appropriate biopsy site is guided transcutaneous determined on t he basis of clinical examination. Traditionally used in practice.
Transthoracic, imageguided	The most appropriate biopsy site is determined or confirmed usually by ultrasound imaging before the biopsy
Subcostal, image-guided	This biopsy is accomplished in almost identical fashion as above, except that the approach is subcostal rather than transthoracic
Transjugular	Biopsy is accomplished through a jugular or femoral venous approach under fluoroscopic guidance

Table 5. Liver Biopsy Terminology. From AASLD POSITION PAPER. Liver biopsy.2009

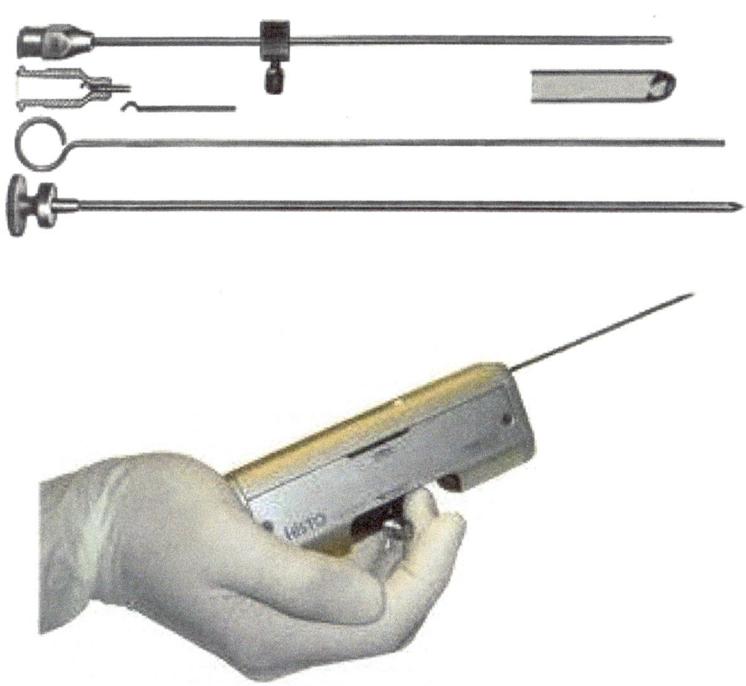

Fig. 5. Menghini needle set (on the top), Tru-cut automatic needle (below)

The transthoracic approach with the routine use of ultrasound scan (US) as a guide to liver biopsy seems to be associated with reduced rate of complications and provides a higher diagnostic yield. Indeed in pediatric liver biopsies and aspirations, US is preferred as a guidance method over CT scan for its versatility, ability to image in real time, decreased cost, portability, and lack of ionizing radiation (36). In spite of the above evidence, some authors question the advantages of a real-time US-guided approach versus blinded biopsy in relation to pain, hypotension, bleeding and rate of subsequent hospitalization (37). Moreover the number of passes should limited to three or fewer whenever possible otherwise the risk of bleeding is higher.

Surgical / laparoscopyc Biopsy. In some circumstances, a surgical approach is utilized because the liver is noted to be abnormal in appearance prior to planned surgery or at the time of surgery. Biopsy in this situation is performed either with typical needle devices or by wedge resection. Notably, the latter has been criticized as producing overestimates of fibrosis due to its proximity to the capsule. This technique of liver biopsy allows adequate tissue sampling under direct vision, with direct (and immediate) control of bleeding. It is generally performed by those with special expertise, typically under general anesthesia. Indeed a typical surgical approach (laparoscopic or open biopsy) for children is considered in case of suspected inherited metabolic liver disease in which more liver tissue is requested for molecular analysis and also muscle and skin biopsies are expected to reach a diagnosis.

Beyond all the different techniques and in order to justify the risk in the procedure, it is essential that the resulting liver biopsy specimen be adequate so as to allow detailed interpretation. This almost always means that thebiopsy should be of large enough size to view a representative amount of parenchyma and number of portal tracts an adequate number of portal tracts has been proposed to be almost 10 for adult patients (38). However it's clear as the sampling variability is almost inevitable due to the patchy distribution of the disease especially in children(39). The size of specimen is essential especially to detect bile ducts or metabolic liver disease whereas less than 10 portal tracts could be enough to allow a diagnosis for viral hepatitis. Biopsy specimen should be obtained for routine histopatology, microbiology, electron microscopy, immunohistochemistry, and copper (if appropriate), and snap-frozen in liquid nitrogen for enzymatic or metabolic investigations. The interpretation of the histology may be difficult and requires considerable specialist expertise.

Transvenous (Transjugular or Transfemoral) Biopsy. A number of specific situations warrant consideration of this approach. Patients with clinically demonstrable ascites; a known or suspected hemostatic defect; a small, hard, cirrhotic liver; morbid obesity with a difficult-to-identify flank site; or those in whom free and wedged hepatic vein pressure measurements are additionally being sought, should be considered candidates to undergo liver biopsy by the transvenous route. Expertise is also important variableswhen considering transvenous biopsy.

The technique has been well described in the literature and should be considered standard for adult patients (40-43) while is not routinely performed for children, therefore availability of local expertise is extremely important when considering transvenous biopsy. Hanafee and collegues first performed transjugular biopsy in 1967. Since that time the technique has been shown to be safe and effective in adults and children.In 1998

Bergey et al demonstrated that specimens of diagnostic quality could be obtained in children of all ages and sizes, even small infants (44). The theory behind transjugular liver biopsy is that instead of making a hole in liver capsule that can bleed externally, the hole is made in the wall of hepatic vein and any bleeding is internal, back to the vein. The risk of bleeding occurs only if somehow the anterior the anterior capsule of the liver is punctured during the transjugular biopsy, which can occur if the liver is small or the needle is placed too pheripherally.

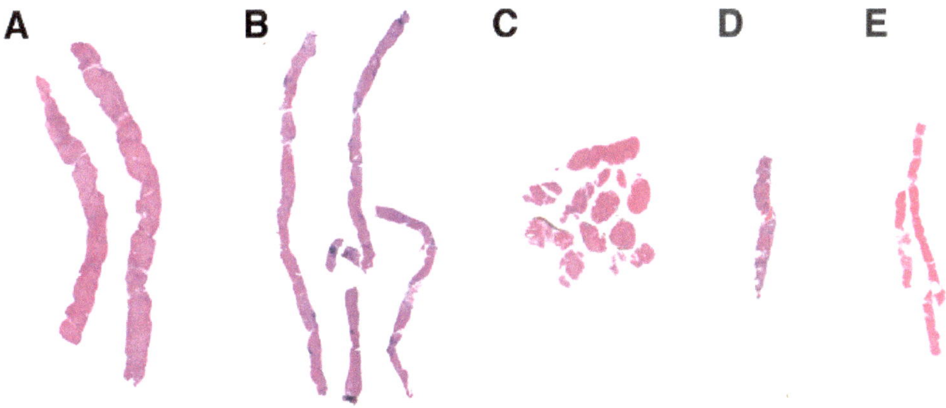

Fig. 6. Specimen of Liver obtained with needles and different techniques. All five biopsies shown in this figure were submitted for grading and staging of chronic hepatitis C. However, only (A) and (B) are felt to provide enough tissue for adequate histologic analysis. (C) is a fragmented specimen. (E) is a biopsy specimen 1.5 cm obtained with a 20-gauge needle. From AASLD POSITION PAPER. Liver biopsy.2009

4. Conclusion

The use of liver biopsy to obtain tissue for histological interpretation play a pivotal role in the practice and science of hepatology and remains a standard for diagnosis and treatment to which numerous other tests are held. Much has been learned about the pitfalls of sampling error and the need to obtain adequate samples so as to minimize this error and about which approaches and devices are most likely to produce good results in different patients.

In terms of safety and comfort, it appears that the ultrasound guided approach improves certain outcomes, particularly in the hands of less experienced operators. This technology, long available in radiology units and increasingly available in liver/endoscopy units, may also reduce the time needed to become proficient in biopsy but likely does not reduce the rate of postprocedure bleeding which, although infrequent, requires careful vigilance.

Perhaps the use of non-invasive markers will be used in the future. For now, liver biopsy is useful andnecessary for the evaluation of chronic hepatopathies, despite the fact that it is not a perfect test.

5. References

[1] Al Knawy B & Shiffman M (2007) Percutaneous liver biopsy in clinical practice. *Liver Int* 27:1166–1173

[2] Balistreri WF (1985) Neonatal cholestasis. *J Pediatr* 106:171–185

[3] Bedossa P et al. (1988) Observer variation in assessment of liver biopsies of alcoholic patients. *Alcohol Clin Exp Res*;12:173-8.

[4] Bedossa P et al. (2003) Sampling variability of liver fibrosis in chronic hepatitis C. *Hepatology*;38:1449-57.

[5] Bergey EA et al. (1998). Pediatric transvenous liver biopsy. *J Vasc Interv Radiol*; 9(5): 829-832.

[6] Bravo AA, et al. (2001) Liver biopsy. *N Engl J Med*;344:495-500.

[7] Bull HJ et al. (1983) Experience with transjugular liver biopsy. *Gut*;24:1057-1060.

[8] Cohen MB et al (1992) Complications of percutaneous liver biopsy in children. *Gastroenterology* 102 (2): 629-32.

[9] Colloredo G et al (2003)Impact of liver biopsy size on histological evaluation of chronic viral hepatitis: The smaller the sample, the milder the disease. *J Hepatol*; 39:239-44.

[10] Crawford AR et al. (1998) The normal adult human liver biopsy: a quantitative reference standard, *hepatology*, 28:323-331

[11] D. C. Rockey et al. Liver biopsy. (2009) AASLD position paper, *hepatology*, vol 49, no 3.

[12] D'antiga L & Mieli Vergani G (2010) La biospia epatica nella pratica clinica, In training and Educational corner, *Bollettino Sigemp*,.

[13] Degos F & Benhamou JP (1999) *Liver biopsy*. In: Bircher J, Benhamou JP, McIntyre N et al Clinical hepatology. Oxford University Press, Oxford, pp 541–548

[14] Firpy RJ, et al. (2004) One year protocol liver biopsy can stratify fibrosis progression in liver transplant recipients with recurrent hepatitis C infections. *Liver trasplan*;10: 1240-47

[15] Furuya K N et al. (1992) Transjugular liver biopsy in children. *Hepatology*; 15:1036-42.

[16] Glaser J&Pausch J (1995) The risk of liver biopsy. *Z Gastroenterol* 33:673–676

[17] Gonzalez-Vallina R et al (1993) Outpatient percutaneous liver biopsy in children.*J PediatrGastroenterol Nutr* 17: 370-5.

[18] Grant A & Neuberger J (1999) Guidelines on the use of liver biopsy in clinical practice. British Society of Gastroenterology. *Gut* 45 Suppl 4: IV1-IV11.

[19] Hevans HN, et al. (2006) Progressive histological damage in liver allograft following pediatric liver transplantation. *Hepatology* may; 43(5): 1109-1117.

[20] Kelly DA, (2008). *Disease of the liver and biliary system in children* (third edition), Wiley-Blackwell, Oxford, Uk

[21] Labayle D et al. (1979) Comparison of the histological lesions in tissue specimens taken from the right and left lobe of the liver in alcoholic liver disease. *Gastroenterol Clin Biol*;3:235-40.

[22] Lachaux A, et al (1995) Complications of percutaneous liver biopsy in infants and children.*Eur J Pediatr*154 (8): 621-3.

[23] Lebrec D et al. Transvenous liver biopsy: an experience based on 1000 hepatic tissue samplings with this procedure. *Gastroenterology* 1982;83:338-340.
[24] Lichtman S, Guzman C, Moore D, Weber JL, Roberts EA (1987) Morbidity after percutaneous liver biopsy.*Arch Dis Child* 62 (9): 901-4.
[25] Lindor KD et al (1996) The role of ultrasonography and automatic-needle biopsy in outpatient percutaneous liver biopsy. *Hepatology* 23:1079–108
[26] MacSween. (2007) Pathology of the Liver, Fifth edition, Churchill Livingstone Elsevier.
[27] McGill DB et al. (1990) A 21-year experience with major haemorrhage after percutaneous liver biopsy. *Gastroenterology* 99:1396–1400
[28] McHutchison J et al (2006) International Fibrosis Group Meeting Participants. Fibrosis as an end point for clinical trials in liver disease: A report of the international fibrosis group. *Clin Gastroenterol Hepatol*;4:1214-20.
[29] Menghini G (1958) One second needle biopsy of the liver. *Gastroenterology* 35 :190 -199
[30] Nobili V, et al (2009) Performance of ELF serum markers in predicting fibrosis stage in pediatric nonalcoholic fatty liver disease. *Gastroenterology* 136:160–167
[31] Nobili Vet al (2003) Blind and ultrasound-guided percutaneous liver biopsy in children. *Pediatr Radiol* 33:772–775
[32] Piccinino F et al (1986) Complications following percutaneous liver biopsy. A multicentre retrospective study on 68276 biopsies. *J Hepatol* 2:165–173
[33] Pietrobattista A et al (2009). Is juvenile liver biopsy unsafe? Putting an end to a common misapprehension. *Pediatr Radiol* 39: 959
[34] Poynard T et al. (2000) Appropriateness of liver biopsy. *Can J Gastroenterol*;14:543-8.
[35] Poynard T et al. (2005) Biomarkers as a first-line estimate of injury in chronic liver diseases: Time for a moratorium on liver biopsy? *Gastroenterology*; 128:1146-8.
[36] Ratziu Vet al . (2005) Sampling variability of liver biopsy in nonalcoholic fatty liver disease. *Gastroenterology*;128:1898-906.
[37] Regev A, et al .(2002) Sampling error and intraobserver variation in liver biopsy in patients with chronic HCV infection. *Am J Gastroenterol*; 97:2614-8.
[38] Rivera-Sanfeliz G et al (2005) Single-pass percutaneous liver biopsy for diffuse liver disease using an automated device: experience in 154 procedures. *Cardiovasc Intervent Radiol* 28 (5): 584-8.
[39] Scheenstra R, et al. (2009) Graft fibrosis after liver transplantation: ten years of follow up. *Hepatology* mar; 49 (3) 880-886.
[40] Schiemann AO, et al (2000) Percutaneous liver biopsy in children: impact of ultrasonography and spring-loaded biopsy needles. *J Pediatr Gastroenterol Nutr* 31 (5): 536-9.
[41] Sebastiani G & Alberti A. (2006) Non invasive fibrosis biomarkers reduce but not substitute the need for liver biopsy. *World J Gastroenterol* 21;12:3682-94.
[42] Sherlock S & Dooley J (eds) (1997) *Diseases of the liver and biliary system*, 10th edn. Blackwell, London

[43] Smith TP et al. (2003) Transjugular biopsy of the liver in pediatric and adult patients using an 18-gauge automated core biopsy needle: a retrospective review of 410 consecutive procedures. *Am J Roentgenol.* Jan;180(1):167-72
[44] Suchy F J, (2007). *Liver disease in children* (third edition), Cambridge University press, New York, USA

18

Bile Duct Paucity in Infancy

Consolato Sergi, Wesam Bahitham and Redha Al-Bahrani
Department of Laboratory Medicine and Pathology,
University of Alberta, Edmonton, AB,
Canada

1. Introduction

Approach to an infant with jaundice and persistent conjugated hyperbilirubinemia includes several pediatric investigations with a different spectrum of invasiveness ranging from clinical biochemistry to liver biopsy. The broad and intense level of investigation needs to be set up soon to exclude surgical conditions that would prompt the child to a beneficial - at least temporary - solution. Paucity of the interlobular bile ducts (PIBD) is defined as a low ratio of interlobular bile ducts to portal tract ratios. However, obtaining adequate tissue for a definitive diagnosis can be a problem in young children. The interlobular bile duct to portal tract ratio is a value that has been considered differently from several authors, but major consensus and discussion platforms among pathologists and hepatologists seem indicate a cut-off value of 0.6 as highly likely for PIBD. PIBD may occur in a non-syndromic setting with various conditions or in genetic syndromes with a peculiar association with simple or complex congenital heart disease. Two well-established syndromes have been identified as genetic syndromes with a PIBD, although the list of the syndromes may be growing in the future. The first syndrome described in the literature is Alagille syndrome (AGS) or arteriohepatic dysplasia with pulmonary stenosis as the most common cardiac single finding and tetralogy of Fallot as the most common complex cardiac defect. Alagille syndrome can be caused by either mutation in the Jagged-1 gene (JAG1) mutation or in the NOTCH2 gene (Bauer et al. 2010). The second syndrome is Williams-Beuren syndrome (WBS), which is a neurodevelopmental disorder with supravalvular aortic or pulmonary stenosis. The WBS is associated with a microdeletion within the 7q11.23 chromosomal band, which encompasses 28 genes and specific low copy repeats serve as substrate for non-allelic homologous recombination leading to the deletion. The most common deletion, which occurs in about 95% of cases, involves a 1.5 megabase DNA segment (Henrichsen et al. 2011). Interestingly, in both genetic syndromes an abnormality of the outlet tract of the ventricular pump of the heart represents one of the most salient feature.

2. Development of intrahepatic biliary system

Understanding the development of the intrahepatic biliary system is crucial to interpret categories of neonatal and infantile cholangiopathies, particularly if infants are preterm or small for gestational age. At the 3rd postovulation week, endodermal cells sprout from the cranial portion of the primitive foregut and grow towards a loosely arranged mesoderm in the direction of the plexus vitellinus of the embryo. Caudally, a bud arises from the foregut and precisely form the anlage of the extrahepatic biliary system (Hammar,1926; Van Eyken et al, 1988; Nakanuma et al, 1997; Desmet,1985; Sergi et al, 2000b). The ductular reaction observed after sub-massive through massive liver necrosis in individuals with fulminant hepatitis supports the theory proposing the presence of common progenitor cells that may differentiate in bile duct cells along the portal vein branches (Desmet,1985; Sergi et al, 2000b; Dorn et al, 2009). At the hilum hepatis between the 6th and the 9th postovulation week, progenitor cells in contact with the mesenchyme surrounding the portal vein form first mono- and later double-layered cell cords with a slit-like lumen. This structure represents indeed the primitive intrahepatic biliary structure, which is also called "ductal plate". From 12 weeks of intrauterine gestation on, a continuous and progressive remodeling of the ductal plate occurs. A few parts of the primitive intrahepatic biliary structures dilate and slightly migrate toward the center of the portal tract, which are called "peripheral tubular or ductular structures" and represent the immature form of the interlobular bile ducts. Subsequently, one or two immature, mostly peripherally located ductular structures transform into mature interlobular bile ducts, while most of them gradually disappear (Sergi et al, 2008a). The transformation of the ductal plate into mature interlobular bile ducts is accompanied by the expression of specific intermediate filaments of the cytoskeleton, the cytokeratins (CK) (Van Eyken et al, 1988; Sergi et al, 2008b; Sergi et al, 2000a). Epithelial cells forming bile ducts express CK-7 and CK-19 in addition to CK-8 and CK-18, the latter two being also positive in normal adult hepatocytes. Quantification of biliary structures and their maturity may be useful in the evaluation of the maturation of the intrahepatic biliary tree in neonatal and infantile cholangiopathies. The ratio between the number of bile ducts and portal tracts during human fetal development has been extensively studied and morphometric and quantitative studies elaborating the dynamics of the remodeling of the primitive fetal biliary structures have been reported using a computer-based image-analysis system as well (Sergi et al, 2000b).

3. Liver biopsy

The liver biopsy is still the gold standard for the diagnosis of neonatal surgical conditions with cholestasis, e.g. biliary atresia (BA), which is the most important surgically correctable form of persistent conjugated hyperbilirubinemia. Liver biopsy is accurate in more than nine cases out of ten, provided that the hepatic tissue contains more than five portal tracts. However, in the routine practice of many pathology services liver biopsy interpretation at neonatal and infantile age is also a true challenge and difficulties can arise not only from atypical presentations, but also from abnormal maturation of the intrahepatic bile duct system (IBDS). In fact, sometimes the initial injury is more severe in the intrahepatic biliary tree rather than the extrahepatic one, and this can result in ductopenia as a first manifestation. Thus, the concept of a neonatal obstructive cholangiopathy as a pathology continuum with a single underlying cause has been proposed, despite it is still being a matter of controversy (Sergi et al, 2008a). According to our previously published data, patterns of ductular reactions may confound the pathologist and ductal plate remnants may indeed recapitulate the embryonic anlage, which can be a true challenge for the pathologist interpreting the liver biopsy (Sergi et al, 2008a). In fact, there are biliary structures that may represent a form of ductular proliferation, which seems to be peculiar to the neonate. It is highly likely that there are probably only limited ways of response to different disorders in the neonatal liver and all of them may record the development of the primitive intrahepatic biliary system or ductal plate.

4. Ductal plate malformation

In the liver, the ductal plate is the protostructure of the intrahepatic biliary system and consists of a double-layered cylinder of biliary-type cells with a slit-like lumen forming around the portal vein and its surrounding mesenchyme (stage of ductal plate). The remodeling of the ductal plate is characterized by the incorporation of a few ductal plate cells into the mesenchyme surrounding the portal vein to form bile ducts as well as by the disappearance of nonmigrating ductal plate cells (stage of remodeling ductal plate and stage of remodeled bile ducts). The development of intrahepatic bile ducts proceeds from the hilar to peripheral portions. Two or more of these developmental stages may be present in the same liver specimen and this should be taken into account in evaluating the maturation of the IBDS. The complete or partial persistence of the primitive double-layered cylinder of biliary-type cells in the developing liver gives rise to portal tracts with an increased number of bile duct structures. The term "ductal plate malformation of the liver" was coined to label this complex biliary plexus with an excess of primitive bile duct structures (Sergi et al. 2000a; Sergi et al. 2000b; Sergi et al. 2000c). Previously, we examined the patterns of cytokeratin 7 (CK7) expressing biliary structures of liver biopsies of infants aged less than one year and found specific patterns in biliary atresia, neonatal hepatitis (a category of inflammation of the liver probably including several conditions showing lobular disarray of the hepatocytes and giant cell transformation as well as presence of extramedullary hematopoiesis) and paucity of the intrahepatic bile duct system or paucity of the interlobular bile ducts (PIBD). Cytokeratins are intermediate filaments of the cytoskeleton and ductal plate remnants have been demonstrated to be present, recapitulating the primitive stages of the IBDS. We also found that the lack of intrahepatic bile ducts in infants aged less than one year is an adverse prognostic factor, which was independent from the etiology of neonatal liver disease (Sergi et al, 2008a) and this is supported by the expression of polyductin or fibrocystin, the gene product of the autosomal recessive polycystic kidney disease (Dorn et al, 2009). Ductal plate malformation may be quite variable, but represents altogether a common way to show a disorder of the correct development of the intrahepatic biliary system in which the apoptosis may play a major role (Sergi et al, 2000a). Studying the models of response to liver injury we found a unimodal distribution of the developmental stages, with many remodeling bile ducts seen in surgically correctable cholangiopathies. The major power of our studies was the blind evaluation of the physiological developmental stages of the intrahepatic bile duct formation through a schematic representation of the stages. This emphasizes how consecutive liver biopsies of patients with biliary atresia (BA) may show characteristic changes in singular cases. In our study, we found an increase of the immunoreactivity of the ductal plate cells in BA and PIBD, but this was a factor that was also observed in other infantile cholangiopathies (neonatal hepatitis, NH; other liver disease, OLD). In the routine practice, it is important to apply a strict definition of interlobular bile duct. The interlobular bile duct should not be confused with neoductules. Indeed, although immunostaining for CK7 is an advance to identify even minute or hypoplastic bile duct radicles that might well be missed in routinely stained sections, an interlobular bile duct is a defined structure with more or less round, well-developed lumen, and is accompanied by an arteriole usually within three arteriolar diameters of distance. In all biopsies an arteriolar to portal tract was calculated to justify the absence of the interlobular bile ducts. Thus, PIBD may be only one aspect or manifestation of a disease primarily characterized by other features and prognosis may be highly variable. Our study aimed to identify a prognostic factor independent from etiology of neonatal liver disease. We chose CK7 instead of CK19 to better highlight the reactive patterns. The ductular proliferation in infants with BA is frequently encompassed in the enlarged and inflamed portal tracts where on-going bile duct destruction takes place. BA affects the development of the intrahepatic and extrahepatic biliary system and results in the progressive fibrotic obstruction of the pre-formed bile ducts. The rapid advances in the understanding of the cellular and molecular physiology of bile secretion have led to a better knowledge of the pathophysiology of cholangiopathy and structural cell damage caused by various hereditary and acquired cholestatic disorders.

5. Developmental Immaturity of the biliary tract

Hepatic haematopoiesis extends from 5 to 6 weeks of embryogenesis to shortly before the time of birth, although at the mid-term the bone marrow begins to take over. Erythropoiesis decreases from a diffuse to an insular pattern (mid-gestation) in the hepatocellular plates, whereas periportal granulopoiesis increases at mid-gestation and correlates with the slow-down of the intrahepatic biliary system development. Besides haematological disorders, fetal haematopoiesis may return to a lesser degree in the form of extra-medullary hematopoiesis (EMH) with insular pattern, during various insults to the intrahepatic biliary system in the young child. In fact, in previous studies, we frequently found EMH in a more or less similar distribution of the four disease classes, which was studied in the CK7-based study. The granulopoietic periportal phase does not seem to be reactivated, because the neutrophils seen in typical or atypical ductular reaction are not accompanied by the presence of periportal myeloblasts. The results of this investigation further defined the important role of liver biopsy in identifying abnormality of the development of the intrahepatic biliary system and correlate it to the development of the hepatic hematopoiesis. This is extremely determining for the outcome in infants presenting with liver disease and to identify "immaturity" in the development of the biliary tract, which can be mis-interpreted as true PIBD (Sergi et al. 2000b). The results of our investigations indicate that early recognition of BD/PT = 0 is clinically significant and is highly likely a harbinger of later worse outcome. The more close and efficient the liaison between histopathologist and clinician, the higher the possibility to rank possible disorders as more or less likely among the set that other observations suggest. We were not able to identify other independent prognostic factors, such as the portal fibrosis and gamma-glutamyl transpeptidase (GGT) levels, in our sample of 87 subjects younger than 1 year of age and undergoing a liver biopsy. Most probably, this was due to the heterogeneity of our cases. The heterogeneity of our cases and the presence of different diagnoses under the heading of NH may also be a limitation in the interpretation of the 'abnormal reactive patterns' and biliary patterns. To date, the sensitivity of liver biopsy in diagnosing BA is greater than 90% and the specificity probably approaches 80% in several centers of excellence for health care. However, the variety of clinical presentation and the associations with congenital defects in other organs have suggested that BA is a heterogeneous disorder. It is plausible that various injuries may damage the normal pathway of development of the intrahepatic biliary system by infections, toxic iatrogenic, immunorelated or ischemic, depending on the presence of specific genetic or other factors. GGT is a molecule located on canalicular and luminal surfaces of liver cells. Bile is a detergent and elutes GGT into the biliary-tract lumen as it travels along the biliary tree and in our double-blind investigation represents the only clinical-biochemistry analyte differing in a statistically significant manner between groups. Thus, biliary epithelial cell patterns do recapitulate the primitive stages of IBDS, which seems to represent a form of ductular proliferation that is peculiar to the neonate. Abnormal reaction patterns occur mainly in NH, and most remarkably with reference to the clinical impact, the lack of intrahepatic bile ducts in infants aged less than 1 year is an adverse prognostic factor independent from etiology of neonatal liver disease.

6. Causes of paucity of interlobular bile ducts in infants

Bile duct paucity or ductopenia may arise in a syndromic or non syndromic setting. For long time "syndromic" bile duct paucity was considered synonymous with arteriohepatic dysplasia, or Alagille syndrome (AGS), which includes congenital heart disease, ocular posterior embryotoxon, and vertebral anomalies (the so-called "butterfly vertebrae"). Alagille syndrome (AS) is an autosomal dominant disorder associated with abnormalities of the liver, heart, skeleton, eye, and kidneys and a characteristic facial appearance (hypertelorism, prominent forehead, flattened nose, and small mandible with pointed chin) and paucity of the interlobular bile ducts or ductopenia (Kamath et al, 2010). Alagille syndrome is characterized by a variable expression and this should be taken into account from both the clinician and the pathologist. The intimate relationship of Notch signaling with the intrahepatic biliary system seems to be fascinating and novel aspects will probably create a platform for future studies (Zanotti et al, 2010). Some patients are diagnosed with AS after prolonged jaundice at neonatal or perinatal age or when liver biopsy findings reveal ductopenia when the children are a little older (Figure 1). Others may be diagnosed during evaluation for right-sided heart disease and congenital heart disease with disturbances of development of the outflow tract of the right heart. Some patients with Alagille syndrome (AS) start to lose interlobular bile ducts in the first months of life, although it seems that in other patients with AS the ductopenia does not appear until 3 years of age. Thus, the morphologic diagnosis of AS cannot be ruled out on the basis of a normal number of ducts in a single liver biopsy early in life. A mild lymphocytic infiltrate with or without an increase of the periductular fibrous tissue accompany the damaged interlobular bile ducts. Moreover, there may be some degree of bile ductular proliferation, canalicular cholestasis, a mild degree of giant cell transformation of hepatocytes, and some degree of hepatocellular necrosis with or

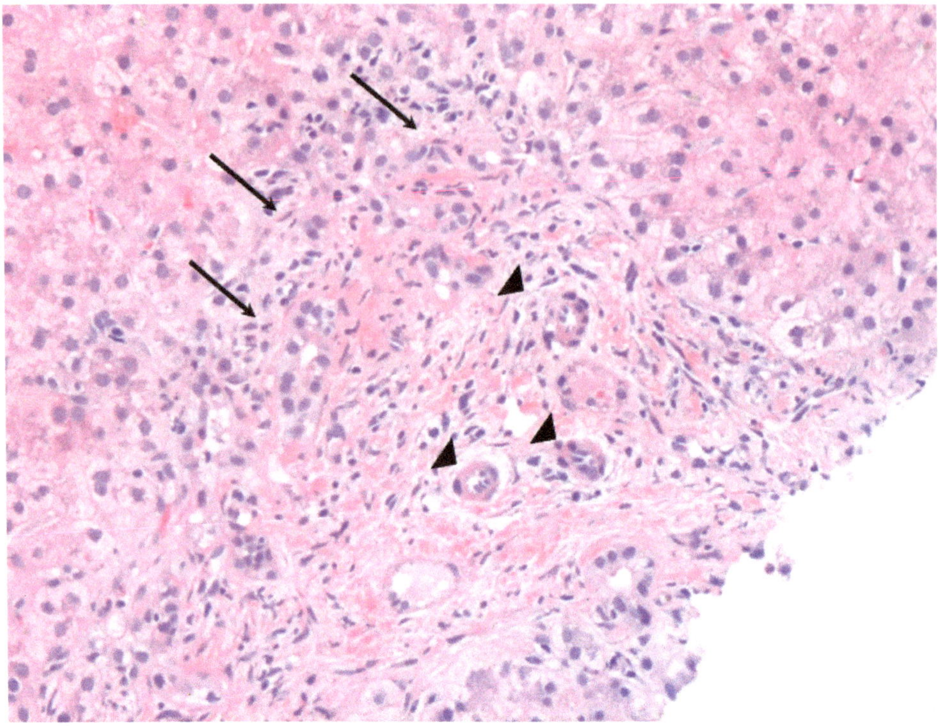

Fig. 1. Paucity of intrahepatic bile ducts in a portal tract of the liver biopsy of a 6-month old male child with Alagille syndrome with tetralogy of Fallot as congenital heart disease. Note the presence of arterioles (arrowheads) and venules (close to the center of the microphotograph) but no accompanying interlobular bile duct. Some biliary ductular proliferation with mononuclear cell inflammation is present at the periphery of the portal tract (arrows) (hematoxylin and eosin staining, x200 original magnification).

without bridging fibrosis and/or cirrhosis. To date, syndromic PIBD is not any more synonymous with AS, but PIBD may be found in at least an additional genetic syndrome, which is the Williams-Beuren or Williams syndrome (WBS). WBS is a rare neuro-developmental disorder caused by a large deletion encompassing about 26 genes localized in the long arm of chromosome 7 (Pober, 2010). Typically, WBS features include a distinctive, "elfin" facial appearance with a low nasal bridge, a cheerful character with strangers as well as delay in the language development, feeding difficulties, and cardiovascular defects, including supravalvular aortic stenosis and more or less transient endocrine abnormalities (hypercalcemia, hypercalciuria, hypothyroidism, and early puberty). Other cardiovascular defects found most often in association with WBS are ventricular septal defect, patent ductus arteriosus, stenosis of supracardiac arteries (cerebral, carotid, coronary, brachiocephalic, and subclavian) but also stenosis of renal and mesenteric aretries, coarctation of the aorta, mitral valve incompetence, tetralogy of Fallot (TOF), and vascular ring. An additional syndrome is Ivemark syndrome or heterotaxy (Cohen et al,

2007). Ivemark syndrome (IS) is a rare disorder that affects multiple organ systems of the body. In most patients the phenotype includes absence (asplenia) or underdevelopment (hypoplasia) of the spleen, congenital heart malformation, and an abnormal arrangement of the internal organs of the chest and abdomen, which is also called "situs viscerum inversus". It is known, however, that the symptoms of IS can vary greatly depending upon the specific abnormalities present. The complex arrangement of the visceral organs indicates how life-threatening complications may occur during infancy. The exact cause of Ivemark syndrome is under investigation. The nonsyndromic category of bile duct paucity includes metabolic disorders, perinatal infections, chromosomal anomalies, abnormalities in bile metabolism and transport, and a large miscellaneous group (Table 1). The histology of early biopsies in nonsyndromic paucity mimics AS in many ways, typically showing cholestasis and giant cell transformation. However, though specific histologic features reflect the etiologic heterogeneity, it has been reported that early portal and perisinusoidal fibrosis seem to be more frequently observed in nonsyndromic PIBD than in AS. Identification of nonsyndromic disorders relies on detailed and collaborative clinical and pathology evaluation, which may include cytogenetics, serologic and biochemical blood tests, molecular studies, special histochemical stains, immunohistochemistry, and transmission electron microscopy. The ultrastructural examination of the bile canaliculus and its lumen is central and is performed for all cases with neonatal, infantile and pediatric cholangiopathy in our centre. There is a significant amount of overlap between the clinical manifestations of WBS and AS. Both syndromes have distinct facies, congenital heart disease of the outflow tract of one or both ventricles, musculo-skeletal anomalies, growth and developmental delay, and occasional renal involvement, but both have different genetic implications. In AS, mutations in the JAG1 gene on chromosome 20p12 are identified in 70% of the cases, whereas 96% of patients affected with Williams syndrome show elastin gene deletion. At the end of the chapter table 1 summarizes the etiology of PIBD.

7. Conclusion

In summary, bile duct paucity or ductopenia can be classified as syndromic or nonsyndromic. Syndromic paucity was originally described as being specific for AS, but it is not true anymore. In addition to bile duct paucity of patients with AS present with characteristic facial appearance and developmental abnormalities affecting the heart, eyes, and vertebrae, a couple of other syndromes have been discovered to have ductopenia and the list will probably grow in the future. A caveat to histologic diagnosis in the young child is that ductopenia may not be present on initial biopsy in as many as 20% to 40% of infants with AS. To further complicate matters, ductular biliary proliferation is identified in a small number of infants with AS, leading to potential diagnostic confusion with biliary atresia, which is a surgical condition. In fact, it is important to remember that the porto-enterostomy or Kasai procedure is not a marker for an underlying severe liver disease and may have a detrimental effect on outcome (Kaye et al. 2010). The normal liver in a term infant and older individual demonstrates an interlobular bile duct to portal tract ratio of 0.9 to 1.8, but it should be emphasized that in a preterm infant or in a small-for-gestational age infant the intrahepatic biliary system may still be developing and this ratio may not be applicable with certainty.

Furthermore, obtaining adequate tissue for diagnosis can be a problem in infants. Repeated liver biopsies should be considered as a guideline in cases where the diagnosis is clinically suspected but not confirmed on histology of the first biopsy. A strict liaison between pediatric hepatologist, pediatric cardiologist and pediatric pathologist is crucial. "Primum non nocere", i.e. the Latin words for the medical professional sentence "First do no harm," are still up to date and remain a fundamental medical precept of Hippocrates (ca. 460-ca. 377 B.C.).

Syndromic	Alagille syndrome Williams syndrome Ivemark syndrome or Heterotaxy syndrome
Nonsyndromic	- Congenital infections Rubella Virus Cytomegalovirus Hepatitis Virus Treponema pallidum - Metabolic Alpha-1-Antitrypsin deficiency Cystic fibrosis (Mucoviscidosis) Niemann-Pick type C Cerebro-hepato-renal syndrome or Zellweger syndrome - Endocrine Disorders Hypopituitarism - Chromosomal Defects Trisomy 21 Monosomy X0 or Turner syndrome - Progressive intrahepatic familial cholestasis (PFIC) - Immunologic disorders - Graft-versus-host disease - Chronic hepatic allograft rejection - Neonatal sclerosing cholangitis - Miscellaneous Maternal use of progesterone during α pregnancy, Norwegian cholestasis, cholestasis with some non-specific familiarity, familial α hemophagocytic lymphohistiocytosis, congenital pancreatic hypoplasia, and renal microcystic disease - Idiopathic

Table 1. Causes of Paucity of Interlobular Bile Ducts in Infants

8. References

Bauer RC, Laney AO, Smith R, Gerfen J, Morrissette JJ, Woyciechowski S, Garbarini J, Loomes KM, Krantz ID, Urban Z, Gelb BD, Goldmuntz E, Spinner NB (2010). Jagged1 (JAG1) mutations in patients with tetralogy of Fallot or pulmonic stenosis. Hum Mutat. 2010 May;31(5):594-601.

Cohen MS, Anderson RH, Cohen MI, Atz AM, Fogel M, Gruber PJ, Lopez L, Rome JJ, Weinberg PM. (2007). Controversies, genetics, diagnostic assessment, and outcomes relating to the heterotaxy syndrome. Cardiology in the young, Vol.17, No.2, (Septemper 2007), pp.29-42.

Dorn L, Menezes LF, Mikuz G, Otto HF, Onuchic LF, Sergi C. (2009). Immunohistochemical detection of polyductin and co-localization with liver progenitor cell markers during normal and abnormal development of the intrahepatic biliary system and in adult hepatobiliary carcinomas. Journal of Cellular and Molecular Medicine, Vol.13, No.7, (July 2009), pp. 1279-90.

Hammar JA. Uber die erste Entstehung der nicht kapillaren intrahepatischen Gallengenge beim Menschen. (1926). Zeitschrift für mikroskopisch-anatomische Forschung, Vol.5, (n.d.), pp. 59-89.

Henrichsen CN, Csárdi G, Zabot MT, Fusco C, Bergmann S, Merla G, Reymond A. (2011) Using transcription modules to identify expression clusters perturbed in Williams-Beuren syndrome. PLoS Comput Biol. 2011 Jan 20;7(1):e1001054.

Kamath BM, Schwarz KB, Hadzić N. Alagille syndrome and liver transplantation. (2010). Journal of Pediatric Gastroenterology and Nutrition. Vol,50, No.1, (January 2010), pp. 11-15.

Kaye AJ, Rand EB, Munoz PS, Spinner NB, Flake AW, Kamath BM. Effect of Kasai procedure on hepatic outcome in Alagille syndrome. (2010). Journal of Pediatric Gastroenterology and Nutrition. 2010 Vol.51, No.3, (Septemper 2010), pp.319-21.

Pober BR. Williams-Beuren syndrome. (2010). The New England Journal of Medicine. Vol.362, No.2, (January 2010), pp.239-52.

Nakanuma Y, Hoso M, Sanzen T, Sasaki M. Microstructure and development of the normal and pathologic biliary tract in humans, including blood supply.(1997). Microscopy Research and Technique. Vol.38,(n.d.), pp.552-70.

Desmet VJ.(1985). Intrahepatic bile ducts under the lens. Journal of Hepatology. Vol.1,(n.d.), pp.545-59.

Sergi C, Benstz J, Feist D, Nutzenadel W, Otto HF, Hofmann WJ. (2008a). Bile duct to portal space ratio and ductal plate remnants in liver disease of infants aged less than 1 year. Pathology. Vol.40, No.3, (April 2008), pp.260-7.

Sergi C, Gross W, Mory M, Schaefer M, Gebhard MM. (2008b) Biliary-type cytokeratin pattern in a canine isolated perfused liver transplantation model. (2008b). Journal of Surgical Research. Vol.146, No.2, (May 2008), pp.146-71.

Sergi C, Adam S, Kahl P, Otto HF. Study of the malformation of ductal plate of the liver in Meckel syndrome and review of other syndromes presenting with this anomaly. (2000a). Pediatric and Development Pathology. Vol.3, No.6, (November- December 2000), pp.568-83.

Sergi C, Adam S, Kahl P, Otto HF. The remodeling of the primitive human biliary system. (2000b). Early Human Development. Vol.58, No.3, (June 2000), pp.167-78.

Sergi C, Kahl P, Otto HF. Contribution of apoptosis and apoptosis-related proteins to the malformation of the primitive intrahepatic biliary system in Meckel syndrome. (2000c). Am J Pathol. 2000 May;156(5):1589-98.

Van Eyken P, Sciot R, Callea F, Van der Steen K, Moerman P, Desmet VJ. The development of the intrahepatic bile ducts in man: a keratin-immunohistochemical study.(1988). Hepatology. Vol.8, (n.d.), pp.1586-95.

Zanotti S, Canalis E.(2010). Notch and the skeleton. Molecular Cell Biology. Vol.30, No.4, (February 2010), pp.886-96.

Part 4

Viral Hepatitis

19

Occult Hepatitis C Virus Infection: Where are We Now?

Florence Nicot[1], Nassim Kamar[2], Lionel Rostaing[2] and Jacques Izopet[1]
[1]*Virology Laboratory, Toulouse University Hospital,*
[2]*Department of Nephrology, Dialysis and Multiorgan Transplantation, Toulouse University Hospital, France*

1. Introduction

Hepatitis C virus (HCV) is the major cause of chronic liver disease worldwide. Up to 30% of infected individuals spontaneously resolve their acute infection, while others develop chronic hepatitis C and replicate the virus seemingly indefinitely, but the features of the host and virus that are responsible for this difference are not yet clear. The persistence of the virus in the liver can lead to cirrhosis and hepatocellular carcinoma. End-stage liver disease due to a chronic HCV infection is currently the number one reason for liver transplantation in many parts of the world. No prophylactic vaccine is presently available and the current antiviral therapy successfully suppresses HCV replication in fewer than 50% of patients with a chronic infection. Until recently, patients who had eliminated HCV spontaneously or after treatment were considered to be definitively cured. But reports of low HCV RNA concentrations in the plasma, peripheral blood mononuclear cells and livers of patients who had cleared HCV has led to uncertainty in both patients and physicians. This new form of HCV infection is called occult HCV infection. This chapter summarises the data presently available on occult HCV infections and discusses its significance and reality.

1.1 HCV infection

1.1.1 HCV virus

Hepatitis C is a member of the *Flaviviridae* family. Its genome of approximately 9.5 kb is a positive RNA strand that encodes a large polyprotein of more than 3000 amino acid residues. The open reading frame is flanked by untranslated regions, the 5′ UTR and 3′ UTR. The 5′UTR region contains the internal ribosomal entry site (IRES). Processing and cleavage of the polyprotein yields structural and non-structural proteins (Figure 1). HCV has great genetic variability, with six genotypes and more than 70 subtypes (Simmonds et al., 2005).

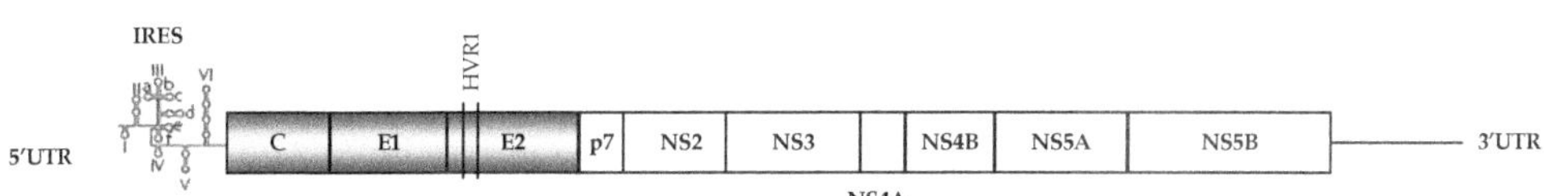

Fig. 1. Organisation of the HCV genome. The region in gray encodes structural proteins and the white one non-structural proteins.

1.1.2 Natural history of HCV infection

Patients infected with HCV virus first develop an acute disease that is usually asymptomatic. Diagnosis is confirmed by the detection of HCV genomic RNA in the plasma, which may also contain anti-HCV antibodies (Figure 2a). About 30% of infected patients spontaneously clear the virus, generally in the 3 months following clinical symptoms (Corey et al., 2006, Gerlach et al., 2003, Micallef et al., 2006)

Unfortunately, 70% of infected patients develop a chronic HCV infection (Figure 2b). The plasma of these patients contains anti-HCV antibodies and HCV RNA. These patients can be divided into two groups. One group has normal liver enzyme activities, while the other has abnormal liver enzyme activities. Thus, 7 - 53% of patients with a chronic HCV infection have normal alanine aminotransferase activities (Alter, 2005, Mathurin et al., 1998, Persico et al., 2000). Hepatic lesions are moderate, but liver biopsies have shown that 90% of patients suffering from chronic hepatitis have lesions (Marcellin et al., 1997b). Analysis of liver biopsies indicates that most patients with a chronic HCV infection have elevated liver enzymes and moderate to severe lesions. About 25% of them develop liver cirrhosis, and this results in hepatocellular carcinoma in 2% of them (Alberti et al., 1999). Liver transplantation is the only treatment available to these patients.

(a)

(b)

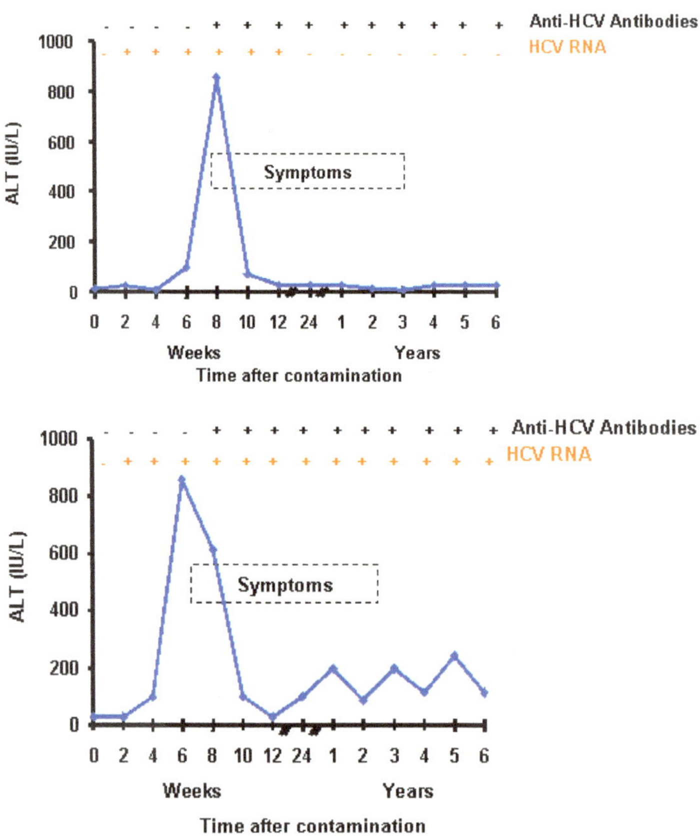

Fig. 2. Natural history of acute (a) and chronic (b) HCV infections.

The natural history of an HCV infection can be modified by anti-HCV therapy. The current antiviral therapy for a chronic HCV infection is pegylated interferon plus ribavirin. It is recommended for patients with a liver fibrosis score of F2 or more. A sustained virological response, defined as undetectable HCV RNA in the serum 6 months after the end of treatment, is achieved in 40-70% of treated patients, depending on the HCV genotype. Patients infected with HCV genotype 1 have a lower sustained virological response (40%) than patients infected with HCV genotypes 2 or 3 (80%). New antiviral therapies targeting directly the HCV genome, anti-protease and anti-polymerase, will improve the sustained virological rate in HCV genotype 1 infected patients (Legrand-Abravanel et al., 2010, McHutchison et al., 2009). Recently, one genetic marker, interleukin 28B, was identified as a factor influencing the natural history of HCV infection and the treatment success of patients chronically infected: patients with a CC genotype clear the virus more easily (Ge et al., 2009, Thomas et al., 2009).

1.1.3 HCV infection in particular populations

The progression of HCV infections in patients with impaired immune systems differs from that in immunocompetent patients. We will focus on patients with end-stage renal disease and patients with an HIV coinfection.

The blood of patients undergoing regular dialysis is much more likely to contain anti-HCV antibodies (7 to 40%) than that of the general population (Rahnavardi et al., 2008), although the percentage has been lower in the past few years because of improved prevention measures, like using gloves, single-use material, and the isolation of HCV-infected people in dialysis units. But it still occurs in French hemodialysis units and requires appropriate management, even though the prevalence of HCV infection has decreased by 7.7% (Saune et al., 2010). It is difficult to evaluate the natural history of HCV in hemodialysis patients because the exact date of contamination is often unknown and the infection can be silent for several years. The liver enzyme activities cannot be used to predict the development of fibrosis in these patients; they can have hepatic lesions with normal liver enzyme activities (Furusyo et al., 2000, Martin et al., 2000). HCV infection is a significant cause of morbidity and mortality in patients with end-stage liver disease, and particularly in renal transplanted recipients. Death is generally due to liver dysfunction and loss of the renal graft. HCV infection has been linked to shorter allograft survival and more acute rejection episodes and virus-related glomerulonephritis (Pereira et al., 1998). Interferon-based treatment after renal transplantation is associated with graft loss and so is not recommended. It has been recommended that all kidney-transplant candidates be treated with alpha-interferon because of the relatively high rate of sustained virological response in HCV-positive dialysis patients given anti-HCV therapy (Izopet et al., 1997, Rostaing et al., 1998).

About 30% of patients infected with HIV are also infected with HCV. HCV infections have become the main cause of morbidity and mortality due to faster development of cirrhosis and hepatocellular carcinoma. These patients are less likely to spontaneously clear their HCV infection and their HCV virus load is often higher than average (Thomas et al., 2000). The virus load is especially increased in patients with low CD4+ T cells counts, probably due to loss of immune control. The rate of sustained virological response is lower in these patients than in those infected with HCV alone. Only 14-38% of patients infected with HCV genotypes 1 or 4 and HIV achieve a sustained virological response, while 44-73% of patients infected with HIV and HCV genotype 2 or 3 do so (Carrat et al., 2004, Chung et al., 2004, Laguno et al., 2004, Torriani et al., 2004).

1.2 HCV tropism

HCV mainly replicates in the liver but there are other extra-hepatic replication sites.

1.2.1 The liver

The liver is the major replication site and contains high concentrations of HCV RNA (about 10^8-10^{11} copies per g tissue) (Sugano et al., 1995). HCV particles, free or associated with serum apolipoproteins, interact with multiple cell surface proteins on hepatocytes (Boonstra et al., 2009). The initial interaction involves glycosaminoglycans (GAGs) and lipoprotein receptors (LDLR), as well as scavenger receptor class B type I (SR-BI), followed by the recruitment of tetraspanin, CD81, and the later use of the tight junction proteins claudin-1 and occludin (OCLN).

In situ hybridization studies found HCV RNA in 5 to 50% of the liver cells of patients chronically infected with HCV genotype 1 (Pal et al., 2006). The proportion of hepatic cells with detectable negative strand HCV RNA (a marker of HCV replication) was closely correlated with the liver enzyme activities and histological changes. Histological damages observed in HCV infection are the results of productive infection of some liver cells.

1.2.2 Extra-hepatic sites

HCV RNA has been detected in the peripheral blood mononuclear cells of chronically infected patients (Blackard et al., 2005, Laskus et al., 2000, Lerat et al., 1996, Lerat et al., 1998, Muller et al., 1993, Navas et al., 1998), in the central nervous system (Forton et al., 2004, Morsica et al., 1997), and other tissues like pancreas, thyroid, spleen (Laskus et al., 1998), seminal fluid (Bourlet et al., 2002, Pasquier et al., 2000). Negative strand HCV RNA was also detected, suggesting HCV replication.

HCV compartmentalization has been described in lymphocytes B cells and dendritic cells (Ducoulombier et al., 2004). The HVR1-E2 sequences found in cells were different from those found in the plasma. Some of the 109 patients tested had very different strains in their peripheral blood mononuclear cells that was undetectable in their plasma (Roque-Afonso et al., 2005). The sequences found in the peripheral blood mononuclear cells of 9 patients were different enough to be classified as another genotype, distinct from the sequences found in the plasma. These strains could have been acquired during co-infection or super-infection. A significant proportion of patients with hepatitis C are infected with two or more HCV variants with distinct IRES sequences and distinct cellular tropism (Di Liberto et al., 2006, Durand et al., 2010). HCV compartmentalization was an independent predictor of treatment response in this study. They also found a correlation between the cellular tropism of HCV variants for liver or B cells *in vivo* and the translational efficiency of their IRES. The IRES of the B cell-specific strains all had a common activity profile and were consistently less efficient than paired plasma IRES in hepatocytes. These findings suggest that HCV replicates extra-hepatically in chronically infected patients. As HCV genotype 1 was more frequently detected than HCV genotypes 2 or 3, this genotype could be better adapted to mononuclear cells (Lerat et al., 1998). Some patients developed a cellular T cells response against a virus whose genotype differed from that of the one detected in plasma (Sugimoto et al., 2005). Patients with HCV compartmentalization in mononuclear cells could develop a stronger immune response, so facilitating virus elimination.

2. Virological tools

The diagnosis of an HCV infection (acute and/or chronic) is based on the detection of serological and molecular markers in serum and plasma. They are also used to initiate treatment and to monitor treatment efficacy.

2.1 Serological assays

Anti-HCV antibodies in the blood plasma or serum are detected using third-generation enzyme immunoassays, which are specific for antibodies against various HCV epitopes. Recombinant antigens are used to capture circulating anti-HCV antibodies. Third-generation enzyme immunoassays are better than 99% specific for anti-HCV antibodies. Their sensitivity is more difficult to determine, given the lack of a reference (gold standard) method, but it is excellent in HCV-infected immunocompetent patients. Detection systems for serum HCV antibodies are insensitive in the acute phase because of long serological window. Immunoassays combining detection of anti-HCV antibodies and HCV antigen reduce the serological window of over 25 days (Laperche et al., 2005). Recently, quantitative immunoassays detecting HCV core antigen were developed. The HCV Ag level correlates the HCV RNA concentration. It can reduce the serological window of over 35 days and is highly specific to detect acute HCV infection in haemodialysis patients (Miedouge et al., 2010).

2.2 HCV RNA detection and quantification

The presence of HCV RNA in serum or plasma is first used to diagnose an HCV infection. The presence of HCV RNA alone, with no anti-HCV antibodies, strongly indicates an acute HCV infection, which must then be confirmed by seroconversion (the appearance of anti-HCV antibodies) a few days or weeks later. Acutely infected patients can also have both HCV RNA and anti-HCV antibodies at the time of diagnosis. It is difficult in this case to distinguish acute hepatitis C from an acute exacerbation of chronic hepatitis C. A patient with clinical or biological signs of chronic liver disease will have chronic hepatitis C if both the anti-HCV antibodies and the HCV RNA are present for at least 6 months. Description of HCV replication in the absence of anti-HCV antibodies is rare with the current enzyme immunoassays, but occurs in profoundly immunodepressed patients, hemodialysis patients or agammaglobulinemic subjects.

The presence of HCV RNA is checked regularly during anti-HCV treatment and treatment is stopped or continues depending on the result. The end-of-treatment and sustained virological responses should be assessed with a sensitive HCV RNA assay, with a lower detection limit of 50 IU/mL or less, according to Consensus Conference recommendations (Anonymous, 2002). The detection of HCV RNA at the end of therapy is highly predictive of a post-treatment relapse, whereas the absence of HCV RNA at the end of treatment indicates a virological response. Patients showing a virological response must be retested for HCV RNA with a sensitive method 24 weeks later to identify a sustained virological response, the endpoint of therapy.

Both qualitative and quantitative assays can be used to detect HCV RNA. Qualitative assays use the principle of target amplification with a "classic" polymerase chain reaction

(PCR), "real-time" PCR or "transcription-mediated amplification" (TMA). Quantitative assays are based on target amplification techniques (competitive PCR or real-time PCR) or signal amplification techniques (branched DNA (bDNA) assays). The commercial assays for HCV RNA are summarized in Table 1. Their ranges of quantification vary considerably.

	Supplier	Detection limit IU/mL	Quantification range IU/mL	
			Lower limit	Upper limit
Qualitative assays				
TMA-based assay Versant	Siemens	5-10	NA	NA
Cobas Amplicor v2.0	Roche	50	NA	NA
APTIMA® HCV RNA	Genprobe	5.3	NA	NA
Quantitative assays				
LCx®HCV RNA Quantitative Assay	Abbott	10	12	100 000 000
Cobas Ampliprep/Cobas TaqMan	Roche	10	43	69 000 000
Cobas Amplicor Monitor v2.0	Roche	600	600	500 000
ARN HCV versant 3.0	Siemens	615	615	7 700 000

Table 1. Detection limits and quantification ranges of commercial techniques for detecting HCV RNA. NA = not applicable

2.3 HCV genotyping

The HCV genotype is routinely determined before treating because the treatment duration, ribavirin dose and virological monitoring procedures depend on the HCV genotype.

The reference method for HCV genotyping is direct sequencing of the NS5B or E1 regions of the HCV genome by means of "in-house" techniques, followed by sequence alignment with prototype sequences and phylogenetic analysis (Sandres-Saune et al., 2003, Simmonds et al., 2005). In clinical practice, HCV genotype can be determined by various commercial kits that use direct sequence analysis of the 5'UTR region (Halfon et al., 2001) or reverse hybridization analysis with genotype-specific probes located in the 5'UTR region (Verbeeck et al., 2008). Unfortunately, analysis of this region tends to misclassify a significant number of HCV subtypes. For example, 20-30% of subtype 1a are not correctly identified (Chen and Weck, 2002). Real-time PCR methods and DNA biochip methods are now available (Gryadunov et al., 2010, Mao et al., 2010, Martro et al., 2008, Nakatani et al., 2010, Park et al., 2009, Verbeeck et al., 2008). Methods based on analysis of the NS5B region are better for discriminating between HCV subtypes (Table 2) (Gryadunov et al., 2010, Sandres-Saune et al., 2003).

Analysis of HCV heterogeneity can be used to determine the source of contamination in cases of nosocomial transmission. The tools should be based on regions of the HCV genome that are variable enough to discriminate between HCV subtypes and even different clusters within a subtype. The best are the NS5B and hypervariable 1 (HVR1)-E2 regions (Figure 1). These are different enough to clearly indicate whether the viruses circulating in different people have a common source (Bracho et al., 2005, Izopet et al., 1999). These regions can also be analysed to determine whether a patient who suffers a late relapse does so because of reactivation of the former virus or because of a new infection with a virus belonging to the same subtype.

Assay	HCV region	Genotype identification	Subtype identification
Line Probe Assay	5'NC (I)	1-6 (mis-typing of G6)	Mis-subtyping
	5'NC+core (II)	1-6 (better idenfication of G6)	Subtype 1a/1b
Sequencing	NS5B or core/E1	1-6	Reference method
	5'NC	1-6 (false idenfication of G6)	Mis-subtyping
Real time PCR	5'NC or NS5B	1-6	Only subtypes 1a, 1b, 2a, 2b, 2c
DNA biochip	5'NC	1-6	Only subtypes 1a, 1b
	NS5B	1-6	More than 30 subtypes

Table 2. Performance of HCV genotyping methods.

3. Definition of an occult HCV infection

The clinical resolution of a hepatitis C infection, either spontaneous or therapy-induced, has conventionally been deemed to reflect the complete eradication of HCV. However, the past 5 years have seen an emergence of several studies documenting the presence of HCV RNA in the liver or peripheral blood mononuclear cells of patients whose serum samples tested negative for HCV RNA by conventional PCR assays, with or without the presence of anti-HCV antibodies. This defined a new form of HCV infection, called occult HCV infection. Occult HCV infections were described using highly sensitive nucleic acid amplification assays with a sensitivity < 3 IU/mL. There are two forms of occult HCV infections: cryptogenic and secondary (Table 3).

Description	Cryptogenic occult HCV infection	Secondary occult HCV infection
HCV RNA detection		
Plasma (conventional PCR assay) *	-	-
Plasma (ultrasentive PCR assay) **	+/-	+/-
Peripheral blood mononuclear cells	+/-	+/-
Liver biospy	+	+/-
Anti-HCV antibodies	-	+
Elevated liver enzymes	yes	no

* Detection limit 50-600 UI/mL, ** detection limit ≤ 3 IU/mL

Table 3. Markers of occult HCV infection.

3.1 Cryptogenic occult HCV infection

Occult HCV infections are termed cryptogenic if the patient has (1) no anti-HCV antibodies and (2) elevated liver enzyme activities (Table 3).

Castillo et al (Castillo et al., 2004) first described "occult HCV infections" in patients with hepatic disorders of unknown origin; they appeared to have no anti-HCV antibodies or HCV RNA by conventional techniques. All other known causes of liver disease were excluded (viruses, autoimmune hepatitis, alcoholism, drugs, metabolic and genetic liver disorders). They used very sensitive PCR methods to detect genomic HCV RNA in the livers of 57 of the 100 patients tested. This rate of positive sample was unexpectedly high. Negative strand HCV RNA was detected in 84% of these 57 patients by *in situ* hybridization. The peripheral blood mononuclear cells from 70% of these patients were also positive for HCV RNA.

Another study detected the HCV RNA genome in the hepatocytes of 27 of 31 patients, none of whom had markers of HCV infection or any abnormal liver function test (Idrees et al., 2010). Both positive and negative strand HCV RNA were found in the livers of 8 (25.8%) patients, suggesting ongoing virus replication in hepatocytes. The main studies describing cryptogenic occult HCV infections are shown in Table 4.

3.2 Secondary occult HCV infection

Occult HCV infections have also been described in patients (1) with anti-HCV antibodies and (2) with normal liver enzyme activities who had cleared their HCV infections, either spontaneously or after treatment. This defined cases of secondary occult HCV infection (Table 3).

The persistence of HCV after hepatitis C had been resolved spontaneously or by treatment was first described in 16 patients (Pham et al., 2004). A very sensitive method (detection limit: 10 copies/mL) revealed HCV RNA in the plasma of 88% of them and in the peripheral blood mononuclear cells of 81% of patients; it was also found in 86% of the monocytes tested. Similar results were obtained in 17 patients whose hepatitis C had been resolved by treatment: 24% had HCV RNA in their serum, 53% in peripheral blood mononuclear cells, 41% in lymphocytes and 65% in macrophages (Radkowski et al., 2005a). Castillo et al detected positive and negative-strand HCV RNA in liver biopsy specimens and cells of 20 sustained responders (Castillo et al., 2006). Positive-strand HCV RNA was detected in 95% of liver biopsy specimens and negative-strand HCV RNA (the replication intermediate) was found in 79% of liver biopsy samples that had positive-strand HCV RNA. Thirteen (65%) samples of peripheral blood mononuclear cells had positive-strand HCV RNA; and 12 of these (92%) also had negative-strand HCV RNA. This suggested that virus replication was taking place in the liver of these patients, which could explain the persistence of intrahepatic HCV years after successful antiviral therapy. In another study, HCV RNA was detected in the serum of 54% of patients who had spontaneously cleared their HCV infection; it was also found in the peripheral blood mononuclear cells of 50 to 64% of them (Carreno et al., 2006, Radkowski et al., 2005b). The main studies describing secondary occult HCV infections are shown in Table 4.

3.3 Diagnosis of occult HCV infections

As the first definition of an occult HCV infection was based on detecting HCV RNA in hepatocytes (Castillo et al., 2004), the presence of HCV RNA in the liver is the reference method. However, liver biopsies are not readily available and the newly available non-invasive methods for evaluating fibrosis will make biopsy-based methods less common. Carreño et al (Carreno et al., 2004) showed that HCV RNA can be detected in the peripheral blood mononuclear cells of 70% of patients with an occult HCV infection. So an alternative for diagnosing an occult HCV infection could be to look for HCV RNA in peripheral blood mononuclear cells. Ultrasensitive PCR assay can also detect HCV RNA in the plasma or serum, although it is undetectable by conventional PCR assay. Thus, HCV RNA concentrations of 60 - 160 copies/mL can be detected in the plasma of patients with an occult HCV infection using an ultrasensitive PCR assay (Bartolome et al., 2007)

All the groups that have described occult HCV infections used different methods to increase the chance of detecting low concentrations of HCV RNA (Pham et al., 2010).

- The first were highly sensitive molecular biological methods with a detection limit of about 3 IU/mL. They were based on nested PCR after reverse transcription targeting the 5'UTR region of the HCV genome. Amplification was often improved by nucleic acid hybridization (Southern blotting).

- The second method consisted of stimulating peripheral blood mononuclear cells *ex vivo* by culturing them with mitogens (interleukin-2 and phytohemaglutinin). This increased the detection of the HCV genome in cells apparently not infected with HCV (Pham et al., 2004, Pham et al., 2005). HCV RNA was detected in the peripheral blood mononuclear cells of about 30% of patients who had cleared HCV, but this percentage can increase up to 75% if the mononuclear cells are cultured with mitogens.
- The third method used an unconventional amount of plasma and number of cells, with plasma volumes of 1 - 4 mL and large numbers of cells ($5x10^5$ - $4x10^6$ cells) (Bartolome et al., 2007, Castillo et al., 2009, Radkowski et al., 2005a). This improved the diagnosis of an occult HCV infection by 10-15%.
- Finally, it is also important to repeat tests on successive samples of plasma and peripheral blood mononuclear cells because HCV RNA detection is rarely permanent. Repeated testing leads to the detection of occult HCV infections in 100% of cases (Pham et al., 2004, Pham et al., 2008, Radkowski et al., 2005a).

Unfortunately, while these techniques seem to be necessary for detecting an occult HCV infection, they are not really suitable for clinical diagnosis.

Study	Patient number	Negative HCV RNA		HCV RNA detection (ultrasensitive PCR assay)			HCV genotype
		Anti HCV antibodies	Hepatic cytolysis	Liver biopsy	Peripheral blood mononuclear cells	Plasma	
(Castillo et al., 2004)*	100	-	Yes	57/100 (57%)	40/57 (70%)	NA	1b
(Bartolome et al., 2007)*	106	-	Yes	106/106 (100%)	69/106 (65%)	62/106 (58%)	1b
(Barril et al., 2008)*	109	-	Yes	NA	49/109 (45%)	NA	1b
(Idrees et al., 2010)	31	-	Yes	23/31 (74%)	NA	NA	3a, 3b, 1a
(Pham et al., 2004)*†	16	+	No	NA	13/16 (81%)	15/17 (88%)	1a, 1b, 2a
(Radkowski et al., 2005a)*†	17	+	No	3/11 (27%)	9/17 (53%)	4/17 (24%)	1a, 1b, 2a, 3a
(Radkowski et al., 2005b)*†	11	+	No	NA	7/11 (64%)	6/11 (54%)	1a, 1b
(Carreno et al., 2006)*	12	+	No	10/12 (83%)	6/12 (50%)	NA	1b
(Castillo et al., 2006)	20	+	No	19/20 (95%)	13/20 (65%)	NA	1b, 2, 3
(Gallegos-Orozco et al., 2008)†	25	+	No	NA	5/25 (20%)	0/25 (0%)	1, 2

* Southern blot detection, † stimulation of cells in culture with mitogens, NA= not applicable

Table 4. Detection of HCV genomic RNA in different compartments in studies on occult HCV infections.

4. Clinical significance of occult HCV infections

To date, only one study had investigated the clinical characteristics of an occult HCV infection (Pardo et al., 2007). Two groups of patients were compared. One group of 68 patients had a cryptogenic occult HCV infection while the second group of 69 patients had a chronic HCV infection. The groups were matched for age, gender, body mass index and the estimated duration of abnormal liver function tests. Patients with an occult HCV infection had significantly higher plasma cholesterol and triglycerides that patient with a chronic HCV infection. But the activities of their alanine aminotransferases and gamma glutamyl transpeptidases were lower. Liver biopsies showed that patients with chronic HCV infections had higher necro-inflammatory activities (96%) and fibrosis scores (75%) than did patients with an occult HCV infection (31% and 15%). However, the two groups had similar proportions of patients with cirrhosis or hepatic steatosis. Patients with an occult HCV infection had fewer HCV-infected hepatocytes (5.3%) than patients with a chronic HCV infection (10.1%). Therefore, an occult HCV infection results in fewer hepatic lesions than a chronic HCV infection. This could be due to the slow replication of HCV RNA observed in occult HCV infections.

Another study evaluated the efficacy of anti-HCV treatment in occult HCV infections (Pardo et al., 2006). They treated 10 patients with a cryptogenic HCV infection with pegylated interferon and ribavirin for twenty-four weeks. These patients had HCV RNA in their livers and peripheral blood mononuclear cells, and all had elevated liver enzymes activities. At treatment withdrawal, eight patients had normal liver enzyme activities and the peripheral blood mononuclear cells of eight tested negative for HCV RNA. Twenty-four weeks after treatment withdrawal, six patients still had normal liver enzymes and seven had peripheral blood mononuclear cells that were negative for HCV RNA. Two biopsies were taken from five patients, one before and one after treatment. HCV RNA was found in the second liver biopsy of all five patients. However, the HCV RNA concentrations in the liver biopsy taken after treatment were lower than in the pre-treatment samples and the number of infected hepatocytes was also lower (2.2%) after treatment than before (3.5%). The necro-inflammatory activity and fibrosis scores had also decreased in three of the five patients. Thus treating patients with a cryptogenic occult HCV infection can improve their liver histology.

5. HCV infectivity in occult HCV infection

The crucial questions are, first, whether detecting HCV RNA fragments, even from the negative strand, should be interpreted as ongoing virus replication, or as molecular residues of a resolved HCV infection and, second, whether patients with low concentrations of HCV RNA can transmit an infectious virus. The presence of negative stranded HCV RNA in peripheral blood mononuclear cells and in the liver of more than 50% of patients with occult HCV infection indicated virus replication. The virus detected in the plasma of patients with an occult HCV infection was identified in particles with densities of 1.03-1.04 to 1.08-1.19 g/mL (Bartolome et al., 2007). These densities are similar to those of the HCV viruses found in chronically infected patients.

Cultures of lymphoid cells established by treating peripheral blood mononuclear cells from healthy individuals with a T cell inducing mitogen *ex vivo* are susceptible to wild-type HCV and capable of supporting its complete replication cycle (MacParland et al., 2006). This system was used to investigate the infectious capacity of low concentrations of HCV RNA, derive from the blood plasma or from the supernatant of peripheral blood mononuclear cells of patients with a sustained virological response. The residual virus in the plasma of patients with an occult HCV infection can be infectious *in vitro* (MacParland et al., 2009). The HCV carried by three of the nine individuals studied produced an infection *in vitro*. Thus, the HCV RNA detected in the plasma of patients with an occult HCV infection was found to be infectious, however the number of experiments was small. If these data are confirmed, an occult HCV infection could facilitate the clinical reactivation of an HCV infection, especially in patients with a damaged immune system. The public health impact and significance for blood and organ donation of such a situation could be very serious.

However, the infection of peripheral blood mononuclear cells is surprising because they do not have some of the membrane receptors that are essential for HCV entry into hepatocytes. They have no SR-BI, claudin-1 or occludin receptors. Moreover, cell-culture produce HCV (HCVcc) could not replicate in peripheral blood mononuclear cells, whatever the cells are (Marukian et al., 2008).

6. Immunology in occult HCV infections

Adaptive cellular immune response mechanisms, especially T cell responses, are believed to play a key role in the recovery from an HCV infection as well as in chronic hepatitis C. Proliferative CD4+ and CD8+ T cell responses are more efficient in patients with an occult HCV infection than in patients with a chronic HCV infection.

6.1 Humoral immune response

Patients with a classical HCV infection develop specific anti-HCV antibodies against virus structural and non-structural proteins. The antibodies appear late after the HCV infection and can never be detected in some cases. HCV can easily evade control by the humoral immune system. The titer of anti-HCV antibodies decrease rapidly in recovered chronically HCV infected patients given interferon-based therapy (Maylin et al., 2009, Toyoda et al., 2005) and can sometimes completely disappear about two decades after HCV recovery (Takaki et al., 2000). Loss of anti-HCV antibodies can be observed in 6 to 20% of immunocompetent patients (Kondili et al., 2002, Lefrere et al., 2004) and in hemodialysis and immunocompromised patients. Patients with a cryptogenic occult HCV infection could be patients who have lost their anti-HCV antibodies.

An immunoenzymatic test targeting the core protein has been developed recently. It detects immunoglobulin G that targets an immunodominant epitope of the HCV capsid (amino acids 5 to 19) that is not detected by other tests. Anti-HCV core antibodies are detected in 98.6% of chronically infected individuals. This test was used to examine the plasma of 145 serological silent patients with a cryptogenic occult HCV infection; 45 of them tested positive for anti-HCV antibodies (Quiroga et al., 2009). This IgG anti-HCV core test identifies occult HCV infections in seronegative, non-viremic patients and may be useful for tracking infections in patients who test negative for anti-HCV antibodies.

6.2 Cellular immune response

Specific T-cell responses alone can control an HCV infection even without an efficient humoral immune response (Post et al., 2004). The cellular immune response can still be detected decades after recovery from a chronic or acute HCV infection (Semmo et al., 2005, Takaki et al., 2000). The authors found that HCV-specific T helper cells and cytotoxic T-cell responses with an interferon-gamma phenotype persisted. HCV specific T-CD8+ cells have been detected in people who were not infected with HCV but were in continuous contact with chronically infected HCV patients (Scognamiglio et al., 1999). This suggests that an immune response can be constructed in response to a subclinical HCV infection. The persistence of a T-specific immune response could be the result of low concentrations of HCV RNA that are undetectable by present techniques. One study compared the cellular immune responses of 50 patients with a cryptogenic occult HCV infection, 141 patients with a chronic HCV infection and 21 patients with cryptogenic liver pathology (Quiroga et al.,

2004). Fifty-two per cent of the patients with a cryptogenic occult HCV infection had a specific proliferative CD4+ T cell response to HCV. Significantly fewer patients with a chronic HCV infection (26%) had this CD4+ T cell response. The specific HCV T cells detected targeted non-structural proteins and produced gamma interferon. The specific proliferative CD8+ T anti-HCV response in patients with an occult HCV infection was also stronger than in chronically infected patients. The cellular immune response may be more efficient in patients with an occult HCV infection, but it is not strong enough to definitively eliminate the virus. The same team demonstrated that HCV-specific CD4+ and CD8+ proliferative responses were observed more frequently in patients who have spontaneously eliminated the virus than in those whose chronic infection was eliminated by treatment (Quiroga et al., 2006).

The peripheral blood mononuclear cells like dendritic cells, monocytes, CD4+ and CD8+ T cells, and B cells of chronically infected patients can contain HCV virus particles. Pham et al found that the same cells were infected in patients with an occult HCV infection (Pham et al., 2008). However, the cytokine profiles differed depending on the type of infection (Pham et al., 2009). The peripheral blood mononuclear cells of patients with occult HCV infection produced more alpha-interferon, gamma interferon and tumor necrosis factor alpha than did those of patients with a chronic HCV infection. But transcription of the interleukin 10 gene was lower in patients with an occult HCV infection. Clearly, the impact of an occult HCV infection on the immunological function of T cells seems to be different from that of a chronic HCV infection, and needs further investigation.

7. Populations at risk of an occult HCV infection: hemodialysis and immunocompromised patients

Genomic HCV RNA was very recently found in the peripheral mononuclear cells of 45% of a group of serum HCV antibody-negative/HCV RNA-negative hemodialysis patients with elevated liver enzyme activities (Barril et al., 2008). This could have a big impact on the management of hemodialysis patients in dialysis units. But these results should be interpreted with caution for several reasons (Kamar et al., 2009). First, they found that the liver enzyme activities of patients with an occult HCV infection were abnormal, whereas the liver enzyme activities of dialysis patients with a chronic active HCV infection were often within the normal range. Second, they reported a very high percentage of deaths (39%) during the short follow-up, but these deaths were not due to HCV liver disease. This suggests that there was another underlying disease, other than an HCV infection, that was responsible for the increased liver enzyme activities. Third, seven of these hemodialysis patients had received a kidney transplant, but their serum remained HCV RNA-negative after kidney transplantation. There is usually a significant increase in the serum HCV RNA concentration of HCV RNA-positive patients after transplantation because of the loss of immune control under immunosuppression (Gane et al., 1996, Pereira and Levey, 1997, Rostaing et al., 2000). Hence, it is surprising that no HCV RNA was detected in the serum of the seven kidney transplant patients who had an occult HCV infection before transplantation.

HCV reactivation should readily occur in immunocompromised patients if HCV really does persist, due to the loss of immune control caused by the regimen of immunosuppressive drugs. We monitored 26 kidney-transplant patients for 10.5 years (range 2–16) after they had eliminated their HCV while on hemodialysis. We search for the presence of HCV RNA in liver biopsies, blood plasma and peripheral blood mononuclear cells (Nicot et al., 2010). The peripheral blood mononuclear cells were stimulated with a mitogen in culture to increase the chance of detecting low concentrations of HCV RNA. We repeated the tests using a very sensitive RT-PCR assay with Southern blotting detection (detection limit, 2 IU/ml). We found no residual HCV RNA in samples tested at the last follow-up. Half the patients were given rabbit antithymocyte globulins and anti-CD3 monoclonal antibodies during induction therapy and for biopsy-proven acute rejection, twenty patients were given mycophenolic acid. These drugs increase HCV viremia in HCV-infected patients (Nelson et al., 2001, Rostaing et al., 2000, Zekry et al., 2004), but none of the kidney-transplant patients tested had any detectable HCV RNA in their plasma. And none of them developed any HCV-related glomerulopathy or liver disease during this long follow-up. No patients who underwent a post-treatment liver biopsy showed any deterioration of their liver histology. The fact that formerly HCV-infected immunocompromised patients did not suffer a relapse suggests the complete eradication of HCV after its elimination while on dialysis.

8. Occult hepatitis C virus infection: the controversy

The data that are presently available on occult HCV infections are conflicting. Studies carried out by three different groups are in favor of occult HCV infection (Carreno et al., 2006, Castillo et al., 2004, Castillo et al., 2005, Castillo et al., 2006, Radkowski et al., 2005a, Radkowski et al., 2005b), while those of many others support the recovery of an HCV infection (Bernardin et al., 2008, George et al., 2009, Maylin et al., 2008, Maylin et al., 2009, Nicot et al., 2010, Swain et al., 2010, Wiegand et al., 2004). Several arguments are in favor of the absence of persistent HCV RNA. HCV is an RNA virus that has no latent stage in its replication cycle and its genome cannot persist as DNA, unlike viruses like HIV, HBV and herpes viruses. It is therefore unclear how low concentrations of HCV can persist.

8.1 Relapse rate is low in patients successfully treated

Relapse rate is extremely low. However, for patients who experienced late relapse, it is not clear whether they suffer a true relapse or are re-infected.

8.1.1 Results of long-term follow-up studies

Long-term follow-up studies have indicated that patients achieving a sustained virological response are at little risk of a late virologic relapse. One conducted on more than 1300 patients given peginterferon alfa-2a, alone or in combination with ribavirin assessed whether a sustained virological response was synonymous with HCV elimination (Swain et al., 2010). It included HCV infected patients alone or co-infected with HIV, with elevated or persistently normal liver enzyme activities. They found that 99.1% of the patients who achieved a sustained virological response after treatment still had undetectable HCV RNA in their serum after a mean follow-up of 3.9 years (range, 0.8 -7.1 years). Another large review of more than 4000 patients derived from studies conducted between 1994 and 2008 concluded that only 3% of sustained virological responders showed evidence of a late recurrence of HCV RNA (between 6 months and 7 years) (Welker and Zeuzem, 2009). Immunocompetent and immunocompromised patients (liver or renal transplanted patients) treated with interferon or pegylated interferon alone or associated with ribavirin were included. Smaller studies reported similar findings: serum HCV RNA remained undetectable in 92% to 100% of patients who achieved a sustained virological response after 2 to 13 years of follow-up (Desmond et al., 2006, Formann et al., 2006, Marcellin et al., 1997a, Veldt et al., 2004).

The description of occult HCV infections was followed by several large cohort studies looking for trace amounts of HCV in the plasma, peripheral blood mononuclear cells and/or liver of various populations. HCV RNA was not detected in the plasma or peripheral blood mononuclear cells of 156 of 344 successfully treated immunocompetent patients followed-up for a median of 3.3 years. While none of these patients suffered a virologic relapse, HCV RNA was detected in 2 of the 114 liver biopsies tested (Maylin et al., 2008). A study on 69 aviremic blood donors found no detectable HCV RNA in their peripheral blood mononuclear cells (Bernardin et al., 2008). Another on aviremic and viremic patients with cryptogenic liver disease HCV-associated systemic vasculitis, or connective tissue disease detected HCV RNA only in the peripheral blood mononuclear cells of patients with viremic HCV RNA (Halfon et al., 2008). These results were obtained using appropriate sample processing and highly sensitive methods; they do not support the idea of HCV persistence.

8.1.2 Improvement of liver histology after successful anti-HCV treatment

The vast majority of patients achieving sustained virological response demonstrate histologic improvements on post-treatment liver biopsies relative to pretherapy (Pearlman and Traub, 2011). The fibrosis scores of 82-88% patients were improved and cirrhosis regressed in 64% of patients. Only a small percentage of liver specimens taken after an interferon-induced sustained virological response contained persistent HCV RNA. For example, only 7 (2%) of 400 sustained virologic responders had detectable HCV RNA in post-treatment liver biopsies (McHutchison et al., 2002). And two of them had a virological relapse 12 months following completion of treatment. Histological studies showed that reduced liver inflammation and improved fibrosis scores in patients with a chronic HCV infection and advanced fibrosis or cirrhosis often accompanies a histological improvement (Formann et al., 2006, George et al., 2009, Marcellin et al., 1997a). This supports the idea of HCV elimination.

8.1.3 Few virological relapse in immunocompromised patients

A few cases of HCV recurrence have been reported in immunocompromised patients, supporting the hypothesis of HCV persistence. One patient was reinfected by the same HCV genotype after chemotherapy for lymphoma (Thomopoulos et al., 2008). The re-emergence of HCV was described in a patient who had been given a short course of prednisolone seven months after the end of HCV therapy, and in another who underwent a kidney transplantation seven months after the end of HCV therapy (Lin et al., 2008). Studies on larger cohorts of patients with an impaired immune system due to HIV coinfection (Page et al., 2010) or immunosuppressive treatment following renal transplantation (Kamar et al., 2003, Nicot et al., 2010) found no HCV RNA persisting in either the serum or peripheral blood mononuclear cells. If HCV really does persist, we should find a greater percentage of relapse in HIV coinfected patients and renal transplanted patients. These data point to the definitive elimination of HCV in patients with undetectable HCV RNA.

8.2 How explain disagreement between studies?

The disagreement between reports of the definitive elimination of HCV or its persistence may be linked to differences in the criteria used to defined plasma viremia in apparently recovered patients. The standard techniques used to classify patients as sustained virological responders in studies describing occult HCV infections ranged from 50-600 IU/mL (135 - 1000 copies/mL), whereas sensitive techniques with detection limits of < 50 IU/mL have been recommended since 2002. About 60% of patients with an occult HCV infection had detectable HCV RNA in the plasma and their mean virus load was 71 HCV RNA copies/mL (range 18-192) (Bartolome et al., 2007). Therefore, HCV genomic RNA should have been detected by conventional tests if sensitive commercial RT-PCR methods had been used to screen the patients. This is supported by the demonstration that serum samples from 6.1% of 184 sustained virological responders that were HCV RNA negative with a standard PCR assay (detection limit 100 IU/mL) tested positive with the TMA assay (detection limit: 5 IU/mL) (Morishima et al., 2008). It is therefore important to use sensitive methods to determine the virological response after anti-HCV treatment.

New HCV infection cannot be excluded in studies showing persistent HCV infections because detailed viral molecular analysis was not used. The patients in these studies were often infected by intravenous drug use or unknown routes and so possibly became re-exposed to the same source of contamination. Most analyses were done on the conserved 5'UTR region, which do not discriminate well subtypes. No accurate phylogeny was done on the NS5B or HVR1-E2 region of the HCV genome. It is therefore difficult to be sure that it was exactly the same virus that reappeared or to exclude re-infection with a common source and a similar virus. This must be borne in mind in studies describing late relapses.

8.3 Kinetics of HCV RNA in cells under treatment

Analysis of the kinetics of HCV RNA in compartments other than the plasma may help us to understand HCV replication and identify clinically significant patterns of response to treatment. The declines in the concentrations of HCV RNA in the peripheral blood mononuclear cells and plasma of patients treated with pegylated interferon and ribavirin were comparable during the initial 12 weeks of therapy (Pugnale et al., 2008). The decrease in HCV RNA in the peripheral blood mononuclear cells started as early as in plasma in many patients, while the kinetics in the two compartments differed markedly for some of them, hinting at compartment-specific HCV replication and response to treatment. HCV RNA was undetectable in the peripheral blood mononuclear cells in 0% of patients on day 0, in 5% on day 1, in 15% on day 4, in 23.6% on day 8, in 48.6% on day 22, in 58% on day 43, in 73% on day 71, and in 81% on day 85. This progression reflects the overall decay of HCV RNA in these cells. The rapid loss of virus from peripheral blood mononuclear cells was associated with a sustained virological response. Another study explored the presence of HCV RNA in different cell subsets (CD4+, CD8+, NK and B cells) of 34 HIV-HCV coinfected patients (23 sustained virological responders and 11 relapsers) at the end of antiviral therapy (de Felipe et al., 2009). HCV RNA was detected in cell subsets of 9 patients: two who achieved a sustained virological response and 7 who relapsed. There is thus a significant association between the presence of HCV RNA in cell subsets at the end of treatment and viral relapse. In the light of the high proportion of HCV-infected cells in cases of occult HCV infection, it is rather surprising that no more cases of HCV relapse were observed in this population.

8.4 Immune control of residual HCV RNA?

A recent study provides data that could resolve this controversy. It seems that low concentrations of HCV RNA reappear sporadically after successful therapy in a small proportion of patients and that this is associated with stimulation of the cellular immune response that controls HCV infection (Veerapu et al., 2011). The plasma and peripheral blood mononuclear cells of 117 patients who had recovered from an HCV infection (tested with Cobas Amplicor HCV test, limit of detection: 100 IU/mL or 270 copies/mL) were re-tested for HCV RNA with a more sensitive method (detection limit: < 40 copies/mL). The plasma of none of the 19 spontaneously recovered patients contained detectable HCV RNA. The cells of one of them tested positive for HCV RNA. The intensity of the PCR band decreased in cells collected later until complete clearance of HCV RNA from the cell compartment by week 93. This suggests that the persistence of a low concentration of HCV RNA is not a common feature of spontaneous HCV clearance. Plasma samples of 15 of 98 (15%) recovered treated patients tested positive for HCV RNA and the peripheral blood mononuclear cells of 3 of 76 patients tested were positive. All the samples obtained later tested negative. The time that had passed since the cessation of therapy differed between those patients with detectable HCV RNA and those without. HCV RNA was mostly detected in the first 8 years after the end of therapy. All later samples tested were HCV RNA negative. The HCV-specific T cell response was more vigorous at the HCV RNA-positive time points than at HCV RNA-negative ones. It triggered non-structural proteins, which are not part of the virus particle but are present only when the virus infects cells and virus RNA is translated into proteins. There could therefore be a correlation between an increased antiviral T-cell response and persistent low concentrations of virus, with the T-cell response stimulated by antigen from the newly translated HCV RNA. These data suggest that trace amounts of HCV RNA may persist for a limited but not indefinite time after successful therapy and may sporadically reappear in the circulation. The residual virus is perpetually kept in check by the immune response. This may be missed in standard clinical evaluations, which typically assess the presence of HCV RNA at a single time point 6 months after cessation of therapy. Moreover, this study shows that peripheral blood mononuclear cells are unlikely to be a long-lived reservoir of HCV in aviremic patients.

9. Conclusion

Most reports of HCV RNA sequences in cell or liver specimens despite HCV RNA being undetectable have come from a relatively few teams studying small cohorts of patients, but none of these patients experienced a real virological relapse. The clinical impact of low levels of HCV replication is not yet well defined. It is not clear whether these findings are replication-competent virus, have any clinical significance, or whether the situation predisposes to virus breakthrough. However, the majority of data from long-term follow-up studies on large cohorts of patients have failed to confirm occult HCV infection. Patients achieving a sustained virological response are very unlikely to suffer a relapse. Very few of them had detectable HCV RNA in their livers, the main replication site, and the liver histology of the majority of them improved. Further well-designed, multicenter, prospective trials are necessary for interferon-based therapies and also in the future for antiviral therapies based on specifically targeted antiviral therapy for HCV to finally resolved these conflicting data.

Waiting new results, we must therefore conclude that a sustained virological response should be considered to be a durable marker of virus eradication because there is limited evidence for occult HCV infection. The patients can be considered not infectious and cured from a virological standpoint.

10. References

Alberti, A., Chemello, L.& Benvegnu, L. (1999). Natural history of hepatitis C. *J Hepatol*, Vol. 31 Suppl 1, No., and 1999), pp. (17-24), 0168-8278

Alter, H.J. (2005). HCV natural history: the retrospective and prospective in perspective. *J Hepatol*, Vol. 43, No. 4, (Oct and 2005), pp. (550-552), 0168-8278

Anonymous. (2002). NIH Consensus Statement on Management of Hepatitis C: 2002. *NIH Consens State Sci Statements*, Vol. 19, No. 3, (Jun 10-12 and 2002), pp. (1-46), 1553-0957

Barril, G., Castillo, I., Arenas, M.D., Espinosa, M., Garcia-Valdecasas, J., Garcia-Fernandez, N., Gonzalez-Parra, E., Alcazar, J.M., Sanchez, C., Diez-Baylon, J.C., Martinez, P., Bartolome, J.& Carreno, V. (2008). Occult hepatitis C virus infection among hemodialysis patients. *J Am Soc Nephrol*, Vol. 19, No. 12, (Dec and 2008), pp. (2288-2292), no ISSN

Bartolome, J., Lopez-Alcorocho, J.M., Castillo, I., Rodriguez-Inigo, E., Quiroga, J.A., Palacios, R.& Carreno, V. (2007). Ultracentrifugation of serum samples allows detection of hepatitis C virus RNA in patients with occult hepatitis C. *J Virol*, Vol. 81, No. 14, (Jul and 2007), pp. (7710-7715), no ISSN

Bernardin, F., Tobler, L., Walsh, I., Williams, J.D., Busch, M.& Delwart, E. (2008). Clearance of hepatitis C virus RNA from the peripheral blood mononuclear cells of blood donors who spontaneously or therapeutically control their plasma viremia. *Hepatology*, Vol. 47, No. 5, (May and 2008), pp. (1446-1452), no ISSN

Blackard, J.T., Smeaton, L., Hiasa, Y., Horiike, N., Onji, M., Jamieson, D.J., Rodriguez, I., Mayer, K.H.& Chung, R.T. (2005). Detection of hepatitis C virus (HCV) in serum and peripheral-blood mononuclear cells from HCV-monoinfected and HIV/HCV-coinfected persons. *J Infect Dis*, Vol. 192, No. 2, (Jul 15 and 2005), pp. (258-265), 0022-1899

Boonstra, A., van der Laan, L.J., Vanwolleghem, T.& Janssen, H.L. (2009). Experimental models for hepatitis C viral infection. *Hepatology*, Vol. 50, No. 5, (Nov and 2009), pp. (1646-1655), 0270-9139

Bourlet, T., Levy, R., Maertens, A., Tardy, J.C., Grattard, F., Cordonier, H., Laurent, J.L., Guerin, J.F.& Pozzetto, B. (2002). Detection and characterization of hepatitis C virus RNA in seminal plasma and spermatozoon fractions of semen from patients attempting medically assisted conception. *J Clin Microbiol*, Vol. 40, No. 9, (Sep and 2002), pp. (3252-3255), 0095-1137

Bracho, M.A., Gosalbes, M.J., Blasco, D., Moya, A.& Gonzalez-Candelas, F. (2005). Molecular epidemiology of a hepatitis C virus outbreak in a hemodialysis unit. *J Clin Microbiol*, Vol. 43, No. 6, (Jun and 2005), pp. (2750-2755), 0095-1137

Carrat, F., Bani-Sadr, F., Pol, S., Rosenthal, E., Lunel-Fabiani, F., Benzekri, A., Morand, P., Goujard, C., Pialoux, G., Piroth, L., Salmon-Ceron, D., Degott, C., Cacoub, P.&

Perronne, C. (2004). Pegylated interferon alfa-2b vs standard interferon alfa-2b, plus ribavirin, for chronic hepatitis C in HIV-infected patients: a randomized controlled trial. *Jama*, Vol. 292, No. 23, (Dec 15 and 2004), pp. (2839-2848), no ISSN

Carreno, V., Castillo, I., Bartolome, J., Rodriguez-Inigo, E., Ortiz-Movilla, N., de Lucas, S.& Pardo, M. (2004). Comparison of hepatitis C virus RNA detection in plasma, whole blood and peripheral blood mononuclear cells of patients with occult hepatitis C virus infection. *J Clin Virol*, Vol. 31, No. 4, (Dec and 2004), pp. (312-313), 1386-6532

Carreno, V., Pardo, M., Lopez-Alcorocho, J.M., Rodriguez-Inigo, E., Bartolome, J.& Castillo, I. (2006). Detection of hepatitis C virus (HCV) RNA in the liver of healthy, anti-HCV antibody-positive, serum HCV RNA-negative patients with normal alanine aminotransferase levels. *J Infect Dis*, Vol. 194, No. 1, (Jul 1 and 2006), pp. (53-60), no ISSN

Castillo, I., Pardo, M., Bartolome, J., Ortiz-Movilla, N., Rodriguez-Inigo, E., de Lucas, S., Salas, C., Jimenez-Heffernan, J.A., Perez-Mota, A., Graus, J., Lopez-Alcorocho, J.M.& Carreno, V. (2004). Occult hepatitis C virus infection in patients in whom the etiology of persistently abnormal results of liver-function tests is unknown. *J Infect Dis*, Vol. 189, No. 1, (Jan 1 and 2004), pp. (7-14), no ISSN

Castillo, I., Rodriguez-Inigo, E., Bartolome, J., de Lucas, S., Ortiz-Movilla, N., Lopez-Alcorocho, J.M., Pardo, M.& Carreno, V. (2005). Hepatitis C virus replicates in peripheral blood mononuclear cells of patients with occult hepatitis C virus infection. *Gut*, Vol. 54, No. 5, (May and 2005), pp. (682-685), no ISSN

Castillo, I., Rodriguez-Inigo, E., Lopez-Alcorocho, J.M., Pardo, M., Bartolome, J.& Carreno, V. (2006). Hepatitis C virus replicates in the liver of patients who have a sustained response to antiviral treatment. *Clin Infect Dis*, Vol. 43, No. 10, (Nov 15 and 2006), pp. (1277-1283), no ISSN

Castillo, I., Bartolome, J., Quiroga, J.A., Barril, G.& Carreno, V. (2009). Presence of HCV-RNA after ultracentrifugation of serum samples during the follow-up of chronic hepatitis C patients with a sustained virological response may predict reactivation of hepatitis C virus infection. *Aliment Pharmacol Ther*, Vol. 30, No. 5, (Sep 1 and 2009), pp. (477-486), 1365-2036

Chen, Z.& Weck, K.E. (2002). Hepatitis C virus genotyping: interrogation of the 5' untranslated region cannot accurately distinguish genotypes 1a and 1b. *J Clin Microbiol*, Vol. 40, No. 9, (Sep and 2002), pp. (3127-3134), 0095-1137

Chung, R.T., Andersen, J., Volberding, P., Robbins, G.K., Liu, T., Sherman, K.E., Peters, M.G., Koziel, M.J., Bhan, A.K., Alston, B., Colquhoun, D., Nevin, T., Harb, G.& van der Horst, C. (2004). Peginterferon Alfa-2a plus ribavirin versus interferon alfa-2a plus ribavirin for chronic hepatitis C in HIV-coinfected persons. *N Engl J Med*, Vol. 351, No. 5, (Jul 29 and 2004), pp. (451-459), no ISSN

Corey, K.E., Ross, A.S., Wurcel, A., Schulze Zur Wiesch, J., Kim, A.Y., Lauer, G.M.& Chung, R.T. (2006). Outcomes and treatment of acute hepatitis C virus infection in a United States population. *Clin Gastroenterol Hepatol*, Vol. 4, No. 10, (Oct and 2006), pp. (1278-1282), 1542-3565 de Felipe, B., Leal, M., Soriano-Sarabia, N., Gutierrez, A., Lopez-Cortes, L., Molina-Pinelo, S.& Vallejo, A. (2009). HCV RNA in peripheral blood cell subsets in HCV-HIV coinfected patients at the end of PegIFN/RBV treatment is associated with virologic relapse. *J Viral Hepat*, Vol. 16, No. 1, (Aug 28 and 2009), pp. (21-27), no ISSN

Desmond, C.P., Roberts, S.K., Dudley, F., Mitchell, J., Day, C., Nguyen, S.& Pianko, S. (2006). Sustained virological response rates and durability of the response to interferon-based therapies in hepatitis C patients treated in the clinical setting. *J Viral Hepat*, Vol. 13, No. 5, (May and 2006), pp. (311-315), no ISSN

Di Liberto, G., Roque-Afonso, A.M., Kara, R., Ducoulombier, D., Fallot, G., Samuel, D.& Feray, C. (2006). Clinical and therapeutic implications of hepatitis C virus compartmentalization. *Gastroenterology*, Vol. 131, No. 1, (Jul and 2006), pp. (76-84), 0016-5085

Ducoulombier, D., Roque-Afonso, A.M., Di Liberto, G., Penin, F., Kara, R., Richard, Y., Dussaix, E.& Feray, C. (2004). Frequent compartmentalization of hepatitis C virus variants in circulating B cells and monocytes. *Hepatology*, Vol. 39, No. 3, (Mar and 2004), pp. (817-825), no ISSN

Durand, T., Di Liberto, G., Colman, H., Cammas, A., Boni, S., Marcellin, P., Cahour, A., Vagner, S.& Feray, C. (2010). Occult infection of peripheral B cells by hepatitis C variants which have low translational efficiency in cultured hepatocytes. *Gut*, Vol. 59, No. 7, (Jul and 2010), pp. (934-942), 1468-3288

Formann, E., Steindl-Munda, P., Hofer, H., Jessner, W., Bergholz, U., Gurguta, C.& Ferenci, P. (2006). Long-term follow-up of chronic hepatitis C patients with sustained virological response to various forms of interferon-based anti-viral therapy. *Aliment Pharmacol Ther*, Vol. 23, No. 4, (Feb 15 and 2006), pp. (507-511), no ISSN

Forton, D.M., Karayiannis, P., Mahmud, N., Taylor-Robinson, S.D.& Thomas, H.C. (2004). Identification of unique hepatitis C virus quasispecies in the central nervous system and comparative analysis of internal translational efficiency of brain, liver, and serum variants. *J Virol*, Vol. 78, No. 10, (May and 2004), pp. (5170-5183), 0022-538X

Furusyo, N., Hayashi, J., Kanamoto-Tanaka, Y., Ariyama, I., Etoh, Y., Shigematsu, M.& Kashiwagi, S. (2000). Liver damage in hemodialysis patients with hepatitis C virus viremia: a prospective 10-year study. *Dig Dis Sci*, Vol. 45, No. 11, (Nov and 2000), pp. (2221-2228), 0163-2116

Gallegos-Orozco, J.F., Rakela, J., Rosati, M.J., Vargas, H.E.& Balan, V. (2008). Persistence of Hepatitis C Virus in Peripheral Blood Mononuclear Cells of Sustained Viral Responders to Pegylated Interferon and Ribavirin Therapy. *Dig Dis Sci*, Vol. 53, No. 9, (Sep and 2008), pp. (2564-2568), no ISSN

Gane, E.J., Naoumov, N.V., Qian, K.P., Mondelli, M.U., Maertens, G., Portmann, B.C., Lau, J.Y.& Williams, R. (1996). A longitudinal analysis of hepatitis C virus replication following liver transplantation. *Gastroenterology*, Vol. 110, No. 1, (Jan and 1996), pp. (167-177), no ISSN

Ge, D., Fellay, J., Thompson, A.J., Simon, J.S., Shianna, K.V., Urban, T.J., Heinzen, E.L., Qiu, P., Bertelsen, A.H., Muir, A.J., Sulkowski, M., McHutchison, J.G.& Goldstein, D.B.

(2009). Genetic variation in IL28B predicts hepatitis C treatment-induced viral clearance. *Nature*, Vol. 461, No. 7262, (Sep 17 and 2009), pp. (399-401), 1476-4687

George, S.L., Bacon, B.R., Brunt, E.M., Mihindukulasuriya, K.L., Hoffmann, J.& Di Bisceglie, A.M. (2009). Clinical, virologic, histologic, and biochemical outcomes after successful HCV therapy: A 5-year follow-up of 150 patients. *Hepatology*, Vol. 49, No. 3, (Mar and 2009), pp. (729-738), no ISSN

Gerlach, J.T., Diepolder, H.M., Zachoval, R., Gruener, N.H., Jung, M.C., Ulsenheimer, A., Schraut, W.W., Schirren, C.A., Waechtler, M., Backmund, M.& Pape, G.R. (2003). Acute hepatitis C: high rate of both spontaneous and treatment-induced viral clearance. *Gastroenterology*, Vol. 125, No. 1, (Jul and 2003), pp. (80-88), 0016-5085

Gryadunov, D., Nicot, F., Dubois, M., Mikhailovich, V., Zasedatelev, A.& Izopet, J. (2010). Hepatitis C virus genotyping using an oligonucleotide microarray based on the NS5B sequence. *J Clin Microbiol*, Vol. 48, No. 11, (Nov and 2010), pp. (3910-3917), 0095-1137

Halfon, P., Trimoulet, P., Bourliere, M., Khiri, H., de Ledinghen, V., Couzigou, P., Feryn, J.M., Alcaraz, P., Renou, C., Fleury, H.J.& Ouzan, D. (2001). Hepatitis C virus genotyping based on 5' noncoding sequence analysis (Trugene). *J Clin Microbiol*, Vol. 39, No. 5, (May and 2001), pp. (1771-1773), 0095-1137

Halfon, P., Bourliere, M., Ouzan, D., Sene, D., Saadoun, D., Khiri, H., Penaranda, G., Martineau, A., Oules, V.& Cacoub, P. (2008). Occult hepatitis C virus infection revisited with ultrasensitive real-time PCR assay. *J Clin Microbiol*, Vol. 46, No. 6, (Jun and 2008), pp. (2106-2108), no ISSN

Idrees, M., Lal, A., Malik, F.A., Hussain, A., Rehman, I.U., Akbar, H., Butt, S., Ali, M., Ali, L.& Malik, F.A. (2010). Occult hepatitis C virus infection and associated predictive factors: The Pakistan experience. *Infect Genet Evol*, Vol., No., (Dec 22 and 2010), pp. 1567-7257

Izopet, J., Rostaing, L., Moussion, F., Alric, L., Dubois, M., That, H.T., Payen, J.L., Duffaut, M., Durand, D., Suc, J.M.& Puel, J. (1997). High rate of hepatitis C virus clearance in hemodialysis patients after interferon-alpha therapy. *J Infect Dis*, Vol. 176, No. 6, (Dec and 1997), pp. (1614-1617), no ISSN

Izopet, J., Pasquier, C., Sandres, K., Puel, J.& Rostaing, L. (1999). Molecular evidence for nosocomial transmission of hepatitis C virus in a French hemodialysis unit. *J Med Virol*, Vol. 58, No. 2, (Jun and 1999), pp. (139-144), 0146-6615

Kamar, N., Toupance, O., Buchler, M., Sandres-Saune, K., Izopet, J., Durand, D.& Rostaing, L. (2003). Evidence that clearance of hepatitis C virus RNA after alpha-interferon therapy in dialysis patients is sustained after renal transplantation. *J Am Soc Nephrol*, Vol. 14, No. 8, (Aug and 2003), pp. (2092-2098), no ISSN

Kamar, N., Nicot, F., Izopet, J.& Rostaing, L. (2009). Occult hepatitis C virus infection in hemodialysis patients: examining the evidence. *Am J Kidney Dis*, Vol. 54, No. 1, (Jul and 2009), pp. (10-12), no ISSN

Kondili, L.A., Chionne, P., Costantino, A., Villano, U., Lo Noce, C., Pannozzo, F., Mele, A., Giampaoli, S.& Rapicetta, M. (2002). Infection rate and spontaneous seroreversion of anti-hepatitis C virus during the natural course of hepatitis C virus infection in the general population. *Gut*, Vol. 50, No. 5, (May and 2002), pp. (693-696), 0017-5749

Laguno, M., Murillas, J., Blanco, J.L., Martinez, E., Miquel, R., Sanchez-Tapias, J.M., Bargallo, X., Garcia-Criado, A., de Lazzari, E., Larrousse, M., Leon, A., Lonca, M., Milinkovic, A., Gatell, J.M.& Mallolas, J. (2004). Peginterferon alfa-2b plus ribavirin compared with interferon alfa-2b plus ribavirin for treatment of HIV/HCV co-infected patients. *Aids*, Vol. 18, No. 13, (Sep 3 and 2004), pp. (F27-36), no ISSN

Laperche, S., Le Marrec, N., Girault, A., Bouchardeau, F., Servant-Delmas, A., Maniez-Montreuil, M., Gallian, P., Levayer, T., Morel, P.& Simon, N. (2005). Simultaneous detection of hepatitis C virus (HCV) core antigen and anti-HCV antibodies improves the early detection of HCV infection. *J Clin Microbiol*, Vol. 43, No. 8, (Aug and 2005), pp. (3877-3883), 0095-1137

Laskus, T., Radkowski, M., Wang, L.F., Vargas, H.& Rakela, J. (1998). Search for hepatitis C virus extrahepatic replication sites in patients with acquired immunodeficiency syndrome: specific detection of negative-strand viral RNA in various tissues. *Hepatology*, Vol. 28, No. 5, (Nov and 1998), pp. (1398-1401), 0270-9139

Laskus, T., Radkowski, M., Piasek, A., Nowicki, M., Horban, A., Cianciara, J.& Rakela, J. (2000). Hepatitis C virus in lymphoid cells of patients coinfected with human immunodeficiency virus type 1: evidence of active replication in monocytes/macrophages and lymphocytes. *J Infect Dis*, Vol. 181, No. 2, (Feb and 2000), pp. (442-448), 0022-1899

Lefrere, J.J., Girot, R., Lefrere, F., Guillaume, N., Lerable, J., Le Marrec, N., Bouchardeau, F.& Laperche, S. (2004). Complete or partial seroreversion in immunocompetent individuals after self-limited HCV infection: consequences for transfusion. *Transfusion*, Vol. 44, No. 3, (Mar and 2004), pp. (343-348), 0041-1132

Legrand-Abravanel, F., Nicot, F.& Izopet, J. (2010). New NS5B polymerase inhibitors for hepatitis C. *Expert Opin Investig Drugs*, Vol. 19, No. 8, (Aug and 2010), pp. (963-975), 1354-3784

Lerat, H., Berby, F., Trabaud, M.A., Vidalin, O., Major, M., Trepo, C.& Inchauspe, G. (1996). Specific detection of hepatitis C virus minus strand RNA in hematopoietic cells. *J Clin Invest*, Vol. 97, No. 3, (Feb 1 and 1996), pp. (845-851), 0021-9738

Lerat, H., Rumin, S., Habersetzer, F., Berby, F., Trabaud, M.A., Trepo, C.& Inchauspe, G. (1998). In vivo tropism of hepatitis C virus genomic sequences in hematopoietic cells: influence of viral load, viral genotype, and cell phenotype. *Blood*, Vol. 91, No. 10, (May 15 and 1998), pp. (3841-3849), 0006-4971

Lin, A., Thadareddy, A., Goldstein, M.J.& Lake-Bakaar, G. (2008). Immune suppression leading to hepatitis C virus re-emergence after sustained virological response. *J Med Virol*, Vol. 80, No. 10, (Aug 19 and 2008), pp. (1720-1722), no ISSN

MacParland, S.A., Pham, T.N., Gujar, S.A.& Michalak, T.I. (2006). De novo infection and propagation of wild-type Hepatitis C virus in human T lymphocytes in vitro. *J Gen Virol*, Vol. 87, No. Pt 12, (Dec and 2006), pp. (3577-3586), no ISSN

MacParland, S.A., Pham, T.N., Guy, C.S.& Michalak, T.I. (2009). Hepatitis C virus persisting after clinically apparent sustained virological response to antiviral therapy retains infectivity in vitro. *Hepatology*, Vol. 49, No. 5, (May and 2009), pp. (1431-1441), no ISSN

Mao, H., Zhang, H., Zhang, H., Zhao, J., Lu, Z., Jin, G., Gu, S., Wang, H.& Wang, Y. (2010). Clinical evaluation of a colorimetric oligonucleotide chip for genotyping hepatitis C virus. *Clin Biochem*, Vol. 43, No. 1-2, (Jan and 2010), pp. (214-219), 0009-9120

Marcellin, P., Boyer, N., Gervais, A., Martinot, M., Pouteau, M., Castelnau, C., Kilani, A., Areias, J., Auperin, A., Benhamou, J.P., Degott, C.& Erlinger, S. (1997a). Long-term histologic improvement and loss of detectable intrahepatic HCV RNA in patients with chronic hepatitis C and sustained response to interferon-alpha therapy. *Ann Intern Med*, Vol. 127, No. 10, (Nov 15 and 1997a), pp. (875-881), no ISSN

Marcellin, P., Levy, S.& Erlinger, S. (1997b). Therapy of hepatitis C: patients with normal aminotransferase levels. *Hepatology*, Vol. 26, No. 3 Suppl 1, (Sep and 1997b), pp. (133S-136S), 0270-9139

Martin, P., Carter, D., Fabrizi, F., Dixit, V., Conrad, A.J., Artinian, L., Peacock, V., Han, S., Wilkinson, A., Lassman, C.R.& Danovitch, G. (2000). Histopathological features of hepatitis C in renal transplant candidates. *Transplantation*, Vol. 69, No. 7, (Apr 15 and 2000), pp. (1479-1484), 0041-1337

Martro, E., Gonzalez, V., Buckton, A.J., Saludes, V., Fernandez, G., Matas, L., Planas, R.& Ausina, V. (2008). Evaluation of a new assay in comparison with reverse hybridization and sequencing methods for hepatitis C virus genotyping targeting both 5' noncoding and nonstructural 5b genomic regions. *J Clin Microbiol*, Vol. 46, No. 1, (Jan and 2008), pp. (192-197), 1098-660X

Marukian, S., Jones, C.T., Andrus, L., Evans, M.J., Ritola, K.D., Charles, E.D., Rice, C.M.& Dustin, L.B. (2008). Cell culture-produced hepatitis C virus does not infect peripheral blood mononuclear cells. *Hepatology*, Vol. 48, No. 6, (Dec and 2008), pp. (1843-1850), 0270-9139

Mathurin, P., Moussalli, J., Cadranel, J.F., Thibault, V., Charlotte, F., Dumouchel, P., Cazier, A., Huraux, J.M., Devergie, B., Vidaud, M., Opolon, P.& Poynard, T. (1998). Slow progression rate of fibrosis in hepatitis C virus patients with persistently normal alanine transaminase activity. *Hepatology*, Vol. 27, No. 3, (Mar and 1998), pp. (868-872), 0270-9139

Maylin, S., Martinot-Peignoux, M., Moucari, R., Boyer, N., Ripault, M.P., Cazals-Hatem, D., Giuily, N., Castelnau, C., Cardoso, A.C., Asselah, T., Feray, C., Nicolas-Chanoine, M.H., Bedossa, P.& Marcellin, P. (2008). Eradication of Hepatitis C Virus in Patients Successfully Treated for Chronic Hepatitis C. *Gastroenterology*, Vol. 135, No. 3, (Sep and 2008), pp. (821-829), no ISSN

Maylin, S., Martinot-Peignoux, M., Ripault, M.P., Moucari, R., Cardoso, A.C., Boyer, N., Giuily, N., Castelnau, C., Pouteau, M., Asselah, T., Nicolas-Chanoine, M.H.& Marcellin, P. (2009). Sustained virological response is associated with clearance of hepatitis C virus RNA and a decrease in hepatitis C virus antibody. *Liver Int*, Vol. 29, No. 4, (Apr and 2009), pp. (511-517), 1478-3223

McHutchison, J.G., Poynard, T., Esteban-Mur, R., Davis, G.L., Goodman, Z.D., Harvey, J., Ling, M.H., Garaud, J.J., Albrecht, J.K., Patel, K., Dienstag, J.L.& Morgan, T. (2002). Hepatic HCV RNA before and after treatment with interferon alone or combined with ribavirin. *Hepatology*, Vol. 35, No. 3, (Mar and 2002), pp. (688-693), no ISSN

McHutchison, J.G., Everson, G.T., Gordon, S.C., Jacobson, I.M., Sulkowski, M., Kauffman, R., McNair, L., Alam, J.& Muir, A.J. (2009). Telaprevir with peginterferon and ribavirin for chronic HCV genotype 1 infection. *N Engl J Med*, Vol. 360, No. 18, (Apr 30 and 2009), pp. (1827-1838), 0028-4793

Micallef, J.M., Kaldor, J.M.& Dore, G.J. (2006). Spontaneous viral clearance following acute hepatitis C infection: a systematic review of longitudinal studies. *J Viral Hepat*, Vol. 13, No. 1, (Jan and 2006), pp. (34-41), 1352-0504

Miedouge, M., Saune, K., Kamar, N., Rieu, M., Rostaing, L.& Izopet, J. (2010). Analytical evaluation of HCV core antigen and interest for HCV screening in haemodialysis patients. *J Clin Virol*, Vol. 48, No. 1, (May and 2010), pp. (18-21), 1386-6532

Morishima, C., Morgan, T.R., Everhart, J.E., Wright, E.C., Apodaca, M.C., Gretch, D.R., Shiffman, M.L., Everson, G.T., Lindsay, K.L., Lee, W.M., Lok, A.S., Dienstag, J.L., Ghany, M.G.& Curto, T.M. (2008). Interpretation of positive transcription-mediated amplification test results from polymerase chain reaction-negative samples obtained after treatment of chronic hepatitis C. *Hepatology*, Vol. 48, No. 5, (Nov and 2008), pp. (1412-1419), no ISSN

Morsica, G., Bernardi, M.T., Novati, R., Uberti Foppa, C., Castagna, A.& Lazzarin, A. (1997). Detection of hepatitis C virus genomic sequences in the cerebrospinal fluid of HIV-infected patients. *J Med Virol*, Vol. 53, No. 3, (Nov and 1997), pp. (252-254), 0146-6615

Muller, H.M., Pfaff, E., Goeser, T., Kallinowski, B., Solbach, C.& Theilmann, L. (1993). Peripheral blood leukocytes serve as a possible extrahepatic site for hepatitis C virus replication. *J Gen Virol*, Vol. 74 (Pt 4), No., (Apr and 1993), pp. (669-676), 0022-1317

Nakatani, S.M., Santos, C.A., Riediger, I.N., Krieger, M.A., Duarte, C.A., Lacerda, M.A., Biondo, A.W., Carilho, F.J.& Ono-Nita, S.K. (2010). Development of hepatitis C virus genotyping by real-time PCR based on the NS5B region. *PLoS One*, Vol. 5, No. 4, and 2010), pp. (e10150), 1932-6203

Navas, S., Martin, J., Quiroga, J.A., Castillo, I.& Carreno, V. (1998). Genetic diversity and tissue compartmentalization of the hepatitis C virus genome in blood mononuclear cells, liver, and serum from chronic hepatitis C patients. *J Virol*, Vol. 72, No. 2, (Feb and 1998), pp. (1640-1646), 0022-538X

Nelson, D.R., Soldevila-Pico, C., Reed, A., Abdelmalek, M.F., Hemming, A.W., Van der Werf, W.J., Howard, R.& Davis, G.L. (2001). Anti-interleukin-2 receptor therapy in combination with mycophenolate mofetil is associated with more severe hepatitis C recurrence after liver transplantation. *Liver Transpl*, Vol. 7, No. 12, (Dec and 2001), pp. (1064-1070), no ISSN

Nicot, F., Kamar, N., Mariame, B., Rostaing, L., Pasquier, C.& Izopet, J. (2010). No evidence of occult hepatitis C virus (HCV) infection in serum of HCV antibody-positive HCV RNA-negative kidney-transplant patients. *Transpl Int*, Vol. 23, No. 6, (Jun and 2010), pp. (594-601), 0934-0874

Page, E.E., Cox, A., Atkins, M.& Nelson, M.R. (2010). Clearance of hepatitis C virus RNA from serum in HIV/hepatitis C virus coinfection indicates eradication from peripheral blood mononuclear cells. *Aids*, Vol. 24, No. 9, (Jun 1 and 2010), pp. (1267-1271), 0269-9370

Pal, S., Shuhart, M.C., Thomassen, L., Emerson, S.S., Su, T., Feuerborn, N., Kae, J.& Gretch, D.R. (2006). Intrahepatic hepatitis C virus replication correlates with chronic hepatitis C disease severity in vivo. *J Virol*, Vol. 80, No. 5, (Mar and 2006), pp. (2280-2290), 0022-538X

Pardo, M., Lopez-Alcorocho, J.M., Castillo, I., Rodriguez-Inigo, E., Perez-Mota, A.& Carreno, V. (2006). Effect of anti-viral therapy for occult hepatitis C virus infection. *Aliment Pharmacol Ther*, Vol. 23, No. 8, (Apr 15 and 2006), pp. (1153-1159), 0269-2813

Pardo, M., Lopez-Alcorocho, J.M., Rodriguez-Inigo, E., Castillo, I.& Carreno, V. (2007). Comparative study between occult hepatitis C virus infection and chronic hepatitis C. *J Viral Hepat*, Vol. 14, No. 1, (Jan and 2007), pp. (36-40), no ISSN

Park, J.C., Kim, J.M., Kwon, O.J., Lee, K.R., Chai, Y.G.& Oh, H.B. (2009). Development and clinical evaluation of a microarray for hepatitis C virus genotyping. *J Virol Methods*, Vol., No., (Oct 23 and 2009), pp. 1879-0984

Pasquier, C., Daudin, M., Righi, L., Berges, L., Thauvin, L., Berrebi, A., Massip, P., Puel, J., Bujan, L.& Izopet, J. (2000). Sperm washing and virus nucleic acid detection to reduce HIV and hepatitis C virus transmission in serodiscordant couples wishing to have children. *Aids*, Vol. 14, No. 14, (Sep 29 and 2000), pp. (2093-2099), 0269-9370

Pearlman, B.L.& Traub, N. (2011). Sustained virological response to antiviral therapy for chronic Hepatitis C Virus infection: a cure and so much more. *Clin Infect Dis*, Vol. 52, No. 7, and 2011), pp. (889-900), 1058-4838

Pereira, B.J.& Levey, A.S. (1997). Hepatitis C virus infection in dialysis and renal transplantation. *Kidney Int*, Vol. 51, No. 4, (Apr and 1997), pp. (981-999), no ISSN

Pereira, B.J., Natov, S.N., Bouthot, B.A., Murthy, B.V., Ruthazer, R., Schmid, C.H.& Levey, A.S. (1998). Effects of hepatitis C infection and renal transplantation on survival in end-stage renal disease. The New England Organ Bank Hepatitis C Study Group. *Kidney Int*, Vol. 53, No. 5, (May and 1998), pp. (1374-1381), 0085-2538

Persico, M., Persico, E., Suozzo, R., Conte, S., De Seta, M., Coppola, L., Palmentieri, B., Sasso, F.C.& Torella, R. (2000). Natural history of hepatitis C virus carriers with persistently normal aminotransferase levels. *Gastroenterology*, Vol. 118, No. 4, (Apr and 2000), pp. (760-764), 0016-5085

Pham, T.N., MacParland, S.A., Mulrooney, P.M., Cooksley, H., Naoumov, N.V.& Michalak, T.I. (2004). Hepatitis C virus persistence after spontaneous or treatment-induced resolution of hepatitis C. *J Virol*, Vol. 78, No. 11, (Jun and 2004), pp. (5867-5874), no ISSN

Pham, T.N., Macparland, S.A., Coffin, C.S., Lee, S.S., Bursey, F.R.& Michalak, T.I. (2005). Mitogen-induced upregulation of hepatitis C virus expression in human lymphoid cells. *J Gen Virol*, Vol. 86, No. Pt 3, (Mar and 2005), pp. (657-666), no ISSN

Pham, T.N., King, D., Macparland, S.A., McGrath, J.S., Reddy, S.B., Bursey, F.R.& Michalak, T.I. (2008). Hepatitis C virus replicates in the same immune cell subsets in chronic hepatitis C and occult infection. *Gastroenterology*, Vol. 134, No. 3, (Mar and 2008), pp. (812-822), no ISSN

Pham, T.N., Mercer, S.E.& Michalak, T.I. (2009). Chronic hepatitis C and persistent occult hepatitis C virus infection are characterized by distinct immune cell cytokine expression profiles. *J Viral Hepat*, Vol.16, No.8, (Aug and 2009), pp. (547-856), 1352-0504

Pham, T.N., Coffin, C.S.& Michalak, T.I. (2010). Occult hepatitis C virus infection: what does it mean? *Liver Int*, Vol. 30, No. 4, (Apr and 2010), pp. (502-511), 1478-3223

Post, J.J., Pan, Y., Freeman, A.J., Harvey, C.E., White, P.A., Palladinetti, P., Haber, P.S., Marinos, G., Levy, M.H., Kaldor, J.M., Dolan, K.A., Ffrench, R.A., Lloyd, A.R.& Rawlinson, W.D. (2004). Clearance of hepatitis C viremia associated with cellular immunity in the absence of seroconversion in the hepatitis C incidence and transmission in prisons study cohort. *J Infect Dis*, Vol. 189, No. 10, (May 15 and 2004), pp. (1846-1855), 0022-1899

Pugnale, P., Herrmann, E., Neumann, A.U., Pawlotsky, J.M., Schalm, S.W., Ferrari, C., Homburger, Y., Zeuzem, S.& Negro, F. (2008). Hepatitis C viral kinetics in plasma and peripheral blood mononuclear cells during pegylated interferon-alpha2a/ribavirin therapy. *J Hepatol*, Vol. 48, No. 6, (Jun and 2008), pp. (932-938), 0168-8278

Quiroga, J.A., Castillo, I., Rodriguez-Inigo, E., Pardo, M.& Carreno, V. (2004). HCV-specific cellular immune responses in patients with occult HCV infection in the liver. *Hepatology*, Vol. 40, No. Suppl 1, and 2004), pp. (278A), no ISSN

Quiroga, J.A., Llorente, S., Castillo, I., Rodriguez-Inigo, E., Lopez-Alcorocho, J.M., Pardo, M.& Carreno, V. (2006). Virus-specific T-cell responses associated with hepatitis C virus (HCV) persistence in the liver after apparent recovery from HCV infection. *J Med Virol*, Vol. 78, No. 9, (Sep and 2006), pp. (1190-1197), 0146-6615

Quiroga, J.A., Castillo, I., Llorente, S., Bartolome, J., Barril, G.& Carreno, V. (2009). Identification of serologically silent occult hepatitis C virus infection by detecting immunoglobulin G antibody to a dominant HCV core peptide epitope. *J Hepatol*, Vol. 50, No. 2, (Feb and 2009), pp. (256-263), 0168-8278

Radkowski, M., Gallegos-Orozco, J.F., Jablonska, J., Colby, T.V., Walewska-Zielecka, B., Kubicka, J., Wilkinson, J., Adair, D., Rakela, J.& Laskus, T. (2005a). Persistence of hepatitis C virus in patients successfully treated for chronic hepatitis C. *Hepatology*, Vol. 41, No. 1, (Jan and 2005a), pp. (106-114), no ISSN

Radkowski, M., Horban, A., Gallegos-Orozco, J.F., Pawelczyk, A., Jablonska, J., Wilkinson, J., Adair, D.& Laskus, T. (2005b). Evidence for viral persistence in patients who test positive for anti-hepatitis C virus antibodies and have normal alanine aminotransferase levels. *J Infect Dis*, Vol. 191, No. 10, (May 15 and 2005b), pp. (1730-1733), no ISSN

Rahnavardi, M., Hosseini Moghaddam, S.M.& Alavian, S.M. (2008). Hepatitis C in hemodialysis patients: current global magnitude, natural history, diagnostic difficulties, and preventive measures. *Am J Nephrol*, Vol. 28, No. 4, and 2008), pp. (628-640), 1421-9670

Roque-Afonso, A.M., Ducoulombier, D., Di Liberto, G., Kara, R., Gigou, M., Dussaix, E., Samuel, D.& Feray, C. (2005). Compartmentalization of hepatitis C virus genotypes between plasma and peripheral blood mononuclear cells. *J Virol*, Vol. 79, No. 10, (May and 2005), pp. (6349-6357), no ISSN

Rostaing, L., Chatelut, E., Payen, J.L., Izopet, J., Thalamas, C., Ton-That, H., Pascal, J.P., Durand, D.& Canal, P. (1998). Pharmacokinetics of alphaIFN-2b in chronic hepatitis C virus patients undergoing chronic hemodialysis or with normal renal function: clinical implications. *J Am Soc Nephrol*, Vol. 9, No. 12, (Dec and 1998), pp. (2344-2348), no ISSN

Rostaing, L., Izopet, J., Sandres, K., Cisterne, J.M., Puel, J.& Durand, D. (2000). Changes in hepatitis C virus RNA viremia concentrations in long-term renal transplant patients after introduction of mycophenolate mofetil. *Transplantation*, Vol. 69, No. 5, (Mar 15 and 2000), pp. (991-994), no ISSN

Sandres-Saune, K., Deny, P., Pasquier, C., Thibaut, V., Duverlie, G.& Izopet, J. (2003). Determining hepatitis C genotype by analyzing the sequence of the NS5b region. *J Virol Methods*, Vol. 109, No. 2, (May and 2003), pp. (187-193), no ISSN

Saune, K., Kamar, N., Miedouge, M., Weclawiak, H., Dubois, M., Izopet, J.& Rostaing, L. (2010). Decreased prevalence and incidence of HCV markers in haemodialysis units: a multicentric French survey. *Nephrol Dial Transplant*, in press, 0931-0509

Scognamiglio, P., Accapezzato, D., Casciaro, M.A., Cacciani, A., Artini, M., Bruno, G., Chircu, M.L., Sidney, J., Southwood, S., Abrignani, S., Sette, A.& Barnaba, V. (1999). Presence of effector CD8+ T cells in hepatitis C virus-exposed healthy seronegative donors. *J Immunol*, Vol. 162, No. 11, (Jun 1 and 1999), pp. (6681-6689), 0022-1767

Semmo, N., Barnes, E., Taylor, C., Kurtz, J., Harcourt, G., Smith, N.& Klenerman, P. (2005). T-cell responses and previous exposure to hepatitis C virus in indeterminate blood donors. *Lancet*, Vol. 365, No. 9456, (Jan 22-28 and 2005), pp. (327-329), 0140-6736

Simmonds, P., Bukh, J., Combet, C., Deleage, G., Enomoto, N., Feinstone, S., Halfon, P., Inchauspe, G., Kuiken, C., Maertens, G., Mizokami, M., Murphy, D.G., Okamoto, H., Pawlotsky, J.M., Penin, F., Sablon, E., Shin, I.T., Stuyver, L.J., Thiel, H.J., Viazov, S., Weiner, A.J.& Widell, A. (2005). Consensus proposals for a unified system of nomenclature of hepatitis C virus genotypes. *Hepatology*, Vol. 42, No. 4, (Oct and 2005), pp. (962-973), no ISSN

Sugano, M., Hayashi, Y., Yoon, S., Kinoshita, M., Ninomiya, T., Ohta, K., Itoh, H.& Kasuga, M. (1995). Quantitation of hepatitis C viral RNA in liver and serum samples using competitive polymerase chain reaction. *J Clin Pathol*, Vol. 48, No. 9, (Sep and 1995), pp. (820-825), 0021-9746

Sugimoto, K., Kaplan, D.E., Ikeda, F., Ding, J., Schwartz, J., Nunes, F.A., Alter, H.J.& Chang, K.M. (2005). Strain-specific T-cell suppression and protective immunity in patients with chronic hepatitis C virus infection. *J Virol*, Vol. 79, No. 11, (Jun and 2005), pp. (6976-6983), 0022-538X

Swain, M.G., Lai, M.Y., Shiffman, M.L., Cooksley, W.G., Zeuzem, S., Dieterich, D.T., Abergel, A., Pessoa, M.G., Lin, A., Tietz, A., Connell, E.V.& Diago, M. (2010). A sustained virologic response is durable in patients with chronic hepatitis C treated with peginterferon alfa-2a and ribavirin. *Gastroenterology*, Vol. 139, No. 5, (Nov and 2010), pp. (1593-1601), 0016-5085

Takaki, A., Wiese, M., Maertens, G., Depla, E., Seifert, U., Liebetrau, A., Miller, J.L., Manns, M.P.& Rehermann, B. (2000). Cellular immune responses persist and humoral responses decrease two decades after recovery from a single-source outbreak of hepatitis C. *Nat Med*, Vol. 6, No. 5, (May and 2000), pp. (578-582), no ISSN

Thomas, D.L., Astemborski, J., Rai, R.M., Anania, F.A., Schaeffer, M., Galai, N., Nolt, K., Nelson, K.E., Strathdee, S.A., Johnson, L., Laeyendecker, O., Boitnott, J., Wilson, L.E.& Vlahov, D. (2000). The natural history of hepatitis C virus infection: host, viral, and environmental factors. *Jama*, Vol. 284, No. 4, (Jul 26 and 2000), pp. (450-456), 0098-7484

Thomas, D.L., Thio, C.L., Martin, M.P., Qi, Y., Ge, D., O'Huigin, C., Kidd, J., Kidd, K., Khakoo, S.I., Alexander, G., Goedert, J.J., Kirk, G.D., Donfield, S.M., Rosen, H.R., Tobler, L.H., Busch, M.P., McHutchison, J.G., Goldstein, D.B.& Carrington, M. (2009). Genetic variation in IL28B and spontaneous clearance of hepatitis C virus. *Nature*, Vol. 461, No. 7265, (Oct 8 and 2009), pp. (798-801), 1476-4687

Thomopoulos, K., Giannakoulas, N.C., Tsamandas, A., Mimidis, K., Fragopanagou, E., Pallasopoulou, M.& Lampropoulou-Karatza, C. (2008). Recurrence of HCV Infection in a Sustained Responder After Chemotherapy for Non-Hodgkin's Lymphoma: Successful Retreatment. *Am J Med Sci*, Vol. 336, No. 1, (Jul and 2008), pp. (73-76), no ISSN

Torriani, F.J., Rodriguez-Torres, M., Rockstroh, J.K., Lissen, E., Gonzalez-Garcia, J., Lazzarin, A., Carosi, G., Sasadeusz, J., Katlama, C., Montaner, J., Sette, H., Jr., Passe, S., De Pamphilis, J., Duff, F., Schrenk, U.M.& Dieterich, D.T. (2004). Peginterferon Alfa-2a plus ribavirin for chronic hepatitis C virus infection in HIV-infected patients. *N Engl J Med*, Vol. 351, No. 5, (Jul 29 and 2004), pp. (438-450), no ISSN

Toyoda, H., Kumada, T., Kiriyama, S., Sone, Y., Tanikawa, M., Hisanaga, Y., Kuzuya, T., Honda, T., Hayashi, K., Nakano, I., Katano, Y.& Goto, H. (2005). Changes in hepatitis C virus (HCV) antibody status in patients with chronic hepatitis C after eradication of HCV infection by interferon therapy. *Clin Infect Dis*, Vol. 40, No. 6, (Mar 15 and 2005), pp. (e49-54), 1058-4838

Veerapu, N.S., Raghuraman, S., Liang, T.J., Heller, T.& Rehermann, B. (2011). Sporadic reappearance of minute amounts of hepatitis C virus RNA after successful therapy stimulates cellular immune responses. *Gastroenterology*, Vol. 140, No. 2, (Feb and 2011), pp. (676-685 e671), 0016-5085

Veldt, B.J., Saracco, G., Boyer, N., Camma, C., Bellobuono, A., Hopf, U., Castillo, I., Weiland, O., Nevens, F., Hansen, B.E.& Schalm, S.W. (2004). Long term clinical outcome of chronic hepatitis C patients with sustained virological response to interferon monotherapy. *Gut*, Vol. 53, No. 10, (Oct and 2004), pp. (1504-1508), no ISSN

Verbeeck, J., Stanley, M.J., Shieh, J., Celis, L., Huyck, E., Wollants, E., Morimoto, J., Farrior, A., Sablon, E., Jankowski-Hennig, M., Schaper, C., Johnson, P., Van Ranst, M.& Van Brussel, M. (2008). Evaluation of Versant hepatitis C virus genotype assay (LiPA) 2.0. *J Clin Microbiol*, Vol. 46, No. 6, (Jun and 2008), pp. (1901-1906), 1098-660X

Welker, M.W.& Zeuzem, S. (2009). Occult hepatitis C: how convincing are the current data? *Hepatology*, Vol. 49, No. 2, (Feb and 2009), pp. (665-675), 0270-9139

Wiegand, J., Jackel, E., Cornberg, M., Hinrichsen, H., Dietrich, M., Kroeger, J., Fritsch, W.P., Kubitschke, A., Aslan, N., Tillmann, H.L., Manns, M.P.& Wedemeyer, H. (2004). Long-term follow-up after successful interferon therapy of acute hepatitis C. *Hepatology*, Vol. 40, No. 1, (Jul and 2004), pp. (98-107), no ISSN

Zekry, A., Gleeson, M., Guney, S.& McCaughan, G.W. (2004). A prospective cross-over study comparing the effect of mycophenolate versus azathioprine on allograft function and viral load in liver transplant recipients with recurrent chronic HCV infection. *Liver Transpl*, Vol. 10, No. 1, (Jan and 2004), pp. (52-57), no ISSN

20

New Aspects of Natural History and Pathogenicity of Hepadnaviral Infection and Hepatocyte Function Revealed by the Woodchuck Model of Hepatitis B

Patricia M. Mulrooney-Cousins and Tomasz I. Michalak
Molecular Virology and Hepatology Research Group, Faculty of Medicine, Health Sciences Center, Memorial University of Newfoundland, St. John's, Newfoundland and Labrador, Canada

1. Introduction

The application of modern molecular biology and immunological techniques exponentially increased the utilization of liver biopsy material collected from either patients or animal models for diagnostic and research purposes. In the areas of our direct research interest, which is focused on delineation of the molecular immunopathogenesis of hepatocellular injury in hepatitis B virus (HBV) infection and hepadnaviral persistence, the mechanisms of hepadnaviral infection of the immune system and elucidation of the hepatocyte immune effector function, we routinely investigate liver biopsy specimens obtained from woodchucks infected with woodchuck hepatitis virus (WHV). The woodchuck-WHV infection system is not only the closest natural animal model of hepatitis B and HBV-induced hepatocellular carcinoma (HCC), but also is unparalleled for the evaluation of novel therapeutic and preventive strategies against HBV and its long-term pathological outcomes, such as chronic hepatitis (CH) and HCC.

The aim of this chapter is to review the findings from investigations of liver biopsy material acquired from the woodchuck model of hepatitis B, as well as primary or cultured hepatocytes derived from WHV-infected and healthy animals. Since some research areas in which the woodchuck model is applied are almost exclusive domains of this laboratory, we will describe these areas in more detail.

1.1 HBV and its pathological significance

Despite the availability of effective prophylactic vaccines, HBV occurs in an estimated 400 million people worldwide as a serologically evident chronic infection (Lia & Liaw, 2010; Liaw *et al.*, 2010; Romano *et al.*, 2011). Many of these individuals succumb after years of CH to liver failure due to cirrhosis and development of HCC. Recent statistics indicate that up to one-third of the global population has evidence of exposure to HBV (WHO, 2008). This may indicate that over 90% of those exposed carry HBV asymptomatically, at levels which are not readily detectable by the current clinical laboratory tests, but which can be often identified by analysis of appropriately prepared samples using research assays of greater sensitivity. This has potential implications for blood transfusion, transplantation, as well as therapy with immunosuppressive and anti-cancerous toxic agents which reactivate silently persisting infection (Feray *et al.*, 1990; Chazouilleres *et al.*, 1994; Dickson *et al.*, 1997; Yotsuyanagi *et al.*, 1998; Grob *et al.*, 2000; Carpenter *et al.*, 2002; Hu, 2002; Yuki *et al.*, 2003; Pollicino *et al.*, 2004; Mulrooney-Cousins & Michalak, 2007; Kao, 2008; De Mitri *et al.*, 2010; Coffin *et al.*, 2011a, 2011b; Morisco *et al.*, 2011; Villadolid *et al.*, 2011).

HBV is a circular 3.2 kilobase-long, partially double-stranded DNA virus whose genome contains four overlapping open reading frames (ORF) named surface (S), core (C), polymerase (P) and X. There are three envelope proteins encoded by the S ORF, designated as large (preS1), middle (preS2), and major or small (S). They have a common carboxy-terminus, but they differ at their amino-termini. The C ORF encodes the virus nucleocapsid protein carrying HBV core antigen (HBcAg) reactivity and a protein which, due to post-translational modifications of HBcAg, displays e antigen (HBeAg) specificity. Transcription of the P ORF results in formation of a multidomain polypeptide with viral reverse transcriptase, RNase, and DNA polymerase activities which are essential for virus replication (Nassal, 2008; Wei *et al.*, 2010). The X protein is derived from the smallest X ORF. It has transcriptional trans-activating properties and plays a role in virus oncogenicity. In terms of the replication strategy, the virus nucleocapsid migrates to the nucleus following entry and removal of envelope. There, HBV relaxed circular DNA (rcDNA) is converted to covalently closed circular DNA (cccDNA) by host DNA polymerases and ligases. This event is the first step in the viral replication cycle and detection of cccDNA serves as the marker of hepadnaviral replication. Four HBV mRNA transcripts, *i.e.*, 3.5, 2.4, 2.1, and 0.7 kb, are transcribed from the cccDNA. The mature nucleocapsid particles containing rcDNA are either packaged into virions, which are exported from the cell, or recycled to the nucleus. HBV and related viruses, known as the hepadnaviral family, are the only DNA viruses that use reverse transcription in their replication cycle.

In regard to pathogenicity, hepadnaviruses are considered to be essentially noncytopathic. Symptoms of hepatitis are a consequence of hepatocyte damage induced primarily by the host's immune responses directed against viral peptides presented on infected cells in the context of major histocompatibility complex (MHC) molecules, particularly class I (Chisari & Ferrari, 1996; Michalak, 2004; Bertoletti *et al.*, 2010; Chisari *et al.*, 2010). The subsequent release of proinflammatory cytokines, such as interferon gamma (IFNγ) and tumor necrosis factor alpha (TNFα), by activated cytotoxic T cells (CTL) are the main mediators of liver injury (reviewed in Michalak, 2004; Bertoletti *et al.*, 2010; Chisari *et al.*, 2010). One of the unique characteristics of hepadnaviruses is their stealth nature during the incubation period with no evidence of T cell recognition for approximately two months after exposure. However, the data from the woodchuck model of hepatitis B indicate that immediately after invasion, WHV induces virus-nonspecific lymphocyte activation (Gujar *et al.*, 2008), as well the cells of the innate immune system recognize virus shortly after its invasion, although they are not able to control virus replication or promptly induce virus-specific T cell responses (Guy *et al.*, 2008a).

One of the mechanisms of viral immune evasion, frequently utilized by viruses capable of long-term persistence, is their ability to infect immune cells (Alacami & Koszinowski, 2000). The lymphotropic nature of HBV has been shown in both in vivo and in vitro conditions (Korba *et al.*, 1987; Blum *et al.*, 1991; Chemin *et al.*, 1992; Calmus *et al.*, 1994; Michalak *et al.*,

1994; Bläckberg & Kigg-Ljunggren, 2001; reviewed in Michalak 2000; Michalak *et al.*, 2007; Pontisso *et al.*, 2008; Coffin *et al.*, 2011a, 2011b). On the other hand, the ability of WHV, which is a close relative of HBV, to infect and propagate in cells of the immune system has been well documented (Korba *et al.*, 1988; Michalak *et al.*, 1999; Michalak *et al.*, 2004, 2007; reviewed in Michalak 2000, 2004; Mulrooney-Cousins & Michalak, 2007). Overall, hepadnaviruses have developed multiple mechanisms to avoid immune elimination allowing them to persist within an infected host independent of whether infection is symptomatic or clinically and serologically silent (occult).

2. The woodchuck model of hepatitis B

2.1 Woodchuck hepatitis virus (WHV)

WHV was discovered in a colony of eastern North American woodchucks in the Philadelphia Zoological Garden, where a high rate of CH and HCC was observed (Summers *et al.*, 1978). The WHV infection in this subspecies of woodchucks *(Marmota monax)* is acknowledged as the most accurate natural model for the study of the natural course of HBV infection, the pathogenesis of hepatitis B and HCC, as well as for preclinical evaluations of new antiviral agents and preventive methods against HBV. WHV and HBV share the same genome organization, significant antigenic cross-reactivity, the same range of targeted organs, and comparable sequelae of liver disease. Thus, both viruses cause hepatitis that progresses from acute hepatitis (AH) to CH and finally HCC (Summers & Mason, 1982; reviewed in Michalak, 1998, 2004; Menne & Tennant, 1999; Menne & Cote, 2007; Roggendorf *et al.*, 2010). Nonetheless, the outbred nature of woodchucks and the relative shortage of WHV- and species-specific reagents and assays limit a wider utilization of the model. On the other hand, the woodchuck-WHV infection system is significantly more accessible and substantially less expensive than a chimpanzee model of hepatitis B, and liver disease and immunological processes in woodchucks are more closely compatible to a human disease situation than those in the avian models of HBV infection or in bioengineered mice. Considering the main differences between WHV and HBV-induced disease, HCC develops in almost all animals which have serum WHV surface antigen (WHsAg)-reactive CH (Popper *et al.*, 1981; Korba *et al.*, 1989). It is believed that the activation of cellular oncogenes, particularly *c-myc* and N-*myc*, through the integration of viral promoter sequences near these genes or through rearrangements of the genes, is responsible for the higher rates of HCC in woodchucks than in humans. However, WHV DNA can also integrate randomly into the hepatocyte genome, similarly to HBV DNA in human and chimpanzee hepatocytes (Feitelson & Lee, 2007; Mason *et al.*, 2009). Another difference is that CH type B in humans frequently advances to cirrhosis, while this is not the case during CH in woodchucks.

2.2 Serological and molecular markers of WHV infection

The profile of serological markers of WHV infection closely mirrors that in HBV infection (Mulrooney-Cousins & Michalak, 2009). The detection of serum WHsAg is indicative of a high virus replication rate and persistence of WHsAg in the circulation for longer than 6 months is indicative of CH, similarly to serum HBsAg in humans. In woodchucks that resolve AH, serum WHsAg falls to undetectable levels. However, concentration of plasma by ultracentrifugation may allow detection of WHsAg long after resolution of AH (Coffin *et al.*, 2004). Further, antibodies to WHV antigens detectable in woodchucks also are similar to their counterparts in HBV infection in terms of the time of their emergence, duration and diagnostic significance. Thus, antibodies to WHV core antigen (anti-WHc) are indicative of exposure to virus and, if they occur alone, they reflect the existence of occult WHV infection in which low levels of circulating WHV DNA can be also detected (Michalak *et al.*, 1999; Coffin *et al.*, 2004). In the case of HBV infection, the detection of IgM or IgG classes of anti-HBc is indicative of a recent or a past exposure to the virus, respectively. However, identification of anti-WHc of IgM class is not yet routinely feasible in woodchucks. Antibodies to WHsAg (anti-WHs) are detectable after resolution of AH or seemingly asymptomatic infection and they confer protection from re-infection. However, as it will be explained later (Section 6.2), this is by no means an indication of total eradication of virus or normal liver histology. In recent years, the development of highly sensitive nucleic acid amplification assays detecting hepadnavirus DNA and its genome replicative intermediates, such as cccDNA and mRNA, have led to the delineation of new forms of hepadnaviral infection. These findings will be summarized below (Sections 6.2 and 6.3). The detection of WHV genome and serological (immunovirological) markers in different stages and forms of infection is summarized in Table 1.

Status	WHsAg	Anti-WHc	Anti-WHs	WHV DNA Serum	WHV DNA Immune cells*	WHV DNA Liver
Pre-acute infection	-	+	-	+	+	+ or -
Acute serologically apparent infection	+	+	-	+	+	+
Chronic serologically apparent infection	+	+	-	+	+	+
Secondary occult infection (SOI)	-	+	+ or -	+	+	+
Primary occult infection (POI)	-	-	-	+	+	- **

* Based on WHV DNA detection in peripheral blood mononuclear cells (PBMC).
** Low levels of WHV DNA and its replication intermediates can be detected after 3 or more years of follow-up of POI (Mulrooney-Cousins *et al.*, manuscript in preparation).

Table 1. Serological markers of WHV infection and WHV DNA detection in serum, cells of the immune system and liver as detected by research assays in various stages and forms of WHV infection

3. Liver biopsy acquisition and histological grading of WHV hepatitis

The significant advantage of the woodchuck model is access to serial liver biopsies from virologically and immunologically well-defined stages of infection, including samples prior to initiation of infection experiments which are essential for base line measurements. In addition, due to the size of the woodchuck liver, a sufficient amount of tissue can be secured via laparotomy for both diagnostic and experimental purposes, including isolation of hepatocytes and intrahepatic immune cells. In this laboratory, the protocols for collection of liver biopsies and preservation of liver tissue samples from woodchucks are highly standardized. Briefly, animals are immobilized under general inhalant anaesthesia in a surgical suite under aseptic conditions. Liver tissue fragments (2-3 if required) are obtained by surgical laparotomy using a 7-mm wide-edge Schmeden No. 2 triangular punch (Churchill & Michalak, 2004). The liver bleeding is stopped with sterile absorbant hemostat cellulose (Surgicel; Ehicon Inc., USA). The tissue sample is divided into at least 3 portions. One is snap frozen in liquid nitrogen for nucleic acid isolations, another fixed in 10% buffered formaldehyde for histological examination, and a third cryopreserved for immunohistochemical investigations (Michalak, 1978). Depending on the nature of the experiment, small tissue fragments are also preserved for ultrastructural and other investigations.

Histological examination of hepatic tissue remains the gold standard for determining the dynamic of progression of liver damage in viral hepatitis. Woodchuck liver specimens are processed exactly as those from patients. Thus, formalin-fixed tissue is embedded in paraffin and thin serial sections (4 μm) are stained with hematoxylin-eosin (H&E), Masson trichrome, periodic acid-Schiff and impregnated with silver. Upon double-blinded microscopic analysis, morphological alterations encountered in hepatocellular, extrahepatocellular intralobular and portal compartments of hepatic parenchyma are graded on a numerical scale from 0 to 3. The overall grade of disease severity from 0 to 3 with 0.5-score intervals, defined as histological degree of hepatitis, is assigned taking into consideration the grades given for each category of liver lesions and the global impression on the pathological picture as a whole (Michalak *et al.*, 1990, 1999, 2000). The pivotal significance of histological examination in uncovering new aspects of natural history of hepadnaviral infection has been illustrated when serial liver biopsies obtained over the lifespan of woodchucks convalescent from AH were analyzed. It was found that although the animals cleared serum WHsAg, mounted anti-WHs and normalized liver enzymes, they persistently carried low levels of replicating virus and their livers showed an intermittent minimal to moderate liver inflammation up to the end of their lives. This documented that liver lesions did not subside completely despite apparent complete serological and biochemical resolution of hepatitis. Importantly, approximately 20% of the animals ultimately developed HCC (Michalak *et al.*, 1999). This finding was consistent with a similar observation made by others (Korba *et al.*, 1989). Accumulating clinical evidence indicates that the same may happen in humans convalescent from an episode of self-limited AH (Pollicino *et al.*, 2004; Simonetti *et al.*, 2010).

4. Isolation of hepatocytes from liver biopsy

Hepatocytes are the site of the most robust virus replication in serologically evident, symptomatic hepadnaviral infection. However, during the pre-acute phase and in the course of persistent low level WHV infection continuing after recovery from AH, termed as secondary occult infection (SOI) (see Section 6.3), the levels of WHV replication are comparable in hepatocytes and in infected immune cells (Michalak *et al.*, 1999, 2004). Up to this point, it has been virtually impossible to mimic the vigorous HBV or WHV replication seen in vivo in cell culture systems. It is for this reason that the derivation of primary hepatocytes from liver biopsies or during autopsy and establishment of cell lines from them are valuable tools in the attempts to understand hepatocyte engagement in different forms of hepadnaviral infection, to uncover mechanisms of hepadnaviral cell-to-cell spread and to assess hepadnavirus influence on hepatocyte function on the single cell level.

In most instances, primary hepatocytes can be isolated by microperfusion with a collagenase buffer under aseptic conditions from as little as 100-150 mg of liver tissue (Churchill & Michalak, 2004). After gentle teasing of the cells through a sieve, the cells are collected by low-speed centrifugation and are extensively washed until a high purity preparation of hepatocytes (>97%) is obtained. Cells are allowed to attach in culture flasks for 4 hours and after culture for 24 hours, hepatocytes from virus-naïve animals can be exposed to WHV for infection experiments, whereas those from WHV-infected woodchucks examined for viral genome and protein expression and/or used for assessing antiviral potential of test agents (Churchill & Michalak, 2004). Using this approach, a hepatocyte cell line, designated as WCM-260, was established from liver biopsy of a healthy woodchuck (Churchill & Michalak, 2004). The hepatocyte origin of the line was confirmed by gene expression analysis and identification of proteins specifically produced by hepatocytes. The studies carried out using this cell line significantly contributed to recognition of different aspects of WHV and hepatocyte biology, including studies on WHV cell tropism (Lew & Michalak, 2001; Mulrooney-Cousins & Michalak, 2008), hepadnavirus effect on the class I MHC expression (Wang *et al.*, 2006), mechanisms of hepatocyte cytotoxicity and their modulation by hepadnaviral infection (Guy *et al.*, 2010, 2011).

5. WHV-cell interactions in vitro

The WCM-260 hepatocyte line was found to be susceptible to WHV infection, regardless of whether the WHV inoculum was derived from serum of WHV-infected woodchucks or from in vitro infected hepatocytes or lymphocytes (Lew & Michalak, 2001; Mulrooney-Cousins & Michalak, 2008). WHV obtained after serial passage in WCM-260 cells caused classical AH in virus-naïve woodchucks (Lew & Michalak, 2001) and the virus genome sequence remained unchanged after multiple passages (Mulrooney-Cousins & Michalak, 2008), indicating that the cells supported replication of the biologically competent virus under conditions favorable to virus growth.

Although hepatocytes and lymphoid cells are known targets of WHV and HBV, there is still very little knowledge in regard to the receptor/s mediating the highly restricted cell tropism characterizing these viruses. However, it has been shown that there is a protease-activated cell recognition site in the preS1 (large) protein of WHV that mediates strictly host-specific binding to woodchuck hepatocytes and lymphoid cells (Jin *et al.*, 1996). The crucial determinant of this site was mapped to amino acids 10-13 at the amino-terminus of the large envelope protein. Synthetic peptides comprising the site sequence bound woodchuck hepatocytes and lymphoid cells with characteristics of a specific ligand-receptor interaction, although their ability to interact with lymphocytes was significantly greater (approximately 1000-fold) than that for hepatocytes. Interestingly, this binding site was protected within the tertiary structure of the virus preS1 envelope protein and was not identifiable unless the protein was treated with proteases. When animals experimentally infected with WHV were examined for the presence of antibodies directed against the site, the antibodies were found to appear as the first immunological indicator of virus infection, suggesting that proteolytic cleavage of the preS1 protein also occurs in vivo (Jin *et al.*, 1996).

6. Findings regarding natural history

Much of our understanding regarding the natural history and pathogenesis of HBV infection has come from investigations of the woodchuck-WHV model. The subsequent sections will be focused on new aspects of the natural history of hepadnaviral infection that have come to light by analyzing the liver and other natural compartments of WHV replication in woodchucks experimentally infected with various virus doses.

6.1 Symptomatic serologically evident hepadnaviral infection

The transmission of WHV through blood and body fluids, as well as vertically from mother to offspring, parallels that of HBV. Most neonates infected with WHV before 3 days after birth or those born to mothers with serum WHsAg-positive infection develop serologically evident CH that almost invariably progresses to HCC. This suggests that the maturity of the immune system at the time of infection is an important element determining establishment of CH. The role of virus dose and a possible influence of virus strain in the rate of CH development have been considered (Cote *et al.*, 2000a, 2000b; Michalak *et al.*, 2004). In adult animals, serum WHsAg-positivity accompanied by AH is usually self-limiting and is followed by the apparent complete antigen clearance; however molecular indicators of residual WHV infection remain (Michalak, 1998; Michalak *et al.*, 1999, 2004; reviewed in Michalak, 2000, 2004; Guy *et al.*, 2008a). The same happens in patients with self-limited AH (Michalak *et al.*, 1994; Grob *et al.*, 2000; Marusawa *et al.*, 2000; Chemin *et al.*, 2001; Murakami *et al.*, 2004; De Mitri *et al.*, 2010; Raimondo *et al.*, 2010). Similarly, approximately 10% of serum WHsAg-positive adult woodchucks and 5-10% of serum HBsAg-positive humans develop CH. However, suppression of the immune responses by administration of cyclosporin A dramatically increases the rate of progression to CH in experimentally infected woodchucks (Cote *et al.*, 1992). This supports the concept that the competence of the immune system plays a pivotal role in CH development.

Lymphotropism is an inherent property of many viruses capable of establishing persistent infection (Alcami & Koszinowski, 2000). There is a long history of findings indicating that both HBV and WHV can persist and actively replicate at extrahepatic locations, specifically in the cells of the lymphatic (immune) system, in the course of serologically evident chronic infection (Pontisso *et al.*, 1984, 2008; Yoffe *et al.*, 1986; Korba *et al.*, 1987, 1988; Ogston *et al.*, 1989). Studies in the woodchuck model significantly contributed to identification of hepadnavial lymphotropism and characterization of virus replication in cells of the immune system. Overall, although WHV replicates at approximately 50 to 100-fold lower levels (per cell) in immune cells than in hepatocytes in chronic symptomatic infection, the size of the reservoir is very large considering the total number of cells which constitute the immune system.

Hepadnavirus clearance without massive immune-mediated destruction of infected hepatocytes occurs in both HBV and WHV infections (Guidotti *et al.*, 1999; Guidotti & Chisari, 2001). In one study, hepatocytes were labeled during the peak of AH, when nearly all liver cells are infected (Kajino *et al.*, 1994). After immunohistochemically evident elimination of WHV antigens from the liver, many labeled hepatocytes were still present, suggesting that non-cytopathic viral clearance occurs in infected woodchucks. Other studies investigating the role of anti-viral cytokines, such as IFNγ and TNFα, as determinants of progression of AH to CH or recovery, demonstrated that the hepatic cytokine milieu during the acute phase of infection is important in determining the outcome of hepatitis in both neonatally acquired and adult WHV infections (Cote *et al.*, 2000b; Hodgson and Michalak, 2001). Thus, elevated intrahepatic levels of IFNγ, TNFα, and CD3 expression, together with a lower hepatic viral load and augmented liver inflammation, preceded recovery from AH, while the opposite coincided with progression of AH to CH (Hodgson & Michalak, 2001). Although cells of the innate immune system sense WHV within the liver as early as an hour after intravenous injection of virus and cause a significant decrease in virus hepatic load within 3 hours post-inoculation, this response is impaired and unable to eliminate virus or promptly induce effective anti-virus T cell response (see Section 9) (Guy *et al.*, 2008a).

Symptomatic hepatitis B is commonly accompanied by autoimmune phenomena clinically appearing as circulating organ non-specific and organ-specific autoantibodies. Although the pathogenic relevance of these responses to liver injury remains unclear in humans, it is generally accepted that their presence coincides with a more severe course of hepatitis (Poralla *et al.*, 1991; Cacoub & Terrier, 2009). In the woodchuck model, WHV infection usually induces organ non-specific autoantibodies, such anti-smooth muscle antibodies (SMA) and anti-nuclear antibodies (ANA) (Dzwonkowski & Michalak, 1990), as well as liver-specific antibodies directed against hepatocyte asialoglycoprotein receptor (ASGPR) (Diao & Michalak, 1996, 1997). It has been found that circulating autoantibodies to ASGPR (anti-ASGPR) induced by WHV infection are capable of causing complement-mediated lysis of hepatocytes and inhibit binding of desialylated glycoproteins to hepatocyte ASGPR, which mediates their clearance (Diao *et al.*, 1998). It has been also shown that the induction of anti-ASGPR prior to infection with a liver pathogenic dose of WHV tended to modulate infection toward CH outcome, and that the occurrence of anti-ASGPR in woodchucks with ongoing CH was associated with exacerbated histological severity of hepatitis. These findings raised the possibility that the liver compromised by CH might be prone to anti-ASGPR directed complement-mediated hapatocellular injury due to formation of the ASGPR-anti-ASGPR immune complexes at hepatocyte plasma membranes (HPM) (Diao *et al.*, 2003). Based on these findings, it is expected that the host's immune response mounted against ASGPR may contribute to both the outcome and the severity of hepadnaviral hepatitis (Diao *et al.*, 1998, 2003).

6.2 Primary occult WHV infection

Primary occult infection (POI) was originally identified in offspring born to woodchuck dams convalescent from AH, including those which developed anti-WHs antibodies after an episode of serum WHsAg-positive infection (Coffin & Michalak, 1999). All offspring from these dams demonstrated low levels of WHV genomes and WHV cccDNA and mRNA in the lymphatic system, while the liver was infected only in some of them. Importantly, no serological markers of infection, such as WHsAg, anti-WHc or anti-WHs, could be detected. In addition, WHV DNA-reactive particles displaying biophysical characteristics of complete virions were found in the circulation of the offspring. Thus, they migrated with comparable velocity in sucrose and had the buoyant density of intact WHV virions. Histological examination of serial liver biopsies showed normal liver morphology in all animals. Furthermore, the inocula prepared from serum or supernatants of cultured lymphoid cells acquired from these offspring induced serologically evident WHV infection and hepatitis in virus-naive adult animals, confirming the pathogenic competence of the virus. Interestingly, the offspring were not protected from challenge with a liver pathogenic dose of WHV (*i.e.*, 1.1×10^{10} vge), indicating that this low level infection did not induce virus-specific protective immunity (Coffin & Michalak, 1999). This study was the first to identify that hepadnaviral infection can be restricted to the lymphatic system and does not engage the liver, indicating that at low infectious doses hepadnavirus could be primarily lymphotropic.

This finding was followed by another study in which the amount of WHV required to establish serologically silent, lymphatic system-restricted infection was determined using intravenous inoculations of woodchucks with serial 10-fold dilutions of a well characterized WHV inoculum (Michalak *et al.*, 2004). The WHV genome was detected in the circulation and its replicative intermediates in cells of the immune system but not in the liver, while anti-viral antibodies were consistently absent. The liver biopsies collected from these animals over 3 years of follow-up showed normal morphology. The study not only confirmed the existence of POI and uncovered that this form of infection is induced by virus doses lower than 10^3 virions, but also established a reproducible model of POI. In the same study, it was uncovered that the inoculum that induced POI at doses greater than 10^3 virions caused classical serum WHsAg-positive AH. Taken together, the results from this study revealed that the amount of invading virus determines whether infection is serologically apparent or silent, that only virus doses greater than 10^3 virions are liver pathogenic, and that the cells of the lymphatic system are primary targets when virus invade a susceptible host at small doses ($<10^3$ virions) (Michalak *et al.*, 2004).

Currently, the long-term pathological consequences of POI are under investigation. In this regard, liver biopsies collected at approximately yearly intervals from animals followed for over 5 years are examined for virus presence and morphological alterations. During this observation period, all animals showed molecular evidence of WHV infection in the absence of the infection serological markers. As expected, the infection was restricted to the lymphatic system. However, after approximately 3 years post-infection, WHV DNA and WHV mRNA became detectable in the liver, even though viral load in serum of these animals rarely exceeded 100 vge/mL. The pathogenic competence of the persisting virus was documented by demonstrating its ability to induce classical AH in virus-naïve animals. This ability was observed regardless of whether serum was collected at the time of lymphatic system-restricted infection or when infection also involved the liver (Mulrooney-Cousins *et al.*, manuscript in preparation). Liver histology remained normal up to 4 years post-infection. However, minimal necroinflammatory alterations were found after 5 years post-infection. The most important finding was that HCC had developed in some of the animals, indicating that the persisting virus retained its oncogenic potency and, therefore, that this form of infection is of a direct pathological relevance (Mulrooney-Cousins *et al.*, manuscript in preparation). In another study, intrahepatic injection of small amounts of recombinant complete WHV DNA has also induced POI, whereas high doses of the same WHV DNA similarly administered can induce typical AH (Will *et al.*, 1982; Chen *et al.*, 1998; Mulrooney-Cousins & Michalak, manuscript in preparation).

The characteristics of WHV-specific T cell immune responses and cytokine expression profiles in circulating lymphoid cells were also examined in the course of experimental POI and subsequent challenge with liver pathogenic dose ($>10^3$ virions) or liver non-pathogenic dose (50 virions) of the same inoculum (Gujar & Michalak, 2009). The data revealed that POI was accompanied by the appearance of a strong WHV-specific T cell proliferative response directed against multiple viral epitopes which intermittently persisted at low levels for up to 10 months of follow-up. Moreover, immediately after exposure to a liver-nonpathogenic dose of WHV, lymphocytes acquired a heightened capacity to proliferate in response to mitogenic stimuli and displayed augmented expression of IFNα, interleukin-12 (IL-12) and IL-2, but not TNFα and the profile of that response was closely comparable to that seen in infection induced with liver-pathogenic viral doses (Gujar *et al.*, 2008; Gujar & Michalak, 2009). The data also showed that virus-specific T cell proliferative reactivity is a very sensitive indicator of exposure to hepadnavirus, even to very small amounts that induce serologically silent infection. They demonstrated that POI is not only identifiable molecularly but it is also a distinctive immunological entity.

The existence of POI in humans has not yet been clearly established, however existence of HBV-specific CD8+ T cell response in the absence of HBV-specific antibodies and the presence of detectable HBV DNA (Zerbini *et al.*, 2008), strongly suggest that this form of infection may occur. On the other hand, the consequences of HBV infection in infants born to mothers with resolved hepatitis B have never been investigated. One of the constraints in this type of study is the difficulty in acquisition of serial samples from different compartments of virus occurrence, i.e., serum or plasma, lymphoid cells (PBMC) and liver, and their proper standardized preparation to secure recovery of small amounts of viral material. Another important limitation is the sensitivity of the clinical assays currently applied for detection of HBV genome, which are at least 100-times less sensitive than the research assays applied for this purpose. The strong similarities between WHV and HBV suggest that the persistence of small amounts of the virus could have a significant impact in terms of transmission of infection and pathogenesis of disorders which are not yet considered to be a consequence of persistent hepadnavirus infection. POI initiated by minute amounts of the virus transmitted from mothers may induce occult infection in neonates, similar to the chronic infection induced in newborns to mothers with symptomatic CH (Beasley, 2009). Also, transmission of virus from unknowingly HBV infected individuals via blood transfusion and organ donation remains a relative risk until clinical laboratory assays reach a sensitivity that is now only obtained by research assays (Lok *et al.*, 1991; Uemoto *et al.*, 1998; Conjeevaram & Lok, 2001; Mulrooney-Cousins & Michalak, 2007, 2009; De Mitri *et al.*, 2010; Schmeltzer & Sherman, 2010).

6.3 Secondary occult hepadnaviral infection

Residual hepadnaviral infection continuing after resolution of HBV and WHV hepatitis, *i.e.*, secondary occult infection or SOI, have been documented in both humans and woodchucks (Liang *et al.*, 1990; Blum *et al.*, 1991; Mason *et al.*, 1992, 1998; Michalak *et al.*, 1994; Michalak *et al.*, 1999; Michalak, 2000; Bläckberg & Kidd-Ljunggren, 2001; Mulrooney-Cousins & Michalak, 2007; Tong *et al.*, 2009; Gerlich *et al.*, 2010; Hollinger & Sood, 2010; Raimondo *et al.*, 2010; Lledo *et al.*, 2011; Said, 2011). It is now evident that the anti-viral immunity established after an encounter with WHV or HBV at doses that cause hepatitis is not able to completely eradicate the virus and replication of virus persists in both hepatocytes and cells of the lymphatic system (Chemin *et al.*, 1992, 1993; Michalak *et al.*, 1994, 1999; Cabrerizo *et al.*, 2000; Mulrooney & Michalak, 2003; Murakami *et al.*, 2004). In this form of infection, the virus can persist for many years without apparent variations in its sequence or emergence of cell type-specific mutants (Laskus *et al.*, 1999; Bläckberg & Kidd-Ljunggren, 2001; Mulrooney-Cousins & Michalak, 2008).

In the woodchuck model, persistence of WHV replication and production of small amounts of infectious virions after resolution of self-limiting AH is life-long when highly sensitive PCR-based assays coupled with detection of amplicons via nucleic acid hybridization (PCR/NAH) are used (Michalak *et al.*, 1999). This life-long carriage involves the liver and is not restricted to the lymphatic organs and PBMC like in POI. As already mentioned (Section 3), animals that have serologically resolved AH show transient minimal to moderate liver inflammatory alterations through their lifespan (Michalak *et al.*, 1999), as has also been reported for individuals with self-limited AH type B (Yuki *et al.*, 2003). Moreover, up to one

fifth of the recovered animals develop HCC (Michalak *et al.*, 1999). Taken together, virus persisting at very low levels as SOI retains its liver pathogenic and oncogenic potentials.
SOI is always accompanied by anti-WHc and frequently by anti-WHs (Michalak *et al.*, 1999; Michalak *et al.*, 2007). It has also been shown that the persistence of isolated anti-WHc is indicative of SOI, even in the absence of prior evidence of serologically evident, i.e., serum WHsAg reactive infection (Coffin *et al.*, 2004). In such animals, low levels of WHV DNA are detectable in the serum, PBMC and liver by PCR/NAH (Coffin *et al.*, 2004). This form of infection is also accompanied by the persisting ability of T cells to respond to virus-specific stimuli (Gujar *et al.* 2008), which also characterize T cell proliferative and cytotoxic responses in patients with a past history of self-limiting AH (Rehermann *et al.*, 1995, 1996a, 1996b; Penna *et al.*, 1996).
The importance of SOI has also been highlighted in the study in which woodchucks were immunized with a bicistronic DNA vaccine carrying WHV core and woodchuck IFNγ in an attempt to enhance induction of protective immunity against virus. It has been postulated that the immunity elicited against nucleocapsid of HBV or WHV could be important in treatment of CH and protection from infection (Murray *et al.*, 1987; Garcia-Navarro *et al.*, 2001). It was found that the animals receiving high doses of the vaccine successfully produced anti-WHc (Wang *et al.*, 2007). However, molecular analysis of liver biopsies revealed that although the animals were protected from hepatitis, as confirmed by histological examination, they were not entirely sheltered from WHV infection since WHV DNA and RNA remained detectable in the livers at levels comparable to those seen in SOI. The results implied that vaccination with DNA encoding hepadnaviral core protein may not be sufficient to mount sterilizing immunity against the virus or prevent establishment of occult infection, although it can protect against development of symptomatic hepatitis.

7. WHV-hepatocyte plasma membrane interactions in the course of hepatitis

As already indicated, the development of hepadnaviral hepatitis is a direct consequence of the cytopathic immune responses directed against infected hepatocytes. However, minimal inflammatory alterations or their absence and essentially normal liver function tests are observed in patients with very high hepatic loads of HBV envelope material where essentially all hepatocytes carry the antigen, as is observed in a healthy chronic HBV carrier state. This and other observations raised questions as to whether there is a relationship between the status of hepadnaviral protein incorporation into HPM structure and immunomorphological forms of hepatitis. This was based on the postulate that hepadnaviral proteins exposed on hepatocytes can modulate immunopathogenic reactions causing liver damage. In a series of studies, highly purified HPM isolated from woodchucks with different stages of WHV hepatitis or HCC were analyzed for the amounts of the HPM-associated WHV proteins, the protein molecular profiles and the nature of their association with the HPM bilayer. Comparative analysis revealed that the HPM levels and molecular profiles of WHV nucleocapsid (core) protein were not related to the duration or histological severity of liver damage. In contrast, quantities of the virus envelope material (WHsAg) were significantly greater in HPM derived from CH than from AH or HCC. Interestingly, although the envelope preS1, preS2 and S polypeptides were detected in all infected HPM, expression of WHV pre-S2 polypeptides was always dominant (Michalak & Lin, 1994) (also see Section 8). Furthermore, in CH, WHV envelope proteins was found to be very tightly bound to HPM and behaved as integral membrane proteins, implying its irreversible incorporation into the plasma membrane structure and suggesting that they could be eliminated only by lysis of infected hepatocytes (Michalak & Churchill, 1988). In addition, HPM from woodchucks with CH or from nontumor parenchyma of animals with HCC, but not HPM from AH or healthy animals, showed an inability to bind an exogenous WHsAg (Michalak & Lin, 1994). The same was also observed for plasma membranes purified from livers of chronic carriers of WHV with minimal hepatitis (Michalak, 1988). Taken together, the extent and the characteristics of WHV envelope interaction with HPM undergo significant variations in the natural course of hepatitis and distinct forms of WHV-induced liver disease display specific properties of that association. The accumulation of WHV envelope proteins in HPM is a prominent characteristic of CH, but is not connected with histological activity of liver inflammation (Michalak *et al.*, 1990). This event may contribute to the maintenance of chronic disease by creating an immune resistant barrier preserving infected hepatocytes. In this regard, the augmented display of WHV envelope proteins, particularly pre-S2 peptides, in CH coincides with a significant inhibition of class I MHC display on hepatocyte surface. This may profoundly impact the effectiveness of the elimination of infected hepatocytes by virus-specific CTL (Michalak *et al.*, 2000).

It should also be noted that anti-WHc and antibodies recognizing WHV e antigen (anti-WHe) reactivity were also detected in association with HPM (Michalak *et al.*, 1990). However, while anti-WHc antibodies were readily identifiable, anti-WHe could only be detected in eluates from HPM of animals that had recovered from AH (Michalak *et al.*, 1990). This suggested that a humoral response against e antigen may contribute to the resolution of acute infection, presumably by the elimination of infected hepatocytes through antibody-mediated cytolysis, as was suggested for chimpanzees vaccinated with HBeAg (Schlicht *et al.*, 1991).

8. WHV inhibition of hepatocyte class I MHC in chronic hepatitis

As previously mentioned, the utilization of such a unique animal model as the WHV-infected woodchucks has certain disadvantages; they are, among others, related to the lack of commercially available reagents and assays. This laboratory has made a significant effort over the years in developing tools essential for research on different aspects of hepadnaviral infection, and the liver and the immune system biology in this model. One of the important antibodies generated was a monoclonal antibody (mAb) against the heavy chain of woodchuck class I MHC (Michalak *et al.*, 1995). Employment of this woodchuck-specific mAb, as well as flow cytometry and immunoblotting analyses, revealed that normal woodchuck hepatocytes express class I MHC, although at a low level, in contrast to the previous assumptions based on immunohistochemical staining. With this new tool in hand, class I MHC expression was examined on hepatocytes and HPM isolated from different stages of experimentally induced WHV hepatitis (Michalak *et al.*, 2000). It was found that AH is characterized by a significantly enhanced hepatocyte surface display of class I MHC. This coincided with the augmented hepatocyte gene expression for class I MHC heavy chain, IFNγ and class I MHC-associated genes, such as β_2-microglobulin and transporters associated with antigen processing (TAP1 and TAP2). However, despite the similarly augmented transcription of class I MHC heavy chain and the associated genes in hepatocytes from woodchucks with CH, there was no evidence of class I MHC protein presence on the hepatocyte surface. This indicated a profound posttranscriptional inhibition in the class I MHC display in hepatocytes chronically infected with WHV (Michalak *et al.*,

2000). Since, the cell surface class I MHC is paramount to the efficient presentation of viral peptides to virus-specific CTLs, this finding was of high importance to our understanding of mechanisms underlying development and perpetuation of CH in hepadnaviral infection.
Further investigations have focused on the elucidation of which of the WHV proteins are specifically responsible for the inhibition of class I MHC display on hepatocytes (Wang & Michalak, 2006). In this study, WCM-260 hepatocytes (see Section 4) transfected with WHV genes encoding individual viral proteins as well as the entire WHV genome were employed. It was found that hepatocyte presentation of class I MHC was significantly inhibited following transfection with the complete WHV genome or with viral subgenomic fragments encoding envelope preS2 (middle) or preS1 (large) protein, which also encompasses the preS2 amino acid sequence. In contrast, hepatocytes transfected with the WHV X gene demonstrated a significant augmentation in the class I MHC protein display. Further, treatment of hepatocytes with recombinant woodchuck IFN-γ (Wang & Michalak, 2005) restored the inhibited presentation of the class I antigen induced by total WHV and preS2 and preS1 sequences. It is of note that the class I antigen suppression was not associated with down-regulation of hepatocyte genes for class I MHV heavy chain, $ß_2$-microglobulin, TAP1, TAP2 and proteasome subunits. Taken together, these findings indicated that the defective presentation of class I MHC on hepatocytes transcribing WHV is a consequence of posttranscriptional suppression exerted by the virus pre-S2 envelope protein and that this defect can be fully reversed by treatment with IFNγ (Wang & Michalak, 2006).

9. Intrahepatic immune response in pre-acute WHV infection

One of the impediments to understanding the pathogenesis of HBV infection is the lack of the delineation of virological and immunological events occurring in the liver immediately after hepadnavirus invasion and during the pre-acute phase of infection, since identification of patients in during this asymptomatic phase of infection is extremely difficult and acquisition of liver biopsy material is practically impossible due to the lack of clinically sound indications. For these types of investigations, the woodchuck model of hepatitis B is particularly well suited. Using woodchucks with experimentally induced AH, the hepatic kinetics of hepadnavirus replication and the profiles of activated genes encoding cytokines, cytotoxic effector molecules and immune cell markers were quantified in sequential liver biopsies from one hour post-inoculation outward using real-time amplification assays (Guy *et al.*, 2008a). To achieve the most complete recognition of the events investigated, over 110 liver biopsies were collected starting from the time when animals were healthy to up to 36 months after virus infection when SOI was established. The study showed that WHV replication is detectable in the liver within one hour after infection. In 3 to 6 hours, significantly augmented hepatic transcription of IFNγ and IL-12 were evident, implying activation of antigen presenting cells. In 48 to 72 hours, natural killer (NK) cells and NK T cells were activated and WHV replication was transiently but significantly inhibited, indicating that this early innate immune response is at least partially successful in limiting virus propagation in the liver. Despite this, T cells were activated 4 to 5 weeks later when hepatitis became histologically apparent. Overall, these data demonstrated that hepadnaviral replication is initiated and the innate response is activated in the liver soon after exposure to a liver pathogenic dose of virus. Nonetheless, this response is unable to prompt a timely virus-specific T cell reactivity which is a characteristic of infections with other viral pathogens (Guy *et al.*, 2008a).

10. New insights into hepatocyte function

It is now acknowledged that the liver plays an important role in immunity, particularly in maintenance of peripheral tolerance and pathogen surveillance. Although the involvement of liver cells, such as Kupffer cells and sinusoidal endothelial cells, is relatively well recognized (Bertolino *et al.*, 2002; Warren *et al.*, 2006; Crispe, 2009), a contribution of hepatocytes to the intrahepatic immunological process was entirely unknown. By using woodchuck and human primary hepatocytes, as well as woodchuck WCM-260 hepatocyte line, novel and unexpected properties of hepatocytes were uncovered (Guy & Michalak, 2008).

10.1 Hepatocyte as cytotoxic effector cells

Initially, in contrast to the previous opinion, it was found that normal primary and cultured hepatocytes constitutively express CD95 ligand (CD95L, formerly called Fas ligand) and are capable of inducing death of CD95-bearing cells (Guy *et al.*, 2006). Cytokines, such as IFNγ and TNFα, can upregulate hepatocyte expression and usage of CD95L. Then, we also documented that hepatocytes express perforin and can kill cells brought into contact with their surface via an exocytic pathway. However, this cytotoxic potency of hepatocytes is not modified by the cytokine milieu (Guy *et al.*, 2008b). We concluded that hepatocytes, similar to lymphocytes, are endowed in two distinct cytotoxic effector mechanisms. The relevance of these findings may pertain not only to fratricidal cell death during the development and progression of liver disease, but implicate an active cytotoxic role for hepatocytes as they may interact with other cells either trafficking through or residing in the liver. In this regard, our recent study showed that hepatocytes are capable of eliminating activated autologous T lymphocytes utilizing both CD95-CD95L and perforin-granzyme B dependent pathways (Guy *et al.*, 2011). Despite that the ability of hepatocytes to eliminate contacted cells was documented and the underlying cytopathic mechanisms were delineated, it remained unknown whether hepatocyte-mediated cell killing is indiscriminant or if hepatocytes are capable of discerning which cells are to be eliminated. Furthermore, the cell surface molecules involved in hepatocyte recognition of cells targeted for killing were recently investigated. In the course of this study, it was identified that the hepatocyte specific protein, ASGPR (as mentioned already in Section 6.1), which plays a central role in the clearance of circulating desialylated glycoproteins, is involved in the recognition and removal of cells by hepatocytes (Guy *et al.*, 2011).

10.2 WHV infection augments hepatocyte cytotoxicity

To recognize if hepadnaviral infection modifies the cytotoxic potency of hepatocytes, we investigated primary hepatocytes isolated from woodchucks with progressing CH and those which resolved AH (Guy *et al.*, 2010). It was found that the hepatocyte potential to kill contacted cells is significantly augmented both during CH and after resolution of AH when compared to hepatocytes from healthy animals. Furthermore, hepatocytes exposed to exogenous IFNγ, but not those transfected with the complete WHV genome or individual virus genes, except the WHV X gene, demonstrated enhanced CD95L and perforin-mediated cytotoxicity. This argued that augmented intrahepatic production of IFNγ rather than virus replication itself increased the killing. In this regard, an increased intrahepatic expression of IFNγ was reported not only in CH but also during SOI continuing after resolution of AH (Hodgson & Michalak, 2001). It was also observed that hepatocytes transfected with the

WHV X gene alone transcribed significantly more CD95L and perforin and killed cell targets more efficiently, suggesting that under certain circumstances, albeit probably very rare, the virus may directly augment hepatocyte cytotoxicity (Guy *et al.*, 2010). This was the first study that demonstrated that the cytotoxic phenotype of hepatocytes can be modified by virus infection and that this occurred irrespective whether liver inflammation is active or progresses quiescently. Although hepatocyte cell killing may not be apparent in the normal liver, it is reasonable to expect that inflammation and other forms of liver damage may heighten the ability of hepatocytes to cause death of other cells residing or passing through the liver and, in consequence, influence progression and outcomes of diseases engaging this organ (Guy *et al.*, 2008).

11. Conclusions

Liver biopsy material is invaluable for determination of the progression of viral hepatitis and assessment of the outcome of antiviral therapy, as well as for investigations into the pathogenesis of hepatocellular injury and perpetuation of hepatitis. Many of the mechanisms of liver disease, the elements of the natural course of hepadnaviral infection, the basic biological properties of hepadnaviruses as well as hepatocyte biology were delineated by utilizing liver biopsy material from the woodchuck model of hepatitis B. This overcame impediments imposed by difficulties in obtaining hepatic tissue specimens from patients with different stages of hepatitis B and from seemingly healthy individuals with silently progressing infection. The ability to obtain sequential liver biopsies prior to and over the course of experimentally induced WHV infection has led to the discovery of previously unknown characteristics and consequences of hepadnaviral infection which are only recently being recognized in the clinical setting. The woodchuck-WHV infection model retains a significant potential to generate new knowledge which should be even more vigorously explored in years to come.

12. Acknowledgements

The authors thank current and former graduate students, post-doctoral fellows and staff of the Molecular Virology and Hepatology Research Group and the Woodchuck Hepatitis Research Facility at the Faculty of Medicine, Memorial University of Newfoundland for their contributions to the research summarized in this review. The studies were supported by operating grants MOP-14818, MT-11262 and RO-15174 awarded to T.I.M. by the Canadian Institutes of Health Research (formerly Medical Research Council of Canada). P.M.M-C. is the Manager of the Woodchuck Hepatitis Research Facility at Memorial University. T.I.M. is the Senior Canada Research Chair in Viral Hepatitis/Immunology supported by the Canadian Institutes of Health Research and Canada Foundation for Innovation.

13. References

Alcami A. & Koszinowski U.H. (2000). Viral mechanisms of immune evasion. *Immunol. Today* 21:447-455

Beasley R.P. (2009). Roadblocks along the road to the control of HBV and HCC. *Ann. Epidemiol.* 19:231-234

Bertoletti A., Maini M.K. & Ferrari C. (2010). The host-pathogen interaction during HBV infection: immunological controversies. *Antivir. Ther.* 15:15-24

Bertolino P, McCaughan G.W. & Bowen DG. (2002). Role of primary intrahepatic T-cell activation in the 'liver tolerance effect'. *Immunol. Cell. Biol.* 80:84-92

Bläckberg J. & Kidd-Ljunggren K. (2001). Occult hepatitis B virus after acute self-limited infection persisting for 30 years without sequence variation. *J. Hepatol.* 33:992-997

Blum H.E., Liang E., Galun E. & Wands J.R. (1991). Persistence of hepatitis B virus DNA after serological recovery from hepatitis B virus infection. *Hepatology* 14: 56-63

Cabrerizo M., Bartolomé J., Caramelo C., Barril G. & Carreño V. (2000). Molecular analysis of hepatitis B virus DNA in serum and peripheral blood mononuclear cells from hepatitis B surface antigen-negative cases. *Hepatology* 32:116-123

Cacoub P. & Terrier B. (2009). Hepatitis B-related autoimmune manifestations. *Rheum. Dis. Clin. North Am.* 35:125-137

Calmus Y., Marcellin P., Beaurain G. & Brechot C. (1994). Distribution of hepatitis B virus DNA sequences in different peripheral blood mononuclear cell subsets in HBs antigen-positive and -negative patients. *Eur. J. Clin. Invest.* 24:548-552

Carpenter P.A., Huang M.L. & McDonald G.B. (2002). Activation of occult hepatitis B from a seronegative patient after hematopoietic cell transplant: a cautionary tale. *Blood* 99:4245-4246

Chazouilleres O., Mamish D., Kim M., Carey K., Ferrell L., Roberts J.P., Ascher N.L. & Wright T.L. (1994). "Occult" hepatitis B virus as a source of infection in liver transplant recipients. *Lancet* 343:142-146

Chemin I., Vermot-Desroches C., Baginski I., Saurin J.C., Laurent F., Zoulim F., Bernard J., Lamelin J.P., Hantz O., Rigal D., & Trepo C. (1992). Selective detection of human hepatitis B surface and core antigen in peripheral blood mononuclear cells subsets by flow cytometry. *J. Clin. Lab. Immunol.* 38:63-71

Chemin I., Vermot-Desroches C., Baginski I., Lamelin J.P., Hantz O., Jacquet C., Rigal D. & Trepo C. (1993). Monitoring of early events of experimental woodchuck hepatitis infection: studies of peripheral blood mononuclear cells by cytofluorometry and PCR. *FEMS Immunol. Med. Microbiol.* 7:241-249

Chemin I., Zoulim F., Merle P., Arkhis A., Chevallier M., Kay A., Cova L., Chevallier P., Mandrand B. & Trepo C. (2001). High incidence of hepatitis B infection among chronic hepatitis cases of unknown aetiology. *J. Hepatol.* 34:447-454

Chen H.S., Miller R.H., Hornbuckle W.E., Tennant B.C., Cote P.J., Gerin J.L. & Purcell R.H. (1998). Titration of recombinant woodchuck hepatitis virus DNA in adult woodchucks. *J. Med. Virol.* 54:92-94

Chisari F.V. & Ferrari C. (1995). Hepatitis B virus immunopathogenesis. *Ann. Rev. Immunol.* 13:29-60

Chisari F.V. & Ferrari C. (1996). Viral hepatitis. In: *Viral Pathogenesis,* R. Ahmed, K.V. Holmes, F. Gonzalez-Scarano, F.A. Murphy, D.E. Griffin, H.L. Robinson, (eds.), pp. 745-778, Lippincott-Raven Publishers, Philadelphia, Pensylvania, USA

Chisari F.V., Isogawa M. & Wieland S.F. (2010). Pathogenesis of hepatitis B infection. *Pathologie Biologie* 58:258-286

Churchill N.D. & Michalak T.I. (2004). Woodchuck hepatitis virus hepatocyte culture models. In: *Methods in Molecular Medicine: Hepatitis B and D Protocols,* R.K.,

Hamatake and J.Y.N. Lau (eds.), vol. 2. pp. 175-187, Humana Press Inc., Totowa, New Jersey, USA

Coffin C.S. & Michalak T.I. (1999). Persistence of infectious hepadnavirus in the offspring of woodchuck mothers recovered from viral hepatitis. *J. Clin. Invest.* 104:203–212

Coffin C.S., Pham T.N.Q., Mulrooney P.M., Churchill N.D. & Michalak T.I. (2004). Persistence of isolated antibodies to woodchuck hepatitis virus core antigen is indicative of occult virus infection. *Hepatology* 40:1053-1061

Coffin C.S., Mulrooney-Cousins P.M., Peters M.G., van Marle G., Roberts J.P., Michalak T.I. & Terrault N.A. (2011a). Molecular characterization of intrahepatic and extrahepatic hepatitis B virus (HBV) reservoirs in patients on suppressive antiviral therapy. *J. Viral Hepat.* 18:415-423

Coffin C.S., Mulrooney-Cousins P.M., van Marle G., Roberts J.P., Michalak T.I. & Terrault N.A. (2011b). Hepatitis B virus (HBV) quasispecies in hepatic and extrahepatic viral reservoirs in liver transplant recipients on prophylactic therapy. *Liver Transpl* 17:955-962.

Conjeevaram H. & Lok A. S. (2001). Occult hepatitis B virus infection: a hidden menace? *Hepatology* 34:204-206

Cote P.J., Korba B.E., Baldwin B., Hornbuckle W.E., Tennant B.C. & Gerin J L. (1992). Immunosuppression with cyclosporin during the incubation period of experimental woodchuck hepatitis virus infection increases the frequency of chronic infection in adult woodchucks. *J. Infect. Dis.* 166:628-631

Cote P.J., Korba B.E., Miller R.H., Jacob J.R., Baldwin B.H., Tennant B.C. & Gerin J.L. (2000a). Effects of age and viral determinants on chronicity as an outcome of experimental woodchuck hepatitis virus infection. *Hepatology* 31:190-200

Cote P.J., Toshkov I., Bellezza C., Ascenzi M., Roneker C., Ann Graham L., Baldwin B.H., Gaye K., Nakamura I., Korba B.E., Tennant B.C. & Gerin J.L. (2000b). Temporal pathogenesis of experimental neonatal woodchuck hepatitis virus infection: increases initial viral load and decreased severity of acute hepatitis during the development of chronic viral infection. *Hepatology* 32:807-817

Crispe I.N. (2009). The liver as a lymphoid organ. *Annu. Rev. Immunol.* 27:147-163

De Mitri M.S., Cassini R. & Bernardi M. (2010). Hepatitis B virus-related hepatocarcinogenesis: molecular oncogenic potential of clear or occult infections. *Eur. J. Cancer 46*:2178-2186

Diao J. & Michalak T.I. (1996). Composition, antigenic properties and hepatocyte surface expression of the woodchuck asialoglycoprotein receptor. *J. Recept. Signal Transduct. Res.* 16:243-271

Diao J. & Michalak T.I. (1997). Virus-induced anti-asialoglycoprotein receptor autoimmunity in experimental hepadnaviral hepatitis. *Hepatology* 25:689-696

Diao J., Churchill N.D. & Michalak T.I. (1998). Complement-mediated cytotoxicity and inhibition of ligand binding to hepatocytes by woodchuck virus-induced autoantibodies to asialoglycoprotein receptor. *Hepatology* 27:1623-1631

Diao J., Slaney D.M. & Michalak T.I. (2003). Modulation of the outcome and severity of hepadnaviral hepatitis in woodchucks by antibodies to hepatic asialoglycoprotein receptor. *Hepatology* 38:629-638

Dickson R.C., Everhart J.E., Lake J.R., Wei Y., Seaberg E.C., Wiesner R.H., Zetterman R.K., Pruett T.L., Ishitani M.B. & Hoofnagle J.H. (1997). Transmission of hepatitis B by transplantation of livers from donors positive for antibody to hepatitis B core antigen. The National Institute of Diabetes and Digestive and Kidney Diseases Liver Transplantation Database. *Gastroenterology* 113:1668-1674

Dzwonkowski P. & Michalak T.I. (1990). Autoantibody pattern in a woodchuck model of hepatitis B. *Clin. Invest. Med.* 13: 322-328

Feitelson M.A. & Lee J. (2007). Hepatitis B virus integration, fragile sites and hepatocarcinogenesis. *Cancer Letters* 252:157-70

Feray C., Zignego A.L., Samuel D., Bismuth A., Reynes M., Tiollais P., Bismuth H. & Brechot C. (1990). Persistent hepatitis B virus infection of mononuclear blood cells without concominant liver infection: the liver transplantation model. *Transplantation* 49: 1155-1158

Garcia-Navarro R., Blanco-Urgoito B., Berraondo P., Sanchez de la Rosa R., Vales A., Hervas-Stubbs S., Lasarte J.J., Borras F., Ruiz J. & Prieto J. (2001). Protection against woodchuck hepatitis virus (WHV) infection by gene gun coimmunization with WHV core and interleukin-12. *J. Virol.* 75:9068-9076

Gerlich W.H., Bremer C., Saniewski M., Schuttler C.G., Wend U.C., Willems W.R. & Glebe D. (2010). Occult hepatitis B virus infection: detection and significance. *Dig. Dis.* 28:116-125

Grob P., Jilg W., Bornhak H., Gerken G., Gerlich W., Gunther S., Hess G., Hudig H., Kitchen A., Margolis H., Michel G., Trepo C., Will H., Zanetti A. & Mushahwar I. (2000). Serological pattern "anti-HBc alone": report on a workshop. *J. Med. Virol.* 62: 450-455

Guidotti L.G., Rochford R., Chung J., Shapiro M., Purcell R. & Chisari F.V. (1999). Viral clearance without destruction of infected cells during acute HBV infection. *Science* 284:825–829

Guidotti L.G. & Chisari F.V. (2001). Non-cytolytic control of viral infections by the innate and adaptive immune response. *Annu. Rev. Immunol.* 19:65-91

Gujar S.A., Jenkins A.K., Guy C.S., Wang J. & Michalak T.I. (2008). Aberrant lymphocyte activation preceded delayed virus-specific T cell response after both primary infection and secondary exposure to hepadnavirus in the woodchuck model of hepatitis B infection. *J. Virol.* 82:6992-7008

Gujar S. A. & Michalak T.I. (2009). Primary occult hepadnavirus infection induces virus-specific T-cell and aberrant cytokine responses in the absence of antiviral antibody reactivity in the woodchuck model of hepatitis B virus infection. *J. Virol.* 83:3861-3876

Guy C.S., Wang J. & Michalak T.I. (2006). Hepatocytes as cytotoxic effector cells can induce cell death by CD95 ligand-mediated pathway. *Hepatology* 43:1231-1240

Guy C.S. & Michalak T.I. (2008). Hepatocytes as cytotoxic effector cells. *Curr. Immunol. Rev.* 4:215-220

Guy C.S., Mulrooney-Cousins P.M., Churchill N.D. & Michalak, T.I. (2008a). Intrahepatic expression of genes affiliated with innate and adaptive immune responses immediately after invasion and during acute infection with woodchuck hepadnavirus. *J. Virol.* 82:8579-8591

Guy C.S., Rankin S.L., Wang J. & Michalak T.I. (2008b). Hepatocytes can induce death of contacted cells via perforin-dependent mechanism. *Hepatology* 47:1691-1701

Guy C.S. & Michalak T.I. (2010). Hepadnaviral infection augments hepatocyte cytotoxicity mediated by both CD95 ligand and perforin pathways. *Liver Int* 30:396-405

Guy C.S., Rankin S.L. & Michalak T.I. (2011). Hepatocyte cytotoxicity is facilitated by asialoglycoprotein receptor. *Hepatology* (in press; e-pub ahead of print Jun 7; doi: 10.1002/hep.24477)

Hodgson P.D. & Michalak T.I. (2001). Augmented hepatic interferon gamma expression and T-cell influx characterize acute hepatitis progressing to recovery and residual lifelong virus persistence in experimental adult woodchuck hepatitis virus infection. *Hepatology* 34:1049-1059

Hollinger F.B. & Sood G. (2010). Occult hepatitis B virus infection: a covert operation. *J. Viral Hepat.* 17:1-15

Hu K.Q. (2002). Occult hepatitis B virus infection and its clinical implications. *J. Viral Hepatitis* 9:243-257

Jin Y.-M., Churchill N.D. & Michalak T.I. (1996). Protease-activated lymphoid cell and hepatocyte recognition site in the preS1 domain of the large woodchuck hepatitis virus envelope protein. *J. Gen. Virol.* 77:1837-1846

Kajino K., Jilbert A.R., Saputelli J., Aldrich C.E., Cullen J. & Mason W.S. (1994). Woodchuck hepatitis virus infections: very rapid recovery after a prolonged viremia and infection of virtually every hepatocyte. *J. Virol.* 68: 5792-5803

Kao J.H. (2008). Diagnosis of hepatitis B virus infection through serological and virological markers. *Expert. Rev. Gastroenterol. Hepatol.* 2:553-562

Korba B.E., Wells F., Tennant B.C., Cote P.J. & Gerin J. L. (1987). Lymphoid cells in the spleens of woodchuck hepatitis virus-infected woodchucks are a site of active viral replication. *J. Virol.* 61:1318-1324

Korba B.E., Cote P.J. & Gerin J.L. (1988). Mitogen-induced replication of woodchuck hepatitis virus in cultured peripheral blood lymphocytes. *Science* 241:1213-1216

Korba B.E., Wells F.V., Baldwin B., Cote P.J., Tennant B.C., Popper H. & Gerin J.L. (1989). Hepatocellular carcinoma in woodchuck hepatitis virus infected woodchucks. Presence of viral DNA in tumor tissue from chronic carriers of animals serologically recovered from acute infections. *Hepatology* 9:461–470

Laskus T., Radkowski M., Wang L.F., Nowicki M. & Rakela J. (1999). Detection and sequence analysis of hepatitis B virus integration in peripheral blood mononuclear cells. *J. Virol.* 73: 1235-1238

Lew Y-Y. & Michalak T.I. (2001). *In vitro* and *in vivo* infectivity and pathogenicity of the lymphoid cell-derived woodchuck hepatitis virus. *J. Virol.* 75:1770-1782

Lia M. & Liaw Y.F. (2010). Chronic hepatitis B: past, present, and future. *Clin. Liver Dis.* 14:531-546

Liang T.J., Blum H. E. & Wands J. R. (1990). Characterization and biological properties of a hepatitis B virus isolated from a patient without hepatitis B virus serologic markers. *Hepatology* 12:204-212

Liaw Y.F., Brunetto M. R. & Hadziyannis S. (2010). The natural history of chronic HBV infection and geographical differences. *Antiviral Therapy* 15:25-33

Lledo J.L., Fernandez C., Gutierrez M.L. & Ocana S. (2011). Management of occult hepatitis B virus infection: An update for the clinician. *World J. Gastro.* 17:1563-1568

Lok A.S., Liang R.H., Chiu E. K., Wong K. L., Chan T. K. & Todd D. (1991). Reactivation of hepatitis B virus replication in patients receiving cytotoxic therapy: report of a prospective study. *Gastroenterology* 100:1432-1434

Marusawa H., Uemoto S., Hijikata M., Ueda Y., Tanaka K., Shimotohno K. & Chiba T. (2000). Latent hepatitis virus infection in healthy individuals with antibodies to hepatitis B core antigen. *Hepatology* 31:488-495

Mason A., Yoffe B., Noonan C., Mearns M., Campbell C., Kelley A. & Perrillo R. P. (1992). Hepatitis B virus DNA in peripheral-blood mononuclear cells in chronic hepatitis B after HBsAg clearance. *Hepatology* 16:26-41

Mason A.L., Xu L., Guo L., Kuhns M. & Perrillo R.P. (1998). Molecular basis for persistent hepatitis B virus infection in the liver after clearance of serum hepatitis B surface antigen. *Hepatology* 27:1736-1742

Mason W.S., Jilbert A.R. & Summers J. (2005). Clonal expansion of hepatocytes during chronic woodchuck hepatitis virus infection. *Proc. Natl. Acad. Sci. USA* 102:1139-1144

Mason W.S., Low H.C., Xu C., Aldrich C.E., Scougall C.A., Grosse A., Clouston A., Chavez D., Litwin S., Peri S., Jilbert A.R. & Lanford R.E. (2009). Detection of clonally expanded hepatocytes in chimpanzees with chronic hepatitis B virus infection. *J. Virol.* 83:8396-8408

Menne S. & Tennant B.C. (1999). Unravelling hepatitis B virus infection of mice and men (and woodchucks and ducks). *Nature Med.* 5:1125-1126

Menne S. & Cote P.J. (2007). The woodchuck as an animal model for pathogenesis and therapy of chronic hepatitis B virus infection. *World J. Gastro.* 13:104-124

Michalak T. (1978). Immune complexes of hepatitis B surface antigen in the pathogenesis of periarteritis nodosa. A study of seven necropsy cases. *Am. J. Pathol.* 90:619-632

Michalak T.I. (1988). Woodchuck hepatitis virus surface antigen association with purified liver plasma membranes from chronic carriers of woodchuck hepatitis virus. In: *Viral Hepatitis and Liver Disease,* A. Zuckerman (ed), pp. 476-480, Alan R. Liss, Inc., New York, USA

Michalak T.I. & Churchill N.D. (1988). Interaction of woodchuck hepatitis virus surface antigen with hepatocyte plasma membrane in woodchuck chronic hepatitis. *Hepatology* 8:499-506

Michalak T.I., Lin B., Churchill N.D., Dzwonkowski P. & Desousa J.R. (1990). Hepadnavirus nucleocapsid and surface antigens and the antigen-specific antibodies associated with hepatocyte plasma membranes in experimental woodchuck acute hepatitis. *Lab Invest.* 6:680-689

Michalak T.I. & Lin B. (1994). Molecular species of hepadnavirus core and envelope polypeptides in hepatocyte plasma membrane of woodchucks with acute and chronic viral hepatitis. *Hepatology* 20:275-286

Michalak T.I., Pasquinelli C., Guilhot S. & Chisari F.V. (1994). Hepatitis B virus persistence after recovery from acute viral hepatitis. *J. Clin. Invest.* 93:230-239

Michalak T.I., Churchill N.D., Codner D., Drover S. & Marshall W.H. (1995). Identification of woodchuck class I MHC antigens using monoclonal antibodies. *Tissue Antigens.* 45:333-342

Michalak T. I. (1998). The woodchuck animal model of hepatitis B. *Viral Hepatitis Rev.* 4:139-165

Michalak T.I., Pardoe I.U., Coffin C.S., Churchill N.D., Freake D.S., Smith P. & Trelegan C.L. (1999). Occult life-long persistence of infectious hepadnavirus and residual liver inflammation in woodchucks convalescent from acute viral hepatitis. *Hepatology* 29:928-938

Michalak T.I. (2000). Occult persistence and lymphotropism of hepadnaviral infection: insights from the woodchuck viral hepatitis model. *Immunol. Rev.* 174:98-111

Michalak T.I., Hodgson P.D. & Churchill N.D. (2000). Posttranscriptional inhibition of class I major histocompatibility complex presentation on hepatocytes and lymphoid cells in chronic woodchuck hepatitis virus infection. *J. Virol.* 74:4483-4494

Michalak T.I. (2004). Immunology of hepatitis B virus. In: *Hepatitis Prevention and Treatment,* J.M. Colacino and B.A. Heinz (eds.), pp.87-105, Birkhauser Verlag Publishers, Basel, Switzerland

Michalak T.I., Mulrooney P.M. & Coffin C.S. (2004). Low doses of hepadnavirus induce infection of the lymphatic system that does not engage the liver. *J. Virol.* 78:1730-1738

Michalak T.I. (2007). Characteristics and consequences of experimental occult hepadnavirus infection in the woodchuck model of hepatitis B. *Curr. Topics Virol.* 6:1-13

Michalak T.I., Pham T.N.Q. & Mulrooney-Cousins P.M. (2007). Molecular diagnosis of occult HCV and HBV infections. *Future Medicine* 2:451-465

Morisco F., Castiglione F., Rispo A., Stroffolini T., Vitale R., Sansone S., Granata R., Orlando A., Marmo R., Reigler G., Vecchi M., Biancone L. & Caporaso N. (2011). Hepatitis B virus infection and immunosuppressive therapy in patients with inflammatory bowel disease. *Dig. Liver Dis.* 43:40-48

Mulrooney P.M. & Michalak T.I. (2003). Quantitative detection of hepadnavirus-infected lymphoid cells by *in situ* PCR combined with flow cytometry: implications for the study of occult virus persistence. *J. Virol.* 77:970-979

Mulrooney-Cousins P.M. & Michalak T.I. (2007). Persistent occult hepatitis B virus infection: experimental findings and clinical implications. *World J. Gastro.* 13:5682-5686

Mulrooney-Cousins P.M. & Michalak T.I. (2008). Repeated passage of wild-type woodchuck hepatitis virus in lymphoid cells does not generate cell type-specific variants or alter virus infectivity. *J. Virol.* 82:7540-7550

Mulrooney-Cousins P.M. & Michalak T.I. (2009). Diagnostic assays for hepatitis B virus. *Hot Topics in Viral Hepatitis* 15:7-13

Murakami Y., Minami M., Daimon Y. & Okanoue T. (2004). Hepatitis B virus DNA in liver, serum, and peripheral blood mononuclear cells after the clearance of serum hepatitis B surface antigen. *J. Med. Virol.* 72:203-214

Murray K., Bruce S.A., Wingfield P., van Eerd P., de Reus A, & Schellekens H. (1987). Protective immunisation against hepatitis B with an internal antigen of the virus. *J. Med. Virol.* 23:101-107

Nassal M. (2008). Hepatitis B viruses: reverse transcription in a different way. *Virus Res.* 134:235-49

Ogston C.W., Schechter E.M., Humes C.A. & Pranikoff M.B. (1989). Extrahepatic replication of woodchuck hepatitis virus in chronic infection. *Virology* 169:9-14

Penna A., Artini M., Cavalli A., Levero M., Bertoletti A., Pilli M., Chisari F.V., Rehermann B., Del Prete G., Fiaccadori F. & Ferrari C. (1996). Long-lasting memory T cell responses following self-limited acute hepatitis B. *J. Clin. Invest.* 98:1185-1194

Pollicino T., Squandrito G., Cerenzia G., Cacciola I., Raffa G., Crax A., Farinati F., Missale G., Smedile A., Tiribelli C., Villa E. & Raimondo G. (2004). Hepatitis B virus maintains its pro-oncogenic properties in the case of occult HBV infection. *Gastroenterology* 126:102-110

Pontisso P., Poon M.V., Tiollais P. & Brechot C. (1984). Detection of hepatitis B virus DNA in mononuclear cells. *Br. Med. J.* 288:1563-1566

Pontisso P., Vidalino L., Quarta S. & Gatta A. (2008). Biological and clinical implications of HBV infection in peripheral blood mononuclear cells. *Autoimm. Rev.* 8:13-17

Popper H., Shih W. W-K., Gerin D.C., Wong D.C., Hoyer B.H., London W.T., Sly D.L. & Purcell R.H. (1981). Woodchuck hepatitis and hepatocellular carcinoma: correlation of histologic with virologic observations. *Hepatology* 1:91-98

Poralla T., Treichel U., Lohr H. & Fleischer B. (1991). The asialoglycoprotein receptor as target structure in autoimmune liver diseases. *Semin Liver Dis* 11:215-222

Raimondo G., Allain, J.P., Brunetto, M.R., Buendia M.A., Chen D.-S., Colombo M., Craxi A., Donato F., Ferrari C., Gaeta G.B., Gerlich W.H., Levrero M., Locarnini S., Michalak, T.I., Mondeli M.U., Pawlowsky J.-M., Pollicino T., Prati D., Puoti M., Samuel D., Shouval S., Smedile A., Squadrito G., Trepo C., Villa E., Will H., Zanetti A.R. & Zoulim F. (2008). Statements from the Taormina expert meeting on occult hepatitis B virus infection. *J. Hepatol.* 49:652-657

Rehermann B., Fowler P., Sidney J., Person J., Redeker A., Brown M., Moss B., Sette A. & Chisari F.V. (1995). The cytotoxic T lymphocyte response to multiple hepatitis B virus polymerase epitopes during and after acute viral hepatitis. *J. Exp. Med.* 181:1047–1058

Rehermann B., Lau D., Hoofnagle J.H. & Chisari F.V. (1996a). Cytotoxic T lymphocyte responsiveness after resolution of chronic hepatitis B virus infection. *J. Clin. Invest.* 97:1655–1665

Rehermann B., Ferrari C., Pasquinelli C. & Chisari F.V. (1996b). The hepatitis B virus persists for decades after patients' recovery from acute viral hepatitis despite active maintenance of a cytotoxic T-lymphocyte response. *Nature Med.* 2:1104-1108

Roggendorf M., Yang D. & Lu M (2010). The woodchuck: a model for therapeutic vaccination against hepadnaviral infection. *Pathologie Biologie* 58:308-314

Romano L., Paladini S., Van Damme P. & Zanetti A.R. (2011). The worldwide impact of global vaccination on the control and protection of viral hepatitis B. *Dig. Liver Dis.* 43:S2-7

Said Z.N. (2011). An overview of occult hepatitis B virus infection. *World J. Gastro.* 17: 1927-1938

Schlicht H.J., von Brunn A. & Theilmann L. (1991). Antibodies in anti-HBe-positive patient sera bind to an HBe protein expressed on the cell surface of human hepatoma cells: implications for virus clearance. *Hepatology* 13:57-61

Schmeltzer P. & Sherman K.E. (2010). Occult hepatitis B: clinical implications and treatment decisions. *Dig. Dis. Sci.* 55:3328-3335

Simonetti J., Bulkow L., McMahon B.J., Homan C., Snowball M., Negus S., Williams J. & Livingstone S. E. (2010). Clearance of hepatitis B surface antigen and risk of hepatocellular carcinoma in a cohort chronically infected with hepatitis B virus. *Hepatology* 51:1531-1537

Summers J., Smolec J.M., & Snyder R. (1978). A virus similar to human hepatitis B virus associated with hepatitis and hepatoma in woodchucks. *Proc. Natl. Acad. Sci. USA* 75:4533–4537

Summers J. & Mason W.S. (1982). Replication of the genome of a hepatitis B-like virus by reverse transcription of an RNA intermediate. *Cell* 29:403–415

Tong M. J., Nguyen M.O., Tong L.T. & Blatt L.M. (2009). Development of hepatocellular circinoma after seroclearance of hepatitis B surface antigen. *Clin. Gastroenterol. Hepatol.* 7:889-893

Uemoto S., Sugiyama K., Marusawa H., Inomata Y., Asonuma K., Egawa H., Kiuchi T., Miyake Y., Tanaka K. & Chiba T. (1998). Transmission of hepatitis B virus from hepatitis B core antibody-positive donors in living related liver transplantation. *Transplantation* 65:494-499

Villadolid J., Laplant K.D., Markham M. J., Nelson D.R. & George T.J. Jr. (2011). Hepatitis B reactivation and rituximab in the oncology practice. *Oncologist* 15: 1113-1121

Wang J. & Michalak T.I. (2005). Comparison of biological activity of recombinant woodchuck interferon gamma and tumor necrosis factor alpha produced in baculovirus and *Escherichia coli* expression systems. *Cytokine* 30:22-34

Wang J. & Michalak T.I. (2006). Inhibition by woodchuck hepatitis virus of class I major histocompatibility complex presentation on hepatocytes is mediated by virus envelope pre-S2 protein and can be reversed by treatment with gamma interferon. *J. Virol.* 80:8541-8553

Wang J., Gujar S.A., Cova L. & Michalak T.I. (2007). Biscistronic woodchuck hepatitis virus core and gamma interferon DNA vaccine can protect from hepatitis but does not elicit sterilizing antiviral immunity. *J. Virol.* 81:903-916

Warren A., Le Couteur D.G., Fraser R., Bowen D.G., McCaughan G.W. & Bertolino P. (2006). T lymphocytes interact with hepatocytes through fenestrations in murine liver sinusoidal endothelial cells. *Hepatology* 44:1182-1190

Wei Y., Neuveut C., Tiollais P. & Buendia M.A. (2010). Molecular biology of hepatitis B virus and role of the X gene. *Pathologie Biologie* 58:267-272

Will H., Cattaneo R., Koch H.G., Darai G. & Schaller H. (1982). Cloned HBV DNA causes hepatitis in chimpanzees. *Nature* 299:740-742

World Health Organization. (August, 2008). Hepatitis B fact sheet No. 204, In: World Health Organization/HepatitisB/ Media Centre, April 2011, Available from: http://www.who.int/mediacentre/factsheets/fs204/en/index.html

Yoffe B., Noonan C.A., Melnick J.L. & Hollinger F.B. (1986). Hepatitis virus DNA in mononuclear cells and analysis of cell subsets for the presence of replicative intermediates of viral DNA. *J. Infect. Dis.* 153:471-477

Yotsuyanagi H.,Yasuda K., Iino S., Moriya K., Shintani Y., Fujie H., Tsutsumi T., Kimura S. & Koike K. (1998). Persistent viremia after recovery from self-limited acute hepatitis B. *Hepatology* 27:1377-1382

Yuki N., Nagaoka T., Yamashiro M., Mochizuki K., Kaneko A., Yamamoto K., Omura M., Hikiji K. & Kato M. (2003). Long-term histologic and virologic outcomes of acute self-limited hepatitis B. *Hepatology* 37:1172-1179

Zerbini A., Pilli M., Boni C., Fisicaro P., Penna A., Di Vincenzo P., Giuberti T., Orlandini A., Raffa G., Pollicino T., Raimondo G., Ferrari C. & Missale G. (2008). The characteristics of the cell-mediated immune response identify different profiles of occult hepatitis B virus infection. *Gastroenterology* 134:1470-1481

21

Hepatitis C Virus Proteins Induce Cirrhosis Antigen Expression on Human Hepatoma Cells *In Vitro*: Implications for Viral Mechanisms in Hepatitis C Fibrogenesis

Alka Saxena[1*] et al.,
[1]*University of Washington, Depts. of Laboratory Medicine,*
[2]*Pathology ,*
[3]*Medicine,*
The United States of America

1. Introduction

Hepatitis C virus (HCV), an RNA virus classified within the *Flaviviridae* (12), has a remarkable propensity for persistence in the human host following acute infection. Infections spontaneously resolve in 20-30% of infected individuals, while 70-80% of infections result in long-term persistent viremia. Chronically infected individuals are at an increased risk of developing hepatocellular injury compared to subjects with acute resolved infections (25), with manifestations progressing from mild to severe (bridging) fibrosis, and, ultimately cirrhosis, in 10-30% of chronic infections. Cirrhosis underlies life-threatening complications of end stage liver disease and/or hepatocellular carcinoma, after a long and extremely variable disease incubation period (25, 38). It is presently impossible to predict which persons with chronic hepatitis C are at greatest risk for disease progression, and, likewise, host-virus relationships are most important for driving chronic hepatitis C disease progression have not been defined. *In vitro* evidence supporting the concept of virus-mediated liver injury has recently been reported, including isolation of cytopathic derivatives of HCV infectious clone JFH1 (27), and also in the chimeric mouse (immune deficient mouse with humanized liver) hepatitis C model (18).

Based on experimental data from acute liver injury rodent model systems, where massive hepatic necrosis is experimentally induced by toxins such as carbon tetrachloride (29), the master mediators of hepatic fibrogenic processes are Transforming Growth Factor beta (TGFbeta) and Platelet Derived Growth factor (PDGF) (17). Hepatic Stellate Cells (HSCs) and macrophages appear to be the major cell types regulating hepatic fibrosis (17, 46). HSCs, normally quiescent in the liver, and potentially derived from hepatic oval cells (45), respond to injury by proliferation and secretion of large amounts of extracellular matrix proteins, in addition to pro-fibrogenic cytokines including TGFbeta. During the process, HSCs are transformed into fibrogenic myofibroblasts. A well characterized liver cirrhosis-

---

* Sampa Pal[1], Stephen J. Polyak[1], Sy Nakao[1], Igor Tikonokov[1], Tao Su[1], Thao Tran[1], Wan Chong Qiu[1], Jessica Wagoner[1], Lisa Thomassen[2], Margaret Shuhart[3] and David R. Gretch[1,3*]

associated antigen, Glial Fibrillary Acidic Protein (GFAP), is induced on pro-fibrotic cells such as HSCs, and is a definitive marker of fibrogenic pathway activation in this latter cell type (29). Studies of fibrosis mechanisms in human liver are limited. One longitudinal study, after liver transplantation, reported that increased density of GFAP in liver biopsy specimens predicted subsequent advanced fibrosis or cirrhosis (9). Although cells harboring GFAP were only presumed to be activated HSCs, the study concluded that 30% of cells in cirrhotic livers may be activated HSCs. However, the possibility of a direct effect of HCV on GFAP expression in hepatocytes was not investigated.

The present study therefore examined the effect of HCV on hepatic fibrosis marker expression, using two human hepatoma cell line model systems, capable of supporting either non-productive HCV replication (HCV replicon, (22)), or productive HCV infection (genotype 2a infectious clone JFH1; (44)). The study also examined liver biopsy samples from HCV infected patients for the simultaneous presence of GFAP and HCV replicative intermediate RNA. Finally, microarrays were used to analyze expression of multiple cellular genes linked with liver fibrosis, in human hepatoma cell lines plus or minus HCV. The effect of HCV on differential expression of 153 genes (1, 3, 17, 28, 37) either involved in, or associated with, with the process of liver fibrosis, is reported.

2. Methods

2.1 Human liver biopsy specimens

Thirty-two liver biopsy specimens, obtained under informed consent and per IRB-approved protocol, were available for study. All 32 subjects had chronic, active (viremic) HCV genotype 1 infections. During procurement, the specimens were immediately preserved in OCT buffer and snap frozen at the bedside. Parallel sections of the liver biopsies were reviewed by a single pathologist who was blinded to HCV status and all other data. Liver fibrosis severity, staged as 0 (no fibrosis) through 4 (cirrhosis), was assigned according to the system described by Batts and Ludwig (5). For the present study, the liver specimens were de-identified for all information except HCV replication status and fibrosis severity. Fresh thin sections were obtained for the GFAP immunostaining experiments described below.

Parallel sections of all 32 liver biopsy specimens were assayed for GFAP expression by immunocytochemistry. 29 of the specimens had been previously analyzed for both HCV genomic (G) and replicative intermediate (RI) RNAs by strand-specific *in situ* hybridization (ISH). Details of the ISH assay, and assay results for a larger sample of hepatitis C cases, were previously reported (31). Of 29 specimens with both GFAP and HCV replication data, HCV RNA was determined as either positive (G+RI+; 20 specimens), or negative (G-RI-; 9 specimens), and GFAP staining level (% of cells per biopsy staining positive for GFAP, or %GFAP) was then analyzed as a function of HCV infection/replication status, and fibrosis stage.

2.2 Hepatoma cell infection by JFH1 HCV

Huh7.5.1 cells (48) were generously provided by Francis Chisari (Scripps Institute, La Jolla, CA). Infection of Huh7.5.1 cells with the HCV JFH1 genotype 2a clone was performed as previously described (43), including the preparation of the JFH1 viral stock, cell infection, and titration. Briefly, we inoculated naïve Huh7.5.1 cells with supernatant harvested from JFH1 RNA transfected cells. Naïve Huh7.5.1 cells were seeded 24 h before infection at a density of 1 x 10^6 per 10 cm dish. The cells were incubated with 2.5 ml of the JFH1 inoculum at an multiplicity of infection of 0.01 for 3 h, washed three times with PBS, and supplemented with fresh complete Dulbecco's modified Eagle's medium. Cells were collected 72 hours post infection and assayed for HCV infection and replication by western blot analysis, immunocytochemistry and/or real time PCR.

2.3 Huh7-HCV replicon cells

Huh7 cells containing either full-length genotype 1b HCV replicon, or a Huh 7.5 hepatoma subline with genotype 1a strain H77 replicon (FL-Neo replicon) (7), were obtained from C. Rice, Rockefeller Institute, and maintained in Dulbecco's modified Eagle's medium (Invitrogen) containing 400 μg/ml of G418 (Calbiochem; San Diego, CA) supplemented with 10 % fetal calf serum (FCS) and 1 % penicillin/streptomycin at 37 °C in a 5 % CO_2 atmosphere.

2.4 Transfection of HCV genes

Conditions for transient transfection of genotype 1a HCV core, NS3/4A, and NS5A genes cloned into expression vector pcDNA3.1 were previously described (30). The day prior to transfection, $0.5x10^6$ Huh7.5.1 cells were plated overnight onto chamber slides. Endotoxin-free plasmid DNA (0.5 μg) was purified (Endofree kit; QIAGEN, CA) and transfected with Lipofectamine 2000 according to the manufacturer's recommendations (Invitrogen, CA).

2.5 Transfection of TGF beta siRNA

100pmol of TGFbeta-specific siRNA was transfected in $0.5x10^6$ cells 24 h after HCV gene transfection. Transfection of siRNA was carried out using Ambion si RNA transfection reagent kit (Ambion, TX) according to the manufacturer's protocol. Mock, non-targeting control siRNA, with limited sequence similarity to known genes (Silencer® Negative Control), was used as negative control (Ambion). At 48 h post-transfection, total RNA and protein were harvested for immunoblot assay and real time RT-PCR, respectively. For immunofluorescence assays, cells were grown in chamber slides for transfection, and fixed in 10% neutral buffered formalin at various times post-transfection, as indicated in the Results section.

2.6 Antibodies and immunoblot analysis

Protein concentrations in cell lysates were quantified (BCA Protein Assay; Pierce), and equal amounts of total protein (10-20 μg) were separated on 4 to 20% sodium dodecyl sulfate-polyacrylamide electrophoresis (SDS-PAGE) gels. Immunoblot analysis was performed using a GFAP-specific monoclonal antibody (Dako, CA) followed by secondary antibodies conjugated to horseradish peroxidase (Jackson ImmunoResearch). The relative levels of GFAP protein were quantified in immunoblots using ImageQuant (version 5.1). The signals from the immunoblot were normalized against the signal from a common cellular housekeeping gene (GADPH), and the ratio of GFAP-specific signal to control GADPH signal was determined.

2.7 Immunocytochemistry

Methods for immunocytochemistry (ICC) were as previously described (31, 32). Briefly, snap frozen liver sections, or hepatoma cells from culture, were fixed in 10% neutral buffered formalin and subjected to immunohistochemistry. Mouse monoclonal antibodies against GFAP were used at 1:100 dilution for 60 minutes (Affinity BioReagents, Co), followed by biotinylated goat antimouse immunoglobulins (dilution 1:200) for 30 minutes at room temperature. Samples were incubated with the Vectastain ABC alkaline phosphatase kit (Vector Laboratories, Burlingame, CA) for 30 minutes at room temperature to develop the vector red substrate. For double immmunostaining, anti-HCV core (Affinity

BioReagents, Co) anti-HCV NS3 (Vision Biosystem, MA) or anti-NS5A antibodies were used in combination staining, at 1:100 dilution for 60 minutes, followed by FIT-C conjugated goat antimouse immunoglobulins (dilution 1:200) for 30 minutes at room temperature. Mounting media containing DAPI (Vector laboratories, CA) was used to counter stain.

2.8 RNA extraction

Total cellular RNA was isolated from either HCV replicon, or negative control Huh7.5 cells, using 10^6 cells and an RNeasy miniprep Kit with an on column DNAse treatment following the manufacturer's protocol (Qiagen). The RNA was quantified and quality checked using an Agilent Bioanalyzer platform (Agilent Technologies); using this standard, all RNA preparations were of highest quality and integrity. The RNA Integrity Numbers (RINs) of all the RNA samples were between 9.7 and 10.0. RINs greater than 6 represent RNA of sufficient quality for quantification experiments (13).

2.9 Real-time RT-PCR

Total RNA was extracted from uninfected or infected hepatoma cells, and reverse transcribed into cDNA using the superscript II first strand synthesis system according to the manufacturer's protocol (Invitrogen, CA). Real-time quantitative PCR was carried out with an ABI 7900 Real-time PCR System, using the GAPDH gene as a reference (30). Three independent experiments were performed, and standard deviations calculated.

2.10 Microarray Hybridization

0.5μg of total RNA was used for a linear T7-based amplification step. To produce Cy3 labeled cRNA, the RNA samples were amplified and labeled using the Agilent qucik Amp Labeling kit (Agilent Technologies). Yields of cRNA and dye incorporation rate were measured with a ND-1000 spectrophotometer (Nano-Drop Technologies). Agilent whole Human genome Oligo Microarrays 4X44K (Miltenyi Biotech, Germany) were used to compare RNA samples from genotype 1a HCV replicon and Huh7.5 cells. The hybridization procedure was performed according to the Agilent 60-mer oligo microarray processing protocol using the Agilent Gene Expression hybridization kit (Agilent Technologies). Briefly, 1.65μg Cy3-labeled fragmented cRNA in hybridization buffer was hybridized overnight at 65°C. The microarrays were washed once with the Agilent Gene Expression Wash Buffer 1 for 1 min at room temperature followed by a second wash with preheated Agilent Gene Expression Wash Buffer 2 (37°C) for 1 min. The last washing step was performed with acetonitrile. Fluorescence signals of the hybridized Agilent Microarrays were detected using Agilent's Microarray Scanner System (Agilent Technologies).

2.11 Image and data analysis

The Agilent Feature Extraction Software (FES) was used to process the microarray image files to determine feature intensities (including background subtraction) and reject outliers. All samples were labeled with Cy3. Rosetta Resolver gene expression data analysis system (Rosetta Biosoftware) was used to build pair-wise ratios and for data normalization.

2.12 Statistical analyses

In all experiments, including pixel count for GFAP fluorescence, densitometric scans of Western blots, RT-PCR analysis and GFAP antigen expression in liver biopsies by ICC, results were calculated as the means (±S.D.) of three independent experiments. For liver biopsy specimens, 3 different microscope fields were each read by 3 different trained study investigators, and results were averaged and compared using one-way analysis of variance. P values of 0.05 or less were considered statistically significant.

3. Results

3.1 Detection of GFAP and HCV RNA in parallel sections from HCV-infected human liver biopsies

A previous study correlating intrahepatic HCV replication with liver fibrosis stage suggested a potential involvement of HCV in liver fibrogenesis [31]. Glial fibrillary acidic protein (GFAP) is a well-known marker of hepatic stellate cell (HSC) activation and liver cirrhosis. Therefore, for the present study, GFAP expression was analyzed in parallel sections from *ex vivo* liver biopsy specimens obtained from 32 HCV genotype 1-infected research subjects. All specimens had been scored previously for both liver fibrosis stage, while 29 specimens had been scored for HCV infection and replication status using viral RNA strand-specific *in situ hybridization* (ISH), as described previously (18). GFAP was determined by ICC and counting percentage of positive cells per biopsy. As expected, there was a significant correlation between percentage of liver cells staining positive for GFAP, and liver fibrosis stage ($p<0.005$) (Figure 1A). 20 specimens were positive for both HCV genomes and replicative intermediate RNAs (G+RI+), while 9 specimens were negative for both markers (G-RI-) despite chronic HCV infection confirmed by both enzyme immunoassay for HCV antibodies, and serum PCR for viral RNA. Figure 1B demonstrates that GFAP staining was significantly increased in parallel sections from the HCV replication positive (G+RI+) liver biopsies, compared to the biopsies lacking HCV RNA signal (G-RI-) (mean 55% GFAP positive cells versus 16% GFAP positive, respectively; $p<0.01$).

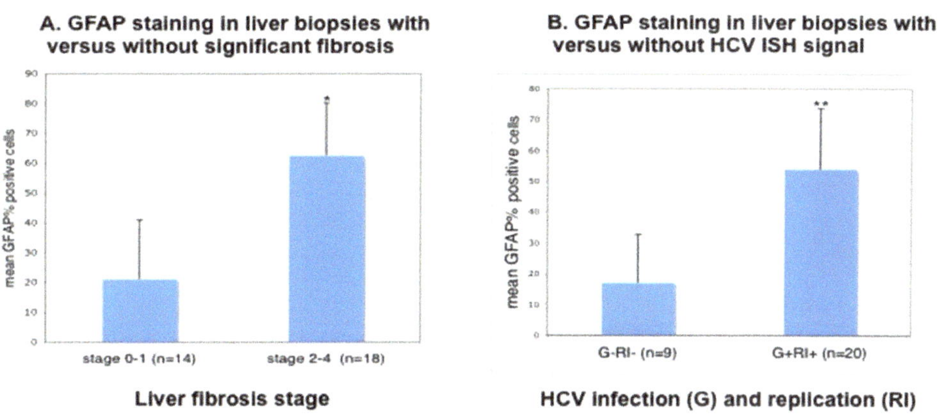

Fig. 1. Relationships between degree of liver fibrosis, GFAP expression, and genotype 1 HCV infection and replication status, in parallel sections of 32 liver biopsy specimens from research subjects. Panel A: GFAP staining according to degree of liver fibrosis in parallel sections from 32 biopsies. Panel B: GFAP staining according to HCV replication status in parallel liver biopsy sections from 29 of the 32 subjects with chronic hepatitis C. * $p<0.005$; ** $p<0.01$.

3.2 HCV induces GFAP expression in cultured human hepatoma cells

To follow up these observations, a series of experiments examined the effect of HCV on cirrhosis antigen (GFAP) expression in well-characterized human hepatoma cell lines. The HCV replicon efficiently replicates, but does not produce progeny virus, in hepatoma Huh 7.5 cells (7, 22). For this experiment, a gentotype 1b replicon was used. Dual immunostaining of negative control Huh7.5 cells showed absence of the HCV core protein, and low or undetectable expression of the liver cirrhosis antigen, Glial Fibrillary Acidic protein (GFAP) (Figures 2A and B, respectively). The presence of the HCV genotype 1b replicon, lead to significant induction of GFAP expression in Huh7.5 cells (Figures 2C and D, respectively). These data were the first suggestion that GFAP expression was up regulated in human liver cells by HCV. To confirm this result, and investigate if the results extend to more than one HCV genotype, GFAP expression was assayed in the human hepatoma cell line Huh7.5.1, in the presence, or absence, of the HCV genotype 2a infectious clone, JFH1 (44, 48). Figures 2E and 1F show negative dual immunostaining of uninfected Huh7.5.1 cells for HCV core and GFAP, respectively, while increased staining of HCV core protein (Figure 2G) and GFAP (Figure 2H) were observed in the presence of JFH1 infection. Quantification of immunofluorescence signals (right hand panel of Figure 2) confirmed highly significant increases in GFAP antigen signal in hepatoma cells in the presence of either HCV replicon, or infectious clone JFH1, respectively (p<0.001 in both cases).

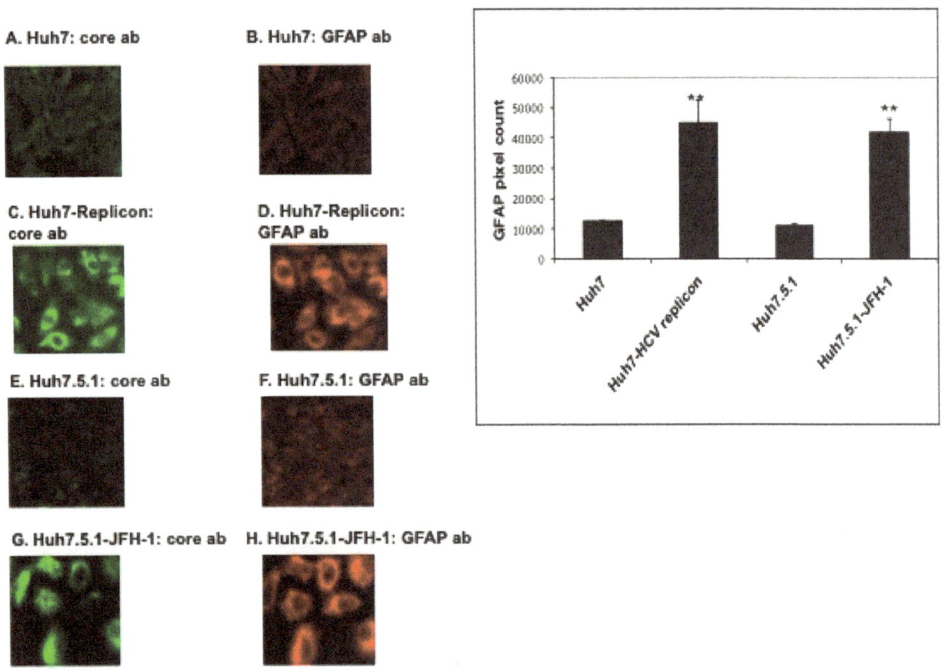

Fig. 2. Induction of GFAP in cultured human hepatoma cells. HCV core and GFAP signals were detected by dual label immunocytochemistry (ICC) using FITC and Texas Red channels, respectively. 40X magnification. In the bar graph, mean GFAP antibody fluorescence from triplicate experiments was quantified by metamorph and expressed as pixel count. ** indicates a significant increase in GFAP fluorescence in the presence of HCV, $p < 0.001$.

3.3 HCV core and NS5A genes both induce GFAP expression in hepatoma cells

The HCV core gene encodes a virion structural component that is known to influence multiple cellular processes (25). Both NS3/4A (helicase and protease) and NS5A (kinase) genetic cassettes also encode cell regulatory functions (14, 23). Thus, these three HCV genes (all derived from genotype 1b HCV) were each tested individually for induction of GFAP protein and RNA. Huh7.5.1 cells were transfected with either empty, or HCV-protein-containing expression vectors, and dual-immunofluorescence was performed to detect GFAP, and the corresponding HCV antigens, 48 hrs after transfection (Figure 3). Figures 3A, B and C illustrate negative immunostaining for HCV core, GFAP and HCV NS5A antigens, respectively, following control vector transfection. Transfection of the NS3/4A cassette also gave negative GFAP signal (data not shown). However, GFAP signal was greatly enhanced in Huh7.5.1 cells transfected with either the HCV core gene (Figure 3E), or the NS5A gene (Figure 3F). Figures 3D and F confirm expression of the HCV core and NS5A proteins in transfected Huh7.5.1 cells, respectively. Interestingly, although HCV core expression was limited to a relatively small subset of transfected cells (Figure 3D), GFAP expression was widespread, and signal was strong even in cells that stained negative for HCV core antigen (compare green and red signals in Figures 3D and E). This result suggested that a diffusible intermediate might be responsible for core-mediated GFAP induction in hepatoma cells. In contrast, NS5A expression was more widespread throughout the transfected cells, the pattern of GFAP expression in response to the NS5A protein was more punctate and discrete than that observed following core transfection, and NS5A staining was observed in the same cells that showed increased GFAP expression (Figure 3F). Quantitative assessment of GFAP immunofluorescence signals, summarized by bar graph in Figure 3, confirmed that the HCV core and NS5A proteins both significantly increased expression of GFAP in cultured hepatoma cells ($p<0.001$ in both cases).

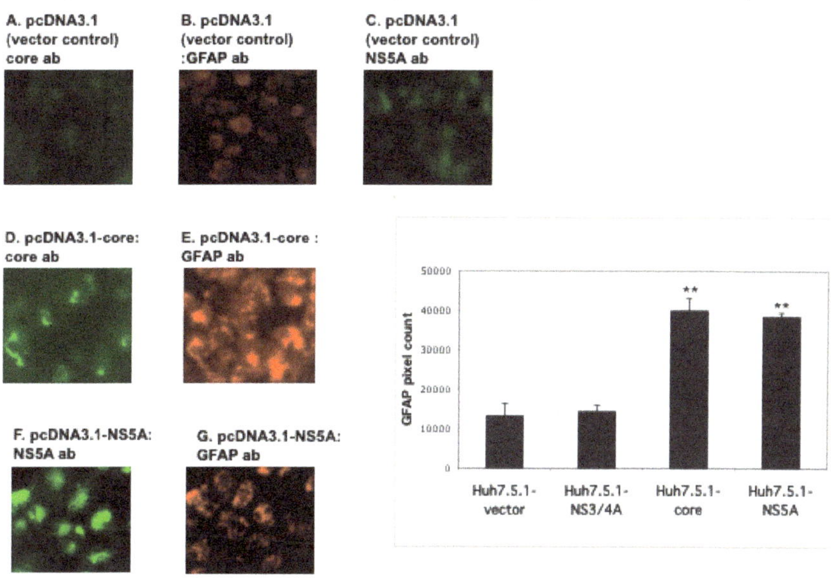

Fig. 3. HCV core and NS5A genes induce GFAP in hepatoma cell lines.HCV antigens and GFAP signals were detected using FITC and Texas Red channels, respectively. 40X magnification. The bar graph compares GFAP signal intensity in the presence of vector or HCV gene products core, NS3/4A, or NS5A.

Experiments using cell extracts, summarized in Figure 4, were performed to confirm the results of cell surface staining. To examine effect of HCV on GFAP protein expression within cells, total cell protein was harvested from Huh7.5 cells, HCV replicon-containing Huh7.5 cells, Huh7.5.1 cells infected with JFH1 virus for 72 hours, and Huh7.5.1 cells following transient transfection with individual HCV core, NS3/4A, or NS5A constructs. Protein extracts were subjected to Western Blot using the same panel of antibodies as used for Figures 2 and 3. GFAP expression was determined by quantification of GFAP pixel intensity in blot images, using GAPDH as control (Figure 4A).

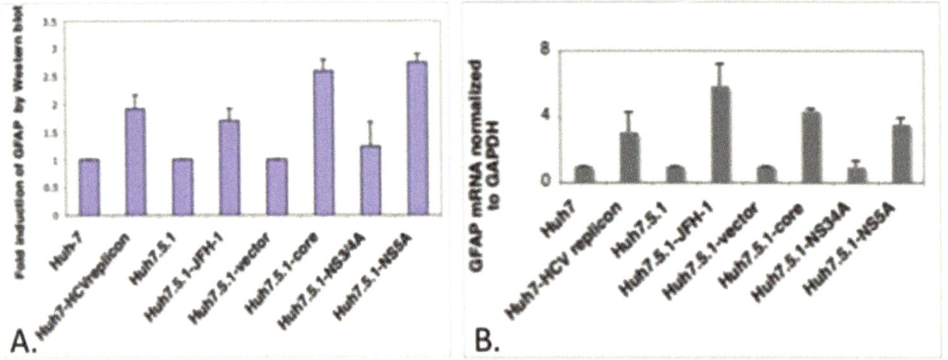

Fig. 4. Quantification of HCV effect on GFAP protein and RNA expression levels, by Western Blot (Panel A) and real time PCR (Panel B), respectively. Experiments were as summarized for Figures 2 and 3. Quantities of GFAP protein or RNA expression were averaged from three experiments. All data were normalized to GAPDH protein (Panel A) or RNA (Panel B) expression levels. * $p < 0.05$; ** $p<0.001$.

GFAP protein levels harvested from culture lysate were increased 1.8-fold in cells containing the HCV replicon, and approximately 1.7-fold in JFH1-infected cells relative to control cells. In cell transfection experiments using Huh7.5.1 cells as control, quantities of GFAP protein expression were increased by either the HCV NS5A gene (approximately 2.8-fold), or the HCV core gene (approximately 2.6-fold), while no significant effect on GFAP expression was observed following NS3/4A transfection. The Western blot experiment confirmed that the genotype 1b HCV replicon, the genotype 2a HCV infectious clone JFH1, the HCV core gene product, and the NS5 gene product were all able to up regulate expression of GFAP protein in cultured hepatoma cells. The effect of HCV on GFAP RNA expression in cultured hepatoma cells is presented in Figure 4B, under identical conditions to that described in Figure 4A. GFAP RNA expression was increased in both HCV replicon cells (approximately 3-fold), and JFH1-infected cells (approximately 6-fold), compared to cultured hepatoma cell line controls. Furthermore, Huh7.5.1 cells transfected with either the core construct, or the NS5A construct, showed approximately 3-fold increases in GFAP RNA expression, while no change in GFAP RNA expression was found following NS3/4A transfection (Figure 4B).

3.4 TGFbeta mediates core induction of GFAP, but not NS5A induction of GFAP

TGF-β is a known modulator of GFAP expression in human astrocytes (35), and the HCV core product is known to induce TGF-β expression *in vitro* (42). Thus, we anticipated that HCV core induction of GFAP in hepatoma cells was TGF-β dependent. As indicated in

Figure 5A, TGF-β RNA expression was increased approximately 3-fold in the presence of either JFH1 infection, or HCV core gene transfection, but not in the presence of either NS3/4A, or NS5A gene transfection. RNA knockdown of TGF-β RNA, using TGF-β -specific siRNA, blocked GFAP induction by the HCV core protein, but had no effect on GFAP induction by the NS5A protein (Figure 5B). The data implicates a TGF-β dependent mechanism for induction of GFAP by the HCV core protein. However, the data argue that the HCV NS5A gene product most likely induces GFAP expression by a TGF-β -independent mechanism.

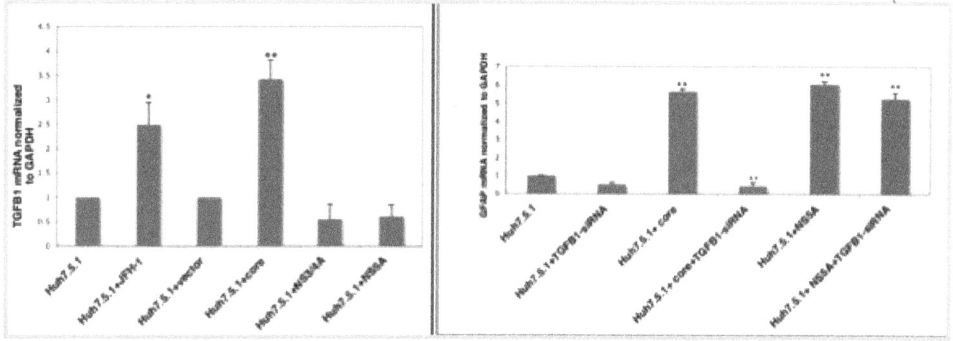

(A) (B)

Fig. 5. Panel A: HCV induction of TGFbeta expression by real-time RT-PCR using cells transfected with either core, NS3/4A, or NS5A in pcDNA3.1 plasmids. Data were normalized to GAPDH RNA. *, $p < 0.05$; **, $p < 0.001$. Panel B: Differential effect of TGFbeta knockdown by siRNA on GFAP induction by HCV core and NS5A. (** Indicates $p < 0.001$).

3.5 Extracellular matrix gene transcriptional responses induced in hepatoma cells by the HCV replicon

To determine the breadth of effect of HCV on the extracellular matrix, microarray analysis was used to analyze, within hepatoma cells, the expression of 153 cellular genes associated with liver fibrosis (1, 3, 17, 28, 37), and to determine the effect of genotype 1a hepatitis C virus replication on matrix gene expression. Genes associated with cell-cell and cell-matrix interactions, along with those implicated in dysregulated tissue remodeling during repair and wound healing, were assessed in Huh7.5 cells in the presence or absence of the HCV replicon. A change in gene expression was considered significant based on two criteria, a greater than 99% probability of being expressed differentially ($P \leq 0.01$), and a fold change of 1.5 or greater, which is conservative. Figure 6 shows the log scatter plot of signal intensities of all spots representing expression levels of individual cellular genes in the presence (Y axis), or absence (X-axis), of the HCV replicon.

The gene panel we analyzed included 20 collagen genes, and 133 non-collagen genes associated with the extracellular matrix (ECM) and cellular adhesion, including remodeling enzymes, cytokines, chemokines, growth factors, and genes involved in signal transduction. From the total of 133 non-collagen genes analyzed, 34 genes were induced by HCV, with induction values ranging from 1.5 fold to 100 fold (Figure 7 and Table I). Another 30 genes were down regulated in the presence of HCV; again with a range of 1.5 fold to 100 fold (Figure 7 and Table I). Finally, 69 non-collagen genes showed no significant change in gene expression in the presence of HCV, relative to control cells (Table II).

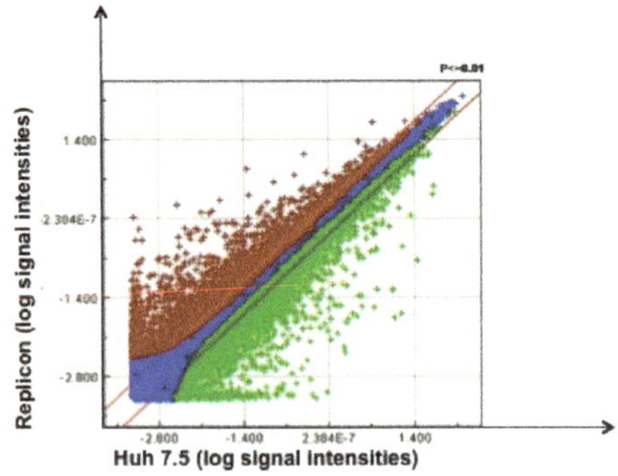

Fig. 6. Pair-wise comparison of signal intensity on DNA microarrays hybridized with RNA from Replicon 1a (Fl-Neo) and Huh 7.5 -control cell lines. The red lines depict the p value cut off (p=0.01), while red and green crosses indicate up and down regulated genes in the Replicon 1a cell line relative to the control cell line.

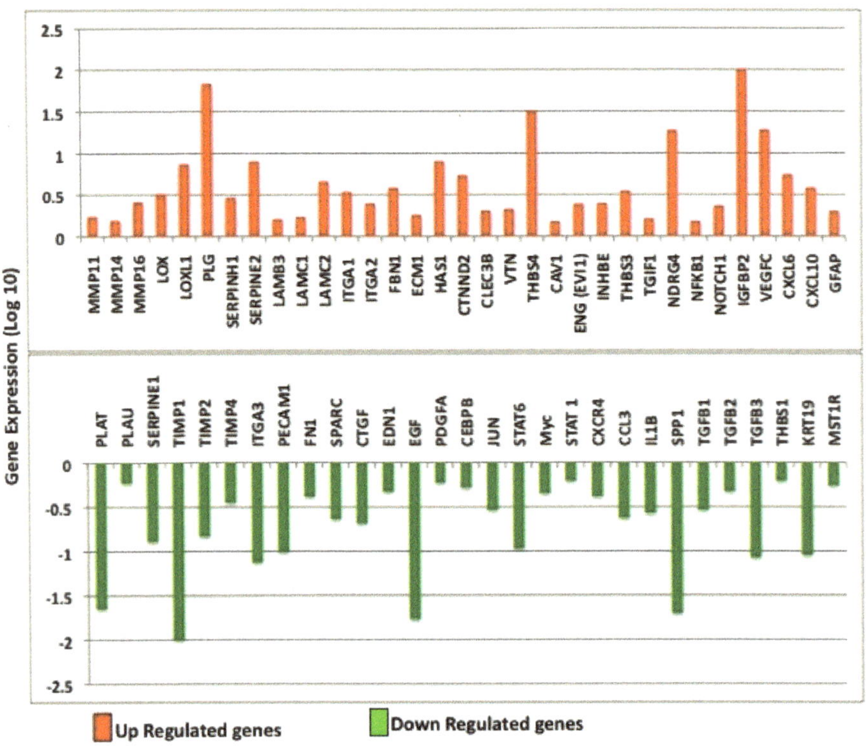

Fig. 7. Regulation of genes linked with hepatic fibrosis, by HCV. The red and green bar graph shows increased or decreased expression (relative to the control Huh 7.5 cells) of various cellular genes linked to liver fibrosis. Expression level, on the vertical axis, refers to the Log-fold change in the transcript abundance of individual genes arranged on the horizontal axis.

Gene Characterization	Gene Symbol	Fold change	P value
Significantly up regulated in Replicon cells			
ECM and Cell adhesion			
Remodeling Enzymes	MMP11	1.73	0.00025
	MMP14	1.54	0.00321
	MMP16	2.57	5 x10-10
	LOX	3.2	0.0
	LOXL1	7.4	0.00005
	PLG	68.079	8x10-6
	SERPINH1	2.9	5x10-10
	SERPINE2	8.0	4x10-18
ECM proteins	LAMB3	1.6	0.003
	LAMC1	1.7	0.0004
	LAMC2	4.5	3x10-14
Cell Adhesion	ITGA1	3.37	1x10-11
	ITGA2	2.46	9x10-7
	FBN1	3.8	1x10-12
	ECM1	1.8	0.007
	HAS1	8.0	0.00004
	CTNND2	5.37	3x10-16
	CLEC3B	2.022	0.00005
	VTN	2.12	1x10-6
	THBS4	32.0	3x10-22
TGFb super family	CAV1	1.5	2x10-21
	ENG (EVI1)	2.43	8x10-6
	INHBE	2.47	3x10-8
	THBS3	3.49	6x10-12
	TGIF1	1.62	0.001
	NDRG4	18.7	3x10-21
Transcription Factors	NFKB1	1.5	5x10-18
	NOTCH1	2.3	0.0
Growth Factors	IGFBP2	100	2x10-23
	VEGFC	19.0	2x10-14
Cytokines	CXCL6	5.5	1x10-9
	CXCL10	3.8	0.0004
	GFAP	2.0	8x10-7
Significantly down regulated in Replicon cells			
ECM and Cell adhesion			
Remodeling Enzymes	PLAT	44.6	0.0
	PLAU	1.7	3x10-29
	SERPINE1	7.7	0.0
	TIMP1	100	3x10-23
	TIMP2	6.7	9x10-19
	TIMP4	2.8	1x10-9

Table 1. Significantly dysregulated transcripts in Replicon Fl-Neo

Gene Characterization	Gene Symbol	Fold change	P value
Significantly down regulated in Replicon cells			
ECM and Cell adhesion			
Cell Adhesion Molecules	ITGA3	13.2	1x10-10
	PECAM1	10.0	3x10-19
	FN1	2.4	2x10-8
Extracellular matrix protein	SPARC	4.3	8x10-14
Growth Factors	CTGF	4.8	8x10-15
	EDN1	2.1	0.0
	EGF	58.3	1x10-22
	PDGFA	1.67	0.0005
Transcription Factors	CEBPB	1.9	0.0006
	JUN	3.4	0.0
	STAT6	9.2	7x10-19
	Myc	2.2	0.0
	STAT 1	1.6	8x10-26
Inflammatory cytokines and chemokines	CXCR4	2.4	3x10-5
	CCL3	4.2	0.0
	IL1B	3.7	1x10-45
	SPP1	50.1	0.0
TGFb super family	TGFB1	3.4	0.0
	TGFB2	2.1	0.001
	TGFB3	11.7	2x10-19
	THBS1	1.6	0.0
Cytoskeletal	KRT19	11.0	1x10-19
Kinase	MST1R	1.8	0.0001

Table 1. Significantly dysregulated transcripts in Replicon Fl-Neo (continuation)

Pro-Fibrotic: ACTA2; SNAI1
Basement Membrane: COL10A1
FACITs : COL19A1, COL20A1
Transmembrane: COL17A1
Multiplexin Collagens: COL13A1, COL15A1, COL18A1
ECM: LAMA1, LAMA2, LAMA3, LAMB1
Remodelling Enzymes: MMP1, MMP2,MMP3, MMP9, MMP13, MMP14, ADAMTS1, ADAMTS8, ADAMTS13, SERPINA1
Cellular Adhesion: ITGB1, ITGB2, ITGB3, ITGB4, ITGB5, ITGB6, ITGB8, ITGAV, ITGA4, ITGA5, ITGA6, ITGA7, ITGAL. ITGAM, CDH1
Inflammatory cytokines and chemokines: CCR2, CXCR4, CCL11, CCL2(MCP-1), IL-13, IL13RA2, IL4, IL5, IFNG, IL13RA2, IL1A, ILK, IL1RN
Growth factors: AGT, PDGFB, VEGFA
TGF beta super family: BMP7, DCN, GREM1, LTBP1, SMAD2, SMAD3, SMAD4, SMAD6, SMAD7, TGFBR1, TGFBR2, THSP2
Transcription Factors: SP1, MITF

Table 2. Transcripts with no significant change in gene expression

Gene Characterization	Gene Symbol	Fold Change	P values
Significantly up-regulated in Replicon cells			
Fibril forming	COL2A1	100	2x10-23
	COL5A2	2.9	8x10-9
	COL11A1	2.8	1x10-9
Non-Fibrillar			
Basement Membrane Collagen	COL4A2	2.2	4x10-7
	COL4A5	1.6	0.008
	COL4A6	1.9	0.00002
	COL8A2	2.0	0.0006
FACITs	COL9A2	2.4	4x10-8
	COL9A3	10.0	3x10-19
	COL12A1	3.2	2x10-8
	COL14A1	53	6x10-18
	COL16A1	15.58	9x10-21
Significantly down regulated in Replicon cells			
Fibril Forming	COL1A1	2.5	3x10-19
	COL1A2	4.6	0.0
	Col3A1	3.8	1.3x10-9
Non-Fibrillar			
Anchoring Filaments Collagen	COL7A1	5.7	4x10-16
Collagen of beaded microfilaments	Col6A1	5.9	3x10-16
	Col6A2	8.4	8.7x10-13

Table 3. Significantly dysregulated Collagen transcripts in Replicon Fl-Neo

The effect of HCV on expression of twenty known collagen genes is presented in Table III. These were grouped into two main molecular classes: the fibril forming species (collagens 1,2,3,5), and non-fibrillar collagens (37). The non-fibrillar collagens were further subdivided. Nine collagen genes had increased transcript abundance in the HCV replicon positive cell line, while four collagen genes showed decreased transcript abundance in the presence of HCV. There was no significant change in the expression of remaining 7 collagen genes when compared to the control Huh 7.5 cells. We observed an increase in fibril forming collagen type 2 and 5. Col2A1 showed an increase of 100-fold. We also found an increase in expression of fibril forming, basement membrane and FACIT collagen molecules in the replicon cell line when compared to the huh7.0 cell line (Table III). However, of interest is the note that the expression of Col1A1 and Col1A2 was down regulated in the presence of HCV (Table I). Col3A1 was also down regulated in the presence of HCV.

There was a 8-fold increase in hyaluronan synthase 1 (Has1) mRNA, along with an increase in transcript abundance of Integrins (ITGA1, ITGA2) and Laminin (LAMC1, LAMC2, LAMB3). Laminin is the main type of adhesive ECM component, and is associated with the basement membrane formation in liver during cirrhosis (Table I).

The expression of fibrosis associated antigen, GFAP, was increased 2-fold in the presence of the genotype 1a HCV replicon, which is very similar to the value observed using real time

PCR analysis of GFAP RNA in the presence of the genotype 1b replicon (Figure 4B). The GFAP data, across multiple HCV genotypes, and different methods of analysis, argue for consistency of the observations of effect of HCV on cell matrix. TGFβ is a known modulator of GFAP in mature glial cells of the CNS, and the major mediator of fibrogenesis in Hepatic Stellate Cells. Surprisingly, TGFβ1, TGFβ2 and TGFβ3 were all down regulated in the presence of HCV replicon, compared to Huh7.5 controls. However, several of the other members of TGFβ super family (CAV1, ENG, INHBE, TGIF1, THBS3 and NDRG4) showed a significant increase in expression in the presence of HCV.

4. Discussion

Why fibrosis and cirrhosis are variable in chronic hepatitis C is unknown. The present study 1) describes a significant relationship between HCV replication and cirrhosis antigen expression *in vivo*, 2) focused on the effect of 3 different HCV genotypes (1a, 1b and 2a) on expression of the liver cirrhosis-associated antigen Glial Fibrillary Acidic Protein (GFAP), and 3) also examined direct effects of hepatitis C virus on 153 cellular genes that contribute to the extracellular matrix (ECM). The data indicate that HCV induces dramatic change in collagens, as well as some known mediators of fibrogenesis, including the cirrhosis antigens GFAP and Smooth Muscle Actin (data not shown). Focus on GFAP revealed two distinct pathways: one TGFbeta dependent, and the other, TGFbeta independent, mediated by two different HCV proteins, core and NS5A. Independent modulation of GFAP expression by two different HCV proteins, via different mechanisms, implies an important function. Two possible implications of the results are: 1) That specific cell surface components play an important role the HCV life cycle; and 2) That HCV may directly accelerate fibrogenesis from within hepatocytes, since many of the molecules induced are profibrogenic in experimental models.

The ECM is a complex molecular network that helps determine the specific architecture of a tissue. During hepatic fibrogenesis, major changes occur in both the quantity and quality of hepatic ECM (*for review, see ref* (37)). Increase in abundance of collagen molecules is the major hallmark of liver fibrosis (6). In the normal liver, the sub-endothelial space of Disse contains both an interstitial and a basement membrane-like ECM of low density. The perisinusoidal matrix is composed of fibrillar collagen types I, III, and V, microfibrillar collagen VI, basement membrane collagens IV and XVIII, traces of FACIT collagens XIV, and small proteoglycans decorin, fibronectin, tensacin-c, laminin and others (36). As the liver becomes fibrotic, significant qualitative and quantitative changes of the ECM occur, predominantly in the periportal and perisinusoidal space, while the total content of collagens and noncollagenous components increases up to tenfold (34). Thus, the perisinusoidal low-density ECM is transformed to a high-density matrix characterized by accumulation of bundles of collagen fibrils and an electron-dense basement membrane.

In the advanced stages of liver fibrosis, Collagens I and II are concentrated in the ECM, to levels elevated 6-fold compared to normal states (6). In our present study, Collagen II A1 mRNA was upregulated 100-fold, while Collagens XII A1 and XIV A1 mRNAs, implicated in stabilizing collagen fibril structure during development and remodeling (24, 47), were up-regulated 3.2 and 53 fold, respectively (Table III). The mRNA for lysyl oxidase (LOX), required for crosslinking of collagens (2, 41), was also upregulated, by 3.2 fold (Table I).

Thus, the effect of HCV on hepatoma cell ECM resembled that observed during liver fibrogenesis. However, the results need to be confirmed in normal liver.

Thrombospondins (THBS3 and THBS4) and chemokines (CXCL10 and CXCL6) were upregulated in Replicon cell line. IGFBP2 gene expression was also significantly upregulated (Table I). IGFBP2 expression is increased in HBV associated HCC (19). In this study, THBS1, TIMP1, TIMP2, TIMP4 were down regulated. Laminin is the main type of adhesive ECM and is associated with the formation of Basement membrane in liver during cirrhosis. Our study shows that LAMB3, LAMC1 and LAMC2 were increased in Replicon cell line (Table I).

The topic of HCV and the cell surface is of high interest, from a receptor standpoint, since the mechanism of HCV infection is rather unique (26). Recent studies have indicated an alternative, claudin-mediated pathway of direct spread of HCV from cell to cell, without an extracellular viral stage (8). Of interest, claudin 6 was significantly upregulated (8.4 fold) (data not shown) in our study, but the significance towards HCV infection dynamics was not assessed.

HCV involvement in hepatic fibrogenesis, through a direct effect on Hepatic Stellate Cells (HSCs), has previously been suggested (39). In separate studies, HCV core isolated from hepatocellular carcinoma cells *ex vivo* was capable of shifting TGF-β responses from cytostatic effects, toward Epidermal Mesenchymal Transition (EMT), in primary mouse or human hepatocytes (4, 33). The present study is the first to describe a potential fibrogenic effect of HCV on hepatocyte-derived hepatoma cells, and potential role of TGFbeta in this effect. Natural variation in HCV core interaction with the TGFbeta pathway has been implicated in liver oncogenesis (4, 33). In the present study, although TGFβ1 was down regulated in Replicon 1a cells, several other genes which interact with TGFβ were upregulated, such as FBN1 (Fibrillin 1) LOXL1, NDRG4, Collagen type XVI type, and several other transcription factors including HOXD1, HOXC10 and CAND2. Since TGFbeta is a pluripotent master regulator of many processes, including injury repair, the overall effect of HCV on TGFbeta regulated mechanisms, and visa versa, needs to be determined.

Induction of GFAP by NS5A, via a TGFbeta-independent mechanism, is a novel finding of the present study. Modulation of cellular gene expression is a well-known function of NS5A (26), and NS5A has been reported to be a negative modulator of the TGF-beta1 signal transduction pathway (11); reduced phosphorylation and nuclear translocation of Smad2, as well as reduced heterodimerization of Smad3 with Smad4, were both observed in the presence of NS5A, and were apparently mediated via direct binding of NS5A to the TGF-beta1 receptor, TbetaR1. Whether or not the NS5A effect was mediated by a soluble factor was not assessed for the present study, and requires further investigation. In the CNS, GFAP is induced by both TGFbeta dependent and independent mechanisms (27), and mediators of TGFbeta independent induction of GFAP have yet to be defined. Determining the mechanism of GFAP induction by NS5A, and determining the overall significance to liver infection by HCV, are important goals of future research.

The present results also raise a diagnostic question: the possibility that increases in GFAP positivity with advanced hepatitis C liver disease may in fact be due to HCV infection of hepatocytes. Evidence for this in the present study included 1) co-localization of GFAP signal with either core or NS5A protein in hepatoma cell culture following gene transfection (in addition to diffuse GFAP signal in cells neighboring core-expressing cells); 2) high correlation between percentage of cells harboring GFAP and HCV replicative intermediate (RI) RNA in serial sections from liver biopsies of HCV-infected study subjects; and 3) high correlation between both markers and degree of hepatic fibrosis in the same liver biopsies. Other lines of human investigation have reveled highly significant associations between HCV genotype 1 infection virology in humans, and hepatitis C disease severity. Both iatrogenic and viral induced immune suppression dramatically accelerates rates and incidence of hepatitis C progression (15, 40). Longitudinal studies have identified genetic evidence of selective outgrowth of high fitness viral variants during disease progression (20, 21). Finally, as alluded to above, intrahepatic HCV replication, as well as nonstructural antigen expression, have been highly correlated with hepatitis C liver disease severity, in the settings of liver transplantation (10, 16), natural infection, and HIV coinfection (31).

These findings collectively support an intriguing hypothesis, that fibrogenesis in hepatitis C may in part be mediated by fibrogenic-like transitions of infected hepatocytes.

In particular, the study draws attention to major cytoskeletal effects of HCV on hepatoma cells, and suggests that such effect may potentially represent a pro-fibrogenic response. The study implicates two HCV proteins as potential mediators of the cytoskeletal changes: HCV core and NS5A. Questions as to the relevance and consequences of HCV modulation of the extracellular matrix remain to be addressed. The potential significance of the observed interaction to HCV life cycle, also needs further investigation.

5. Acknowledgements

This research was supported in part by NIH grants 2 R01 AI 49168-10 and 5 R01 AI 66209-05 to DRG. The authors acknowledge Mr. Matt Maria for assistance with the manuscript.

6. References

[1] Asselah, T., I. Bieche, I. Laurendeau, V. Paradis, D. Vidaud, C. Degott, M. Martinot, P. Bedossa, D. Valla, M. Vidaud, and P. Marcellin. 2005. Liver gene expression signature of mild fibrosis in patients with chronic hepatitis C. Gastroenterology 129:2064-2075.

[2] Bailey, A. J. 2001. Molecular mechanisms of ageing in connective tissues. Mech Ageing Dev 122:735-755.

[3] Bataller, R., and D. A. Brenner. 2005. Liver fibrosis. J Clin Invest 115:209-218.

[4] Battaglia, S., N. Benzoubir, S. Nobilet, P. Charneau, D. Samuel, A. L. Zignego, A. Atfi, C. Brechot, and M. F. Bourgeade. 2009. Liver cancer-derived hepatitis C virus core proteins shift TGF-beta responses from tumor suppression to epithelial-mesenchymal transition. PLoS One 4:e4355.

[5] Batts, K. P., and J. Ludwig. 1995. Chronic hepatitis. An update on terminology and reporting. Am J Surg Pathol 19:1409-1417.

[6] Benyon, R. C., and J. P. Iredale. 2000. Is liver fibrosis reversible? Gut 46:443-446.

[7] Blight, K. J., J. A. McKeating, J. Marcotrigiano, and C. M. Rice. 2003. Efficient replication of hepatitis C virus genotype 1a RNAs in cell culture. Journal of virology 77:3181-3190.

[8] Brimacombe, C. L., J. Grove, L. W. Meredith, K. Hu, A. J. Syder, M. V. Flores, J. M. Timpe, S. E. Krieger, T. F. Baumert, T. L. Tellinghuisen, F. Wong-Staal, P. Balfe, and J. A. McKeating. 2011. Neutralizing antibody-resistant hepatitis C virus cell-to-cell transmission. Journal of virology 85:596-605.

[9] Carotti, S., S. Morini, S. G. Corradini, M. A. Burza, A. Molinaro, G. Carpino, M. Merli, A. De Santis, A. O. Muda, M. Rossi, A. F. Attili, and E. Gaudio. 2008. Glial fibrillary acidic protein as an early marker of hepatic stellate cell activation in chronic and posttransplant recurrent hepatitis C. Liver transplantation : official publication of the American Association for the Study of Liver Diseases and the International Liver Transplantation Society 14:806-814.

[10] Chang, M., A. P. Marquardt, B. L. Wood, O. Williams, S. J. Cotler, S. L. Taylor, R. L. Carithers, Jr., and D. R. Gretch. 2000. In situ distribution of hepatitis C virus replicative-intermediate RNA in hepatic tissue and its correlation with liver disease. J Virol 74:944-955.

[11] Choi, S. H., and S. B. Hwang. 2006. Modulation of the transforming growth factor-beta signal transduction pathway by hepatitis C virus nonstructural 5A protein. The Journal of biological chemistry 281:7468-7478.

[12] Choo, Q. L., K. H. Richman, J. H. Han, K. Berger, C. Lee, C. Dong, C. Gallegos, D. Coit, R. Medina-Selby, P. J. Barr, and et al. 1991. Genetic organization and diversity of the hepatitis C virus. Proc Natl Acad Sci U S A 88:2451-2455.

[13] Fleige, S., and M. W. Pfaffl. 2006. RNA integrity and the effect on the real-time qRT-PCR performance. Mol Aspects Med 27:126-139.

[14] Gale, M., Jr., and E. M. Foy. 2005. Evasion of intracellular host defence by hepatitis C virus. Nature 436:939-945.

[15] Graham, C. S., L. R. Baden, E. Yu, J. M. Mrus, J. Carnie, T. Heeren, and M. J. Koziel. 2001. Influence of human immunodeficiency virus infection on the course of hepatitis C virus infection: a meta-analysis. Clin Infect Dis 33:562-569.

[16] Gretch, D. R., C. E. Bacchi, L. Corey, C. dela Rosa, R. R. Lesniewski, K. Kowdley, A. Gown, I. Frank, J. D. Perkins, and R. L. Carithers, Jr. 1995. Persistent hepatitis C virus infection after liver transplantation: clinical and virological features. Hepatology 22:1-9.

[17] Jiao, J., S. L. Friedman, and C. Aloman. 2009. Hepatic fibrosis. Curr Opin Gastroenterol 25:223-229.

[18] Joyce, M. A., K. A. Walters, S. E. Lamb, M. M. Yeh, L. F. Zhu, N. Kneteman, J. S. Doyle, M. G. Katze, and D. L. Tyrrell. 2009. HCV induces oxidative and ER stress, and sensitizes infected cells to apoptosis in SCID/Alb-uPA mice. PLoS Pathog 5:e1000291.

[19] Lee, C. F., Z. Q. Ling, T. Zhao, and K. R. Lee. 2008. Distinct expression patterns in hepatitis B virus- and hepatitis C virus-infected hepatocellular carcinoma. World J Gastroenterol 14:6072-6077.

[20] Li, H., B. J. McMahon, S. McArdle, D. Bruden, D. G. Sullivan, D. Shelton, H. Deubner, and D. R. Gretch. 2008. Hepatitis C virus envelope glycoprotein co-evolutionary dynamics during chronic hepatitis C. Virology 375:580-591.

[21] Li, H., D. G. Sullivan, N. Feuerborn, S. McArdle, K. Bekele, S. Pal, M. Yeh, R. L. Carithers, J. D. Perkins, and D. R. Gretch. 2010. Genetic diversity of hepatitis C virus predicts recurrent disease after liver transplantation. Virology 402:248-255.

[22] Lohmann, V., F. Korner, J. Koch, U. Herian, L. Theilmann, and R. Bartenschlager. 1999. Replication of subgenomic hepatitis C virus RNAs in a hepatoma cell line. Science 285:110-113.

[23] Macdonald, A., and M. Harris. 2004. Hepatitis C virus NS5A: tales of a promiscuous protein. The Journal of general virology 85:2485-2502.

[24] Marchant, J. K., G. Zhang, and D. E. Birk. 2002. Association of type XII collagen with regions of increased stability and keratocyte density in the cornea. Exp Eye Res 75:683-694.

[25] McMahon, B. J., D. Bruden, M. G. Bruce, S. Livingston, C. Christensen, C. Homan, T. W. Hennessy, J. Williams, D. Sullivan, H. R. Rosen, and D. Gretch. 2010. Adverse outcomes in Alaska natives who recovered from or have chronic hepatitis C infection. Gastroenterology 138:922-931 e921.

[26] Meertens, L., C. Bertaux, L. Cukierman, E. Cormier, D. Lavillette, F. L. Cosset, and T. Dragic. 2008. The tight junction proteins claudin-1, -6, and -9 are entry cofactors for hepatitis C virus. Journal of virology 82:3555-3560.

[27] Mishima, K., N. Sakamoto, Y. Sekine-Osajima, M. Nakagawa, Y. Itsui, S. Azuma, S. Kakinuma, K. Kiyohashi, A. Kitazume, K. Tsuchiya, M. Imamura, N. Hiraga, K. Chayama, T. Wakita, and M. Watanabe. 2010. Cell culture and in vivo analyses of cytopathic hepatitis C virus mutants. Virology 405:361-369.

[28] Nalpas, B., R. Lavialle-Meziani, S. Plancoulaine, E. Jouanguy, A. Nalpas, M. Munteanu, F. Charlotte, B. Ranque, E. Patin, S. Heath, H. Fontaine, A. Vallet-Pichard, D. Pontoire, M. Bourliere, J. L. Casanova, M. Lathrop, C. Brechot, T. Poynard, F. Matsuda, S. Pol, and L. Abel. 2010. Interferon gamma receptor 2 gene variants are associated with liver fibrosis in patients with chronic hepatitis C infection. Gut 59:1120-1126.

[29] Niki, T., P. J. De Bleser, G. Xu, K. Van Den Berg, E. Wisse, and A. Geerts. 1996. Comparison of glial fibrillary acidic protein and desmin staining in normal and CCl4-induced fibrotic rat livers. Hepatology 23:1538-1545.

[30] Pal, S., S. J. Polyak, N. Bano, W. C. Qiu, R. L. Carithers, M. Shuhart, D. R. Gretch, and A. Das. 2010. Hepatitis C virus induces oxidative stress, DNA damage and modulates the DNA repair enzyme NEIL1. J Gastroenterol Hepatol.

[31] Pal, S., M. C. Shuhart, L. Thomassen, S. S. Emerson, T. Su, N. Feuerborn, J. Kae, and D. R. Gretch. 2006. Intrahepatic hepatitis C virus replication correlates with chronic hepatitis C disease severity in vivo. J Virol 80:2280-2290.

[32] Pal, S., D. G. Sullivan, S. Kim, K. K. Lai, J. Kae, S. J. Cotler, R. L. Carithers, Jr., B. L. Wood, J. D. Perkins, and D. R. Gretch. 2006. Productive replication of hepatitis C

virus in perihepatic lymph nodes in vivo: implications of HCV lymphotropism. Gastroenterology 130:1107-1116.

[33] Pavio, N., S. Battaglia, D. Boucreux, B. Arnulf, R. Sobesky, O. Hermine, and C. Brechot. 2005. Hepatitis C virus core variants isolated from liver tumor but not from adjacent non-tumor tissue interact with Smad3 and inhibit the TGF-beta pathway. Oncogene 24:6119-6132.

[34] Rojkind, M., M. A. Giambrone, and L. Biempica. 1979. Collagen types in normal and cirrhotic liver. Gastroenterology 76:710-719.

[35] Romao, L. F., O. Sousa Vde, V. M. Neto, and F. C. Gomes. 2008. Glutamate activates GFAP gene promoter from cultured astrocytes through TGF-beta1 pathways. J Neurochem 106:746-756.

[36] Schuppan, D., and A. Gressner. 1999. Function and metabolism of collagens and other extracellular matrix proteins., p. 381-407. *In* J. Bircher, J. Benhamou, N. McIntyre, M. Rizzetto, and J. Rodes (ed.), Oxford Textbook of Clinical Hepatology, 2nd Edition. Oxford University Press, New York.

[37] Schuppan, D., M. Ruehl, R. Somasundaram, and E. G. Hahn. 2001. Matrix as a modulator of hepatic fibrogenesis. Seminars in liver disease 21:351-372.

[38] Seeff, L. B. 2002. Natural history of chronic hepatitis C. Hepatology 36:S35-46.

[39] Shin, J. Y., W. Hur, J. S. Wang, J. W. Jang, C. W. Kim, S. H. Bae, S. K. Jang, S. H. Yang, Y. C. Sung, O. J. Kwon, and S. K. Yoon. 2005. HCV core protein promotes liver fibrogenesis via up-regulation of CTGF with TGF-beta1. Exp Mol Med 37:138-145.

[40] Shuhart, M. C., M. P. Bronner, D. R. Gretch, L. V. Thomassen, C. F. Wartelle, H. Tateyama, S. S. Emerson, J. D. Perkins, and R. L. Carithers, Jr. 1997. Histological and clinical outcome after liver transplantation for hepatitis C. Hepatology 26:1646-1652.

[41] Smith-Mungo, L. I., and H. M. Kagan. 1998. Lysyl oxidase: properties, regulation and multiple functions in biology. Matrix Biol 16:387-398.

[42] Taniguchi, H., N. Kato, M. Otsuka, T. Goto, H. Yoshida, Y. Shiratori, and M. Omata. 2004. Hepatitis C virus core protein upregulates transforming growth factor-beta 1 transcription. J Med Virol 72:52-59.

[43] Wakita, T., T. Pietschmann, T. Kato, T. Date, M. Miyamoto, Z. Zhao, K. Murthy, A. Habermann, H. G. Krausslich, M. Mizokami, R. Bartenschlager, and T. J. Liang. 2005. Production of infectious hepatitis C virus in tissue culture from a cloned viral genome. Nat Med 11:791-796.

[44] Wakita, T., T. Pietschmann, T. Kato, T. Date, M. Miyamoto, Z. Zhao, K. Murthy, A. Habermann, H. G. Krausslich, M. Mizokami, R. Bartenschlager, and T. J. Liang. 2005. Production of infectious hepatitis C virus in tissue culture from a cloned viral genome. Nature medicine 11:791-796.

[45] Wang, P., T. Liu, M. Cong, X. Wu, Y. Bai, C. Yin, W. An, B. Wang, J. Jia, and H. You. 2009. Expression of extracellular matrix genes in cultured hepatic oval cells: an origin of hepatic stellate cells through transforming growth factor beta? Liver international : official journal of the International Association for the Study of the Liver 29:575-584.

[46] Wynn, T. A., and L. Barron. 2010. Macrophages: master regulators of inflammation and fibrosis. Seminars in liver disease 30:245-257.

[47] Young, B. B., M. K. Gordon, and D. E. Birk. 2000. Expression of type XIV collagen in developing chicken tendons: association with assembly and growth of collagen fibrils. Dev Dyn 217:430-439.

[48] Zhong, J., P. Gastaminza, G. Cheng, S. Kapadia, T. Kato, D. R. Burton, S. F. Wieland, S. L. Uprichard, T. Wakita, and F. V. Chisari. 2005. Robust hepatitis C virus infection in vitro. Proceedings of the National Academy of Sciences of the United States of America 102:9294-9299.

Permissions

The contributors of this book come from diverse backgrounds, making this book a truly international effort. This book will bring forth new frontiers with its revolutionizing research information and detailed analysis of the nascent developments around the world.

We would like to thank Yoshiaki Mizuguchi, MD, PhD, for lending his expertise to make the book truly unique. He has played a crucial role in the development of this book. Without his invaluable contribution this book wouldn't have been possible. He has made vital efforts to compile up to date information on the varied aspects of this subject to make this book a valuable addition to the collection of many professionals and students.

This book was conceptualized with the vision of imparting up-to-date information and advanced data in this field. To ensure the same, a matchless editorial board was set up. Every individual on the board went through rigorous rounds of assessment to prove their worth. After which they invested a large part of their time researching and compiling the most relevant data for our readers. Conferences and sessions were held from time to time between the editorial board and the contributing authors to present the data in the most comprehensible form. The editorial team has worked tirelessly to provide valuable and valid information to help people across the globe.

Every chapter published in this book has been scrutinized by our experts. Their significance has been extensively debated. The topics covered herein carry significant findings which will fuel the growth of the discipline. They may even be implemented as practical applications or may be referred to as a beginning point for another development. Chapters in this book were first published by InTech; hereby published with permission under the Creative Commons Attribution License or equivalent.

The editorial board has been involved in producing this book since its inception. They have spent rigorous hours researching and exploring the diverse topics which have resulted in the successful publishing of this book. They have passed on their knowledge of decades through this book. To expedite this challenging task, the publisher supported the team at every step. A small team of assistant editors was also appointed to further simplify the editing procedure and attain best results for the readers.

Our editorial team has been hand-picked from every corner of the world. Their multi-ethnicity adds dynamic inputs to the discussions which result in innovative outcomes. These outcomes are then further discussed with the researchers and contributors who give their valuable feedback and opinion regarding the same. The feedback is then collaborated with the researches and they are edited in a comprehensive manner to aid the understanding of the subject.

Apart from the editorial board, the designing team has also invested a significant amount of their time in understanding the subject and creating the most relevant covers. They scrutinized every image to scout for the most suitable representation of the subject and create an appropriate cover for the book.

The publishing team has been involved in this book since its early stages. They were actively engaged in every process, be it collecting the data, connecting with the contributors or procuring relevant information. The team has been an ardent support to the editorial, designing and production team. Their endless efforts to recruit the best for this project, has resulted in the accomplishment of this book. They are a veteran in the field of academics and their pool of knowledge is as vast as their experience in printing. Their expertise and guidance has proved useful at every step. Their uncompromising quality standards have made this book an exceptional effort. Their encouragement from time to time has been an inspiration for everyone.

The publisher and the editorial board hope that this book will prove to be a valuable piece of knowledge for researchers, students, practitioners and scholars across the globe.

List of Contributors

Yasuhiko Sugawara, Norihiro Kokudo and Yoji Kishi
University of Tokyo, Japan

Mona H. Ismail
College of Medicine, University of Dammam, Department of Internal Medicine, Division of Gastroenterology, King Fahad Hospital of the University, Saudi Arabia

Andrea Tannapfel and Berenike Flott-Rahmel
Institute of Pathology, Ruhr-University Bochum, Germany

Véronique Miette, Meriem Abdennour, Laurent Sandrin and Magali Sasso
Echosens, France

Mahmoud Rushdi Abd Ellah
Department of Animal Medicine, Faculty of Veterinary Medicine, Assiut University, Assiut Egypt

Annarosa Floreani
Dept. of Surgical and Gastroenterological Sciences, University of Padova, Italy

Heba Mohamed Abdella
Tropical Medicine, Faculty of Medicine, Ain Shams University, Cairo, Egypt

Piero Luigi Almasio, Anna Licata and Claudia Randazzo
University of Palermo, Italy

David Roberge and Tatiana Cabrera
McGill University Health Centre, Canada

Jan Schjøtt
Regional Drug Information Centre (RELIS Vest), Haukeland University Hospital, Norway

Johannes W. Rey
University Hospital of Mainz, Department of Internal Medicine I, Germany

Jochen W.U. Fries
University Hospital of Cologne, Institute of Pathology, Germany

Chen Hao, Xie Junjie, Shen Baiyong, Deng Xiaxing, Tao Ran, Peng Chenghong and Li Hongwei
Center of Organ Transplantation, Ruijin Hospital, Shanghai Jiao Tong University School of Medicine, P.R. China

Marco Carbone and James Neuberger
Liver Unit, Queen Elizabeth Hospital, United Kingdom

Teresa Casanovas, Carme Baliellas and Maria Carmen Peña Cala
Hospital Universitari de Bellvitge, Institut Català de la Salut, IDIBELLL, Hospitalet de Llobregat-Barcelona, Spain

Hiroshi Sadamori, Takahito Yagi and Toshiyosi Fujiwara
Departments of Gastroenterological Surgery, Okayama University Graduate School of Medicine, Dentistry and Pharmaceutical Sciences, Japan

Tetsuya Ogino
Departments of Pathology, Okayama University Graduate School of Medicine, Dentistry and Pharmaceutical Sciences, Japan

Giuseppe Maggiore, Marco Sciveres and Aurelio Sonzogni
Department of Pediatrics University of Pisa, Pediatric Hepatology and Liver Transplant Unit and Pathology Unit, UPMC-Ismett, Italy

A. Pietrobattista, A. Alterio, D. Comparcola, M. R. Sartorelli and V. Nobili
Department of Hepatogastroenterology and Nutrition, Pediatric Hospital Bambino Gesù, Italy

G. Natali and R. Fruhwirth
Radiology Interventional Unit, Pediatric Hospital Bambino Gesù, Italy

Consolato Sergi, Wesam Bahitham and Redha Al-Bahrani
Department of Laboratory Medicine and Pathology, University of Alberta, Edmonton, AB, Canada

Florence Nicot and Jacques Izopet
Virology Laboratory, Toulouse University Hospital, France

Nassim Kamar and Lionel Rostaing
Department of Nephrology, Dialysis and Multiorgan Transplantation, Toulouse University Hospital, France

Patricia M. Mulrooney-Cousins and Tomasz I. Michalak
Molecular Virology and Hepatology Research Group, Faculty of Medicine, Health Sciences Center, Memorial University of Newfoundland, St. John's, Newfoundland and Labrador, Canada

Alka Saxena, Sampa Pal, Stephen J. Polyak, Sy Nakao, Igor Tikonokov, Tao Su, Thao Tran, Wan Chong Qiu and Jessica Wagoner
University of Washington, Depts. of Laboratory Medicine, United States of America

Lisa Thomassen
University of Washington, Dept. of Pathology, United States of America

Margaret Shuhart
University of Washington, Dept. of Medicine, United States of America

David R. Gretch
University of Washington, Depts. of Laboratory Medicine, United States of America
University of Washington, Dept. of Medicine, United States of America